MRI
of the
Foot and Ankle

MRI
of the
Foot and Ankle

Editors

Andrew L. Deutsch, M.D.
Associate Director
Tower Musculoskeletal Imaging Center
Los Angeles, California
Associate Clinical Professor of Radiology
University of California, San Diego

Jerrold H. Mink, M.D.
Director
Tower Musculoskeletal Imaging Center
Los Angeles, California

Roger Kerr, M.D.
Chief, Musculoskeletal Imaging
Department of Radiology
Cedars-Sinai Medical Center
Los Angeles, California
Clinical Professor of Radiology
University of Southern California School of Medicine
Los Angeles, California

Raven Press   New York

Raven Press, Ltd., 1185 Avenue of the Americas, New York, New York 10036

Made in the United States of America

Library of Congress Cataloging-in-Publication Data

MRI of the foot and ankle / editors, Andrew L. Deutsch, Jerrold H.
    Mink, Roger Kerr.
        p. cm.
        Includes bibliographical references and index.
        ISBN 0-88167-899-6
        1. Foot—Magnetic resonance imaging. 2. Ankle—Magnetic resonance
    imaging. I. Deutsch, Andrew L. II. Mink, Jerrold H. III. Kerr,
    Roger.
        [DNLM: 1. Ankle Injuries—diagnosis. 2. Foot—injuries. 3. Foot
    Diseases—diagnosis. 4. Magnetic Resonance Imaging. WE 880 M939]
    RD563.M825 1992
    617.5′8507548—dc20
    DNLM/DLC
    for Library of Congress   92-3457
                                                                                                        CIP

The material contained in this volume was submitted as previously
unpublished material, except in the instances in which some of the illustrative
material was derived.

Great care has been taken to maintain the accuracy of the information
contained in the volume. However, neither Raven Press nor the editors can be
held responsible for errors or for any consequences arising from the use of the
information contained herein.

Materials appearing in this book prepared by individuals as part of their
official duties as U.S. Government employees are not covered by the above-
mentioned copyright.

9 8 7 6 5 4 3 2 1

To the "home team" who make life what it is:
Jeanne, Peter, Phillip, and Dana
and
to four physicians whom I greatly admire:
L. Peter Deutsch, J. Willis Hurst, George R. Leopold, and Donald Resnick

A.L.D.

To Barbara, Justin, Samantha, Sade, and Fletcher

J.H.M.

To my wife, Heidi, and our children, Daniel and Johanna

R.K.

Contents

Contributors

John V. Crues III, M.D. *Medical Director, Medical Imaging Group, Cottage Community Magnetic Resonance Center, Santa Barbara, California; Assistant Clinical Professor of Radiological Sciences, UCLA School of Medicine, Los Angeles, California 90024*

Andrew L. Deutsch, M.D. *Associate Director, Tower Musculoskeletal Imaging Center, 444 South San Vicente Boulevard, Los Angeles, California 90048; Associate Clinical Professor of Radiology, Department of Radiology, University of California, San Diego, California*

Charles L. Dumoulin, Ph.D. *Research Scientist, General Electric Research and Development Center, 1 River Road, Schenectady, New York 12301*

Roger Kerr, M.D. *Chief, Musculoskeletal Imaging, Department of Radiology, Cedars-Sinai Medical Center, 8700 Beverly Boulevard, Los Angeles, California 90048; Clinical Professor of Radiology, University of Southern California School of Medicine, Los Angeles, California*

Roger A. Mann, M.D. *Associate Clinical Professor, Department of Orthopaedic Surgery, University of California, San Francisco, California 94609*

Jerrold H. Mink, M.D. *Director, Tower Musculoskeletal Imaging Center, 444 San Vicente Boulevard, Los Angeles, California 90048*

Donald Resnick, M.D. *Professor of Radiology, University of California, San Diego, and Veterans Affairs Medical Center, 3350 La Jolla Village Drive, San Diego, California 92161*

Mark E. Schweitzer, M.D. *Assistant Professor of Radiology, Thomas Jefferson University Hospital, 111 South 11th Street, Philadelphia, Pennsylvania 19107*

Frank G. Shellock, Ph.D. *Research Scientist, Tower Musculoskeletal Imaging Center, 444 San Vicente Boulevard, Los Angeles, California 90048; Assistant Clinical Professor of Radiology, Department of Radiological Sciences, UCLA School of Medicine, Los Angeles, California 90024*

Fred L. Steinberg, M.D. *Director, Center for Vascular and Advanced Body MRI, Roxsan Radiology Medical Group, Beverly Hills, California 90048*

Preface

During the past decade there has been an explosion of interest in the clinical application of magnetic resonance (MR) to medical imaging. The high soft tissue and spatial resolution of MR, coupled with its multiplanar capability, have proven ideal for the noninvasive depiction of all the principal components (e.g., bone, muscle, ligaments) of the musculoskeletal system. MR imaging (MRI) has provided a window through which we can observe a wide spectrum of abnormalities involving bone and soft tissue. Many of the disorders depicted by MRI have previously eluded diagnosis by other available diagnostic methods, and the technique has afforded us a unique opportunity for increasing our awareness and understanding of many of these disorders. MRI has rapidly become a well established diagnostic technique that in many situations has already displaced previously established methods (e.g., arthrography of the knee) and is posing significant challenges to many others.

The impetus for the development of a text devoted to MRI of the foot and ankle mirrors both the knowledge explosion in musculoskeletal MRI as well as the surge in interest in both clinical and radiological circles in disorders of this anatomic region. The demands placed on the foot and ankle by an ever-increasingly active recreational and sports-minded population has focused previously unparalleled clinical attention toward foot and ankle derangements. The emergence of ankle arthroscopy as a diagnostic and therapeutic technique has further heightened the need for and expectations of diagnostic imaging for early and accurate diagnosis.

This text provides a working reference source for radiologists involved in diagnostic imaging as well as for clinicians caring for individuals with foot and ankle disorders. This work reflects the authors' experience with more than 4,000 MRI examinations of the foot and ankle. It reviews not only the current applications of MRI to this region, but discusses emerging developments that we believe will significantly affect the direction of MRI as applied to the foot and ankle in the coming years.

The opening chapter of the book is devoted to a discussion of the physical basis of MRI. It provides a foundation for understanding the principles underlying the production of MR images as well as the variety of pulse sequence options available for assessment of foot and ankle disorders. Emphasis in this section, as well as where appropriate throughout the book, is on high-resolution imaging, pulse sequence selection, and state-of-the-art techniques for optimizing diagnostic image quality. Also included is a succinct discussion of safety issues germane to clinical MRI. The section on anatomy is presented as a text–atlas and is provided to serve as a reference at the time of image interpretation. A chapter devoted to biomechanics reflects the importance of these considerations in understanding many foot and ankle disorders. The chapter on traumatic injuries to bone emphasizes the entire spectrum of osseous abnormalities demonstrable by MRI and reviews the physical basis for MRI of bone and pulse sequence options available for these purposes. A chapter devoted to osteochondral injuries of the talar dome also provides a detailed background consideration of articular cartilage to provide the interested reader with a sufficient basis for understanding current and future technical developments directed at imaging this structure. The author's initial experience with MR–arthrography for assessment of articular cartilage is also discussed. The section on bone and soft tissue infections emphasizes the rapidly emerging role of MRI in this area and contrasts MRI to existing scintigraphic methods. The formidable challenge provided by the diabetic foot and diabetic neuroarthropathy is considered. The chapter on tendon disorders comprehensively reviews this now well-established application of MRI. In the chapter on ankle ligaments, a detailed consideration of normal anatomy is provided as well as emerging applications in acute and chronic ankle injuries. A chapter on muscle injuries is included and reflects the author's considerable experience in this sports-medicine–related application of MRI. Soft tissue and osseous tumors of the foot and ankle are reviewed in detail. A chapter on MR angiography and venography of the foot and lower extremity is included, reflecting the clinical emergence of this exciting application of MRI. Entrapment syndromes and miscellaneous disorders of the foot and ankle constitute the concluding chapter.

This work should provide a valuable source of reference to radiologists on a practical day to day basis at the view box. Additionally, given the emerging importance of MRI to a number of medical specialties, this text is also intended for clinicians actively involved in the management of patients with foot and ankle problems and for whom a basic working knowledge of MRI is assuming greater importance. It is also our hope that this book will serve to enhance excellence in diagnostic imaging devoted to this area as well as to stimulate further investigation and development of the application of MRI to foot and ankle disorders.

Andrew L. Deutsch

Acknowledgments

The editors wish to thank the many individuals whose efforts significantly contributed to the production of this text. The skill and patience of the MR technology staff at Tower Imaging, including Joe Fraire, Mark Tournie, Kim Fernandez, Gina Slimp, Lisa Edwards, Brenda Tompkins, Kim Thibodeaux, Ernest Fontelera, Claire Alonzo, Art Aguilar, Andy Andrade, and Rosalyn Thomas, are greatly appreciated. The high quality of the reproductions can be credited to the skill and devotion of Francisco Chanes who is responsible for the overwhelming majority of the photography. Finally, the editors wish to thank Julie Sassoon, without whose tireless secretarial and organizational assistance this project could not have been accomplished, and Dr. Kerr would like to thank Sue Solender for her secretarial assistance.

MRI
of the
Foot and Ankle

MRI of the Foot and Ankle,
edited by A.L. Deutsch, J.H. Mink, and R. Kerr,
Raven Press, Ltd., New York © 1992

CHAPTER 1

Technical and Safety Considerations

John V. Crues III and Frank G. Shellock

TECHNICAL CONSIDERATIONS

Magnetic resonance imaging (MRI) represents one more milestone in the prodigious growth in application of magnetic resonance (MR) since the first successful nuclear magnetic resonance (NMR) experiments were performed in 1946 by Purcell and colleagues (1) at Harvard and by Block (2) at Stanford. Purcell and Block received the Nobel Prize in physics in 1952 for their landmark experiments. Throughout the 1950s and 1960s, MR became a key component in the armamentarium of chemists and physicists for evaluation of molecular structures. However, even though Gabillard noted the ability to obtain spatial localization in NMR in 1951 (3), it was not until the 1970s that medical applications of MR were seriously considered. In 1971, Damadian et al. published the first article on medical applications of NMR, and in 1972 he applied for the first patent for field-focusing nuclear magnetic resonance (FONAR) technique for MRI (4). The following year, Lauterbur published an article describing MRI using zeugmatography (5). Other MRI techniques rapidly followed (6–11). Early clinical trials with prototype imaging devices began in the early 1980s.

OVERVIEW OF NMR PHYSICS

A complete discussion of the physics of MRI is beyond the scope of this text. Fortunately for the interested reader, many excellent articles and books have been written on NMR physics and its medical applications (9,12–28). The present discussion will be limited to a minimum of basic concepts that we believe to be most relevant for the MRI medical practitioner. The importance of MRI spatial resolution and contrast resolution, as well as the signal-to-noise ratio, will be addressed. Surface coils will be discussed in general terms, and their importance for MRI of the foot and ankle will be emphasized. This chapter will also include a brief discussion of MRI protocols for foot and ankle imaging. The chapter will end with a discussion of MRI bioeffects and safety considerations.

PHYSICAL CONCEPTS

Much like the earth, although on a much smaller scale, a proton consists of a ball of electrically charged matter that spins about its own axis, generating a magnetic field. Like a compass placed into a magnetic field, it tends to align itself in the direction of a magnetic field. Unlike a compass, however, the proton is constrained by the laws of quantum mechanics to point either roughly in the direction of the magnetic field, the parallel state, or in the opposite direction to the magnetic field, the antiparallel state. A description of the exact motion of the proton is beyond the scope of this chapter and is not required for a practical understanding of MRI (9,12,20,29).

The overall picture of the interactions of the countless protons within the body and the magnetic field can be markedly simplified by using the bulk magnetization vector $\mathbf{M}$, which is the vector sum of the magnetic moments of all of the individual protons in the imaging volume (2,9,25). This quantity can be measured easily and is the essential parameter that generates the NMR signal used in MRI. When the body is initially placed within the magnetic field, the body's $\mathbf{M}$ is stationary and points in the direction of the main magnetic field

J.V. Crues III: Medical Imaging Group, Cottage Community Magnetic Resonance Center, Santa Barbara, California, and Department of Radiological Sciences, UCLA School of Medicine, Los Angeles, California 90024.

F.G. Shellock: Tower Musculoskeletal Imaging Center, Los Angeles, California 90048; Department of Radiological Sciences, UCLA School of Medicine, Los Angeles, California 90024.

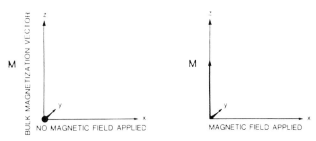

FIG. 1.1. The bulk magnetization vector. With no external magnetic field, the bulk magnetization vector, **M**, is zero. In the presence of an applied magnetic field, **M** is nonzero and points in the direction of the applied field, the z direction.

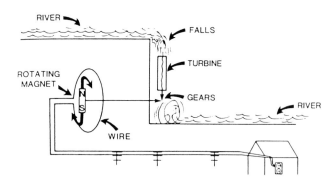

FIG. 1.3. Electricity generation at Niagara Falls. Current is induced in wires by a rotating magnetic field. In MRI the rotating magnetic field is the bulk magnetization vector during resonance.

(Fig. 1.1). This direction, by convention, is called the z direction. By use of radiofrequency energy at a specific frequency given by the Larmor equation:

$$F = \gamma B, \qquad [1.1]$$

where F is frequency, γ is the gyromagnetic ratio (42 megahertz, MHz per tesla), and B is the strength of the main magnetic field, **M** can be rotated away from the z axis. If the proper magnitude and length of the radiofrequency pulse are used, then the bulk magnetization vector can be rotated 90° into the x-y plane (Fig. 1.2). In this position, the z component of **M** is now zero, and the x-y component is maximum. Once in the x-y plane, the bulk magnetization vector rotates around the z axis with the same frequency as given by the Larmor equation. This is the resonant state referred to in the term NMR. This is also referred to as being "in phase," which in physics vernacular means that most of the countless precessing nuclei at any given time are pointing in the same direction in the x-y plane (13,25).

A moment's digression to describe electricity generation at Niagara Falls is instructive (Fig. 1.3). An understanding of the production of electrical current within wires is essential to an understanding of MRI. At Niagara Falls, water flows over the falls into a tur-

bine, causing the turbine to spin. The turbine is connected via mechanical gears to a magnet that is rotated by the rotating turbines. Current is induced within wires placed in the vicinity of the magnet by the rotating magnetic field. The wires are connected through transformers (which vary the voltage) to household electric outlets.

What does this have to do with MRI? Once the bulk magnetization is rotated into the x-y plane, it spins in space with a frequency given by the Larmor equation. Therefore, as with the magnet connected to the turbine at Niagara Falls, if wires are placed near the patient, the electrical current will be induced in those wires. The induced current is then fed to a computer for analysis. Fortunately, though, the nuclei are spinning at 64 MHz, and the patient is not!

So far we have described the 90° pulse; however, pulses at any angle can be and are applied to the nuclei to produce an almost endless variety of images and image contrasts. These pulse sequences have been named by some of the most imaginative physicists of the 20th century and include techniques such as GRASS (gradient recalled acquisition in the steady state), FLASH (fast, low-angle-shot) (18,30–32), STIR (short tau inversion recovery) (33,34), MAVIN (multiple-angle, variable-interval, nonorthogonal) (35), STEAM (stimulated-echo methods) (31,36), CHESS (chemical-shift selective) (37), inversion recovery, RARE (38), and spin echo. Most of the images in this book were produced by the Carr-Purcell spin-echo technique (39); however, the STIR and gradient-echo techniques are also important in musculoskeletal imaging.

The spin-echo technique begins with a 90° pulse and ignores the signal that is immediately created, called the free induction decay (FID) (Fig. 1.4). After a time delay, called tau (τ), a 180° pulse is applied, and at a time τ after the 180° pulse, a signal is generated called the spin echo (12,13,16,19,29,39–41). It is important to note, however, that the initial signal of the FID de-

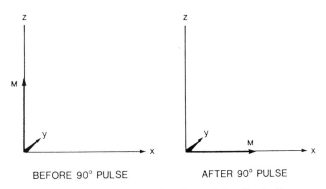

FIG. 1.2. Rf pulses. A 90° rf pulse rotates the bulk magnetization vector from pointing in the z direction to pointing in the x-y plane.

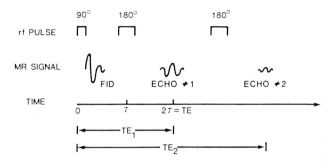

FIG. 1.4. The spin echo. The most frequently used MRI technique involves the Carr-Purcell spin echo. A 90° pulse is followed after a time delay of τ ms by a 180° pulse, which causes rephasing of the nuclei leading to a spin echo. For technical reasons the free-induction decay (FID) is ignored and the signal from the echo is used in calculating the image. The timing parameters τ and TE are shown and discussed in the text.

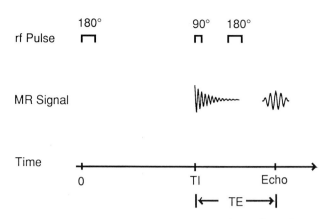

FIG. 1.5. The Inversion Recovery technique. The IR sequence begins with a 180° pulse that inverts **M**. At a time T1 (inversion time) later a standard spin echo 90°–180° sequence is performed. The strength of the resultant signal is proportional to the magnitude of **M** at the time of the 90° pulse.

cays because the individual protons in different regions of a voxel precess at slightly different frequencies because of local magnetic field inhomogeneities. Thus, the nuclei rapidly spin out of phase with one another. This causes the decay in the strength of the bulk magnetization vector, **M**. The 180° rf pulse rephases that component of the dephasing of the nuclei due to static, time-independent magnetic field inhomogeneities. The time between the 90° pulse and the generation of the spin echo is called TE, the echo delay time. This is an important parameter determining image contrast in musculoskeletal imaging and is determined by the radiologist before scanning a patient. The signal from the echo is fed into the computer and is used to generate the image.

The standard spin-echo technique can be modified in many ways to enhance tissue contrast. One technique frequently used in musculoskeletal imaging is the inversion recovery technique. Inversion recovery pulses begin with a 180° inversion pulse (Fig. 1.5), which is followed after a delay of T1 by a standard 90°–180° spin-echo sequence (33,34). The effect of this technique on tissue contrast is discussed below with primary reference to the STIR (short T1 inversion recovery) technique under relaxation mechanisms.

Gradient-echo pulse sequences encompass a large family of pulsing techniques that may display a large spectrum of contrast differences. These sequences have in common replacement of the 180° refocusing rf pulse with a rapid reversal of a magnetic field gradient (Fig. 1.6). The sequence begins by an rf pulse that is typically less than the 90° pulse that initiates spin-echo imaging. The amount the initial pulse rotates the bulk magnetization vector in the direction of the x-y plane is called the flip angle. Varying the flip angle in gradient echoes is important for two reasons. Small flip angles less than 90° do not completely saturate the protons.

If a second pulse sequence is begun in a repetition time (TR) less than the T1 of the protons, significant signal cannot be induced if the flip angle is close to 90° because sufficient time will not have elapsed to allow **M** to regain magnetization along the z direction. When small flip angles are used, **M** is not rotated completely into the x-y plane and sufficient magnetization along z is maintained to allow use of short TRs, which may translate into shorter imaging times (*vide infra*). Second, varying the flip angle changes the inherent contrast in the resultant images. As a rough approximation, the smaller the flip angle, the more T2-like is the image contrast.

The 180° refocusing pulse can be replaced by a gradient reversal because the initial gradient causes dephasing of the nuclei along the direction of the gradient

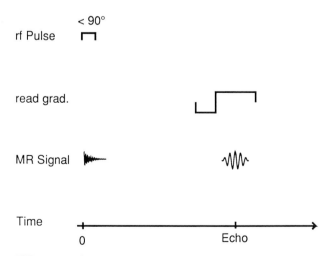

FIG. 1.6. Gradient-echo techniques. Gradient-echo (GRE) techniques are a family of echo techniques that usually begin the sequence with an rf pulse of less than 90° and generate an echo by reversing a magnetic field gradient, rather than using a 180° rf refocusing pulse.

by placing nuclei along the gradient in different magnetic fields. Nuclei in different magnetic fields resonate at different frequencies, thus dephasing the nuclei. Phase-encoding gradients are then placed on the object for spatial localization (*vide infra*). The dephasing is reversed by reversing the magnetic field gradient, which brings the nuclei back into phase, thus producing an echo.

This process is usually performed rapidly with short TEs because static magnetic field inhomogeneities within tissues (magnetic susceptibility effects) can degrade gradient-echo images and these artifacts are minimized with short TE acquisitions. The dephasing due to time-independent magnetic field variations within the tissues are better compensated for using 180° rf pulses (*vide infra*).

The signal used to generate the image using gradient-echo pulse sequences is primarily from the initial free-induction decay, not from an rf-induced spin echo (Fig. 1.6). The decay rate of the free-induction decay is called T2* and is primarily dependent on fixed (non–time-dependent) magnetic field inhomogeneities within the tissues, which are produced by imperfection in the main magnet and fixed magnetic field gradients within tissues due to differing magnetic properties of adjacent body tissues (the magnetic susceptibility effects). Thus, gradient-echo images are often called T2*-weighted images (see contrast below).

Regular spin echo (90°–180°), inversion recovery (180°–90°–180°), and typical gradient echo (<90°–gradient reversal) are three frequently used pulse sequences from an almost endless list of possible techniques. Clearly, the future will continue to unveil newer techniques and enhancement of present techniques that will further improve musculoskeletal imaging in the years ahead. The burden of continued research and development of new techniques and proof of their clinical utility will be a challenge to students of musculoskeletal imaging, who will be richly rewarded by advances in diagnostic sensitivity and accuracy.

SPATIAL LOCALIZATION

Generating a NMR signal is only the beginning of the process of creating a diagnostic study. In order to generate an image, the brightness of each point in the photograph must be proportional to the intensity of the MR signal emanating from the corresponding small volume of tissue (called a voxel). A mechanism to localize the origin of the signal spatially must be used. Many techniques have been attempted, but the technique that is most frequently used in medical MRI is the two-dimensional Fourier-transform technique (7). This technique uses small linear magnetic field gradients along the x' and y' directions to determine spatial localization in the plane of the image. (In this chapter, z refers to direction of the main magnetic field, and x and y refer to directions orthogonal to z; z' refers to the direction perpendicular to the image slice plane of a two-dimensional Fourier-transform image and is the same as z only for an axial image; x' and y' are orthogonal directions to z'.) One direction, x', uses frequency encoding for spatial localization. If a small linear magnetic field in the z direction that varies in magnitude along the x' axis is superimposed on the large uniform static magnetic field in the z direction, then nuclei along the x' axis will vary their frequencies of precession directly proportional to the magnetic field gradient according to Eq. 1.1. Thus, nuclei on one side of the body will precess more rapidly than nuclei on the opposite side. The frequencies of the MR signal can therefore be used to localize its site of origin.

Fullerton masterfully illustrated this technique using the analogy of strings in a harp (16). Consider a harpist in one room and a trained musician in an adjoining room. If the harpist plucks a string, the musician can determine the distance from the harpist to the plucked string by listening to the pitch of the note played. If the pitch is low, then the string is far from the harpist, if high the string is near to the harpist. Therefore, the frequency of the note played encodes the location of the string. The training and talent of the musician allows her to decode the frequency information into the desired position. Similarly, the frequency of the emitted rf from nuclei in a magnetic field gradient encodes spatial location within the body, which can be decoded by a computer using the mathematics of Fourier transforms. It is the mathematical technique of Fourier transforms that gives the computer "perfect pitch" to provide accurate spatial localization. The interested reader is encouraged to read Fullerton's original article for a more detailed discussion of the analogy between frequency encoding and a wonderful musical instrument (16).

Unfortunately, frequency encoding can be used in only one direction. Spatial encoding in the y' direction requires a different technique called phase encoding. A detailed description of this technique is beyond the scope of this chapter (13,20). However, the application of the phase-encoding technique to a simplified example is helpful in developing a qualitative understanding of the technique and in explaining important limitations of this process (15).

Consider imaging a square beaker of water (Fig. 1.7). As described below, slice location in one direction, z', can be determined by a slice selection gradient at the time of the initial 90° pulse. Spatial localization in another direction, the x' direction, can be determined by frequency encoding. The final dimension, y', requires phase encoding. For the beaker of water the correct plot of signal intensity versus distance along the y' direction is depicted in Fig. 1.8. It is 0 outside of the

beaker filled with
water

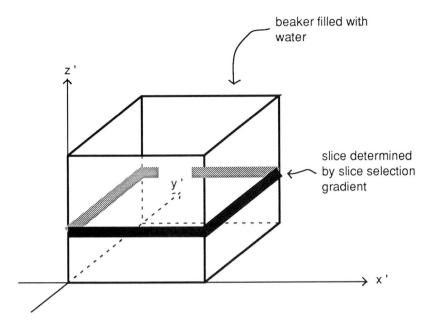

slice determined
by slice selection
gradient

FIG. 1.7. Square beaker of water. Phase encoding as used to generate spatial information in 2-DFT MRI may not be initially intuitively understood. A simple square beaker of water may be helpful in conceptualizing 2-DFT imaging. The beaker is illustrated with the frequency encoding direction along the x' axis. The phase encoding direction is along the y' axis, and the plane of imaging is perpendicular to the z' axis.

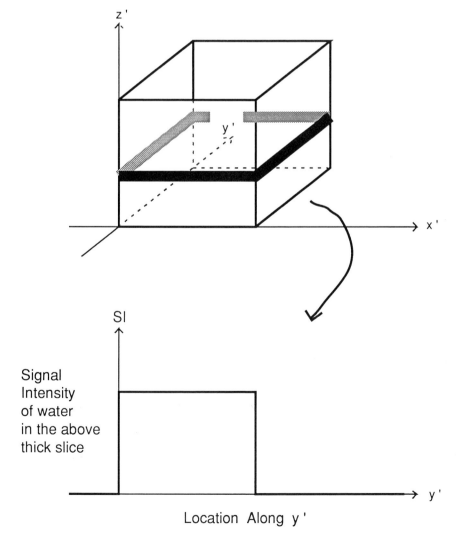

Signal
Intensity
of water
in the above
thick slice

Location Along y'

FIG. 1.8. Plot of signal intensity versus distance along the phase-encoding axis for a square beaker of water. An image of the water in a square beaker should show 0 signal outside of the beaker and a constant high signal within the region in the beaker containing the water. This is plotted above.

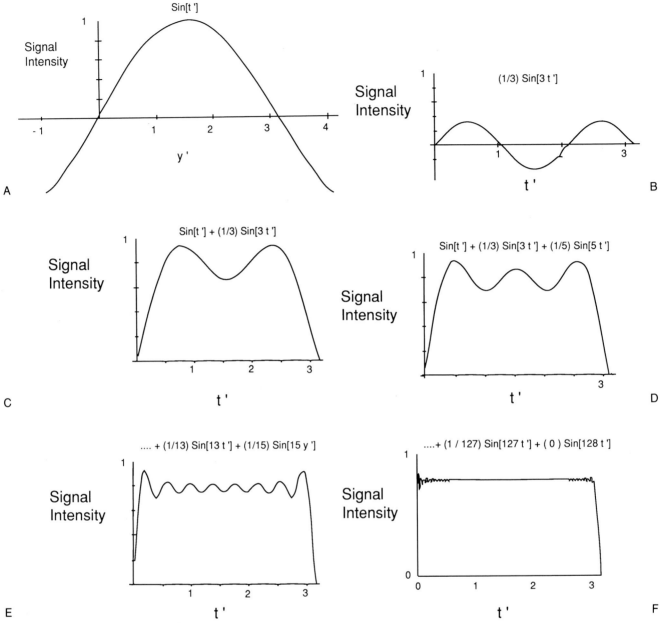

FIG. 1.9. Plot of terms in the Fourier transform of a square beaker of water. **A:** A graph of the first sine term in the Fourier transform depicts a low frequency component of the signal intensity, which is important in displaying large features of the imaged object. **B:** The second term displayed by itself is a higher frequency component of the signal intensity, but does not by itself display a close resemblance to the signal intensity of the beaker of water. **C:** When the higher and lower frequency terms are added together, the resultant graph much more closely resembles the desired signal intensity. **D–F:** As more terms in the Fourier series are added, the resultant signal distribution more closely approaches that shown in Fig. 1.8. Notice, however, that as more terms are added the "wiggles" become higher in frequency and cluster near the edges of the signal distribution. This effect produces the truncation artifact often noted on MR scans near the boundaries between bright and dark objects.

beaker and a constant value within the beaker because the water gives a uniform signal. According to Fourier's theorem any arbitrary, well-behaved mathematical function can be exactly reproduced by an infinite series of sine and cosine functions:

$$F(y') = A(n) \sin(n\ t) + B(n) \cos(n\ t) + \quad [1.2]$$

For the beaker of water this series is calculated as the following:

$$Sl(y') = 1 \sin(t) + \tfrac{1}{3} \sin(3\ t)$$
$$+ \tfrac{1}{5} \sin(5\ t) + \cdots \quad [1.3]$$

This series is schematically diagrammed in Fig. 1.9. Notice that the first sine term (Fig. 1.9A) is a rough approximation of the desired signal intensity function without sharp margins. Higher order (frequency) sine functions [i.e., the sin(3 t) term] by themselves do not reproduce the desired signal intensity well (Fig. 1.9B). However, when higher order terms are added to the lower order terms a much closer approximation to the desired function is obtained (Fig. 1.9C–F). The lower order (lower frequency) terms are necessary for accurate depiction of large anatomical structures. Adding additional higher order terms significantly improves the image, especially edge sharpness, which is necessary for high-resolution images (Fig. 1.9D–F).

Fourier series have their place, but how are the critical coefficients A(n) and B(n) obtained in clinical MRI? Each of these coefficients must be measured by separate pulse sequences. Each coefficient (A or B) that is necessary to multiply times the sine functions must be measured by separate individual phase encodings. For instance, when no phase-encoded gradient along the y' direction is applied, the intensity of returned signal from the strip of nuclei in the y' direction located at a specified x' location (located by frequency encoding) is proportional to the A(0) coefficient. The returned signal when a small phase-encoded gradient is applied is proportional to A(1). Higher order coefficients are proportional to returned signal when stronger gradients are applied. Remember, only one phase-encoded gradient can be applied during any one TR interval when standard imaging techniques are used. Consequently, imaging time is directly proportional to the number of phase encodings used to calculate the image. Since the more phase encodings used, the more higher order terms are included in the calculation, higher spatial resolution requires longer imaging times. Imaging time is given by the following formula:

$$\text{time} = [(\text{NEX}) \times (\text{\# phase encodings})$$
$$\times (\text{TR interval})]/\text{NP}, \quad [1.4]$$

where NEX is the number of times a given phase encoding is repeated to improve the signal-to-noise ratio, \# is the number of different phase encodings used to calculate the image, TR is the time between 90° (or smaller) pulses, and NP is the number of phase encodings per pulse (usually 1). Thus, a 256 matrix in the y' phase-encoded direction requires twice as much imaging time as a 128 matrix. An entire multislice, multiecho spin-echo imaging sequence is illustrated in Fig. 1.10.

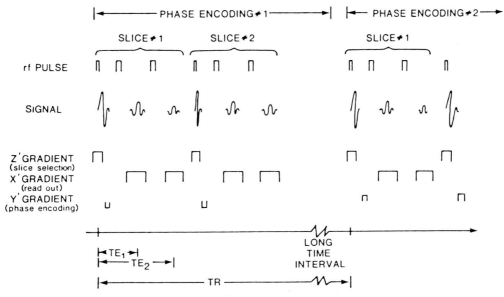

FIG. 1.10. A simplified pulse timing diagram for a multislice, multiecho, spin-echo sequence. The slice-selection gradient is on only during the 90° pulse. The readout or frequency-encoding gradient is on during the spin echoes, and the phase-encoding gradient is turned on after the 90° pulse, but before the spin-echo. The phase-encoding gradient changes for each phase-encoded step.

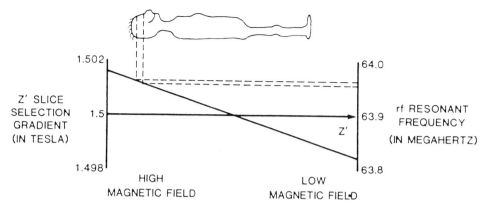

FIG. 1.11. Slice-selection gradient. If a narrow spectrum of radiofrequencies (rf) is used to resonate the nuclei in the presence of a magnetic gradient varying along the z' direction, then only nuclei in a slice through the head will be resonated. Lowering the radiofrequency will select a more caudal slice. A steeper gradient will create a thinner slice. A narrower rf spectrum will also result in a thinner slice.

Although a simple square beaker with water in it was used in the above example, Fourier's theorem is applicable to any well-behaved mathematical function. This means that no matter how complicated signal intensity may be in the y' direction, phase encoding can be used to evaluate it.

Next to image quality, the time required to acquire an image significantly impacts the clinical use of MRI. Consequently, many investigators have attempted to use the information in Eq. 1.4 to modify the length of acquisition time. According to Eq. 1.4 the length of time can be shortened by decreasing several factors. The number of excitations (NEX) is the number of times the data is repeated and averaged together. Decreasing NEX directly reduces the signal-to-noise ratio of the image. Usually the smallest NEX is chosen, which routinely gives diagnostic quality images for the body part, coil, and field strength used. The number of phase encodings performed for a given acquisition field of view (FOV) determines the spatial resolution in the phase-encoding direction. Although decreasing the number of phase encodings decreases imaging time, one pays for the decreased time with poorer spatial resolution and increased truncation artifacts (see Artifacts below). The TR is often shortened to decreased imaging time; however, for spin-echo imaging long TRs are necessary for optimal signal-to-noise ratio and, more importantly, image contrast (*vide infra*). Long TR intervals are less important for image contrast using gradient-echo techniques; thus, these techniques usually use short TR intervals with low flip angle initial pulses to shorten imaging time (18).

According to Eq. 1.4, another way to shorten imaging times is to increase the number of phase encodings per pulse (NP). Mansfield et al.'s echo-planar techniques have performed subsecond imaging times

with good image contrast (42–46). These techniques allow multiple rapidly acquired phase-encoded echoes to be obtained from a single pulse excitation. "Fast spin echo" is a similar technique that allows rapid spin-echo T2-weighted images in $\frac{1}{16}$ or $\frac{1}{32}$ of the usual time by acquiring multiple phase encodings per 90° pulse.

We have yet to describe how the slice location is selected. Notice in Fig. 1.10 that a gradient is located along the z' direction during the initial rf pulse. If a narrow spectrum of radiofrequencies is used in the pulse, then only a narrow band of nuclei at just the right magnetic field strength (Fig. 1.11) will be resonated. All other nuclei will not see the initial pulse and therefore will not be involved in the full spin-echo or gradient-echo sequence and will not generate a signal at the spin echo. The thickness of the slice is determined by the width of the spectrum of the initial rf pulse frequencies as well as the slope of the gradient.

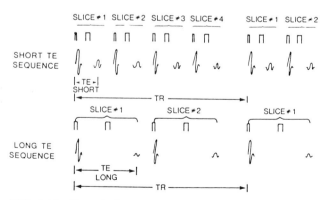

FIG. 1.12. The relationships between TR, TE, and number of obtainable slices. With a given TR, more slices can be obtained with a short TE than with a long TE. Assuming a given TE, more slices can be obtained by lengthening the TR.

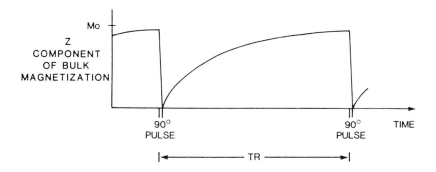

FIG. 1.13. T1 relaxation. After the 90° pulse (or any other pulse), the bulk magnetization vector returns to the baseline value, Mo, in a logarithmic fashion. The time it takes for the z component of **M** to return approximately two-thirds of the way back to Mo is called T1.

The slice location is determined by the relationship between the exact Larmor frequency of nuclei along the z' axis and the center frequency of the initial pulse spectrum. Thus, by decreasing the frequency of the initial pulse, nuclei lower along the z' axis will be excited, and a slice located more caudally can be obtained (Fig. 1.11).

Notice that the TE is typically much shorter than the TR for usual spin-echo sequences. This means that in the interval between the initial rf pulse for one slice location and the next initial rf pulse for that same slice location, initial pulses at other slice locations can be interposed. This is schematically diagrammed in Figs. 1.10 and 1.12 and is the basis for the most frequently used imaging sequence, called the multislice, multiecho two-dimensional Fourier-transform spin-echo pulse sequence. Notice that the longer the delay in TE, the fewer slice locations can be placed in a given TR interval (Fig. 1.12). Also notice that with longer TRs, more slice locations can be simultaneously acquired in a given data acquisition. Frequently in MRI, the choices for TE and TR are as much dependent on the number of slices desired as on image contrast (*vide infra*).

RELAXATION MECHANISMS

Important in understanding the causes of contrast differences between tissues with MRI is an understanding of the T1, T2, and T2* relaxation processes (47–57). Immediately after the 90° pulse the bulk mag-

netization vector begins returning back to its baseline value of magnitude Mo pointing in the z direction (Fig. 1.13). The process is dependent on two basic principles called T1 relaxation and T2 relaxation. T1 relaxation returns the z component of **M** from zero to Mo, and T1 is roughly the time it takes for the z component to go from zero after the 90° pulse up to two-thirds of its maximum value, Mo. T2 relaxation causes the x-y component of **M** to return to zero and is defined as roughly the time it takes for the x-y component of the bulk magnetization vector to decrease from its maximum value right after the 90° pulse to roughly one-third of its maximum value (Fig. 1.14).

A simple understanding of the causes of these two processes is helpful in characterizing tissues by MRI (21,58,59). The z component of the bulk magnetization vector, i.e., the component along the direction of the main magnetic field, is strictly determined by the difference in the number of nuclei pointed in the parallel direction versus the number of nuclei pointed in the antiparallel direction. After the 90° pulse, the number of nuclei pointing parallel and antiparallel are equal. However, soon after the 90° pulse, more nuclei will lodge in the parallel, low-energy state than in the antiparallel state. Thus, more will point in the direction of the magnetic field, and the z component of the bulk magnetization vector will go from zero to a positive quantity along the z axis. Any process within the tissues that speeds up the flipping of nuclei will shorten the time it takes for the z component to rise back up to its baseline value. This occurs when hydrogen nuclei are closely associated with large macromolecules, be-

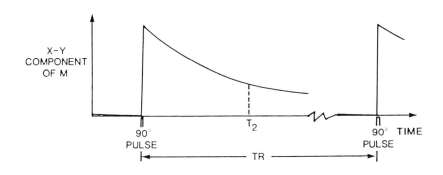

FIG. 1.14. T2 relaxation. After the 90° pulse (or any other rf pulse), the x-y component of the bulk magnetization vector returns toward zero exponentially. The time required to reach approximately one-third of the maximum value is called T2.

cause large macromolecules rotate, and part of their rotation is near the Larmor frequency (21,59,60). The rotations will create local electromagnetic fields that vary at frequencies at or around the Larmor frequency. This will cause rapid switching of nuclei between the parallel and antiparallel states and will shorten T1. A similar process exists in the arms of triglycerides and is responsible for the short T1 of fat. This process can be markedly accelerated if paramagnetic materials are attached to the macromolecules, since they greatly accentuate the intensity of the locally fluctuating electromagnetic field (61). Therefore, tissues with short T1 values include proteinaceous cysts, fat, hemorrhage, and tissues containing infused gadolinium, a paramagnetic agent that can be given intravenously.

T2 relaxation processes are somewhat different from T1 processes (13,25,62). Substances with short T2 values contain hydrogen nuclei that are fixed in position. Tremendous variations in the strength of magnetic fields exist at the atomic level. If fixed in location, nuclei in different magnetic fields will precess at different rates (as described by Eq. 1.1); therefore, nuclei in a given region that begin resonating in phase with each other will soon get out of phase. Substances that are fluid, such as urine or water, have long T2 values, because the nuclei move rapidly throughout the substance. They thus spend part of their time in regions of low magnetic field strength and part of their time in regions of high magnetic field strength. The net effect over a pulse sequence is that the nuclei effectively experience a single average magnetic field. The nuclei stay in phase longer, and the tissue has a long T2. This is a process called "motional narrowing." Liquids tend to have long T2 values, as do tissues that contain excess amounts of free water secondary to edema or neoplastic disease (63,64). Because abnormal states such as inflammation or neoplasm tend to be associated with larger amounts of free water than are found in normal tissues, T2-weighted images are in general more sensitive in detecting many disease processes than sequences that are not T2-weighted.

T2* processes are those magnetic effects that lead to dephasing of nuclei after the initial rf pulse (i.e., the decay of the FID). T2* is defined as roughly the time required for the initial FID to decay to one-third of its peak value (Fig. 1.15). The loss of signal is due to dephasing of the nuclei by all magnetic field inhomogeneities within imaged tissues. In practice for the FID, this process is dominated by fixed (time-independent) magnetic field inhomogeneities within the tissues. Such fixed tissue inhomogeneities are usually independent of primary physicochemical properties of the tissues, but mostly dependent on equipment imperfections and bulk tissue magnetic susceptibility effects. Thus, soft tissue contrast base on the T2* effects is often poor. These constant field inhomogeneities are

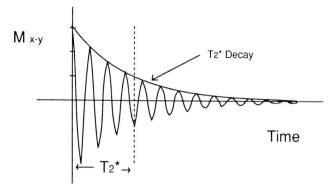

FIG. 1.15. T2* and the free-induction decay (FID). T2* is defined as the time it takes for the FID to decay the roughly one-third of its initial peak value.

mostly reversed by 180° rf-induced spin echoes, but magnetic inhomogeneities that change between the initial rf pulse and the spin echo are not corrected by the 180° pulse, leading to irreversible signal loss (the T2 effects). Magnetic field inhomogeneities that change with time are usually less important in the FID decay, but are strongly dependent on the basic physicochemical properties of tissues. Thus, soft tissue contrast is usually superior on rf spin-echo images than gradient-echo images.

Because of the importance of T1 and T2 in tissue characterization, a thorough understanding of the relationship between the TE and TR selected to produce images and the resultant T1 and T2 weightings of the subsequent images is critical in MRI (13,41,49–47,62, 65,66). Figure 1.16 shows the height of the z component of the bulk magnetization vector as a function of time after the 90° pulse for two tissues with differing T1 values. Notice that a tissue with a short T1 may have a higher bulk magnetization vector at the time of the next 90° pulse. Because the magnitude of the x-y component of the bulk magnetization vector after the 90° pulse is proportional to the value of the z component right before the 90° pulse, a tissue with a short T1 will produce a brighter signal than a tissue with a long T1 if all other factors are equal. Notice also that if the TR is short, there is a large difference between the height of the bulk magnetization vector at the time of the next 90° pulse between long and short T1 tissues (Fig. 1.16). Therefore, in general with spin-echo imaging, the shorter the TR, the more T1-weighted is the image. Conversely, the longer the TR, the less T1-weighted is the image.

Figure 1.17 shows the time course of T2 decay for two tissues, one with a long T2 and one with a short T2. Notice that the x-y component of the bulk magnetization vector, and therefore the intensity of the signal picked up by the receiving wires, is larger for long T2 substances than for short T2 substances. Also

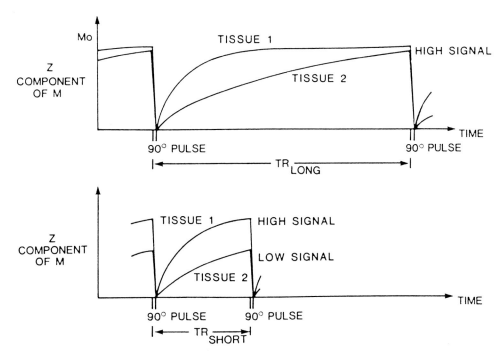

FIG. 1.16. T1 weighting. If two tissues differ in T1 values, then they can best be differentiated by signal intensities with short TR sequences. With a long TR, both tissue 1 (short T1) and tissue 2 (long T1) give high signals. With a short TR, tissue 2 has not regained magnetization and will give a low signal, whereas tissue 1 will have regained magnetization and give a strong signal. The large signal differential will allow easy MR differentiation of the neighboring tissues. Thus, images acquired with short TR values are more T1-weighted than those with long TR values.

note that the longer the TE, i.e., the point at which we sample the signal, the more separation there is between tissues with differing T2 values. As a general rule, sequences with longer TE values are more T2-weighted sequences and conversely, sequences with shorter TE values are less T2-weighted sequences.

A frequent dilemma noted by imagers versed in x-ray techniques is that some tissues, such as joint fluid, may appear darker on some images than surrounding fatty tissues (i.e., on T1- and intermediate-weighted

images), but brighter than surrounding tissues on other images (i.e., T2-weighted images). This occurs when tissues with long T1 and T2 values (fluid) are adjacent to structures with short T1 and T2 values (fat). On T1- and intermediate-weighted images, such as the first echo in Fig. 1.18, fat will be bright because of its short T1. On the second echo, the contrast reverses because of the long T2 of fluid. Therefore, an understanding of the causes of signal intensities in MRI can eliminate

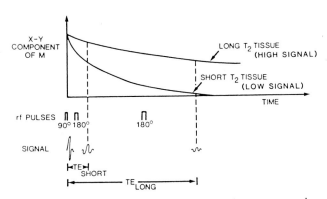

FIG. 1.17. T2 weighting. If other parameters are equal, a long T2 tissue will emit higher signal than a short T2 tissue. The difference in signal intensity will be maximal for long TE values. Therefore, long TE acquisitions yield T2-weighted images.

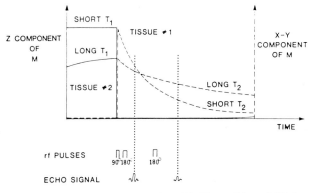

FIG. 1.18. Contrast reversal in MRI. Short T1 and T2 tissues such as fat can be brighter than long T1 and T2 tissues such as joint effusions on first-echo, intermediate-weighted images, but darker than effusions on second echo, T2-weighted images. This can be confusing to radiologists familiar with x-ray–based imaging.

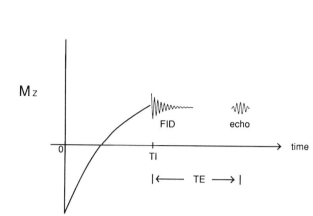

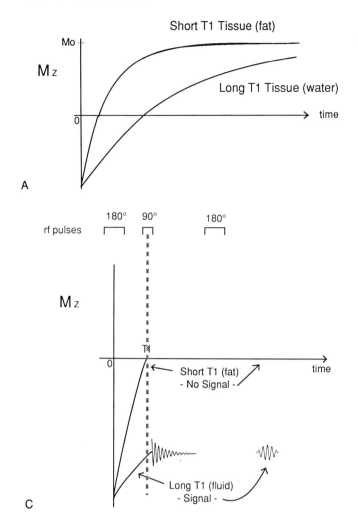

FIG. 1.19. Contrast in the STIR sequence. **A:** After the 180° inverting pulse, tissues with different T1 values will recover magnetization at different rates. Short T1 tissues will recover more rapidly and the magnitude of **M** will decrease to zero before rising back up to Mo more rapidly than long T1 tissues. **B:** The signal intensity of the spin echo used to generate the image is proportional to the magnitude of **M**z at the time of the 90° pulse. **C:** As **M** recovers back to its baseline value, its magnitude decreases to 0 before rising to Mo. If the T1 is selected so that the 90° pulse occurs when **M**z for fat is 0, then fat will not return a signal and will be black on the resultant images. Pathology with a long T1 will generate a signal and be bright; thus, it will be highly conspicuous.

potential confusion and be helpful for tissue characterization.

The STIR technique is a form of inversion recovery sequence. If the T1 is very short (150–200 ms), the 90° pulse of the spin-echo sequence will occur at a time when **M** of fat is near 0, but tissues with longer T1 values will be nonzero (Fig. 1.19) (33,34). The resultant spin-echo signal will be 0 for regions of the body containing tissue with similar T1 values as fat, but higher for regions of the body containing water-based tissues. The contrast in the resultant images depicts low signal in predominantly fatty regions. STIR images are especially useful in evaluating infiltrative disease or edema in high lipid regions, such as bone marrow (67–70). The signal from disease processes may be masked by the high signal from the lipid in standard spin-echo sequences, but the suppression of lipid signal in the STIR images allows improved visualization of underlying abnormal processes. STIR images may also be useful in evaluating articular cartilage (see chapter by Deutsch, Osteochondral Injuries of the Talar Dome) because joint fluid tends to be bright and the articular cartilage slightly darker (*vide infra*). One drawback of

STIR images is that the signal suppression is not specific for fat, but will suppress any tissue that has a short T1 relaxation time. When contrast agents that shorten tissue T1 times, such as gadolinium, are used, STIR images may suppress desired contrast enhancement.

More specific fat suppression using radiofrequency pulses just before the spin-echo sequences can specifically suppress signal from fat (71,72). Rf fat suppression techniques exploit the small differences in resonant frequency of the proton nuclei in lipid versus the higher resonant frequency of protons in water. The narrow rf pulse centered at the lipid resonant frequency "saturates" fat protons, i.e., rotates their **M** into the *x-y* plane, so that subsequent imaging pulses rotate **M** out of the *x-y* plane, thus inhibiting resonance of these selected spins during the subsequent imaging pulse sequence. The water protons are unaffected because the saturation pulse does not contain energy at the resonant frequency of water. Unlike the STIR technique, this technique does not use T1 to determine suppression; therefore, nonlipid short T1 tissues are unaffected and continue to display signal. Rf saturation is an excellent technique to use with gadolinium to suppress high signal intensity from fat, which may mask signal from contrast-enhanced tissues.

Hematomas can be confusing on MRI (73–84). Acute hematomas may appear isointense compared with surrounding soft tissues on T1- and intermediate-weighted images. On T2-weighted images it may be isointense (because of oxyhemoglobin in intact red cells) or of low intensity because of the magnetic susceptibility effect of deoxyhemoglobin contained within intact red cells (78). Subacute hemorrhage appears bright on T1-weighted images because of the paramagnetic effect of iron in methemoglobin (73) and on T2-weighted images because of motional narrowing of free water collected during the degradation process (78). Older hematomas are characterized by a black periphery that is secondary to hemosiderin deposition (78,79,85,86). Knowledge of these characteristic changes is helpful in obviating misinterpretation of findings in acute hematomas that may be isointense with surrounding structures and in dating the ages of old hematomas.

In contrast to hematomas, interstitial hemorrhage into medullary bone and muscle is immediately associated with long T2 relaxation times. This is probably due to separation of the red cells from the serum within the interstitium, which does not occur in a pool of whole blood. The water molecules are then separated from the magnetic susceptibility effects of the red cells, which then display long T2 characteristics typical of free water. Thus, medullary hemorrhage in trabecular fractures of acute bony injuries and interstitial hemorrhage into acute muscle and tendon tears are typically bright on T2-weighted images immediately after the injury (see chapters by Deutsch, Traumatic Injuries of Bone and Necrosis, and by Kerr, Tumors: Soft Tissue and Bone).

Table 1.1 summarizes the foregoing findings concerning T1 and T2 weighting of images. In general, the best T1-weighted image is one with a short TR and a short TE, so that there is good T1 weighting and limited T2 weighting. Conversely, the best T2-weighted image is one with a long TR (so that there is less T1 weighting) and a long TE (so that there is good T2 weighting). Intermediate weighting can be obtained with a long TR and a short TE. This is occasionally referred to as a balanced image, a spin-density image, or a proton-density image; however, the latter terms can be confusing because the TR values are not long enough and the TE values are not short enough in routine imaging to give a truly representative image of proton density. Therefore, I prefer to call these intermediate-weighted images. In general, there is little clinical usefulness for short-TR long-TE images, as the signal-to-noise ratio is generally too poor for good tissue contrast.

SIGNAL-TO-NOISE RATIO

A critical determinant of image quality is the ratio between the strength of the signal coming back from the nuclei and the intensity of the "noise" that comes both from the patient and from the electronics (87,88). A low signal-to-noise ratio (S/N) means that the useful signal is not markedly stronger than the noise. The image appears "grainy," to use a common radiologic term based on standard film screen radiography. Several determinants of the MR system combine to determine the S/N for a given image (89). The patient is the source for the signal to be evaluated and for a significant amount of noise that is received. This component of the S/N is fixed and cannot be readily changed by the operator. The antenna, electronics, and computer also generate significant noise if proper engineering and design of the system are not employed, including the use of surface coils when indicated (vide infra) (90,91). This component of the S/N is manufacture-dependent, and great progress has been made by manufacturers in limiting the noise from this segment of the system. Another determinant of S/N is the magnetic field strength employed for imaging. At present, it is somewhat controversial exactly how S/N varies with field strength; however, an approximate guess at the present time is that S/N increases roughly in direct proportion to the square root of the field strength.

Of significance to users of MRI are the relationships between parameters of the imaging protocols employed and the S/N. Technical factors that can be selected at the time of imaging that affect S/N include the following: (a) the NEX employed, (b) the voxel size, (c) the TR value, (d) the TE value, and (e) the interslice spacing.

The NEX refers to the number of times a set of phase-encoded gradients is averaged together to calculate the image (see Eq. 1.4). In other words, an image could be obtained with one excitation, and if a 128 matrix were used in the y' direction, 128 90° pulses would be performed. This would require 128 times the TR to produce the image. If two excitations were used, then twice as many 90° pulses would be required to produce the image. Therefore, the data acquisition time would be doubled. The S/N improves propor-

TABLE 1.1. Association between pulse parameters and T1 and T2 weighing

| | TE | |
	Short (<30 ms)	Long (>60 ms)
TR		
Short (≤800 ms)	T1 weighted	Ugly
Long (≥2,000 ms)	Intermediate weighted	T2 weighted

tional to the square root of the number of excitations employed (87). Because examination time is an important factor in determining cost, a heavy price must be paid for using increased excitations to decrease the "graininess" of an image.

The S/N is also directly proportional to the square root of the volume of tissue emitting the signal, i.e., the voxel. As the size of the voxel increases, more tissue is available to return a signal. However, there is also more tissue to generate noise. Because the noise is random, it partly cancels itself, and the overall S/N improves proportional to the square root of the voxel size (87). In turn, the voxel size depends on the FOV used and the number of pixels into which the FOV is divided. A pixel is the area of the smallest picture unit that is used to generate the image, i.e., the cross-sectional area of a voxel in the plane of the image. Typical imagers use a 256 matrix along the frequency-encoded direction and either a 128, 192, or 256 matrix along the phase-encoded direction. The depth of the voxel is determined by the slice thickness. Therefore, the voxel size can be doubled by going from a 256 matrix along the y' direction to a 128 matrix, thus improving the S/N by the square root of 2. Alternatively, the voxel size can be doubled by increasing the slice thickness from a 5-mm to 10-mm thick section, with the matrix size being unchanged, and again a factor of the square root of 2 in S/N will be gained. Therefore, there is a strong interrelationship involving the time of imaging, the in-plane resolution, the slice thickness, and the size of the FOV.

The TR and TE values markedly affect S/N. As discussed in the previous section, a long TR allows the z component of $\mathbf{M}$ to relax back to near Mo, allowing the maximum signal to be generated after the next 90° pulse (Fig. 1.16). Because the noise is unchanged, long TR values result in better S/N. Conversely, TE is the time delay after the 90° pulse during which the signal rapidly decays before being sampled (Fig. 1.17). The longer the TE, the smaller the signal and the smaller the S/N.

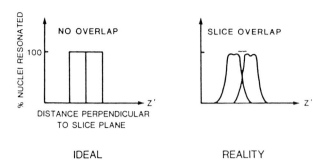

FIG. 1.20. Slice profile. The ideal slice profile would be rectangular. Unfortunately, real profiles have rounded, sloping edges that can overlap and degrade image quality.

The effect of interslice spacing on S/N and image contrast are somewhat more subtle (92–96). The slice selection technique discussed earlier (Fig. 1.11) does not give perfectly sharp edges to the slice. Instead, the edges of the slice are rounded (Fig. 1.20). If the slices abut one another, there is a volume of overlap between slices. In other words, some of the nuclei that resonated with the recent 90° pulse of the adjacent slice will again be resonated by the very next 90° pulse. This markedly shortens the effective TR for these nuclei, leading to less signal and decreased tissue contrast. Optimal image quality often requires a 20% separation between adjacent slices. In some MR imagers, interleaving the acquisition by pulsing every other slice in one sequence and then using a second acquisition immediately following the first to fill in the spaces also eliminates image degradation from slice overlaps. Table 1.2 summarizes the effects that various MRI parameters have on S/N.

In the final image, the most important determinant of diagnostic quality is the contrast resolution (87). Contrast resolution is, in essence, a combination of spatial resolution and contrast differences between adjacent anatomic structures or abnormalities. One of the major advantages of MRI over other cross-sectional

TABLE 1.2. *Factors affecting S/N, imaging time, and spatial resolution*

Factors affecting S/N	↑ Field strength	Number of excitations	↑ Voxel size	↑ TR	↑ TE	Slice spacing	Surface coil
Major effect on S/N	↑	↑ √N	↑ √V	↑	↓	↑	↑
Major effect on imaging time	○	↑ N	↓ (with ↓ number of phase encodings)	↑	○	○	○
Major effect on spatial resolution	○	○	↓	○	○	↓ (decrease in plane perpendicular to slice)	○

↑, Directly increases; ↓, directly decreases; ○, indirect effects only.
N, number of excitations; V, volume of the voxel.

imaging techniques is the increased inherent contrast between different soft tissues. Maximizing contrast resolution in MRI requires proper selection of imaging parameters and knowledge of the anatomy and abnormality to be evaluated.

ACQUISITION FIELD OF VIEW

The importance of the acquisition FOV in joint MRI cannot be overemphasized. High spatial resolution is essential in evaluating the many small anatomic structures that are critical in joint function, such as capsules, ligaments, tendons, etc. The spatial resolution along an axis within the image plane is given by the following equation:

$$\text{resolution (mm)} = \text{FOV (mm)}/\text{matrix} \qquad (1.5)$$

where FOV is the acquisition field of view and matrix is the acquisition matrix in the direction of interest. Therefore, spatial resolution is improved, i.e., is smaller, either by decreasing the acquisition FOV or increasing the acquisition matrix size. Since acquisition time increases with increasing matrix size, as described in Eq. 1.4, the most efficient imaging of joints is obtained using FOVs just large enough to include the body region of interest. Thus, ankle and foot imaging should be performed with acquisition FOVs in the range of 10 to 14 cm (Table 1.3).

ARTIFACTS

Artifacts in MRI of the knee can be divided into three categories: artifacts seen in images secondary to malfunction of the imaging apparatus; artifacts that are

TABLE 1.3. *Protocols used in evaluating the foot and ankle[a]*

Study	Seq.	Plane	FOV	TR	TE	TI	NEX	Sl. Th.	Skip	A. Mtx	Phase O	Comment
Achilles' tendon	1	S	16	500	15		1	3	I	256	+	True sagittal
	2	A	12	2,000	25/80		2	5	1	128 (192)[b]	+	With fast spin echo
	3	S	16	2,200	35	160	1	3	1.5	128	+	
Ankle and hindfoot	1	S	12	500	20		1	3	I	256	+	True sagittal
	2[b]	A	12	2,000	20/80		2	3	1	128	+	
	3	S/C	12	2,200	35	160	1	3	1.5	128		
	4	C/S	12	600	20		2	3	0.5	192	+	FAT SAT [b] For posterior tibial and peroneal tendons angle perpendicular to long axis of the tendon at the level of the malleolus
OCD of the talus	1	S	12	500	20		1	3	I	256	+	Dual 3″ coils
	2	C/S	12	600	20		2	3	0.5	192	+	FAT SAT
	3	S/C	12	2,200	35	160	1	3	1.5	128	+	Choice of S/C depends on lesion location
	4	A	12	2,000	25/80		2	3	0	128 (192)[b]		CS MEMP [b] Fast spin echo
Midfoot	1	S	12	500	20		1	3	I	256	+	
	2	A*	12	2,000	20/80		2	3	1	128	+	
	3	S	12	2,200	35	160	1	3	1.5	128	+	Optional
Forefoot	1	S	10	500	20		1	3	I	256	+	Quad or dual coils
	2	A*	10	2,000	20/80		2	3	1	128	+	
	3	S/C	10	2,200	35	160	1	3	1.5	128	+	Optional

[a] These protocols should only be used as a guide. A given patient's protocol may have to be specifically tailored to the clinical information needed. The surface coil utilized is an extremely important determinant of image quality.

Seq., sequence; Plane, plane of image; FOV, field of view; TR, repetition time; TE, echo delay time; TI, inversion time for inversion recovery images; NEX, number of excitations; Sl. Th., slice thickness; Skip, separation between slices; I, interleaved; A. Mtx, number of phase encodings; Phase O, oversampling in the phase direction; Sup, superior; S, sagittal; A, axial; A*, axial (see below); C, coronal.

For imaging the ankle, the axial plane (A) is considered to be perpendicular to the long axis of the lower leg (e.g., tibia and fibula).

For imaging the foot, the axial plane (A*) is considered to be perpendicular to the long axis of the metatarsals.

produced by properly functioning equipment and are inherent in the two-dimensional Fourier-transform MRI technique; and artifacts secondary to patient motion. This chapter will not address artifacts due to equipment malfunction. However, selected artifacts in the latter two categories that we have observed in MRI of the foot and ankle will be briefly discussed.

The physics and chemistry of chemical-shift artifacts have been discussed elsewhere (89,97–99). Briefly, chemical-shift artifacts are observed because hydrogen nuclei that are embedded in large molecules are surrounded by dense clouds of electrons. Because electrons are negatively charged, they will vary their normal orbits in the presence of a magnetic field such that their motions will induce a local magnetic field that will weakly oppose the main magnetic field. This has been called the diamagnetic effect and has been described by Purcell (100). Thus, hydrogen nuclei embedded in large molecules are "shielded" from the main magnetic field and will actually experience a slightly lower magnetic field strength. Because the frequency at which the nuclei precess is given by the Larmor equation (Eq. 1.1), these nuclei will precess at a slightly lower frequency than surrounding nuclei that are not embedded within the dense electron clouds of large molecules. For example, if one considers fat, in which the hydrogen nuclei along the triglyceride arms are embedded in dense electron clouds, and nearby free water, in which the hydrogen nuclei are essentially unshielded from the main magnetic field, then the hydrogen protons in fat will resonate at a lower frequency than those in surrounding water. As described previously, position along the x' direction is assigned based on frequencies. Therefore, there will be an apparent shift in the location of fat toward the low-frequency x' direction with respect to free water.

The chemical shift is dependent on several technical factors that can also be manipulated (97). The magnitude of the chemical shift increases with increasing field strength. However, the number of pixels involved in the chemical shift will decrease proportional to increasing slope of the frequency-encoding gradient. Therefore, the actual magnitude of the chemical shift in numbers of pixels and prominence on the images is dependent on the combination of the strength of the main magnetic field and the strength of the imaging gradients along the x' direction. A second type of chemical shift artifact is seen in gradient echo images. Since protons embedded in lipid precess slightly more slowly than protons in water, immediately after the initial excitation pulse both will be pointing in the same direction, i.e., "in phase." However, a few milliseconds later the bulk magnetization vector of the water protons will have precessed more rapidly and will be in front of **M** for lipid protons. The rapidity of this process depends on the strength of the main magnetic

field, B$_0$. At 1.5-T these spins go in and out of phase in approximately 4.5 ms. If you consider voxels between fat and water tissues that contain both fat and water, then the signal emanating from these voxels will depend on the TE selected. If the TE is chosen such that the fat and water **M**'s are in phase, the voxel signal will be bright. If the **M**'s are out of phase they will partially cancel each other and the signal from the voxel will be low. Consequently, "out-of-phase" images often show an artificial black line between fat and water tissues, such as between kidneys and retroperitoneal fat. "Out-of-phase" images may be more sensitive to bone marrow disease than "in-phase" images.

Artifacts secondary to arterial pulsation can significantly degrade images. This artifact looks like a "ring-down artifact" seen in ultrasound and is due to periodic ambiguities in assigning spatial location along the phase-encoded direction caused by regular motion of the arterial walls and blood flow (89,98,101–104). Another "ring artifact" occurs due to ambiguities in assigning spatial information when insufficient data have been obtained. This is called the "truncation artifact" and usually is more prominent in the phase-encoded direction (89,105,106). This has been confused with a related artifact, the "Gibb's artifact" (105). This is caused by the "wiggles" produced by the phase-encoding process at edges where there is a large, abrupt transition in tissue signal intensities (Fig. 1.9F). We have found that this only rarely poses a difficulty in diagnostic evaluation of the foot and ankle, especially when phase-encoding matrices of greater than 128 are used.

Wraparound artifact occurs when the computer incorrectly assigns a signal emanating from a body part outside the imaging FOV to a position location within the imaging FOV (89). This may be important when acquisition FOVs smaller than the body are used. Fortunately, wraparound artifact has been virtually eliminated in ankle and foot imaging by two techniques that are now widely used. Local surface coils both improve reception of signal from body nuclei, thus improving the S/N, and decrease wraparound artifact by limiting signal reception from other body tissues. Many scanners now also have the ability to acquire image data from a large region around the body part of interest, but display a high-resolution image of the region of interest without wraparound artifact (i.e., Fourier oversampling). This technique has been termed "no phase wrap" and "no frequency wrap" by some manufacturers. Since this technique of oversampling can be implemented without time or S/N costs, we routinely oversample in both frequency and phase directions to minimize artifacts. With these two techniques in widespread use, wraparound artifact is no longer a common problem in joint imaging.

Implanted metallic devices can produce artifacts in

MR images by two mechanisms. Ferromagnetic objects have their own permanent magnetic fields that can markedly distort a surrounding magnetic field. Because magnetic gradients are used in assigning spatial location in MRI, ferromagnetic implants can markedly distort MR images. Orthopedic implants are rarely ferromagnetic. All metals distort radiofrequency uniformity immediately adjacent to the implant and radiofrequency distortion produces bizarre signal changes (Fig. 1.21). However, the artifact is adjacent to the implant, and structures more than about 1 cm away from the metal usually can be well evaluated. In our experience, orthopedic implants have not posed a threat to patients undergoing MRI.

Artifacts stemming from the patient are predominantly due to motion (101,102,104). Using an interleaved data acquisition series, an interesting phenomenon can be seen with patient motion. Because an interleaved sequence requires two separate data acquisitions that are then interleaved, motion of the patient during only one data acquisition series causes artifact on every other image. Patient motion artifact is minimized by positioning the patient comfortably during the procedure, explaining the entire procedure to the patient before imaging, and limiting imaging time to the shortest period possible.

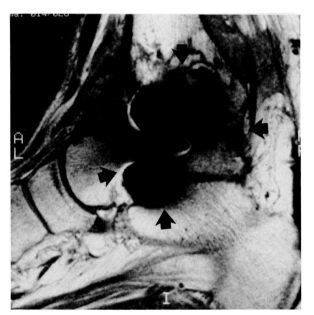

FIG. 1.21. Metal artifact. Because metals conduct electricity they can markedly distort rf fields, causing bizarre artifacts characterized by surrounding of seemingly random regions of very high and low signal intensity. Unlike CT, however, with MRI these artifacts are usually localized to the region of the body immediately surrounding the metal. Ferromagnetic objects will in addition markedly distort the surrounding magnetic field. Since magnetic fields are used for localizing the source of the image, this induces image distortion.

In summary, multiple potential artifacts can degrade MRIs of joints, and an adequate understanding of these artifacts is essential to avoid misinterpretation and to select image acquisition techniques that will maximize image quality.

SURFACE COILS

A surface coil is a radiofrequency antenna designed to be positioned near the surface of a tissue to be imaged to improve S/N when imaging a localized area of the body. The importance of S/N cannot be overemphasized in imaging extremities by MRI (65,90,91, 107,108).

Important anatomic parts in the extremities are small, so voxel sizes must be small to obtain necessary diagnostic spatial resolution. The number of excitations must be limited to minimize imaging time. We believe the use of surface coils is absolutely necessary for ankle and foot imaging with all currently available MR imagers. The sensitivity of the antenna for picking up the signal emanating from the tissues in large part depends on the proximity of the antenna wire to the tissue of interest (65,108–114). By placing the antenna close to the body, the efficiency of recovering the signal is improved without increasing noise to the same extent.

Surface coils are designed in various ways to maximize their efficiency with different types of magnets and different field strengths. Some surface coils are used only to receive the signal from the body part. Other surface coils both transmit the radiofrequency pulse and receive the radiofrequency signals from the tissues. A detailed description of surface coil technology is beyond the scope of this chapter. We have had excellent results using a local coil that both receives signal and transmits rf pulses (Fig. 1.22) (GE Medical Systems, Milwaukee, WI). High-resolution images of the foot and ankle can also be accomplished using a number of different surface coils and configurations. For high resolution, small FOV studies, the authors have used two circular 3-inch coils in a modified Helmholtz configuration (Fig. 1.22). More recently, a currently investigational quadrature coil has been used to produce high quality images of the toes and forefoot (Fig. 1.22) (GE Medical Systems, Milwaukee, WI).

EXAMINATION PROTOCOL

In designing imaging protocols for the foot and ankle, several points must be considered. A technique must be devised to produce images of good spatial and contrast resolution of the bones, tendons, ligaments,

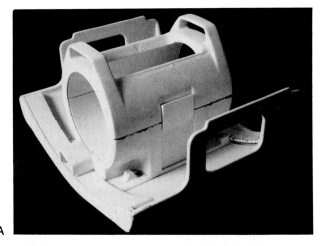

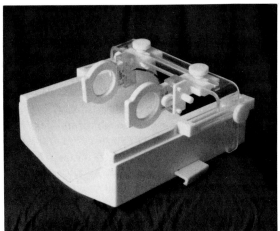

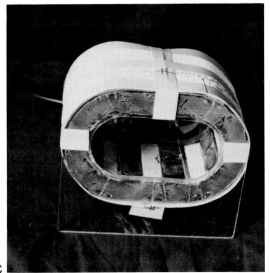

FIG. 1.22. Surface coil. A variety of surface coils and configurations can be used for imaging the ankle and foot. In **A**, a locally placed send-receive surface coil can provide overall excellent images of the ankle and foot. In **B**, two circular 3-inch coils in a modified Helmholtz configuration can provide excellent images for high resolution small FOV work such as the talar dome. In **C**, a currently investigational quadrature coil has produced excellent images of the toes and forefoot. (General Electric Medical Systems, Milwaukee, WI.)

and other relevant structures around the foot and ankle. The image acquisition time must be minimized to improve patient acceptability, decrease patient motion artifact, and limit the cost of the examination. Our goal was to design protocols that could be performed reliably within 30 to 45 min (Table 1.3).

BIOEFFECTS AND SAFETY CONSIDERATIONS OF MRI

Exposure to the three different electromagnetic fields used for MRI (i.e., the static magnetic field, gradient magnetic fields, and radiofrequency electromagnetic fields) are potentially hazardous to the patient if applied at sufficiently high levels (115–122). To date, more than 80 research studies have been conducted to determine whether there are any deleterious bioeffects associated with MRI. The results of these investigations have been summarized by Shellock (116) in a comprehensive review of this topic. The research on

bioeffects of MRI have yielded predominantly negative results, but the data are insufficient to assume absolute safety. Therefore, a number of areas of concern exist with respect to the safe application of this imaging modality.

BIOEFFECTS OF STATIC MAGNETIC FIELDS

The literature on static magnetic field–related bioeffects is contradictory and often confusing. Unfortunately, there is a paucity of data concerning the effects of high intensity static magnetic fields on humans. Some of the original investigations on human subjects exposed to static magnetic fields were performed by Vyalov (124,125), who studied workers involved in the permanent magnet industry. These subjects were exposed to static magnetic fields ranging from 0.015 T to 0.35 T and reported feelings of headache, chest pain, fatigue, vertigo, loss of appetite, insomnia, itching, and other nonspecific ailments (124,125). Exposure to additional potentially hazardous environmental working conditions (i.e., elevated room temperature, airborne metallic dust, chemicals, etc.) may have been partially responsible for the reported symptoms in these study subjects. Since this investigation lacked an appropriate control group, it is difficult to ascertain if there was a definite correlation between the exposure to the static magnetic fields and the reported abnormalities. Subsequent studies performed with more scientific rigor have not substantiated many of the above findings (119–121).

Temperature Effects

There are conflicting statements in the literature regarding the effect of static magnetic fields on body and skin temperatures of mammals. Reports have indicated that static magnetic fields either increase or both increase and decrease temperature depending on the orientation of the organism in the static magnetic fields (126). Other articles state that static magnetic fields have no effect on skin and body temperatures of mammals (121,127,128,129).

A recent investigation indicated exposure to a 1.5-T static magnetic field does not alter skin and body temperatures in humans (129). This study was performed using a special fluoroptic thermometry system demonstrated to be unperturbed by high intensity static magnetic fields (129). Therefore, skin and body temperatures of human subjects are not believed to be effected by exposure to static magnetic fields up to 1.5 T (128,129).

Magnetohydrodynamic Effects

A magnetohydrodynamic effect (i.e., an additional biopotential superimposed on the normal biopotential) may be observed during exposure to static magnetic fields and is caused by blood, a conductive fluid, flowing through a magnetic field. The result is an induced biopotential. This induced biopotential is exhibited by an augmentation of T wave amplitude as well as other nonspecific waveform changes that are apparent on the electrocardiogram and have been observed at static magnetic field strengths of as low as 0.1 T (121,130,131). The increase in T wave amplitude is directly related to the intensity of the static magnetic field, such that at low static magnetic field strengths the effects are not as predominant compared with higher ones. Because there are no other circulatory alterations that appear to coincide with these electrocardiographic changes, no short-term biologic risks are believed to be associated with the magnetohydrodynamic effect that occurs in conjunction with static magnetic field strengths up to 2 T (120,121,130).

Neurological Effects

Theoretically, electrical impulse conduction in nerve tissue may be affected by exposure to static magnetic fields. However, this is another area in the biological effects literature that contains contradictory information. Some researchers have reported remarkable effects on the function as well as the structures of the central nervous system that were associated with exposure to static magnetic fields (132–141), whereas others have failed to show any significant changes (142–145). Further investigations of potential unwanted biological effects are needed because of the relative lack of clinical studies in this field that are directly applicable to MRI. At the present time, exposure to static magnetic fields up to 2.0 T do not appear to influence significantly bioelectric properties of neurons in humans (115,116,120).

In summary, there is no conclusive evidence for irreversible or hazardous biological effects related to acute, short-term exposures of humans to static magnetic fields up to field strengths of 2.0 T. However, as of 1992, there are five 4.0-T MR scanners operating at various research sites around the world. A preliminary study has indicated that workers and volunteer subjects exposed to a 4.0-T MRI system have experienced vertigo, nausea, headaches, a metallic taste in their mouths, and magnetophosphenes (i.e., visual light flashes believed to be caused by gradient magnetic field–induced excitation of the retina) (135). Further research is required to study the mechanisms responsible for these undesirable bioeffects and to determine possible means to counterbalance them.

BIOEFFECTS OF GRADIENT MAGNETIC FIELDS

Gradient magnetic fields can induce electrical fields and currents in conductive media, including biologic tissue, according to Faraday's law of induction. The potential for interaction between gradient magnetic fields and biologic tissue is inherently dependent on the fundamental field frequency, maximum flux density, average flux density, the presence of harmonic frequencies, the waveform characteristics of the signal, the polarity of the signal, the current distribution in the body, and the electrical properties and sensitivity of the particular cell membrane (115–119, 145).

The induction of significant electrical currents in conductive tissues is a potential source of harmful bioeffects associated with MRI. For example, intense currents could directly stimulate electrically excitable cells (i.e., nerve cells, skeletal muscle fibers, blood vessels, cardiac muscle fibers, etc.) to depolarize and alter normal physiologic function. The physiologic reactions to induced electrical currents range from mild cutaneous sensations to involuntary muscle contractions, burns, cardiac arrhythmias, and cardiac fibrillation (116,120,121,122,146,147,148).

The production of magnetophosphenes, which are visual light flashes of flickers, is considered to be one of the most sensitive physiologic responses to gradient magnetic fields (120–122). Magnetophosphenes are supposedly caused by electrical stimulation of the retina and are completely reversible with no associated health effects (120). There has been no report of the occurrence of magnetophosphenes related to the use of clinical MRI scanners up to field strengths of 1.5 T. However, magnetophosphenes have been observed by normal subjects with a 4.0-T MRI scanner (135).

The current recommendation issued by the U.S. FDA for exposure to gradient magnetic fields during MRI is that the rate of change of the magnetic fields should not be sufficient to cause peripheral nerve stimulation by an adequate margin of safety (at least a factor of three) (149). In the event that significant electrical currents are induced during MRI, it is predicted that cutaneous nerves or peripheral skeletal muscle will be stimulated and, thus, give ample warning before the occurrence of a more deleterious response, such as cardiac arrhythmia or fibrillation (115,116,117, 120,150).

The above guidelines are believed to provide a wide margin of safety with respect to exposure to gradient magnetic fields during MRI, but it is imperative to realize that the newer echo planar or imaging techniques that require more rapid and complex applications of gradient magnetic fields may easily exceed the recommended levels and must be thoroughly evaluated for potential health hazards. Preliminary studies performed in human subjects have demonstrated that induced eddy currents have resulted in peripheral nerve stimulation producing muscle twitches or contractions in synchrony with field pulses (151,152).

BIOEFFECTS OF RADIOFREQUENCY ELECTROMAGNETIC FIELDS

Radiofrequency (RF) radiation is capable of generating heat in tissues as a result of resistive losses. Therefore, the main bioeffects associated with exposure to RF radiation are related to the thermogenic qualities of this electromagnetic field (115–118,120, 153–155). Exposure to RF radiation may also cause athermal, field-specific alterations in biological systems that are produced without a significant increase in temperature (118,148,156). This topic is somewhat controversial due to assertions concerning the role of electromagnetic fields in producing cancer and developmental abnormalities, along with the concomitant ramifications of such effects (118,148,156,157). A re-

port from the U.S. Environmental Protection Agency claimed that the existing evidence on this tissue is sufficient to demonstrate a relationship between low-level electromagnetic field exposures and the development of cancer (156). To date, there have been no specific studies performed to study potential athermal biological effects of MRI. However, those interested in a thorough review of this topic, particularly as it pertains to MRI, are referred to the extensive article by Beers (157).

Exposure to RF radiation is typically quantified by means of determining the specific absorption rate (SAR) (122,148,154). SAR is the mass normalized rate at which RF power is coupled to biologic tissue and is indicated in units of watts per kilogram (W/kg). Measurements or estimates of SAR are not trivial, particularly in human subjects, and there are several methods of determining this parameter for RF energy dosimetry (122,148,154,155,158,159).

The SAR that is produced during MRI is a complex function of numerous variables including the frequency (which, in turn, is determined by the strength of the static magnetic field), type of RF pulse (i.e., 90° or 180°), repetition time, pulse width, type of RF coil used, volume of tissue within the coil, resistivity of the tissue, configuration of the anatomical region imaged, and other factors (115,116,120). The actual increase in tissue temperature caused by exposure to RF radiation depends on the duration of exposure, the ambient conditions, and the specific qualities of the subject's thermoregulatory system (i.e., skin blood flow, sweat rate, etc.).

The efficiency and absorption pattern of RF energy are mainly determined by the physical dimensions of the tissue in relation to the incident wavelength (120,122,148,154). Because of the above relationship between RF energy and physical dimensions, studies that are designed to investigate the effects of exposure to RF radiation during MRI that are intended to be applicable to the clinical setting require tissue volumes and anatomical shapes comparable to that of human subjects. Of additional note is that there is no laboratory animal that sufficiently mimics or simulates the thermoregulatory system or responses of humans. For these reasons, results obtained in laboratory animal experiments cannot simply be "scaled" or extrapolated to human subjects (122,148,153–155).

Little quantitative data has been previously available on thermoregulatory responses of humans exposed to RF radiation before the studies performed with MRI. The few studies that existed did not directly apply to MRI because these investigations either examined thermal sensations or therapeutic applications of diathermy, usually involving only localized regions of the body (122,148,154,158). Several studies of RF power absorption during MRI have been performed recently and have yielded useful information about tissue heating. During MRI, tissue heating results primarily from magnetic induction with a negligible contribution from the electric fields, so that ohmic heating occurs greatest at the surface of the body and approaches zero at the center of the body. Predictive calculations and measurements obtained in phantoms and human subjects exposed to MRI support this pattern of temperature distribution (160–166).

An investigation using fluoroptic thermometry probes that are unperturbed by electromagnetic fields (165) demonstrated that human subjects exposed to MRI at SAR levels up to 4.0 W/kg (i.e., 10 times higher than the level currently recommended by the U.S. FDA) have no statistically significant increases in body temperatures and elevations in skin temperatures that are not believed to be clinically hazardous (165). These results imply that the suggested exposure level of 4.0 W/kg for RF radiation during MRI is too conservative for individuals with normal thermoregulatory function (165). Additional studies are needed, however, to assess physiologic responses of patients with conditions that may impair thermoregulatory function (e.g., elderly patients; patients with underlying health conditions such as fever, diabetes, cardiovascular disease, or obesity; and patients taking medications that affect thermoregulation such as calcium blockers, beta blockers, diuretics, vasodilators, etc.) before subjecting them to MRI procedures that require high SARs.

Theoretically, an RF radiation "hot spot" caused by an uneven distribution of RF power may arise whenever current concentrations are produced in association with restrictive conductive patterns (120). There has been the suggestion that RF radiation "hot spots" may generate thermal "hot spots" under certain conditions during MRI (120). Since RF radiation is mainly absorbed by peripheral tissues, thermography has been used to study the heating pattern associated with MRI at high whole-body SARs (161). This study demonstrated that there is no evidence of surface thermal "hot spots" related to MRI of human subjects. The thermoregulatory system apparently responds to the heat challenge by distributing the thermal load, producing a "smearing" effect of the surface temperatures. However, there is a possibility that internal thermal "hot spots" may develop from MRI (167).

CURRENT SAFETY RECOMMENDATIONS FOR MRI

In 1988, the U.S. FDA reclassified MRI scanners from a Class III to a Class II device and revised safety recommendations that were originally issued in 1982 (149). The present recommended FDA guidelines for

exposures to the electromagnetic radiation used during MRI are as follows:

1. *Static magnetic field.* Static magnetic field strengths not exceeding 2.0 T are below the level of concern for the static magnetic field. Should the static magnetic field strength exceed 2.0 T, additional evidence of safety must be provided by the sponsor or manufacturer.

2. *Gradient magnetic field.* The acceptable exposures to gradient magnetic fields are those that are insufficient to induce peripheral neuromuscular stimulation by at least a factor of three. Alternatively, other safety criteria may be implemented by those involved in MRI, as follows: a) demonstrate that the maximum dB/dt of the MRI system is 6 T/sec or less; b) demonstrate that for axial gradients, dB/dt <20 T/s for $r \geq 120$ μs, or dB/dt $< (2,400/r)$ T/s for 12 μs $< r <$ 120 μs, or dB/dt < 200 T/s for $r \leq 12$ μs (r equals the width in μs of a rectangular pulse or the half period of a sinusoidal dB/dt pulse). For transverse gradients, dB/dt is considered to be below the level of concern when it is less than three times the above limits for axial gradients.

3. *RF electromagnetic fields.* The acceptable exposures are a whole-body averaged specific absorption rate (SAR) of ≤ 0.04 W/kg, spatial peak in 1 g of tissue of ≤ 8.0 W/kg, and 3.2 W/kg averaged over the head or, alternatively, those that do not cause a body core temperature greater than 1°C except for inpatients with impaired systemic blood flow and/or perspiration (i.e., patients with compromised thermoregulatory systems), local exposures of less than 38°C in the head, 39° within the trunk, and 40° in the extremities (149). The above exposure levels apply to normal clinical environments where the individual is resting and lightly dressed.

MRI AND PATIENTS WITH ELECTRICALLY, MAGNETICALLY, OR MECHANICALLY ACTIVATED IMPLANTS AND DEVICES

The U.S. FDA requires labeling of MRI scanners to indicate that the device is contraindicated for patients who have electrically, magnetically, or mechanically activated implants because the magnetic and electromagnetic fields produced by the MR device may interfere with the operation of these devices (149). Therefore, patients with internal cardiac pacemakers, implantable cardiac defibrillators, cochlear implants, neurostimulators, bone-growth stimulators, implantable electronic drug infusion pumps, and other similar devices that could be adversely affected by the electromagnetic fields used for MRI should not be examined by this imaging modality (115,116,120,167–171).

Prior *ex vivo* testing of certain of these implants and devices may indicate that they are, in fact, MRI compatible.

The risks associated with scanning patients with cardiac pacemakers are related to the possibility of movement, reed switch closure or damage, programming changes, inhibition or reversion to an asynchronous mode of operation, electromagnetic interference, and induced currents in lead wires (120,171). At least one patient with a pacemaker has been scanned by MRI without incident (172). A letter to the editor recently indicated that a patient who was not pacemaker-dependent underwent MRI knowingly having his pacemaker "disabled" during the procedure (172). Although this patient sustained no apparent discomfort and the pacemaker was not damaged, it is inadvisable to perform this type of maneuver routinely on patients with pacemakers because of the potential to encounter the aforementioned hazards.

Of particular concern is the possibility that the pacemaker lead wire(s) or other similar intracardiac wire configuration could act as an antenna in which the gradient and/or RF electromagnetic fields may induce sufficient current to cause fibrillation, a burn, or other potentially dangerous event (120,173). Because of this theoretically deleterious and unpredicted effect, patients referred to MRI with residual external pacing wires, temporary pacing wires, Swan-Ganz thermodilution catheters, and/or any other type of internally or externally positioned conductive wire or similar device should not undergo MRI because of the possible associated risks (173–175).

Some types of cochlear implants employ a relatively high-field strength cobalt samarium magnet used in conjunction with an external magnet to align and retain a radiofrequency transmitter coil on the patient's head, whereas other types of cochlear implants are electronically activated. Consequently, MRI is strictly contraindicated in patients with these implants because of the high likelihood of injuring the patient and/or the possibility of damaging or altering the operation of the cochlear implant.

Because there is a potential for demagnetizing implants that involve magnets (i.e., certain dental implants, sphincters, stoma plugs, ocular implants, and other similar devices) that may necessitate surgery to replace the damaged device, these should be removed from the patient before MRI, if possible (168,169). Otherwise, MRI should not be performed on a patient with a magnetically activated implant. A patient with any other similar electrically, magnetically, or mechanically activated implant or device should be excluded from examination by MRI unless the particular implant or device has been previously demonstrated to be unaffected by the electromagnetic fields used for MRI (170).

MRI AND METALLIC IMPLANTS, MATERIALS, OR DEVICES

The potential risks associated with performing MRI in patients with ferromagnetic implants, materials, or devices are related to the induction of electric currents, heating, the misinterpretation of an artifact as an abnormality, and the possibility of movement or dislodgement (115,116,120). Electrical currents can be generated in conductive materials by gradient magnetic fields or by movement of conductive materials through the static magnetic field. Conductive implants, materials, or devices may be heated by the induction of electromotive forces subjected to gradient magnetic fields and, under certain conditions, by arcing effects if the object is positioned too close to another conductor and sufficient voltage is generated (120). To date, there have been several incidents of MRI inducing electrical currents in metallic devices that resulted in injuries to patients (175). The majority of these incidents were related to the misuse of monitoring devices, whereby current was induced in the leads or cables of the monitors during MRI, resulting in superficial heating and, in some cases, serious burns (174,175). In regard to temperature elevations produced by MRI of metallic implants, materials, or devices, none of these appear to be clinically significant (176–182).

The various types of artifacts caused by metal, including unusual artifacts arising from tattooed eyeliner and certain types of eye make-up, have been described and are generally well recognized (183,184). The distortion of the image by metallic implants or materials is caused by the disruption of the local magnetic field that perturbs the relationship between position and frequency that is crucial for accurate image reconstruction. Ferromagnetic implants, materials, or devices that incorporate small magnets can produce especially significant artifacts (168,169).

The degree of image distortion depends on the magnetic susceptibility, quantity, shape, orientation, and position of the object in the body as well as the technique used for imaging and image processing (i.e., 2D Fourier transform reconstruction, back projection, etc.) (184). Artifacts caused by MRI of patients with metallic implants, materials, or devices are typically seen as local or regional distortions of the image and/or signal void that is frequently unpredictable. In some instances, a marked hyperintensity may be observed. Certain nonferromagnetic implants, materials, or devices may likewise cause image artifacts because eddy currents can be generated in these objects by gradient magnetic fields that, in turn, disrupt the local magnetic field (120,173,184).

Several important factors influence the relative risk of using MRI in patients with ferromagnetic implants or materials, including the strength of the static and gradient magnetic fields; the degree of ferromagnetism of the implant, material, or device; the mass and geometry of the implant, material, or device; its location and orientation *in situ*; and the length of time it has been in place (115,116,120,173). These factors should be considered carefully before subjecting a patient with a ferromagnetic implant, material, or device to MRI particularly if it is located in a potentially dangerous area of the body where movement or dislodgement could injure the patient.

Numerous studies have assessed the ferromagnetic qualities of various metallic implants, materials, or devices by measuring the deflection forces or movement associated with static magnetic fields used for MRI. The results have indicated that patients with certain metallic implants, materials, or devices that are nonferromagnetic or ferromagnetic ones that are minimally affected by the magnetic fields relative to their *in vivo* applications (i.e., deflection force was considered to be insufficient to move or dislodge the implant or material *in situ*) can safely undergo MRI. Because

TABLE 1.4. *Metallic implants and foreign bodies contraindicated for MRI*

Aneurysm clips
  Drake (DR14, DR24), Edward Weck, Triangle Park, NJ
  Drake (DR16), Edward Weck
  Drake (301 SS), Edward Weck
  Downs multipositional (17-7PH)
  Heifetz (17-7PH), Edward Weck
  Housepian
  Kapp (405 SS), V. Mueller
  Kapp curved (404 SS), V. Mueller
  Kapp straight (404 SS), V. Mueller
  Mayfield (301 SS), Codman, Randolph, MA
  Mayfield (304 SS), Codman
  McFadden (301 SS), Codman
  Pivot (17-7PH), V. Mueller
  Scoville (EN58J), Downs Surgical, Decatur, GA
  Sundt-Kees (301 SS), Downs Surgical
  Sundt-Kees Multi-Angle (17-7PH), Downs Surgical
  Vari-Angle (17-7PH), Codman
  Vari-Angle Micro (17-7PM SS), Codman
  Vari-Angle Spring (17-7PM SS), Codman
Carotid artery vascular clamps
  Poppen-Blaylock (SS), Codman
Dental devices and materials
  [a] Palladium clad magnet, Parkell Products, Farmingdale, NY
  [a] Titanium clad magnet, Parkell Products
  [a] Stainless steel clad magnet, Parkell Products
Heart valves
  Starr-Edwards, Model Pre 6000, American Edwards, Irvine, CA

Intravascular coils, stents and filters
  [b] Gianturco embolization coil, Cook, Bloomington, ID
  [b] Gianturco bird nest IVC filter, Cook
  [b] Gianturco zig-zag Stent, Cook
  [b] Gunther IVC filter, Cook
  [b] New retrievable IVC filter, Thomas Jefferson University, Philadelphia, PA
  [b] Palmaz endovascular stent, Ethicon, Sommerville, NJ
Ocular implants
  [a] Fatio eyelid spring/wire
  Retinal tack (SS-martensitic), Western European
Otologic implants
  Cochlear implant (3M/House)
  Cochlear implant (3M/Vienna)
  Cochlear implant, Nucleus Mini 22-channel, Cochlear, Englewood, CO
  McGee piston stapes prosthesis, (platinum/17Cr-4Ni SS), Richards Medical, Memphis, TN
Pellets, bullets, schrapnel, etc.
  BB's, Daisy
  BB's, Crosman
  Bullet, 7.62 × 39 mm (copper, steel), Norinco
  Bullet, 0.380", (copper, nickel, lead), Geco
  Bullet, 0.45", (steel, lead), North America Ordinance
  Bullet, 9 mm (copper, lead), Norma
Penile implants
  [a] Penile Implant, OmniPhase, Dacomed Corp., Minneapolis, MN
Miscellaneous
  Cerebral ventricular shunt tube, connector (type unknown)
  [c] Swan-Ganz Catheter, Thermodilution, American Edwards, Irvine, CA
  [a] Tissue expander with magnetic port, McGhan Medical, Santa Barbara, CA

[a] The potential for these metallic implants or devices to produce significant injury to the patient is minimal. However, performing MRI in a patient with one of these devices may be uncomfortable for the individual and/or may result in damage to the implant.

[b] Ferromagnetic coils, filters, and stents typically become firmly incorporated into the vessel wall several weeks after placement and, therefore, it is highly unlikely that they will become dislodged by magnetic forces after a suitable period of time has passed.

[c] While there is no magnetic deflection associated with the Swan-Ganz thermodilution catheter, there has been a report of a catheter "melting" in a patient undergoing MRI. Therefore, this catheter is considered contraindicated for MRI.

The relative risks of performing MRI in patients with pellets, bullets, or schrapnel are related to whether or not they are positioned near a vital structure.

Manufacturer information is provided if indicated in previously published references or if, otherwise, known.

SS, stainless steel.

prior knowledge of the interaction between the magnetic fields and the specific type of metallic implant, material, or device is essential for safe screening of patients, the literature on this topic has been compiled and is presented in Table 1.4.

Various types of orthopedic implants, materials, and devices (i.e., hip prostheses, stainless steel mesh, nails, screws, plates, wires, etc.) have been evaluated to determine the presence of ferromagnetic qualities. Of these, only the Perfix interference screw used for reconstruction of the anterior cruciate ligament has significant ferromagnetism. Although the potential for movement or dislodgement of this implant is minimal once it is placed *in vivo*, the substantial artifact created by the presence of the Perfix interference screw prevents an evaluation of the knee by MRI.

Patients may present for MRI with externally applied devices that must also be assessed for safety before undergoing examination by this imaging technique. For example, a halo vest used for fixation of the cervical spine is an example of a metallic device that may or may not be compatible with MRI. Most halo vests are composed of metallic materials that present unwanted risks and produce mild to severe imaging artifacts (185–187). Therefore, patients with

halo vests are not typically regarded as suitable candidates for MRI. This is unfortunate because MRI often provides a useful diagnostic evaluation of the spinal cord and associated soft tissue structures that is unobtainable with other imaging techniques.

A study detailing the effect of various halo vests on image quality has indicated that these devices cause image distortion that is primarily dependent on the type of material used to construct the halo rings and support uprights (185). Halo vests made from stainless steel produced the poorest image quality followed by those made from aluminum, titanium, and graphite (185). This prior study did not assess deflection forces, heating, or induced currents, each of which may present a potential hazard to the patient undergoing MRI if the halo vest is mainly composed of ferromagnetic and/or conductive materials.

Some commercially available halo devices are composed of nonferromagnetic materials, but there is still a theoretical hazard of inducing electric current in the ring portion of any halo device made from conductive materials (187). The current within such a closed loop is of additional concern for eddy current induction and potential image degradation effects (185–187). Furthermore, there is a potential for the patient to be in-

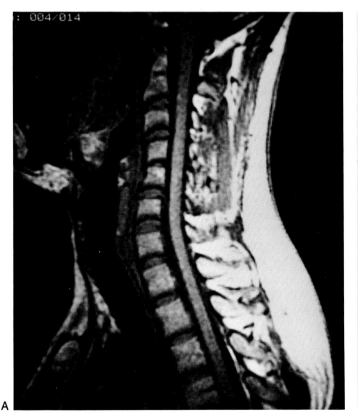
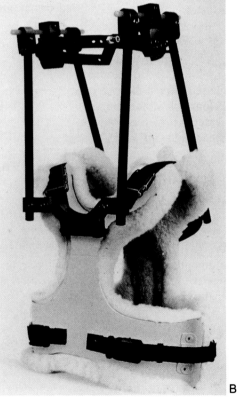

FIG. 1.23. T1-weighted sagittal plane image of the cervical spine (**A**) obtained from a patient wearing an MRI-compatible halo vest (**B**).

volved in part of this closed loop, so that there would be the concern of a possible burn or electric injury to the patient.

Specially designed, commercially available halo vests have now been developed that are made from both nonferromagnetic and nonconductive materials that have little or no interaction with the electromagnetic fields used for MRI (Fig. 1.23). Therefore, there are no associated safety-related problems or imaging artifacts related to the use of these devices during MRI of the cervical spine.

Another possible risk related to MRI and ferromagnetic materials is the "missile effect." The missile effect refers to the capability of the static magnetic field to attract ferromagnetic objects (i.e., oxygen tanks, tools, etc.) within the fringe field that may subsequently be drawn into the magnet by considerable force. This represents one of the greatest potential hazards of the static magnetic field and the occurrence of the missile effect can pose a significant risk to the patient inside the scanner and/or anyone who is in the path of the ferromagnetic missile. In extreme cases, the magnet may need to be "quenched" in order to extract sizable ferromagnetic objects from MRI systems, particularly those with high-field strengths, resulting in considerable financial loss due to replacing cryogens, down-time, etc.

In order to guard against a catastrophe caused by the missile effect, the immediate area around the MRI scanner should be clearly demarcated, labeled with appropriate warning signs, and secured by trained staff that are cognizant of MRI safety. In addition, all patients, visitors, and other individuals who enter the magnet area should be screened, their metallic personal belongings should be removed, and they should be educated about the potential hazards of the magnetic fringe field of the MRI scanner.

SCREENING PATIENTS FOR METALLIC FOREIGN BODIES BEFORE MRI

Patients may present to MRI with a history of metallic foreign bodies such as bullets, shrapnel, or other types of metallic fragments. The relative risk of scanning these patients depends on the possibility of movement or dislodgement of the metallic foreign body as well as whether or not it is positioned in a potentially hazardous site within the body (170).

A patient who encounters the static magnetic field of an MRI scanner with an intraocular metallic foreign body is at a particular risk for significant eye injury. The single reported case of a patient who experienced eye damage resulting in blindness underwent MRI on a 0.35-T scanner and had an intraocular metal fragment dislodged, which was 2.0 × 3.5 mm in size, during the procedure (188). This incident emphasizes the importance of adequately screening patients with suspected intraocular metallic foreign bodies before MRI.

Patients with a high suspicion of having an intraocular metallic foreign body (e.g., a metal worker exposed to metallic slivers with a history of an eye injury) should have radiographs of the orbits to rule out the presence of a metallic fragment before exposure to the static magnetic field. If a patient with a suspected ferromagnetic intraocular foreign body has no symptoms and radiographs of the orbits do not demonstrate a radiopaque foreign body, MRI may be performed safely. If a patient has no history of injury to the eye but was a metal worker or subjected to metallic splinters or fragments, it is highly unlikely that this patient has a metallic foreign body that would cause an injury during MRI. Therefore, MRI may be performed in this instance without obtaining radiographs of the orbits. However, if the patient presents with a history of an eye injury caused by a metal foreign body, radiographs of the orbits are obtained to ascertain whether or not the foreign body was removed. The above is the recommendation of the Safety Committee of the Society for Magnetic Resonance Imaging (170).

Patients referred for examination by MRI may also have foreign bodies from pellets, bullets, or schrapnel. Most of the pellets and bullets that have been previously tested for ferromagnetism are composed of nonferromagnetic materials (181,182). Ferromagnetic ammunition typically comes from foreign countries and/or is used by the military (181,182). Schrapnel usually contains various amounts of steel and, therefore, is ferromagnetic and presents a potential hazard for MRI (181,182). Furthermore, since pellets, bullets, and schrapnel may be contaminated with ferromagnetic materials, these objects represent relative contraindications for MRI (181,182). Patients with these foreign bodies should be regarded on an individual basis with respect to whether the object is positioned near a vital neural, vascular, or soft tissue structure. Using conventional radiography to search for metallic foreign bodies is a sensitive and relatively inexpensive means of identifying patients who are unsuitable for MRI and can also be used to screen patients who may have metal fragments in potentially hazardous sites of the body.

Each imaging center should establish a standardized policy for screening patients with suspected foreign bodies. The policy should include guidelines to which patients require work-up by radiographic procedures, the specific procedure to be performed (i.e., number and type of views, position of the anatomy, etc.), and each case should be considered on an individual basis (170). These precautions should be taken with regard to patients referred to MRI in any MRI system regardless of the field strength, magnet type, and presence or absence of magnetic shielding (170).

POTENTIAL HAZARDS OF ACOUSTIC NOISE ASSOCIATED WITH MRI

A potential risk associated with the use of MRI is related to the acoustic noise produced during the operation of the scanner. Acoustic noise is caused by the activation and deactivation of the gradient magnetic fields. This noise is enhanced with higher gradient magnetic fields, higher gradient duty cycles, and sharper pulse transitions (170,189). Acoustic noise generated during MRI has been demonstrated to cause patient annoyance, interference with oral communication, and reversible hearing loss in patients who did not wear ear protection (190).

Although gradient magnetic field–related noise levels measured on several commercial MRI devices were considered to be within the recommended safety guidelines (189), these safe levels do not take into consideration that MRI is used for a patient population that may be more sensitive to the effects of acoustic noise. In addition, there has not been any research on the effect of the more significant gradient noises associated with the newer echo planar or ultrafast imaging techniques that are significantly louder than conventional pulse sequences. Furthermore, the possibility exists that significant gradient coil–induced noise may produce permanent hearing impairment in certain patients who are particularly susceptible to the damaging effects of relatively loud noises. The safest and least expensive means of preventing problems associated with acoustic noise during MRI is to require the routine use of disposable earplugs or other similar noise reduction device (116,170,173).

THE USE OF MRI IN PREGNANT PATIENTS

The current guidance of the U.S. FDA requires labeling of MRI devices to indicate that the safety of MRI when used to image the fetus and the infant "has not been established" (149). In Great Britain, the National Radiological Protection Board in 1983 in recommending the acceptable limits of exposure for clinical MRI specified that "it might be prudent to exclude pregnant women during the first three months of pregnancy" (191).

Although MRI is not currently considered to be hazardous to the fetus, only a few investigations have examined the teratogenic potential of this imaging modality. By comparison, literally thousands of studies have been performed to examine the possible hazards of ultrasound during pregnancy and controversy still exists concerning the safe use of this diagnostic imaging modality.

MRI is indicated for use in pregnant women if other non-ionizing forms of diagnostic imaging are inadequate or if the examination provides important information that would otherwise require exposure to ionizing radiation (i.e., x-ray, computed tomography, etc.). For pregnant patients, it is recommended that they be informed that, to date, there has been no indication that the use of clinical MRI during pregnancy has produced deleterious effects. However, as noted by the FDA, the safety of MRI during pregnancy has not been proven (170). The above information is detailed in the Policies, Guidelines, and Recommendations for MR Imaging Safety and Patient Management developed by the Safety Committee of the Society for Magnetic Resonance Imaging (170).

Patients who are pregnant or suspect they are pregnant must be identified before undergoing MRI in order to assess the risks versus the benefits of the examination. Since there is a high spontaneous abortion rate in the general population during the first trimester of pregnancy (i.e., >30%), particular care should be exercised with the use of MRI during the first trimester because of associated potential medicolegal implications relative to spontaneous abortions.

MRI AND PATIENTS WITH CLAUSTROPHOBIA

Claustrophobia and a variety of other psychological reactions including anxiety, panic disorders, and emotional distress may occur in patients before or during the MRI examination. These sensations originate from several factors, including the restrictive dimensions of the interior of the MRI scanner, the gradient noises, the duration of the examination, the ambient conditions within the bore of the magnet, etc. Because deleterious psychological responses to MRI usually delay or require cancellation of the examination, several different procedures have been developed and are recommended to avert these problems, including (192–197):

1. educating the patient concerning the specific aspects of the MRI examination including the internal dimensions of the scanner, the level of gradient noise to expect, etc.
2. allowing a relative or friend who has been properly screened to remain with the patient during the procedure
3. maintaining physical or verbal contact with the patient
4. placing the patient in a prone position to alleviate the "closed-in" feelings or introducing the patient feet-first versus head-first into the scanner

5. using a fan in the magnet bore to provide additional air movement
6. providing MRI-compatible headphones to transmit music to the patient
7. using prisms or mirrored glasses or mirrors within the scanner to allow the patient to see out of the scanner
8. using a blindfold so that the patient is not aware of the close surroundings
9. using relaxation strategies such as controlled breathing or mental imagery
10. using hypnotism or psychological "desensitization" techniques
11. providing use of MRI-compatible stereo or television during the procedure.

These aforementioned procedures used either individually or in combination will have varying degrees of success. If all else fails, short-acting sedation or anesthesia may be necessary to accomplish the MRI examination in patients experiencing claustrophobia, anxiety, panic disorders, or emotional distress.

SEDATION AND ANESTHESIA DURING MRI

Choloral hydrate is often used as the primary agent of sedation for MRI performed on children less than 2 years old at a dosage of 80 mg/kg (not to exceed 2,000 mg) (198). Supplemental Nembutal may be used during the MRI examination at a dosage of up to 2 mg/kg and is administered intravenously (198). Sleep deprivation is recommended for a higher success rate when sedating children (198). For adults, intravenous diazapam is typically effective for adequate sedation during MRI. In more difficult cases, general anesthesia may be required and should be administered by an anesthesiologist experienced in working in the MRI environment.

MONITORING PHYSIOLOGIC PARAMETERS DURING MRI

Physiologic monitoring is essential for the safe use of MRI in patients who are sedated, anesthetized, comatose, critically ill, or otherwise unable to communicate with the operator. All of these types of patients should be routinely monitored during MRI and, in view of the variety of currently available MRI-compatible monitoring equipment (Fig. 1.24), there is no reason to exclude these patients from examination by this imaging technique. Virtually every physiologic parameter that may be obtained under normal circumstances in the critical care unit or operating room is capable of being monitored during MRI. These parameters include heart rate, systemic blood pressure, intracardiac

pressure, end-tidal carbon dioxide, oxygen saturation, respiratory rate, skin blood flow, and temperature (198–201). Table 1.5 lists several examples of MRI-compatible monitors that have been tested and operated successfully at static magnetic field strengths up

TABLE 1.5. *Examples of MRI-compatible monitors and respirators[a]*

Device and manufacturer	Function
Omega 1400 In Vivo Laboratories, Inc. Broken Arrow, OK	Blood pressure Heart rate
Fiber-Optic Pulse Oximeter Nonin Medical Plymouth, MI	Oxygen saturation Heart rate
525 Respiratory Rate Monitor Biochem International Waukesha, WI	Respiratory rate
MicroSpan Capnometer 8800 Biochem International Waukesha, WI	Respiratory rate End-tidal carbon dioxide
Aneuroid Chest Bellows Coulbourn Instruments Allentown, PA	Respiratory rate
Laserflow Blood Perfusion Monitor Vasomedics, Inc. St. Paul, MN	Skin blood flow
Medpacific LD 5000 Laser-Doppler Perfusion Monitor Medpacific Corporation Seattle, WA	Skin blood flow
Fluoroptic Thermometry System Model 3000 Luxtron Mountain View, CA	Temperature
Omni-Vent, Series D Columbia Medical Marketing Topeka, KS	Respirator
Ventilator, Model 225 Monaghan Medical Corporation Plattsburgh, PA	Respirator

[a] Note that these devices may require modifications to make them MRI-compatible and none of them should be positioned closer than 8 ft from the entrance of the bore of a 1.5-T MRI scanner. Also, monitors with metallic cables, leads, or probes will cause mild to moderate imaging artifacts if placed near the imaging area of interest. Consult manufacturer to determine compatibility with specific MRI scanners and for additional safety information.

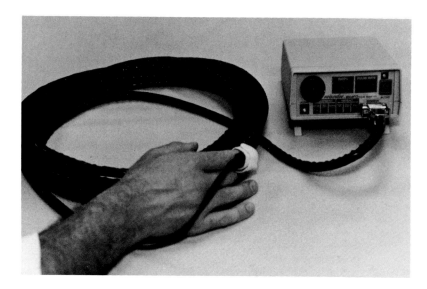

FIG. 1.24. MRI-compatible, fiber optic pulse oximeter used to obtain continuous recordings of heart rate and oxygen saturation.

to 1.5 T. MRI-compatible respirators have also been developed for patients who require ventilatory support and are commercially available from several vendors (198–201).

REFERENCES

1. Purcell EM, Torre HC, and Pound RV, *Resonance absorption by nuclear magnetic moments in a solid.* Physiol Rev, 1946. **69**: p. 37–38.
2. Block F, *Nuclear induction.* Physiol Rev, 1946. **70**: p. 460–473.
3. Gabillard R, *Resonance nucleaire.* Compt Rend, 1951. **232**: p. 1551–1553.
4. Damadian R, *et al., Field focus nuclear magnetic resonance (FONAR): Visualization of a tumor in a live animal.* Science, 1976. **194**: p. 1430–1432.
5. Lauterbur PC, *Image formation by induced local interations: Examples employing nuclear magnetic resonance.* Nature, 1973. **242**: p. 190–191.
6. Andrew ER, *NMR imaging of intact biological systems.* Philos Trans R Soc Lond [Biol], 1980. **289**: p. 471–481.
7. Crooks LE, *Overview of NMR imaging techniques*, in *Nuclear Magnetic Resonance Imaging in Medicine*, L Kaufman, LE Crooks, and AR Margulis, Editors. 1981, Igaku-Shoin: Tokyo, p. 42–50.
8. Edelstein WA, Hutchison J, and Johnson G, *Spin warp NMR imaging and applications to human whole body imaging.* Phys Med Biol, 1980. **25**: p. 751–756.
9. Hinshaw WS and Lent AH, *An introduction to NMR imaging: From the Block equation to the imaging equation.* Proc IEEE, 1983. **71**: p. 338–350.
10. Hoult DI, *Rotating frame Zeugmatography.* Philos Trans R Soc Lond [Biol], 1980. **289**: p. 543–547.
11. Mallard J, *et al., In vitro NMR imaging in medicine: The Aberdeen approach, both physical and biological.* Philos Trans R Soc Lond [Biol], 1980. **289**: p. 519–533.
12. Abragam A, *The Principles of Nuclear Magnetism.* 1983, London: Oxford University Press.
13. Bradley WG, Newton TH, and Crooks L, *Physical principles of nuclear magnetic resonance,* in *Advanced Imaging Techniques.* 1983, p. 15–61.
14. Budinger TF and Lauterbur PC, *Nuclear magnetic resonance technology for medical studies.* Science, 1884. **226**: p. 288–298.
15. Crues JVI and Morgan FW, *Physical and technical consider-ations in magnetic resonance imaging,* in *Magnetic Resonance Imaging in Orthopaedics and Rheumatology,* DW Stoller, Editor. 1989, Lippincott: Philadelphia.
16. Fullerton GD, *Basic concepts for nuclear magnetic resonance imaging.* Magn Reson Imag, 1982. **1**: p. 39–55.
17. Gore JC, *et al., Medical nuclear magnetic resonance imaging: I. Physical principles.* Invest Radiol, 1981. **16**: p. 269–274.
18. Haacke EM and Tkach JA, *Fast MR imaging: Techniques and clinical applications.* AJR, 1990. **155**: p. 951–964.
19. Hahn EL, *Spin echoes.* Physiol Rev, 1950. **50**: p. 580–594.
20. Jones JP, *et al., Principles of magnetic resonance,* in *Magnetic Resonance Annual 1985,* HY Kressel, Editor. 1985, Raven Press: New York. p. 71–111.
21. Koenig SH and Brown RD, *Determinants of proton relaxation rates in tissue.* Magn Reson Imag, 1984. **1**: p. 437–449.
22. Pykett IL, *NMR imaging in medicine.* Sci Am, 1982. **246**: p. 78–88.
23. Pykett IL, *et al., Principles of nuclear magnetic resonance imaging.* Radiology, 1982. **143**: p. 157–168.
24. Young SW, *Magnetic Resonance Imaging: Basic Principles.* 1988, New York: Raven Press.
25. Wolf GL and Popp C, *NMR-A Primer for Medical Imaging: Clear Explanations of Basic Principles for the Radiologist, Orthopedic Surgeon, Internist, Technician.* 1984, Thorofare, NJ: Slack.
26. Budinger TF and Margulis AR, ed. *Medical Magnetic Resonance: A primer—1988.* 1988, The Society of Magnetic Resonance in Medicine: Berkeley, CA. p. 385.
27. Lufkin RB, *The MRI Manual.* 1990, Littleton, MA: Year Book Medical Publishers, Inc.
28. Mettler FA, Jr., Muroff LR, and Kulkarni MV, ed. *Magnetic Resonance Imaging and Spectroscopy.* 1986, Churchill Livingstone: New York.
29. Slichter CP, *Principles of Magnetic Resonance.* 1963, New York: Harper & Row.
30. Frahm J, Haase A, and Matthaei D, *Rapid three-dimensional MR imaging using the FLASH technique.* J Comput Assist Tomogr, 1986. **10**: p. 363–368.
31. Haase A, *et al., MR imaging using stimulated echoes (STEAM).* Radiology, 1986. **160**: p. 787–790.
32. Haase A, *et al., Dynamic digital substraction imaging using fast low-angle shot MR movie sequences.* Radiology, 1986. **160**: p. 537–541.
33. Bydder GM, *et al., MR imaging of the liver using short T1 inversion recovery sequences.* J Comput Assist Tomogr, 1985. **9**(6): p. 1084–1089.
34. Bydder GM, *et al., The short T1 inversion recovery sequence—an approach to MR imaging of the abdomen.* Magn Reson Imag, 1985. **3**(3): p. 251–254.

35. Reicher MA, *et al., Multiple-angle, variable-interval, nonorthogonal MRI.* AJR, 1986. **147**: p. 363–366.
36. Matthaei D, *et al., Multipurpose NMR imaging using stimulated echoes.* Magn Reson Med, 1986. **3**: p. 554–561.
37. Matthaei D, *et al., Multiple chemical shift selective (CHESS) MR imaging using stimulated echoes.* Radiology, 1986. **160**: p. 791–794.
38. Friedburg H, Henning J, and Schumacher M, *RARE-MR myelography in routine clinical practice. Experience with 175 cases.* Rofo, 1987. **146**(5): p. 584–90.
39. Carr HY and Purcell EM, *Effect of diffusion on free precession in nuclear magnetic resonance experiments.* Physiol Rev, 1954. **94**: p. 630–638.
40. Feinberg DA, *et al., Multiple spin-echo magnetic resonance imaging.* Radiology, 1985. **155**: p. 437–442.
41. Kneeland JB, Knowles RJR, and Cahill PT, *Multi-section multi-echo pulse magnetic resonance techniques: Optimization in a clinical setting.* 1985. **155**: p. 159–162.
42. Chrispin A, *et al., Transectional echo planar imaging of the heart in cyanotic congenital heart disease.* Pediatr Radiol, 1986. **16**(4): p. 293–297.
43. Mansfield P, *Real-time echo-planar imaging by NMR.* Br Med Bull, 1984. **40**(2): p. 187–190.
44. Rzedzian R, *et al., Real-time nuclear magnetic resonance clinical imaging in paediatrics.* Lancet, 1983. **2**(8362): p. 1281–1282.
45. Saini S, *et al., Forty-millisecond MR imaging of the abdomen at 2.0 T.* Radiology, 1989. **173**(1): p. 111–116.
46. Stehling MK, *et al., Ultrafast magnetic resonance scanning of the liver with echo-planar imaging.* Br J Radiol, 1990. **63**(750): p. 430–437.
47. Bradley WG, *Effect of relaxation times on magnetic resonance interpretation.* Noninvas Med Imag, 1984. **1**: p. 193–204.
48. Bydder GM and Young IR, *Clinical use of the partial saturation and saturation recovery sequences in MR imaging.* J Comput Assist Tomogr, 1985. **9**: p. 1020–1032.
49. Foster MA, *et al., Nuclear magnetic resonance pulse sequence and discrimination of high- and low-fat tissues.* Magn Reson Imag, 1984. **2**: p. 187–192.
50. Hendrick RE, Nelson TR, and Hendee WR, *Optimizing tissue contrast in magnetic resonance imaging.* Magn Reson Imag, 1984. **2**: p. 193–204.
51. Mitchell MR, *et al., Spin echo technique selection: Basic principles for choosing MRI pulse sequence timing intervals.* Radiographics, 1986. **6**: p. 245–247.
52. Moran PR, *A general approach to T1, T2, and spin-density discrimination sensitivities in NMR imaging sequences.* Magn Reson Imag, 1984. **2**: p. 17–22.
53. Perman WH, *et al., Contrast manipulation in NMR imaging.* Magn Reson Imag, 1984. **2**: p. 23–32.
54. Posin JP, *et al., Variable magnetic resonance imaging parameters: Effect on detection and characterization of lesions.* Radiology, 1985. **155**: p. 719–725.
55. Wehrli FW, *et al., Mechanisms of contrast in NMR imaging.* J Comput Assist Tomogr, 1984. **8**: p. 369–380.
56. Wehrli FW, *et al., The dependence of nuclear magnetic resonance (NMR) image contrast on intrinsic and pulse sequence timing parameters.* Magn Reson Imag, 1984. **2**: p. 3–16.
57. Ziedses des Plantes BG, Falke THM, and den Boer JA, *Pulse sequences and contrast in magnetic resonance imaging.* Radiographics, 1984. **4**: p. 869–883.
58. Amtey SR, *NMR and water proton relaxation in tissues.* Magn Reson Imag, 1982. **1**: p. 63–67.
59. Fullerton GD, Potter JL, and Dornbluth NC, *NMR relaxation of protons in tissues and other macromolecular water solutions.* Magn Reson Imag, 1982. **1**: p. 209–228.
60. Soloman I, *Relaxation processes in a system of two spins.* Physiol Rev, 1955. **99**: p. 559–565.
61. Bloemberg N, *Proton relaxation times in paramagnetic solutions.* J Chem Phys, 1957. **27**: p. 572–573.
62. Ehman RL, *et al., Spin-spin relaxation time (T2) dependence in MR saturation- and inversion-recovery images.* AJR, 1984. **143**: p. 903–906.
63. Davis PL, *et al., NMR characteristics of normal and abnormal rat tissues,* in *Nuclear Magnetic Resonance Imaging in Medicine,* L Kaufman, LE Crooks, and AR Margulis, Editors. 1981. Igaku-Shoin: Toyko, p. 71–100.
64. Shah SS, *et al., Significance of water proton spin-lattice relaxation times in normal and malignant tissues and their subcellular fractions. II.* Magn Reson Imag 1982. **1**: p. 155–164.
65. Bydder GM, *et al., Use of closely coupled receiver coils in MR imaging: Practical aspects.* J Comput Assist Tomogr, 1985. **9**: p. 987–996.
66. Wehrli FW, *Principles of magnetic resonance,* in *Magnetic Resonance Imaging,* DD Stark and WG Bradley, Editors. 1987, Mosby: St. Louis.
67. Baker LL, *et al., Benign versus pathologic compression fractures of vertebral bodies: assessment with conventional spin-echo, chemical-shift, and STIR MR imaging.* Radiology, 1990. **174**(2): p. 495–502.
68. Dwyer AJ, *et al., Short-Ti inversion-recovery pulse sequence: Analysis and initial experience in cancer imaging.* Radiology, 1988. **168**(3): p. 827–836.
69. Golfieri R, *et al., The role of the STIR sequence in magnetic resonance imaging examination of bone tumours.* Br J Radiol, 1990. **63**(748): p. 251–256.
70. Shuman WP, *et al., Comparison of STIR and spin-echo MR imaging at 1.5 T in 90 lesions of the chest, liver, and pelvis [see comments].* Am J Roentgenol, 1989. **152**(4): p. 853–859.
71. Harned EM, *et al., Bone marrow findings on magnetic resonance images of the knee: accentuation by fat suppression.* Magn Reson Imag, 1990, **8**(1): p. 27–31.
72. Totterman S, *et al., MR fat suppression technique in the evaluation of normal structures of the knee.* J Comput Assist Tomogr, 1989. **13**(3): p. 473–479.
73. Bradley WG and Schmidt, PG, *Effect of methemoglobin formation on the MR appearance of subarachnoid hemorrhage.* Radiology, 1985. **156**: p. 99–103.
74. Cohen MD, *et al., MR appearance of blood and blood products: An in vitro study.* AJR, 1986. **146**: p. 1293–1297.
75. De La Paz RL, *et al., NMR imaging of intracranial hemorrhage.* J Comput Assist Tomogr, 1984. **8**: p. 599–607.
76. Di Chiro G, *et al., Sequential MR studies of intracerebral hematomas in monkeys.* AJNR, 1986. **7**: p. 193–199.
77. Dooms GC, *et al., MR imaging of intramuscular hemorrhage.* J Comput Assist Tomogr, 1985. **9**: p. 908–913.
78. Gomori JM, *et al., Intracranial hematomas: Imaging by high-field MR.* Radiology, 1985. **157**: p. 87–93.
79. Gomori JM, *et al., Occult cerebral vascular malformations: High-field MR imaging.* Radiology, 1986. **158**: p. 707–713.
80. Moon KL, *et al., Nuclear magnetic resonance imaging of CT-isodense subdural hematomas.* AJNR, 1984. **5**: p. 319–322.
81. Sipponen JT, Sepponen RE, and Sivula A, *Nuclear magnetic resonance (NMR) imaging of intracerebral hemorrhage in the acute and resolving phases.* J Comput Assist Tomogr, 1983. **7**: p. 954–959.
82. Sipponen JT, *et al., Intracranial hematomas studied by MR imaging at 0.17 and 0.02 T.* J Comput Assist Tomogr, 1985. **9**: p. 698–704.
83. Swensen SJ, *et al., Magnetic resonance of hemorrhage.* AJR, 1985. **145**: p. 921–927.
84. Zimmerman RD and Deck MDF, *Intracranial hematomas: Imaging by high-field MR.* Radiology, 1985. **159**: p. 565.
85. Brasch RC, *et al., Magnetic resonance imaging of transfusional hemosiderosis complicating thalassemia major.* Radiology, 1984. **150**: p. 767–771.
86. Drayer B, *et al., Magnetic resonance imaging of brain iron.* AJNR, 1986. **7**: p. 373–380.
87. Bradley WG, Kortman KE, and Crues JV, *Central nervous system high-resolution magnetic resonance imaging: Effect of increasing spatial resolution on resolving power.* Radiology, 1985. **156**: p. 93–98.
88. Edelstein WA, *et al., The intrinsic signal-to-noise ratio in NMR imaging.* Magn Reson Imag, 1986. **3**: p. 604–618.
89. Bellon EM, *et al., MR artifacts: A review.* AJR, 1986. **147**: p. 1271–1281.
90. Beyer D, *et al., Use of surface coils in magnetic resonance imaging of orbit and knee.* Diagn Imag Clin Med, 1986. **55**: p. 84–91.
91. Harms SE and Muschler G, *Three-dimensional MR imaging of*

the knee using surface coils. J Comput Assist Tomogr, 1986. **10**: p. 773–777.

92. Chui M, Blakesley D, and Mohapatra S. *Test method for MR image slice profile.* J Comput Assist Tomogr, 1985. **9**: p. 1150–1152.

93. Crooks LE, *et al., Thin-section definition in magnetic resonance imaging.* Radiology, 1985. **154**: p. 463–467.

94. Feinberg DA, *et al., Contiguous thin multisection MR imaging by two-dimensional Fourier transform techniques.* Radiology, 1986. **158**: p. 811–817.

95. Fitzsimmons JR and Googe RE, *Multisection-multiecho MR imaging: Effect on image quality.* Radiology, 1985. **157**: p. 813–814.

96. Kneeland JB, Shimakawa A, and Wehrli FW, *Effect of intersection spacing on MR image contrast and study time.* Radiology, 1986. **158**: p. 819–822.

97. Babcock EE, *et al., Edge artifacts in MR images: Chemical shift effect.* J Comput Assist Tomogr, 1985. **9**: p. 252–257.

98. Pusey E, *et al., Magnetic resonance imaging artifacts: Mechanism and clinical significance.* Radiographics, 1986. **6**: p. 891–911.

99. Weinreb JC, *et al., Chemical shift artifact in clinical magnetic resonance images at 0.35 T.* AJR, 1985. **145**: p. 183–185.

100. Purcell EM, *Electricity and Magnetism.* Berkeley Physics Course, Vol. 2. 1963, McGraw-Hill: New York.

101. Ehman RL, *et al., Influence of physiologic motion on the appearance of tissue in MR images.* Radiology, 1986. **159**: p. 777–782.

102. Schultz CL, *et al., The effect of motion on two-dimensional Fourier transformation magnetic resonance images.* Radiology, 1984. **152**: p. 117–121.

103. Wendt RE III, *et al., Phase alterations of spin echoes by motion along magnetic field gradients.* Magn Reson Med, 1985. **2**: p. 527–533.

104. Wood ML and Henkelman RM, *MR imaging artifacts in magnetic resonance imaging.* Med Phys, 1985. **12**: p. 143–151.

105. Lufkin RB, *et al., Boundary artifacts due to truncation errors in MR imaging.* AJR, 1986. **147**: p. 1283–1287.

106. Wood ML and Henkelman RM, *Truncation artifacts in magnetic resonance imaging.* Magn Reson Med, 1985. **2**: p. 517–526.

107. Crues JV, *et al., Meniscal tears of the knee: Accuracy of magnetic resonance imaging.* Radiology, 1987. **164**: p. 445–448.

108. Lufkin RB, *et al., Solenoid surface coils in magnetic resonance imaging.* Radiology, 1986. **146**: p. 409–412.

109. Axel L, *Surface coil magnetic resonance imaging.* J Comput Assist Tomogr, 1984. **8**: p. 381–384.

110. Ehman RL, *MR imaging with surface coils.* Radiology, 1985. **157**: p. 549–550.

111. Fisher MR, *et al., MR imaging using specialized coils.* Radiology, 1985. **157**: p. 443–447.

112. Hyde JS and Kneeland JB, *High-resolution methods using local coils,* in *Biomedical Magnetic Resonance Imaging,* FW Wehrli, JB Kneeland, and D Shaw, Editors. 1987, VCH Publishers: New York.

113. Kneeland JB, *et al., High-resolution MR imaging using loop-gap resonators: Work in progress.* Radiology, 1986. **158**: p. 247–250.

114. Kulkarni MV, Patton JA, and Price RR, *Technical considerations for the use of surface coils in MRI.* AJR, 1986. **147**: p. 373–378.

115. Shellock FG, Crues JV, MRI: *Safety considerations in magnetic resonance imaging.* MRI Decisions, 1988. **2**: p. 25–30.

116. Shellock FG, *Biological effects and safety aspects of magnetic resonance imaging.* Magn Reson Q, 1989. **5**: p. 243–261.

117. Kanal E, Shellock FG, Talagala L, *Safety considerations in MR imaging.* Radiology, 1990. **176**: p. 593–606.

118. Adey WR, *Tissue interactions with nonionizing electromagnetic fields.* Physiol Rev, 1981. **61**: p. 435–514.

119. Barnothy MF, *Biological Effects of Magnetic Fields.* Vols. 1 & 2, 1964, 1969. Plenum Press: New York.

120. Persson BRR, Stahlberg F, *Health and Safety of Clinical NMR Examinations.* 1989, CRC Press, Inc: Boca Raton, FL.

121. Tenforde TS, *Magnetic Field Effects on Biological Systems.* 1979, Plenum Press: New York.

122. Michaelson SM, Lin JV, *Biological Effects and Health Implications of Radiofrequency Radiation.* 1987, Plenum Press: New York.

123. Reid A, Smith FW, Hutchinson JMS, *Nuclear magnetic resonance imaging and its safety implications: Follow-up of 181 patients.* Br J Radiol 1982. **55**: p. 784–786.

124. Vyalov AM, *Magnetic fields as a factor in the industrial environment.* Vestn Akad Med Nauk, 1967. **8**: p. 72–79.

125. Vyalov AM, *Clinico-hygenic and experimental data on the effect of magnetic fields under industrial conditions,* in *Influence of Magnetic Fields on Biological Objects,* Kholodov Y, Editor. Moscow 1971. Translated by the Joint Publications Research Service. JPRS-63-38, pp. 20–35, 1974.

126. Sperber D, Oldenbourg R, Dransfeld K, *Magnetic field induced temperature change in mice.* Naturwissenschaften, 1984. **71**: p. 100–101.

127. Tenforde TS, *Thermoregulation in rodents exposed to high-intensity stationary magnetic fields.* Bioelectromagnetics, 1986. **7**: p. 341–346.

128. Shellock FG, Schaefer DJ, Gordon CJ, *Effect of a 1.5 T static magnetic field on body temperature of man.* Magn Reson Med, 1986. **3**: p. 644–647.

129. Shellock FG, Schaefer DJ, Crues JV, *Effect of a 1.5 Telsa static magnetic field on body and skin temperature of man.* Magn Reson Med, 1989. **11**: p. 371–375.

130. Beischer DE, Knepton JC, *Influence of strong magnetic fields on the electrocardiogram of squirrel monkey (Saimiri sciures).* Aerospace Med, 1964. **35**: p. 939–944.

131. Tenforde TS, Gaffey CT, Moyer BR, Budinger TF, *Cardiovascular alterations in Macaca monkeys exposed to stationary magnetic fields. Experimental observations and theoretical analysis.* Bioelectromagnetics, 1983. **4**: p. 1–9.

132. Garber HJ, Oldendorf WH, Braun LD, Lufkin RB, *MRI gradient fields increase brain mannitol space.* Magn Reson Imaging, 1989. **7**: p. 605–610.

133. Jehenson P, Duboc D, Lavergne T, Guize L, Guerin F, Degeroges M, Syrota A, *Change in human cardiac rhythm by a 2 Tesla static magnetic field.* Radiology, 1988. **166**: p. 227–230.

134. Ossenkopp KP, Innis NK, Prato FS, Sestini E, *Behavioral effects of exposure to nuclear magnetic resonance imaging: I. Open-field behavior and passive avoidance learning in rats.* Magn Reson Imag 1986. **4**: p. 275–280.

135. Redington RW, Dumoulin CL, Schneck JF, Roemer PB, Souza SP, Mueller OM, Eisner DR, Piel JE, Edelstein WA, *MR imaging and bio-effects in a whole body 4.0 Tesla imaging system.* Soc Magn Res Imag, Book of Abstracts, Vol. 1, p. 20, 1988.

136. Shivers RR, Kavaliers M, Tesky CG, Prato FS, Pelletier RM, *Magnetic resonance imaging temporarily alters blood-brain barrier permeability in the rat.* Neurosci Lett, 1987. **76**: p. 25–31.

137. Stojan L, Sperber D, Dransfeld K, *Magnetic-field-induced changes in the human auditory evoked potentials.* Naturwessenschaften, 1988. **75**: p. 622–623.

138. Von Klitzing L, *Static magnetic fields increase the power intensity of EEG of man.* Brain Res, 1989. **483**: p. 201–203.

139. Weiss J, Herrick RC, Taber KH, Plisher GA, *Bio-effects of high magnetic fields: A study using a simple animal model.* Magn Reson Imag, 1990. **8(S1)**: p. 166.

140. Abdullakhozaeva MS, Razykov SR, *Structural changes in central nervous system under the influence of a permanent magnetic field.* Bull Exper Biol Med, 1986. **102**: p. 1585–1587.

141. Hong C-Z, *Static magnetic field influence on human nerve function.* Arch Phys Med Rehabil, 1987. **68**: p. 162–164.

142. Gulch RW, Lutz O, *Influence of strong static magnetic fields on heart muscle contraction.* Phys Med Biol, 1986. **31**: p. 763–769.

143. Hong C-Z, Shellock FG, *Short-term exposure to a 1.5 Tesla static magnetic field does not effect somato-sensory evoked potentials in man.* Magn Reson Imag, 1990. **8**: p. 65–69.

144. Sweetland J, Kertesz A, Prato FS, Nantau K, *The effect of magnetic resonance imaging on human cognition.* Magn Reson Imag, 1987. **5**: p. 129–135.

145. Brown HD, Chattopadhyay SK, *Electromagnetic-field exposure and cancer.* Cancer Biochem Biophys, 1988. **9**: p. 295–342.

146. Bernhardt J, *The direct influence of electromagnetic fields on nerve and muscle cells of man within the frequency range of 1 Hz to 30 MHz*. Radiat Environ Phys, 1979. **16**: p. 309–323.

147. Watson AB, Wright JS, Loughman J, *Electrical thresholds for ventricular fibrillation in man*. Med J Australia, 1973. **1**: p. 1179–1182.

148. NCRP Report No. 86, *Biological Effects and Exposure Criteria for Radiofrequency Electromagnetic Fields*. National Council on Radiation Protection and Measurements. Bethesda, 1986.

149. F.D.A, *Magnetic resonance diagnostic device; Panal recommendation and report on petitions for MR reclassification*. Fed Reg 1988. **53**: p. 7575–7579.

150. Reilly JP, *Peripheral nerve stimulation by induced electric currents: Exposure to time-varying magnetic fields*. Med Biol Eng Comput, 1989. **27**: p. 101–112.

151. Cohen MS, Weisskoff R, Rzedzian R, Kantor H, *Sensory stimulation by time-varying magnetic fields*. Magn Reson Med, 1990. **14**: p. 409–414.

152. Fischer H, *Physiological effects of fast oscillating magnetic field gradient*. Radiology, 1989. **173**: p. 382.

153. Erwin DN, *Mechanisms of biological effects of radiofrequency electromagnetic fields: An overview*. Aviat Space Environ Med, 1988. **59**:(11, Suppl).): p. A21–A3111.

154. Gordon CJ, *Thermal physiology*, in *Biological Effects of Radiofrequency Radiation*. 1981, EPA-600/8-83-026A, Washington, D.C. pp. 4-1 to 4-28.

155. Gordon CJ, *Normalizing the thermal effects of radiofrequency radiation: Body mass versus total body surface area*. Bioelectromagnetics, 1987. **8**: p. 111–118.

156. Pool R, *Electromagnetic fields: The biological evidence*. Science, 1990. **249**: p. 1378–1381.

157. Beers J, *Biological effects of weak electromagnetic fields from 0 Hz to 200 MHz: A survery of the literature with special emphasis on possible magnetic resonance effects*. Magn Reson Imag, 1989. **7**: p. 309–331.

158. Coulter JS, Osbourne SL, *Short wave diathermy in heating of human tissues*. Arch Phys Ther, 1936. **17**: p. 679–687.

159. Bottomly PA, Edelstein WA, *Power deposition in whole body NMR imaging*. Med Phys, 1981. **8**: p. 510–512.

160. Shellock FG, Crues JV, *Temperature, heart rate, and blood pressure changes associated with clinical MR imaging at 1.5 T*. Radiology, 1987. **163**: p. 259–262.

161. Shellock FG, Schaefer DJ, Grundfest W, Crues JV, *Thermal effects of high-field (1.5 Tesla) magnetic resonance imaging of the spine: Clinical experience above a specific absorption rate of 0.4 W/kg*. Acta Radiologica, 1986. **Suppl 369**: p. 514–516.

162. Shellock FG, Gordon CJ, Schaefer DJ, *Thermoregulatory responses to clinical magnetic resonance imaging of the head at 1.5 Tesla: Lack of evidence for direct effects on the hypothalamus*. Acta Radiologica, 1986. **Suppl 369**: p. 512–513.

163. Shellock FG, Crues JV, *Corneal temperature changes associated with high-field MR imaging using a head coil*. Radiology, 1988. **167**: p. 809–811.

164. Shellock FG, Crues JV, *Temperature changes caused by clinical MR imaging of the brain at 1.5 Tesla using a head coil*. AJNR, 1988. **9**: p. 287–291.

165. Shellock FG, Schaefer DJ, Crues JV, *Alterations in body and skin temperatures caused by MR imaging: Is the recommended exposure for radiofrequency radiation too conservative?* Br J Radiol, 1989. **62**: p. 904–909.

166. Shellock FG, Rothman B, Sarti D, *Heating of the scrotum by high-field-strength MR imaging*. AJR, 1990. **154**: p. 1229–1232.

167. Shuman WP, Haynor DR, Guy AW, Wesbey GE, Schaefer DJ, Moss AA, *Superficial and deep-tissue increases in anesthetized dogs during exposure to high specific absorption rates in a 1.5-T MR imager*. Radiology, 1988. **167**: p. 551–554.

168. Shellock FG, *Ex vivo assessment of deflection forces and artifacts associated with high-field MRI of "mini-magnet" dental protheses*. Magn Reson Imag, 1989. **7**(Suppl 1): p. IT-03.

169. Liang MD, Narayanan K, Kanal E, *Magnetic port in tissue expanders: A caution for MRI*. Magn Reson Imag, 1989. **7**: p. 541–542.

170. Shellock FG, Kanal E, *Policies, guidelines, and recommendations for MR imaging safety and patient management*. J Magn Reson Imag, 1991. **1**: p. 97–101

171. Hayes DL, Holmes DR, Gray JE, *Effect of a 1.5 Tesla nuclear magnetic resonance imaging scanner on implanted permanent pacemakers*. JACC, 1987. **10**: p. 782–786.

172. Alagona P, Toole JC, Maniscalco BS, Glover MU, Abernathy GT, Prida XE, *Nuclear magnetic resonance imaging in a patient with a DDD pacemaker*. PACE 1989 (letter). **12**: p. 619.

173. Edelman RR, Shellock FG, Ahladis J, *Practical MRI for the technologist and imaging specialist*, in *Clinical Magnetic Resonance Clinical*, RR Edelman and J Hesselink, Editors. 1990, WB Saunders: Philadelphia.

174. Shellock FG, Slimp G, *Severe burn of the finger caused by using a pulse oximeter during MRI*. AJR, 1989. **153**: p. 1105.

175. Kanal E, Shellock FG, *Burns associated with clinical MR examinations*. Radiology, 1990. **175**: p. 585.

176. Davis PL, Crooks L, Arakawa M, McRee R, Kaufman L, Margulis AR, *Potential hazards in NMR imaging: Heating effects of changing magnetic fields and RF fields on small metallic implants*. AJR, 1981. **137**: p. 857–860.

177. Shellock FG, Crues JV, *High-field MR imaging of metallic biomedical implants: An in vitro evaluation of deflection forces and temperature changes induced in large protheses*. Radiology, 1987. **165**: p. 150.

178. Shellock FG, Crues JV, *High-field MR imaging of metallic biomedical implants: An ex vivo evaluation of deflection forces*. AJR, 1988. **151**: p. 389–392.

179. Shellock FG, Schatz CJ, *High-field strength MRI and otologic implants*. AJNR, 1991. **12**: p. 279–281.

180. Shellock FG, Meeks T, *Ex vivo evaluation of ferromagnetism and artifacts for implantable vascular access ports exposed to a 1.5 T MR scanner*. J Magn Reson Imag 1991. **1**: p. 243.

181. Teitelbaum GP, Yee CA, Van Horn DD, Kim HS, Colletti PM, *Metallic ballistic fragments: MR imaging safety and artifacts*. Radiology, 1990. **175**: p. 855–859.

182. Shellock FG, Curtis JS, *MR imaging and biomedical implants, materials, and devices. An updated review*. Radiology, 1991. **180**: p. 541–550.

183. Sacco DC, Steiger DA, Bellon EM, Coleman PE, Haacke EM, *Artifacts caused by cosmetics in MR imaging of the head*. AJR, 1987. **148**: p. 1001–1004.

184. Pusey E, Lufkin RB, Brown RKJ, et al. *Magnetic resonance imaging artifacts: Mechanism and clinical significance*. RadioGraphics, 1986. **6**: p. 891–911.

185. Ballock RT, Hajek PC, Byrne TP, Garfin SR, *The quality of magnetic resonance imaging, as affected by the composition of the halo arthrosis*. J Bone Joint Surg, 1989. **71-A**: p. 431–434.

186. Malko JA, Hoffman JC, Jarretr PJ, *Eddy-current-induced artifacts caused by an "MR-compatible" halo device*. Radiology, 1989. **173**: p. 563–564.

187. Shellock FG, Slimp G, *MRI-compatible halo vest for cervical spine fixation*. AJR, 1990. **154**: p. 631–632.

188. Kelly WM, Pagle PG, Pearson A, San Diego AG, Soloman MA, *Ferromagnetism of intraocular foreign body causes unilateral blindness after MR study*. AJNR, 1986. **7**: p. 243–245.

189. Hurwitz R, Lane SR, Bell RA, Brant-Zawadzki MN, *Acoustic analysis of gradient-coil noise in MR imaging*. Radiology, 1989. **173**: p. 545–548.

190. Brummett RE, Talbot JM, Charuhas P, *Potential hearing loss resulting from MR imaging*. Radiology, 1988. **169**: p. 539–540.

191. National Radiological Protection Board, *Revised guidelines on acceptable limits of exposure during nuclear magnetic clinical imaging*. Br J Radiol, 1983. **56**: p. 974–977.

192. Granet RB, Gelber LJ, *Claustrophobia during MR imaging*. N J Med, 1990. **87**: p. 479–482.

193. Flaherty JA, Hoskinson K, *Emotional distress during magnetic resonance imaging*. NEJM, 1989. **320**: 467–468.

194. Fishbain DA, Goldberg M, Labbe E, Zacher D, Steele-Rosomoff R, Rosomoff H, *Long-term claustrophobia following magnetic resonance imaging*. Am J Psychiatry, 1988. **145**: p. 1038–1039.

195. Quirk ME, Letendre AJ, Ciottone RA, Lingley JF, *Anxiety in patients undergoing MR imaging*. Radiology, 1989. **170**: p. 463–466.

196. Weinreb JC, Maravilla KR, Peshock R, Payne J, *Magnetic resonance imaging: Improving patient tolerance and safety*. AJR, 1984. **143**: p. 1285–1287.

197. Klonoff EA, Janata JW, Kaufman B, *The use of systematic desensitization to overcome resistance to magnetic resonance imaging (MRI) scanning*. J Behav Ther Exp Psychiatry, 1986. **17**: p.189–192.

198. Holshoulser B, Hinshaw DB, Shellock FG, *Sedation, anesthesia, and physiologic monitoring during MRI*. ARRS Syllabus, AN Hasso and DD Stark, Editors. 1991. p. 9–15.

199. McArdle CB, Nicholas DA, Richardson CJ, Amparo EG, *Monitoring of the neonate undergoing MR imaging: Technical considerations*. Radiology, 1986. **159**: 223–226.

200. Shellock FG, *Monitoring during MRI. An evaluation of the effect of high-field MRI on various patient monitors*. Med Electr, 1986. **Sept.**, p. 93–97.

201. Shellock FG, *Monitoring sedated patients during MRI*. Radiology, 1990 (letter). **177**: p. 586.

MRI of the Foot and Ankle,
edited by A.L. Deutsch, J.H. Mink, and R. Kerr,
Raven Press, Ltd., New York © 1992

CHAPTER 2

Normal Anatomy of the Foot and Ankle

Mark E. Schweitzer and Donald Resnick

SUPERFICIAL TISSUES AND COMPARTMENT ANATOMY

The skin of the foot is thin except for relative thickening over the heel and at the plantar aspect of the heads of the metatarsals. There is little fat dorsally, but significant fat exists in the plantar subcutaneous tissue. This fat is most prominent under the heads of the metatarsals. The dorsal deep fascia is thin and continuous with the extensor retinaculum as well as the fascia of the sole of the foot.

There are three plantar compartments of the foot: medial, central, and lateral. Thin membranous sheets medially and laterally enclose the compartments of the first (medial) and fifth (lateral) digits. The thick longitudinally oriented plantar aponeurosis covers the central compartment. This aponeurosis has five extensions into the digits. The second, third, and fourth digits are continuous with the central compartment.

The superficial transverse metatarsal ligament lies deep to the aponeurosis and reinforces the heads of the metatarsals. Transverse fasciculae act to reinforce the web spaces.

The medial compartment contains the abductor hallucis muscle, the flexor hallucis brevis muscle, the tendon of the flexor hallucis longus muscle, the medial plantar nerve and vessels, and the first metatarsal bone. Within the central component are the flexor digitorum brevis muscle, the quadratus plantae, the four plantar lumbricle muscles, the tendon of the flexor digitorum longus muscle, a portion of the tendon of the flexor hallucis longus muscle, and the lateral plantar nerve and vessels. The lateral compartment contains the abductor digiti minimi and flexor digitorum minimi brevis muscles.

RETINACULA, TENDON SHEATHS, AND BURSAE

With the change in orientation of the tendons from vertical in the leg to horizontal in the foot, five retinacula act to maintain close apposition of tendons to the osseous structures about the ankle and prevent bowstringing of these tendons.

The superior extensor retinaculum reinforces the crucial fascia arteriorly just above the ankle. The inferior extensor retinaculum is a Y-shaped band seen along the dorsum of the foot. The upper limb of the Y is located at the level of the ankle and attaches to the medial malleolus. The lower limb blends into the deep fascia of the sole of the foot.

The flexor retinaculum is seen medially enclosing the tarsal tunnel. Three septae divide the tarsal tunnel into four compartments. The first encloses the tendon of the tibialis posterior, the second encloses the tendon of the flexor digitorum longus, the third encloses the posterior tibial vessels and the tibial nerve, and the last encloses the tendon of the flexor hallucis longus muscle.

The superior and inferior peroneal retinacula are fascial thickenings seen laterally. Contained within these retinacula are the tendons of the peroneal longus and brevis muscles.

Sheaths surround most of the tendons that traverse the ankle joint. Separate sheaths are seen for the tendons of the tibialis anterior, extensor hallucis longus, tibialis posterior, flexor digitorum longus, and flexor hallucis longus. The tendons of the peroneal longus and brevis have a common sheath that divides into separate

M.E. Schweitzer: Thomas Jefferson University Hospital, Philadelphia, Pennsylvania 19107.

D. Resnick: University of California, San Diego, and Veterans Administration Medical Center, San Diego, California 92161.

sheaths just below the level of the ankle joint. The tendons of the extensor digitorum longus and peroneus tertius also share a common sheath. The sheath of the tibialis anterior is the most proximal of the ankle tendon sheaths. The Achilles tendon has no sheath and the intrinsic muscles of the feet lack sheaths as well.

Synovial sheaths enclose the flexor tendons of the toes. They begin at the bases of the distal phalanges and extend to the tendinous insertion.

Several bursae are seen in the foot and ankle. Posteriorly is the subcutaneous calcaneal (retroachilles) bursa lying between the insertion of the Achilles tendon on the calcaneus and the subcutaneous tissue. Deep to the Achilles tendon lies the retrocalcaneal bursa. Subcutaneous bursae also are noted superficial to the medial and lateral malleoli.

Adventitial bursae frequently develop adjacent to the medial aspect of the first metatarsal bone, superficial to the plantar aspect of the calcaneus, adjacent to the lateral aspect of the cuboid, and over the interphalangeal joints.

LEG

The musculature of the lower leg is divided into three compartments: posterior, lateral, and anterior.

Posterior

The deep and superficial layers of the calf muscles are separated by crural fascia. The superficial layer contains the gastrocnemius, soleus, and plantaris muscles. The deep layer consists of the popliteus, tibialis posterior, flexor hallucis longus, and flexor digitorum longus muscles.

The gastrocnemius muscle originates from the posterior aspect of the femoral condyles. Separate origins for each head, one arising from the medial condyle and one arising from the lateral condyle, are seen. In the midcalf the muscle belly ends in a wide, flat tendon, the Achilles tendon. The soleus lies deep to the gastrocnemius muscle, one head originating from the superior portion of the fibula with the other head originating from the posterior and medial aspects of the tibia and the popliteal line. The soleus inserts at the mid-portion of the Achilles tendon. The plantaris is a small muscle originating from the lateral femoral condyle with a small long tendon beginning in the proximal leg. It also usually inserts on the Achilles tendon.

The flexor hallucis longus is the most lateral muscle of the deep compartment. It originates in the posterior aspect of the middle of the fibula and inserts on the distal phalanx of the first digit. Its tendon begins above the medial malleolous and is posterior to the tendons of the tibialis posterior and flexor digitorum longus.

The flexor digitorum longus muscle originates from the posterior aspect of the tibia and inserts with four slips on second to fifth of the distal phalanges. Its tendon begins at the same level as that of the flexor hallucis longus; however, it is anterior to it. The tibialis posterior muscle has a complex origin from the posterior aspects of the tibia and fibula and the interosseous membrane. It inserts on the navicular, cuneiform, calcaneus, and second, third, and fourth metatarsals. The tibialas posterior is the deepest and most central muscle of the posterior compartment. Its myotendinous junction is slightly proximal to that of the flexor hallucis longus and flexor digitorum longus. The tendon of the tibialis posterior lies anterior and medial to the tendons of the flexor hallucis longus and flexor digitorum longus muscles.

Lateral Component

The lateral component consists of the peroneus longus and brevis muscles. Both originate from the lateral portion of the fibula. The origin of the peroneus longus muscle is more superior than that of peroneus brevis muscle. The myotendinous junction of the peroneus longus occurs above the ankle at the level of the soleal insertion into the Achilles tendon. The tendon of the peroneus brevis begins somewhat more distal. These tendons then pass laterally to the ankle with the peroneal brevis inserting on the base of the fifth metatarsal. The peroneal longus tendon subsequently crosses medially to its insertion on the first metatarsal bone and medial cuneiform.

Anterior Component

The muscles of the anterior compartment consist of the extensor digitorum longus, peroneus tertius, extensor hallucis longus, and tibialis anterior.

The extensor digitorum longus is the most lateral muscle of this compartment, originating from the upper portion of the tibia and the fibula as well as the interosseous membrane. The extensor digitorum longus tendon inserts on the lateral four toes. Its tendon begins at the level of the lateral malleolus and continues as the most lateral of the tendons of the anterior compartment. The peroneus tertius muscle is closely associated with the extensor digitorum longus muscle. It originates from the distal portion of the fibula and interosseous membrane and inserts on the base of the fifth metatarsal bone.

The extensor hallicus longus muscle also originates from the distal aspect of the fibula and interosseous membrane, but it inserts on the distal phalanx of the first toe. Its tendon lies between the laterally positioned extensor digitorium longus and medially positioned tibialis anterior tendons. The tibialis anterior muscle originates from the lateral aspect of the tibia and interosseous membrane and inserts on the medial cuneiform and first metatarsal bone. Its tendon begins as the most proximal of the ankle tendons and it is also the most medial of the tendons of the anterior compartment.

Foot

The muscles of the foot are usually described in layers rather than compartments.

The superficial layer of plantar muscles includes the abductor hallucis, flexor digitorum brevis, and abductor digit minimi. The abductor hallucis muscle originates from the medial aspect of the calcaneus, plantar aponeurosis, and flexor retinaculum and inserts on the proximal phalanx of the great toe. The medial and lateral plantar vessels and nerve pass deep to the proximal portion of the abductor hallucis muscle.

The flexor digitorum brevis muscle also originates from the medial portion of the calcaneus as well as the plantar fascia and then passes laterally to insert on the middle phalanges of the second through fifth digits.

The abductor digit minimi muscle originates from the lateral process of the calcaneal tubecle and inserts on the proximal phalanx of the fifth digit.

The second layer of the foot consists of the quadratus plantae and lumbrical muscles as well as the tendons of the flexor hallucis longus and flexor digitorum longus. The quadratus plantae muscle originates from the medial and lateral calcaneal tuberosities with its insertion blending in with the tendon slips of the flexor digitorum longus. The lumbrical muscles originate from the tendon of the flexor digitorum longus while inserting at the second through fifth metatarsophalangeal joints on the flexor aponeurosis.

The third layer includes the flexor hallucis brevis, adductor hallucis, and flexor digiti minimi brevis muscles. The flexor hallucis brevis muscle is the most medial of this layer originating from the cuboid and lateral cuneiform. It inserts at the base of the proximal phalanx of the first toe and the adjacent sesamoids. The adductor hallucis has two heads. The oblique head arises from the second through fourth metatarsal bases and the long plantar ligament. The transverse head originates from the joint capsules of the third, fourth, and fifth metatarsophalangeal joints and the deep transverse ligament. The two heads of the adductor hallucis muscle join and insert with the flexor hallucis brevis tendon. The flexor digiti minimi muscle arises from the cuboid and the base of the fifth metatarsal bone and inserts on the proximal phalanx of the fifth toe.

The fourth layers consists of the seven interosseous muscles. This is the deepest muscle layer in the plantar aspect of the foot. The interosseous muscles originate from the metatarsal bases and consist of four dorsal and three plantar muscles. The dorsal interosseous muscles insert laterally on the proximal phalanges while the plantar interosseous muscles insert medially.

Dorsally, there is only one intrinsic muscle of the foot. The thin extensor digitorum brevis muscle originates in the superior portion of the calcaneus, lateral talocalcaneal ligament, and extensor retinaculum and inserts on the lateral aspect of the first through fourth proximal phalanges.

LIGAMENTS

The ligaments of the ankle will be discussed in detail later in the text. Following is a discussion of the intrinsic ligaments of the foot.

Several intrinsic ligaments act to appose the talus and calcaneus closely and provide congruity at the subtalar joints. The medial talocalcaneal ligament connects the posterior process of the talus medially, with the posterior aspect of the sustentaculum tali. The lateral talocalcaneal ligament extends parallel but deep to the calcaneofibular ligament. The posterior talocalcaneal ligament extends from the lateral tubercle of the talus for a short distance to the upper and medial portions of the calcaneus. The strong interosseous talocalcaneal ligament is seen within the tarsal sinus.

Several ligaments support the talocalcaneonavicular joint. The broad dorsal talonavicular ligament supports the joint capsule. Below the joint is the dense plantar calcaneonavicular ligament (spring) extending from the sustentaculum tali to the inferior part of the navicular bone. Laterally, this joint is also supported by the calcaneonavicular portion of the bifurcate ligament.

The calcaneocuboid joint is supported by the dorsal calcaneocuboid ligaments, as well as the calcaneocuboid band of the bifurcate ligament. In addition, the plantar ligaments, the plantar calcaneocuboid, the spring ligament, and the long plantar support this joint. The long plantar ligament extends from the plantar surface of the calcaneus to the cuboid and to the bases of the third, fourth, and fifth metatarsals.

The dorsal and plantar cuboidonavicular ligaments as well as the strong interosseous cuboidconavicular ligament connect the cuboid and navicular bones. Additional supporting ligaments of the midfoot include dorsal cuneonavicular ligaments, dorsal intercuneiform ligaments, and the dorsal cuneocuboid ligament. In addition, there are plantar cuneonavicular, plantar intercuneiform, and plantar cuneocuboid ligaments. Cuboid interosseous and intercuneiform ligaments also act to support the midfoot joints.

The tarsometatarsal joints are supported by weak dorsal and slightly stronger plantar tarsometatarsal ligaments. The intermetatarsal joints are supported by strong dorsal, plantar, and interosseous ligaments.

The plantar ligament is a dense band crossing each metatarsophalangeal joint and serves as a weightbearing surface because the ball of the foot supports the metatarsophalangeal joints. The plantar ligaments are interconnected by the deep transverse ligament. The hallux lacks a true plantar ligament although the interconnecting ligaments extending between sesamoid bones, first metatarsus, and proximal phalanx function as the continuation of the plantar ligament medially. Strong collateral ligaments connect the medial and lateral aspects of the metatarsal bones and the corresponding portion of the phalanges.

The interphalangeal joints also are supported by collateral ligaments as well as by the tendons of the extensor digitorum longus and brevis, the tendon of the extensor hallucis dorsally, and the tendons of flexor digitorum longus and brevis and of the extensor hallucis longus plantarly. Digital fibrous sheaths begin at the heads of the metatarsal bones and extend to the bases of the distal phalanges enclosing the flexor and extensor tendons and joint capsules.

Vasculature

The dorsalis pedis artery, the continuation of the anterior tibial artery, provides the major blood supply to the dorsum of the foot with frequent contributions from the perforating branch of the peroneal artery. The anterior lateral and anterior medial malleolar arteries are branch vessels and provide the blood supply to the anterior aspect of the ankle. Medial and lateral tarsal arteries are branch vessels and provide the blood supply to the tarsal bones. In most patients the dorsalis pedis artery gives rise to a laterally oriented arcuate artery at the level of the Lis-Franc joint. The arcuate artery branches into second, third, and fourth metatarsal arteries. The first metatarsal artery is the terminal vessel of the dorsalis pedis artery. The metatarsal arteries terminate as the dorsal digital proper arteries providing the blood supply to the toes.

The plantar surface of the foot receives its arterial supply from the two terminal branches of the posterior tibial artery; the medial and lateral plantar arteries. The medial plantar artery has a deep branch in the region of the midfoot with a superficial tibial plantar artery continuing distally. The lateral plantar artery continues medially to form the plantar arch beneath the bases of the metatarsal bones. This plantar arch gives off three or four metatarsal arteries that anastomose with the dorsal metatarsal arteries. Two plantar digital proper arteries are end vessels of the dorsal metatarsal arteries.

The superficial dorsal venous network begins as two dorsal collateral digital veins and one median digital vein on the dorsum of each toe. At the web space these vessels combine to form the four superficial dorsal metatarsal veins. These metatarsal veins then combine to form the dorsal venous arch, which drains into the lesser saphenous vein laterally and the greater saphenous vein medially.

Nerves

The major innervation of the foot is supplied by medial and lateral plantar nerves. The medial plantar nerve is the larger and more anterior of these two plantar nerves. It arises deep to the flexor retinaculum and divides into its terminal branches at the level of the base of the first metatarsal bone. It ends in the medial plantar digital proper nerve and the first three common plantar nerves. These plantar nerves follow the course of the common plantar digital arteries in the web spaces. The lateral plantar nerve is smaller than the medial nerve and follows the course of the lateral plantar artery. Its two terminal branches, one superficial and one deep, arise at the lateral aspect of the quadratous plantar muscle. Other branches continue to innervate the remaining lateral (fourth) web space and the lateral aspect of the fifth digit.

ABBREVIATIONS USED IN FIGURES 1–52

abhm abductor hallucis muscle
ac articular cartilage
admm abductor digiti minimi muscle
admt abductor digiti minimi tendon
ahm abductor hallucis muscle
at achilles tendon
ata anterior tibial artery
atfl anterior talo-fibular ligament
atifl anterior tibio-fibular ligament

attl anterior tibio-talar ligament
bl bifurcate ligament
ccl cuboid cuneiform ligament
cfl calcaneo-fibular ligament
cl collateral ligament
dcl dorsal capsular ligament
dcml dorsal cuneo-metatarsal ligament
dcuml dorsal cuboido-metatarsal ligament
df dorsal fascia

di   dorsal interosseous muscle
dncl   dorsal naviculo-cuboid ligament
dpn   deep peroneal nerve
dtnl   dorsal talo-navicular ligament
edbm   extensor digitorum brevis muscle
edbt   extensor digitorum brevis tendon
edlm   extensor digitorum longus muscle
edlt   extensor digitorum longus tendon
ee   extensor expansion
eehl   extensor expansion hallucis longus
ehbm   extensor hallucis brevis muscle
ehbt   extensor hallucis brevis tendon
ep   eponychium
es   extensor sling
fdbm   flexor digitorum brevis muscle
fdmt   flexor digitorum brevis tendon
fdlm   flexor digitorum longus muscle
fdlt   flexor digitorum longus tendon
fdmb   flexor digiti minimi brevis muscle
fhbm   flexor hallucis brevis muscle
fhbt   flexor hallucis brevis tendon
fhlm   flexor hallucis longus muscle
fhlt   flexor hallucis longus tendon
fht   combined flexor hallucis tendon
fr   flexor retinaculum
fs   fibrous digital sheath
gsv   greater saphenous vein
ier   inferior extensor retinaculum
itcl   interosseous talocalcaneal ligament
jc   joint capsule
kf   karger's fat
lm   lumbricle muscle
lpan   lateral plantar artery and nerve
lpl   long plantar ligament
lsv   lesser saphenous vein

ltcl   lateral talocalcaneal ligament
mf   metatarsal plantar fat pad
mpan   median plantar artery and nerve
mtcl   medial talocalcaneal ligament
n   nail
nb   nail bed
ncl   naviculo-cuboid ligament
pa   plantar aponeurosis
pavb   peroneal arteries and vein branches
pbm   peroneal brevis muscle
pbt   peroneal brevis tendon
pcnl   plantar calcaneal-navicular ligament (spring)
pi   plantar interosseous muscle
pitfl   posterior inferior tibio-fibular ligament
plm   peroneal longus muscle
plt   peroneal longus tendon
pma   plantar metatarsal artery
pp   plantar plate
pr   peroneal retinaculum
pt   peroneus tertius
pta   posterior tibial artery
ptan   posterior tibial artery and nerve
ptfl   posterior talo-fibular ligament
qp   quadratus plantae muscle
sm   soleus muscle
sn   sural nerve
tam   tibialis anterior muscle
tat   tibialis anterior tendon
tcl   tibial calcaneal ligament
tn   tibial nerve
tnl   tibia-navicular ligament
tpm   tibialis posterior muscle
tpt   tibialis posterior tendon
tt   tuftal subcutaneous fat and fibrous tissue

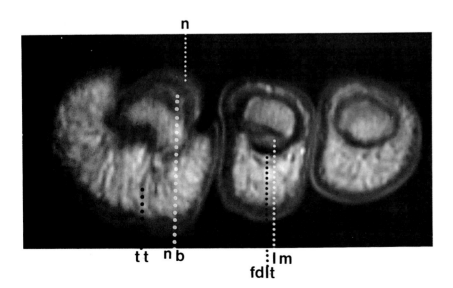

FIG. 2.1. Axial image of the distal aspect of toes.

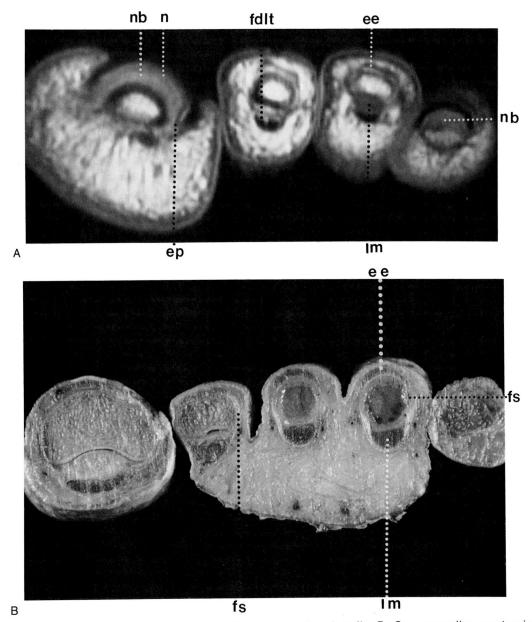

FIG. 2.2. A: Axial image of the level of the first and fourth nails. **B:** Corresponding anatomic section.

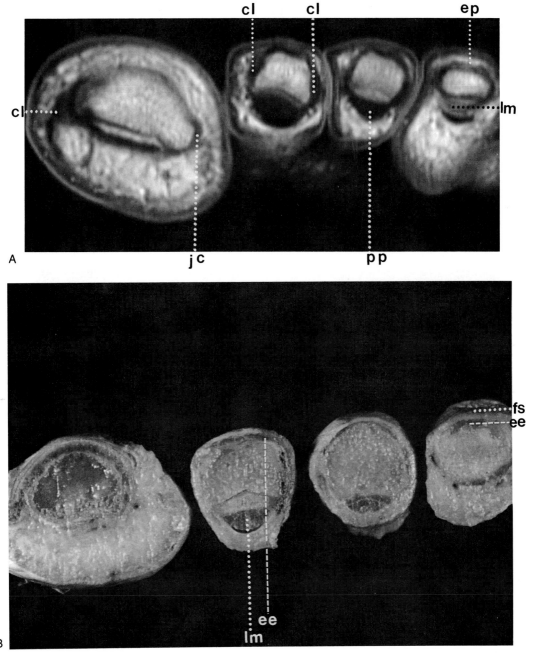

FIG. 2.3. **A:** Axial image of the level of interphalangeal joints. **B:** Corresponding anatomic section.

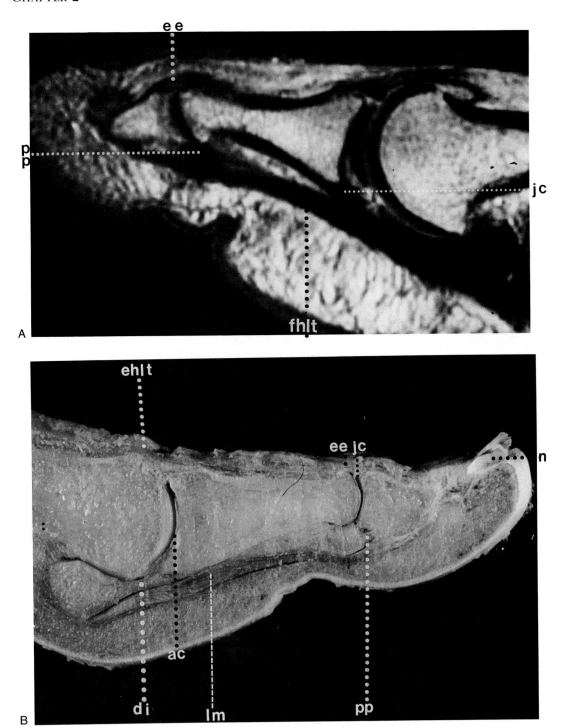

FIG. 2.4. A: Sagittal image of the first toe. **B:** Sagittal image of the mid-first ray.

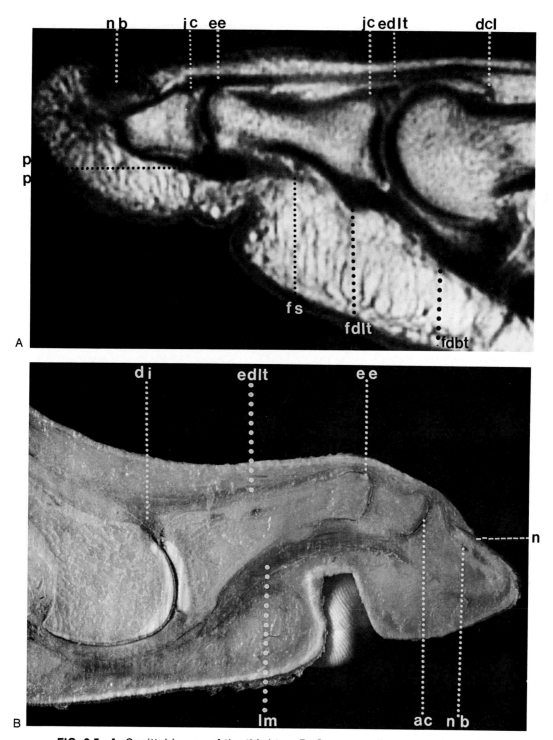

FIG. 2.5. A: Sagittal image of the third toe. **B:** Corresponding anatomic section.

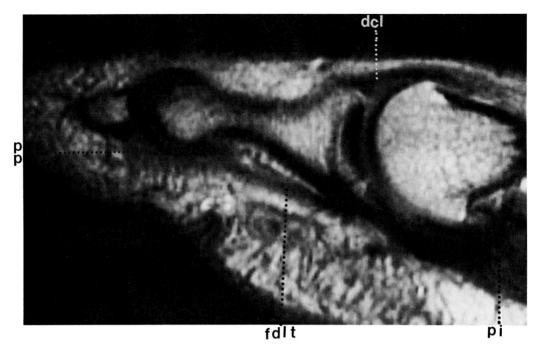

FIG. 2.6. Sagittal image through the lateral aspect of the third toe.

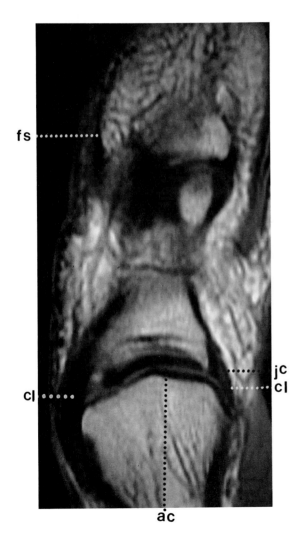

FIG. 2.7. Coronal image through the dorsal aspect of the first toe.

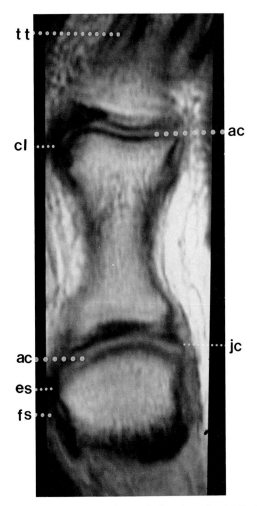

FIG. 2.8. Coronal image through the dorsal mid-first toe.

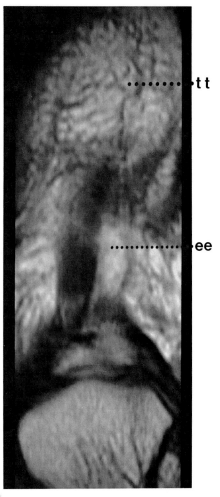

FIG. 2.9. Coronal image through the dorsal plantar aspect of the first toe.

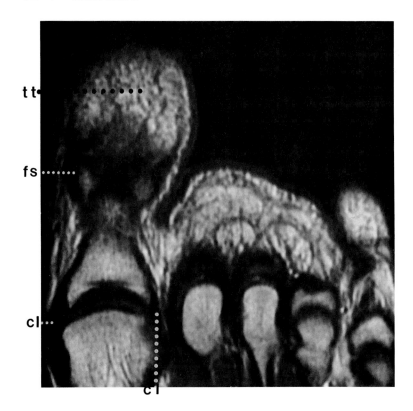

FIG. 2.10. Coronal image of the dorsal toes.

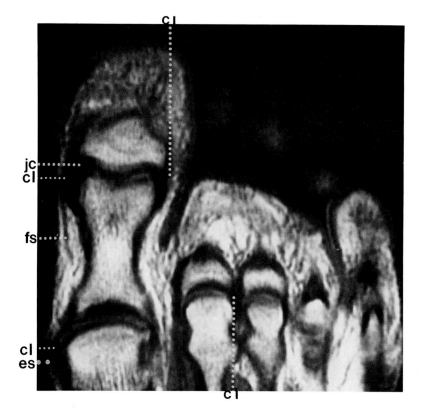

FIG. 2.11. Coronal image, plantar to Fig. 2.10.

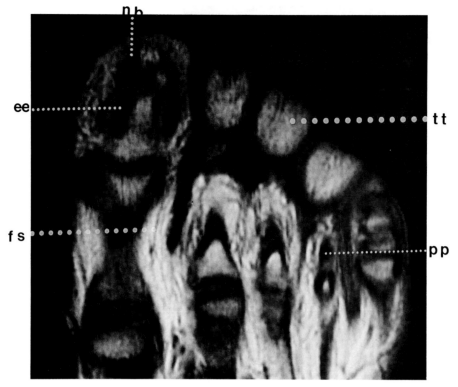

FIG. 2.12. Coronal image of the level of the first extensor expansion.

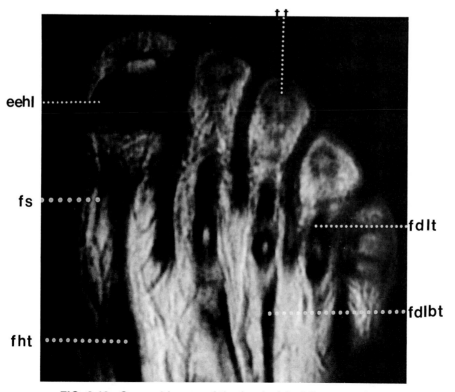

FIG. 2.13. Coronal image of the level of 2–4 flexor tendons.

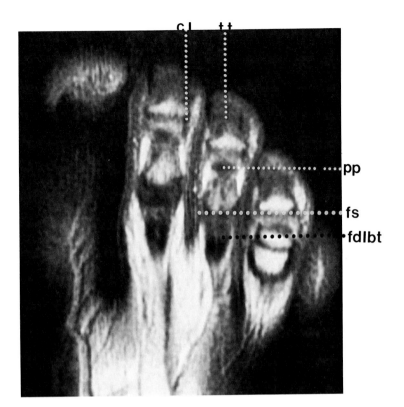

FIG. 2.14. Coronal image of the level of the interphalangeal joints.

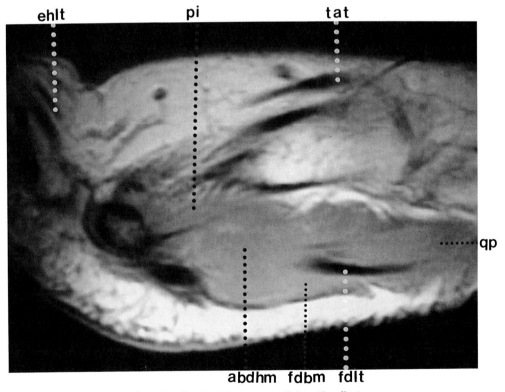

FIG. 2.15. Sagittal image medial to the first ray.

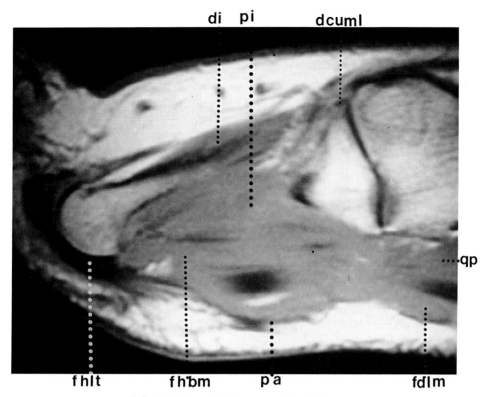

FIG. 2.16. Sagittal image of the first ray.

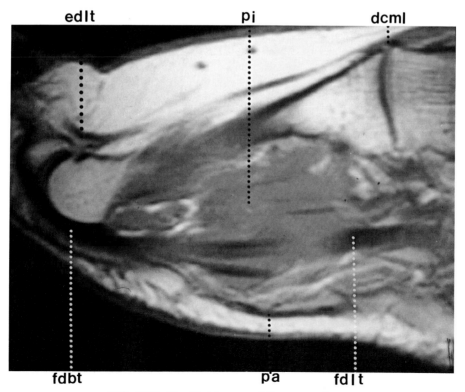

FIG. 2.17. Sagittal image of the second ray.

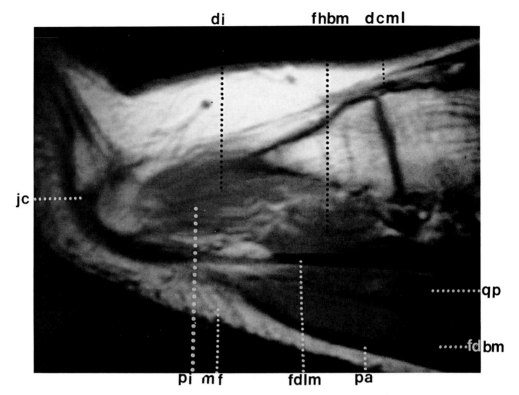

di   fhbm   dcml

jc

qp

fdbm

pi mf   fdlm   pa

FIG. 2.18. Sagittal image of the level of the third ray.

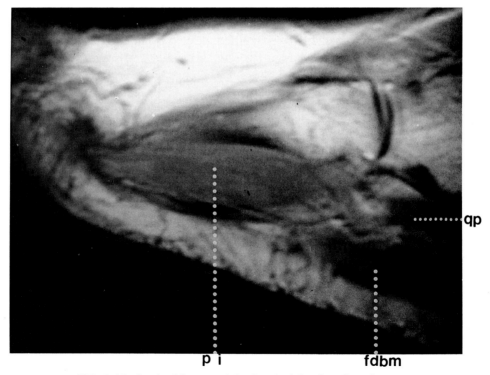

qp

p i   fdbm

FIG. 2.19. Sagittal image of the level of the fourth web space.

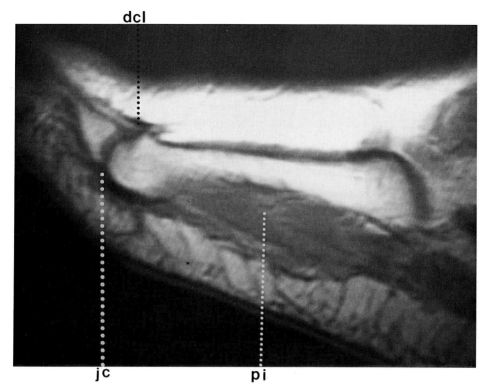

FIG. 2.20. Sagittal image of the fifth ray.

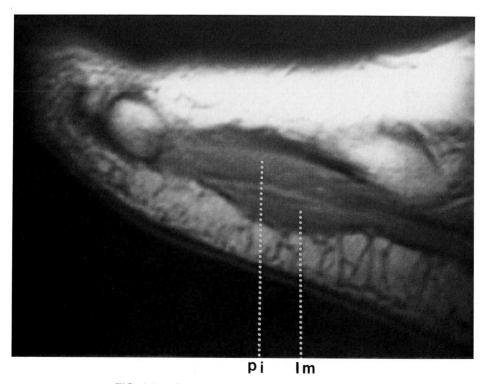

FIG. 2.21. Sagittal image lateral to the fifth ray.

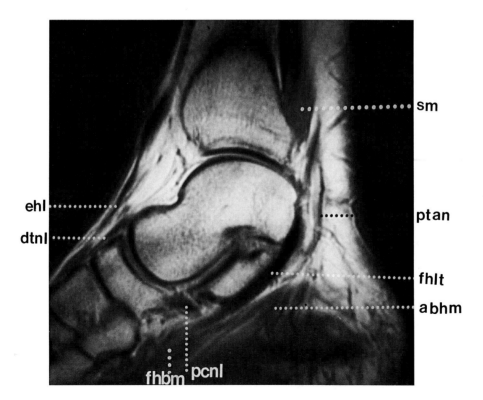

FIGS. 2.22–28. Sagittal images of the ankles beginning medially.

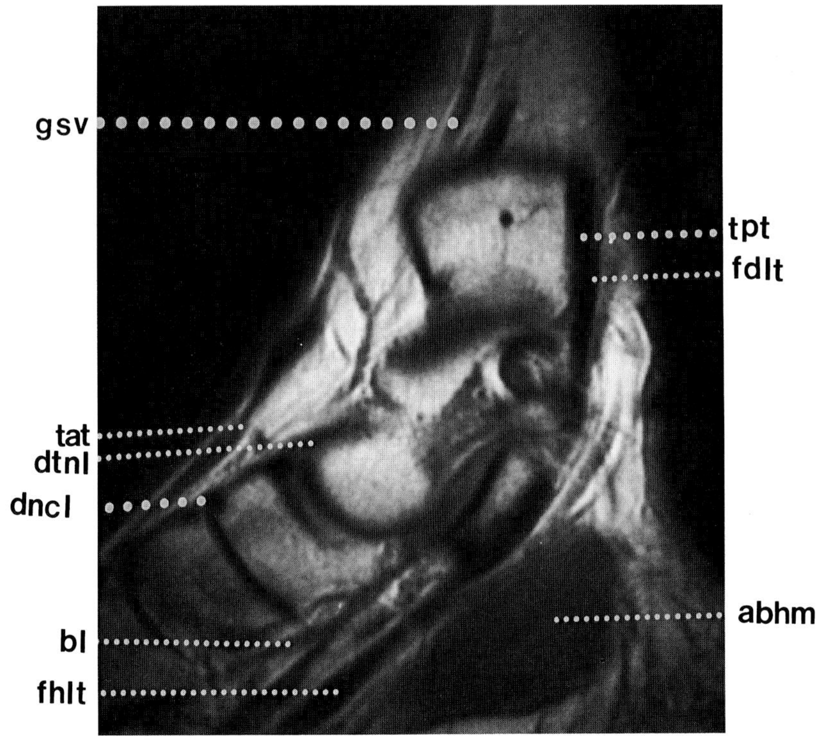

gsv

tpt

fdlt

tat

dtnl

dncl

bl

fhlt

abhm

FIG. 2.22.

sm

ehl

dtnl

ptan

fhlt

abhm

fhbm pcnl

FIG. 2.23.

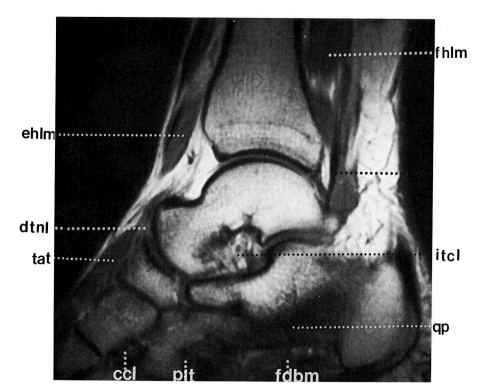

FIG. 2.24.

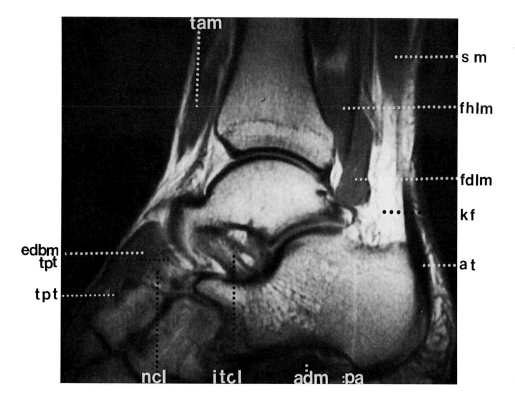

FIG. 2.25.

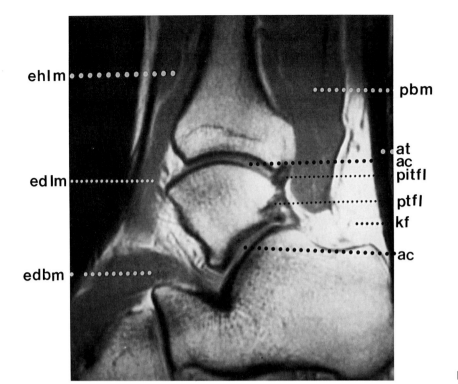

FIG. 2.26.

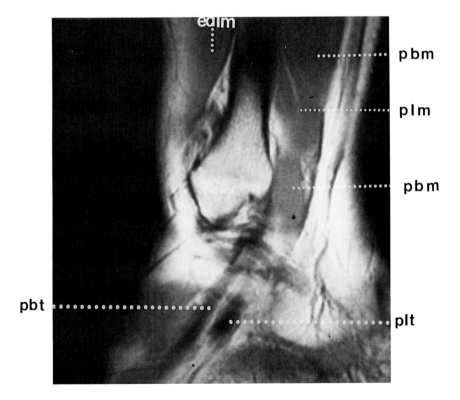

FIG. 2.27.

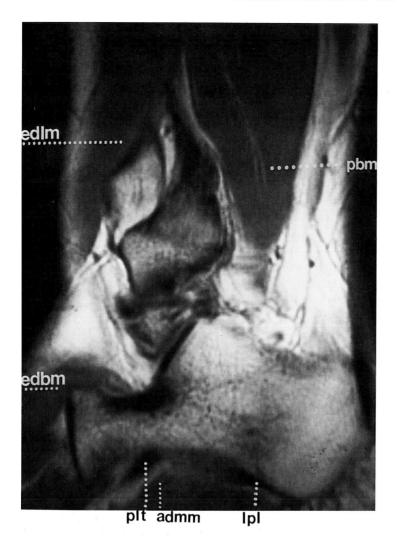

FIG. 2.28.

—40. Axial images beginning just below the ndesmosis.

Tib Ant
Ext hal longus — *Ext dig longus*

peroneus tertius longus tendon

inf. externus retinaculum ↗ *tibialis tendon* ↗ *Anterior tendon* ↗ *Extensor longus digitorum longus* ↗ *Ant tibial Artery*

tat ehlt edlt edlm

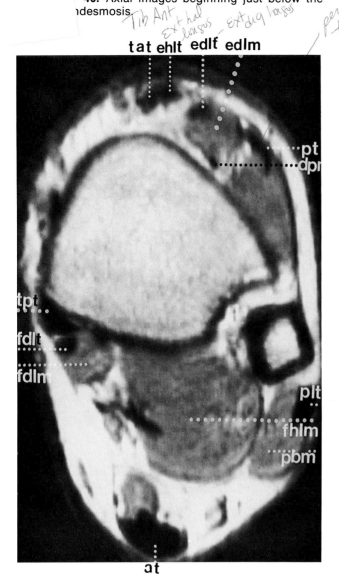

pt
dpn

tpt

fdlt

fdlm

plt

fhlm

pbm

at

FIG. 2.29.

ier tat edl ata

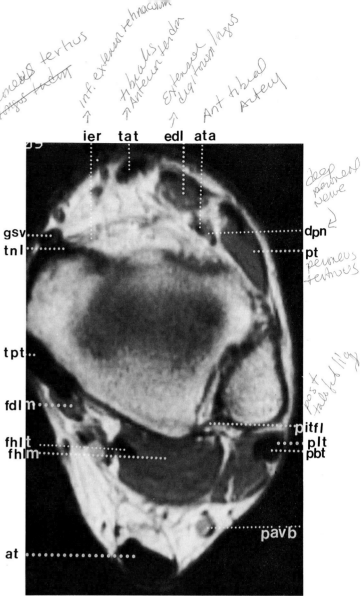

deep peroneal nerve ↙

gsv
tnl

dpn

pt *peroneus tertius*

tpt

fdlm

fhlt
fhlm

pitfl

plt
pbt

post talofibular lig

pavb

at

FIG. 2.30.

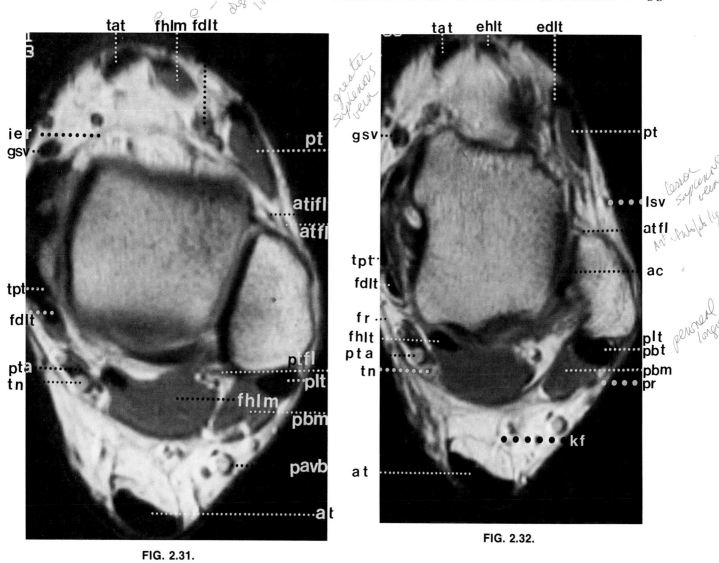

FIG. 2.31.

FIG. 2.32.

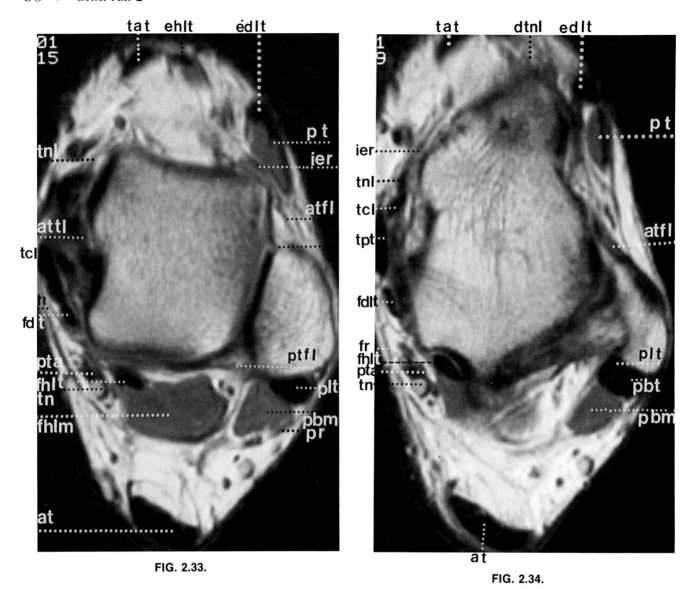

FIG. 2.33.

FIG. 2.34.

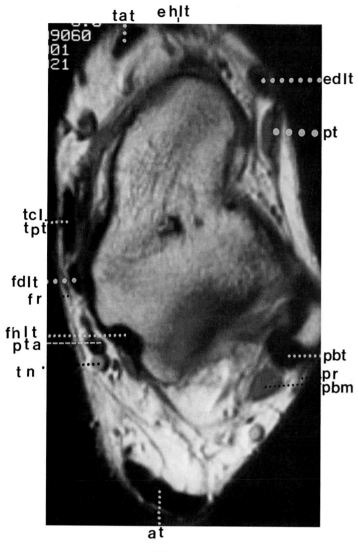

dtnl dorso talonavicular lig

pt peroneus tertius

extensor dychoum Brevis

FIG. 2.35.

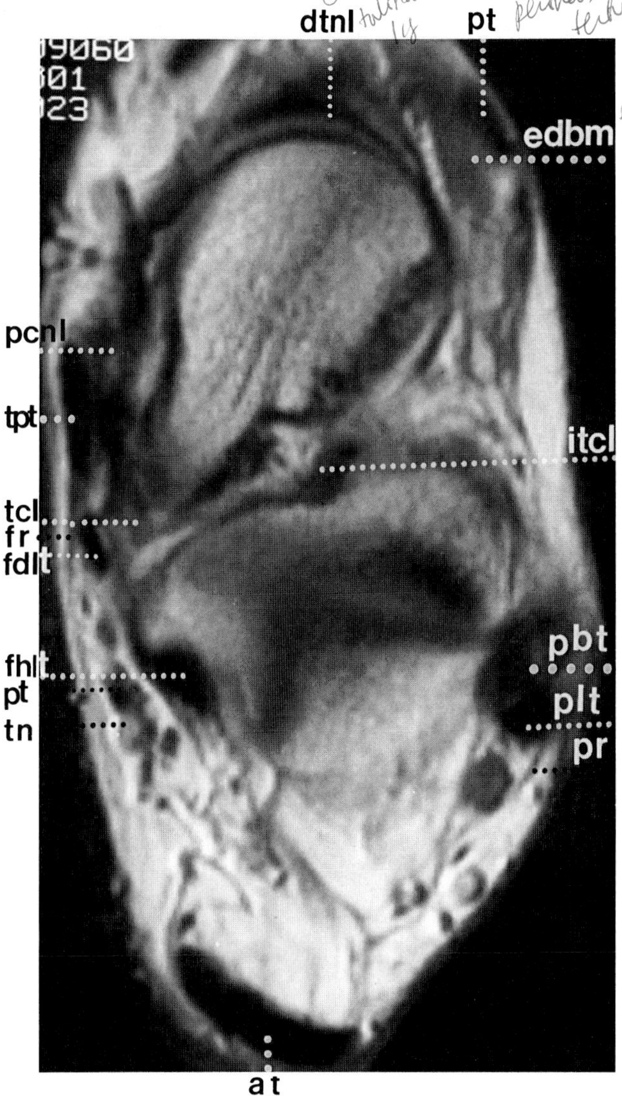

FIG. 2.36.

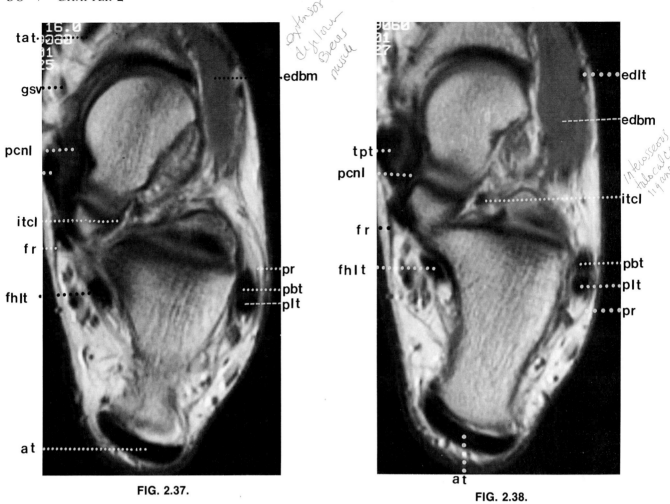

Extensor digitorum Brevis muscle

Interosseous talocalcaneal ligament

tat — gsv — pcnl — itcl — f r — fhlt — at — edbm — pr — pbt — plt

tpt — pcnl — f r — fhlt — at — edlt — edbm — itcl — pbt — plt — pr

FIG. 2.37.

FIG. 2.38.

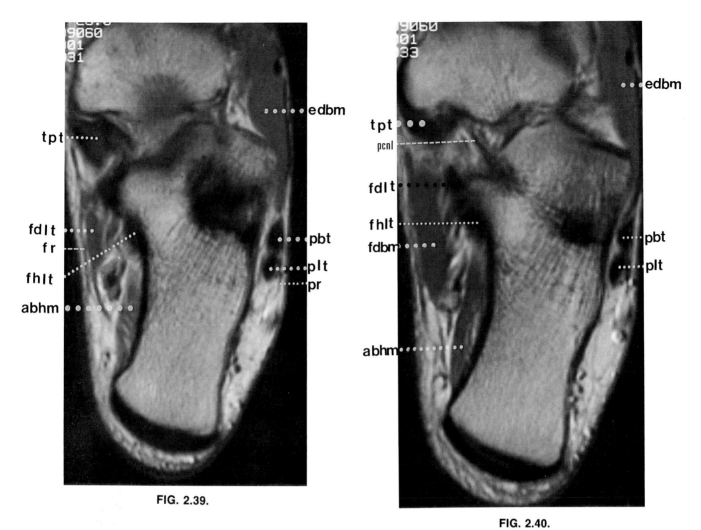

FIG. 2.39.

FIG. 2.40.

FIGS. 2.41–52. Coronal images (perpendicular to long axis of foot) beginning posteriorly at posterior calcaneus.

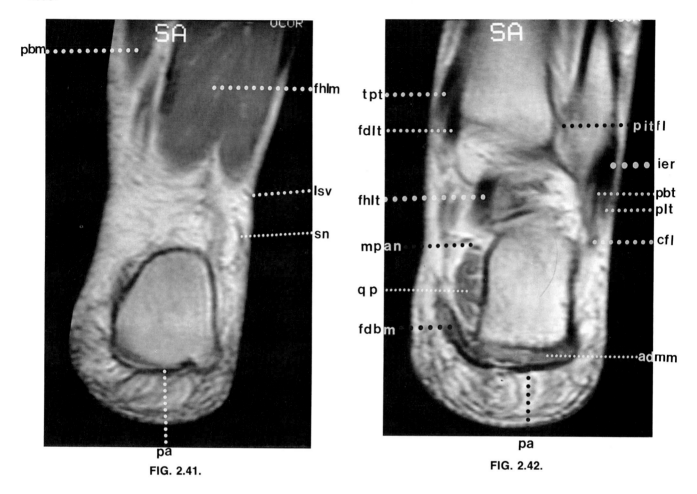

FIG. 2.41.

FIG. 2.42.

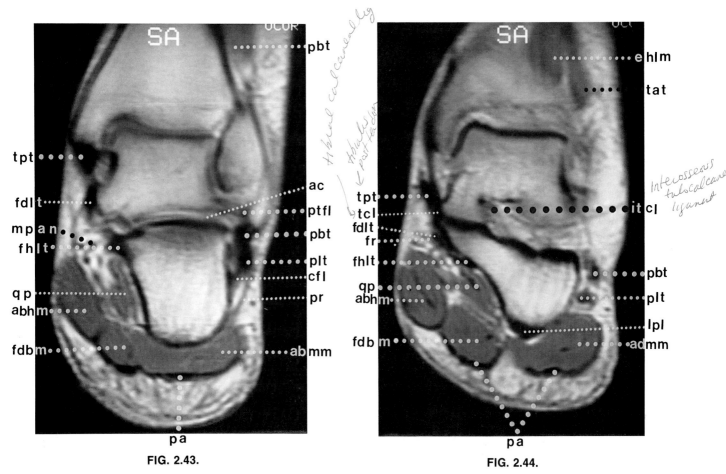

tibial calcaneal lig

tibialis (post tendor)

Interosseous talocalcaned ligament

FIG. 2.43.

FIG. 2.44.

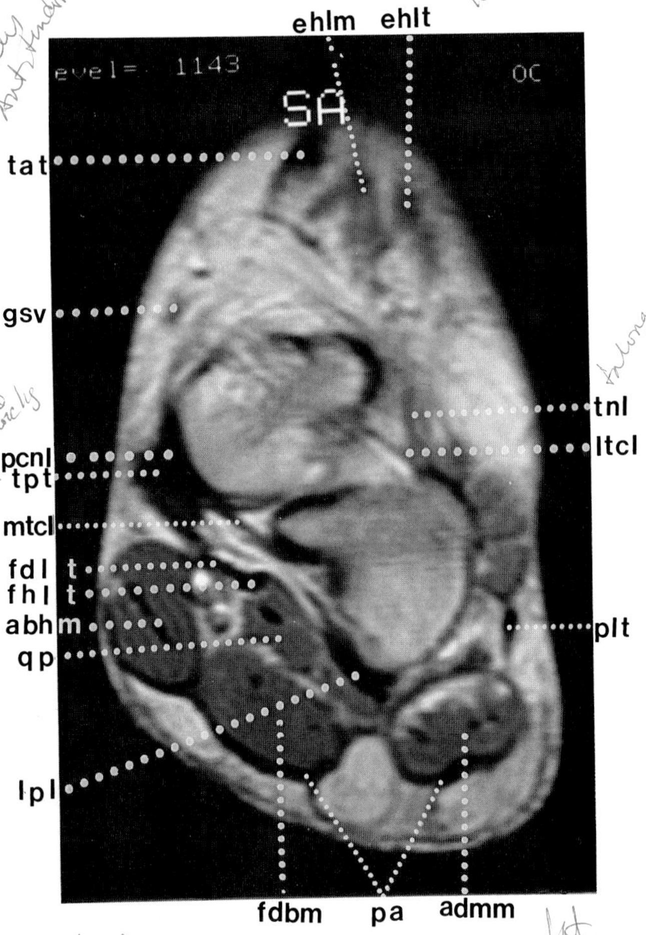

FIG. 2.45.

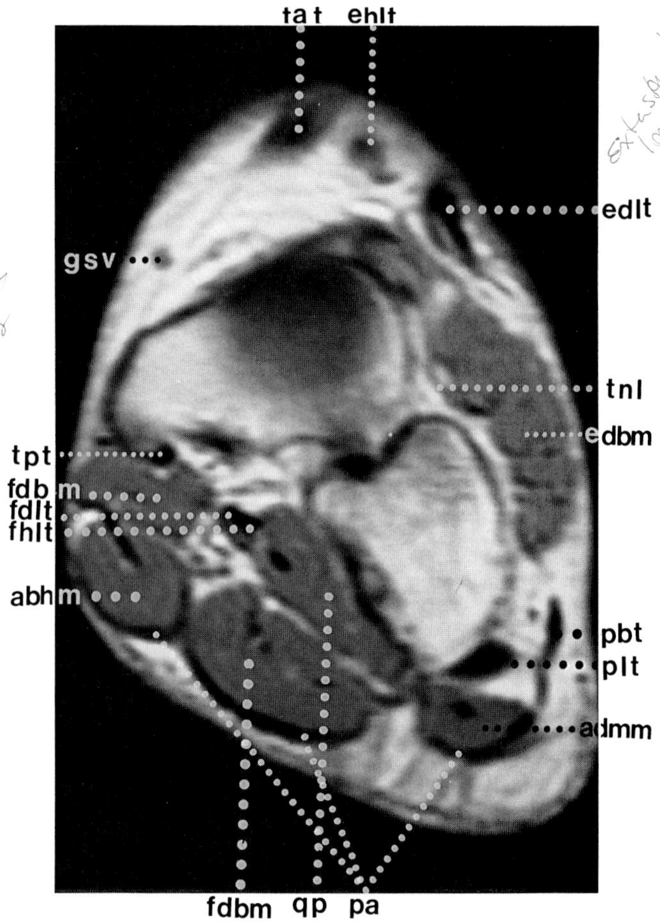

FIG. 2.46.

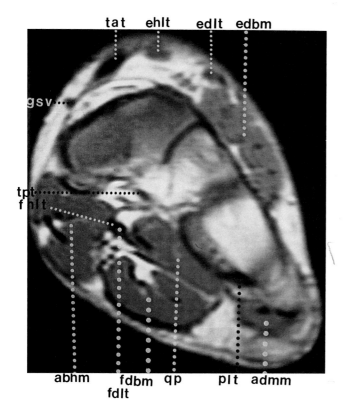

FIG. 2.47.

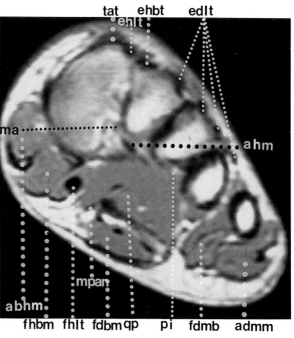

FIG. 2.49.

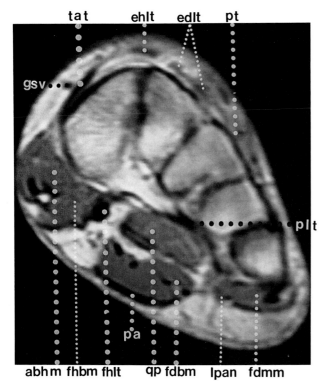

FIG. 2.48.

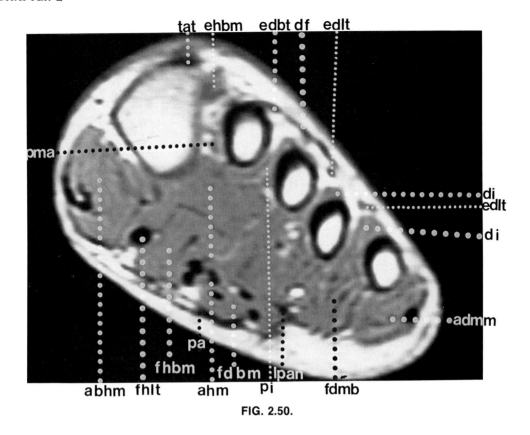

FIG. 2.50.

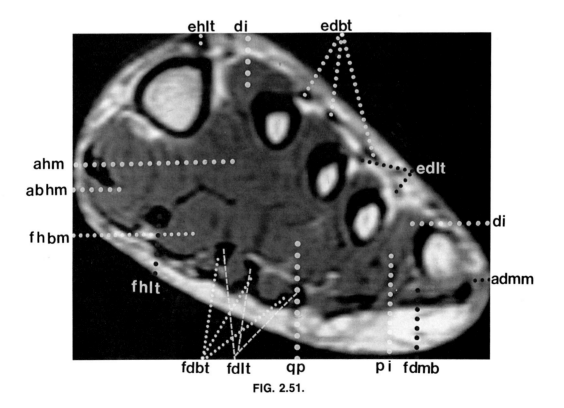

FIG. 2.51.

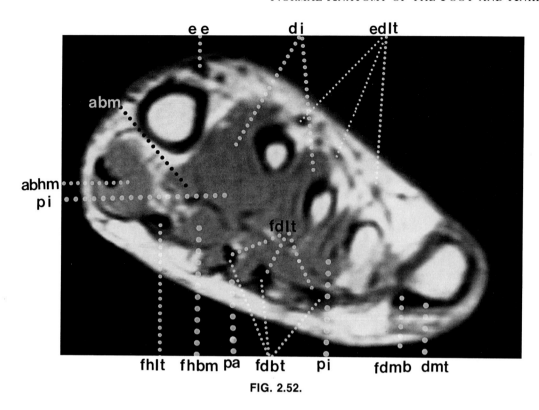

FIG. 2.52.

REFERENCES

1. Draves DJ, *Anatomy of the Lower Extremity*. 1986, Williams and Wilkins: Baltimore.
2. Netter FH, *The CIBA Collection of Medical Illustrations, vol. 8, Musculoskeletal System. Anatomy, Physiology, and Metabolic Disorders*. 1987, CIBA-Geigy: Summit, NJ.
3. Williams PL, Warwick R, Pyston M, and Bannister LH, *Gray's Anatomy 37th Ed*. 1989, Churchill Livingstone: Edinburgh.
4. Kang HS and Resnick D, *MRI of the Extremities: An Anatomic Atlas*. 1991, W.B. Saunders: Philadelphia.
5. Jaffe WL, Garro PJ, and Laitma JF, *Paleontology, embryology, and anatomy of the foot*, in *Disorders of the Foot and Ankle*, MH Jahss Editor. 1991, W.B. Saunders: Philadelphia, p. 3–34.

MRI of the Foot and Ankle,
edited by A.L. Deutsch, J.H. Mink, and R. Kerr,
Raven Press, Ltd., New York © 1992

CHAPTER 3

Biomechanics for Radiology

Roger A. Mann

Human gait permits us to move from place to place with the least expenditure of energy. As we walk, the center of gravity is moved in both a vertical and horizontal plane. During gait, force is exerted against the ground. A person weighing 150 pounds, walking a mile, exerts approximately 60 tons of force per foot per mile at the time of initial ground contact, and during running, approximately 120 tons of force per foot per mile. It thus becomes obvious that probably the most important mechanism of walking must deal with the absorption and dissipation of this force followed by the stabilization of the foot at toe-off. During walking the foot is flexible at the time of initial ground contact in order to absorb the impact of striking the ground, following which through a series of events the foot becomes a rigid lever-arm at the time of toe-off. Many events occur in order to bring about this transition from a flexible to a rigid foot. This chapter briefly outlines the mechanisms that permit this series of events to occur using the least expenditure of energy.

THE WALKING CYCLE

The walking cycle is used to define the events of a step. A step begins and ends with heel strike of the same foot. Normally we walk at a speed of approximately 120 steps/min, which means a normal cycle consumes approximately 1 s. The walking cycle is divided into two basic phases: the stance phase (when the foot is on the ground) and the swing phase (when the foot is off the ground). The stance phase consumes about 62% of the cycle and the swing phase 38%. Throughout each walking cycle there are two periods of double limb support when both feet are on the

ground (0–12% and 50–62%) and a period of single limb support when the swing leg is off the ground (12–50% and 60–100%) (Fig. 3.1).

BIOMECHANICS OF WEIGHTBEARING

As the body passes through space the center of gravity moves, which results in forces being exerted against the ground. These forces consist of a vertical force, which is perpendicular to the ground, a fore and aft shear, a mediolateral shear, and a torque. The vertical

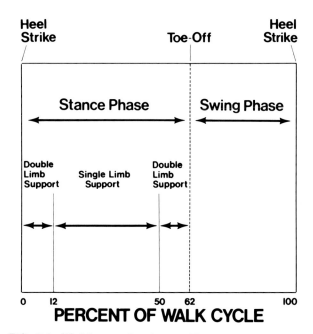

FIG. 3.1. Walking cycle phases. The walking cycle defines the events that occur during a step. Stance phase constitutes 62% of the cycle and swing phase 38%. There are two periods of double limb support when both feet are on the ground, and one period of single limb support when one foot is on the ground.

R.A. Mann: Department of Orthopaedic Surgery, University of California, San Francisco, San Francisco, California 94609.

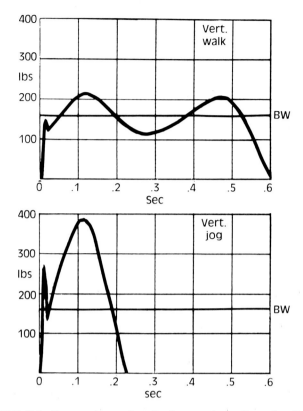

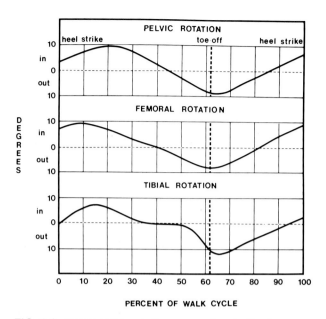

FIG. 3.3. Transverse rotation occurring in the lower extremity during walking. Internal rotation occurs until approximately 15% of the cycle, after which progressive external rotation occurs until toe-off, when internal rotation once again begins. (From ref. 7, with permission.)

FIG. 3.2. Comparison of vertical ground reaction of walking vs. jogging. The vertical force during jogging for a 150-pound individual reaches a maximum of almost 400 pounds as compared to the same person walking, which reaches a maximum of approximately 215 pounds. (From ref. 7, with permission.)

force is the greatest in magnitude and consists of two peaks and a valley. The first peak is related to the upward movement of the center of gravity, and the second, the downward movement. The valley results from the fact that after the center of gravity has moved upward, as it reaches the top of a trajectory it unloads the foot before it starts to fall back toward the ground (Fig. 3.2). During jogging the vertical force increases to almost two and a half times body weight. The other interesting feature of the vertical force curve is the initial spike, which results from the initial force of the foot against the ground. For walking it is about 80% body weight, and for jogging approximately 160% of body weight. The magnitude of this spike may be altered by using various types of heel material.

TRANSVERSE ROTATION

During walking, rotation occurs in the transverse plane in the lower extremity, which consists of the pelvis, femur, and tibia (1). This rotation follows a specific pattern during normal gait. One has only to observe an individual following a stroke to realize how important the normal rotation of the lower extremity is in permitting one to walk in a normal manner (Fig. 3.3).

The rotation begins as the heel strikes the ground, which loads the calcaneus, which in response to this loading undergoes rapid eversion into valgus. This then results in a series of events, some of which pass distally into the foot and others that pass proximally into the lower extremity. The eversion of the calcaneus is translated distally across the transverse tarsal joint (talonavicular and calcaneocuboid), which responds by unlocking, which creates a flexible mid-foot. The eversion of the calcaneus is translated proximally by the subtalar joint into internal rotation, which passes across the ankle joint into the entire lower extremity. It is this passive internal rotation mechanism that is responsible for the "pronation" that occurs in the foot at the time of initial ground contact and is not under the control of any muscle group per se. It is controlled only by the shape of the articular surfaces and their ligamentous support. The pronation reaches a maximum at about 12% of the walking cycle, after which progressive stabilization of the foot occurs.

The stabilization of the foot is brought about from proximal to distal, just the opposite of the internal rotation, which is mediated from distal to proximal. The external rotation is brought about by the contralateral swinging limb imparting an external rotation torque to the stance leg pelvis. This external rotation is passed distally across the knee and ankle joints to the subtalar joint where it is translated from the external rotation above into inversion of the subtalar joint below. Distally, this rotation results in inversion of the subtalar joint, which in turn stabilizes the transverse tarsal joint. This mechanism is aided by the action of the plantar aponeurosis, the oblique placement of the ankle joint, and the oblique metatarsal break. It is this mechanism that converts the foot from a flexible structure at the time of initial ground contact to a rigid lever-arm at the time of toe-off.

THE METATARSAL BREAK

The metatarsal break is the oblique axis that passes across the metatarsal heads in a lateral direction (2) (Fig. 3.4). The obliquity of the break is noted by observing the oblique crease across the top of one's leather shoe. The purpose of the metatarsal break is that it imparts an external rotation force to the lower extremity as the body passes over the toes and probably accounts for the last few degrees of the external rotation, which is initiated proximally.

PLANTAR APONEUROSIS

The plantar aponeurosis is important because it provides stability to the first metatarsophalangeal joint

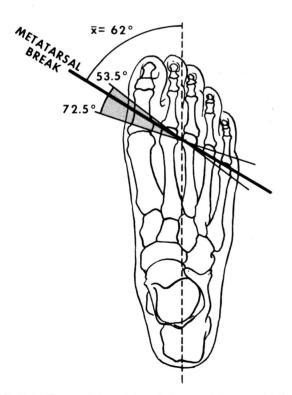

FIG. 3.4. The metatarsal break is an oblique axis that passes across the metatarsophalangeal joints. This obliquely placed axis helps to distribute the body weight across the metatarsals and aid in external rotation of the lower extremity. (From ref. 6, with permission.)

and helps to stabilize the medial longitudinal arch. The plantar aponeurosis arises from the tubercle of the calcaneus and passes forward, inserting into the base of the proximal phalanx. The function of the plantar aponeurosis has been likened to a windlass mechanism so that with dorsiflexion of the metatarsophalangeal joints the plantar aponeurosis is wrapped around the metatarsal heads and depresses them (3). This, in turn, brings about elevation of the longitudinal arch. The mechanism is the strongest for the first metatarsophalangeal joint and becomes less effective as one moves laterally across the foot. The mechanism of the plantar aponeurosis with dorsiflexion of the metatarsophalangeal joints enhances the external rotation that occurs in the lower extremity in the last half of the stance phase.

It thus becomes obvious that none of the mechanisms of the foot function as an isolated entity, but all function together in producing stability of the foot. The mechanics of the foot at the time of initial ground contact are passive, and those just described at the time of toe-off in which the foot becomes a rigid lever-arm are active.

THE ANKLE JOINT

The ankle joint is not simply a hinge joint, but permits gliding of the tibia over the dome of the talus. The trochlear surface of the talus is shaped like a section from a cone whose apex is based medially (3) (Fig. 3.5). The ankle joint is externally rotated in relation to the knee, and the foot is slightly internally rotated in relation to the ankle.

The ligaments about the ankle joint consist medially of the deltoid ligament, which fans out over the narrower aspect of the talus, and laterally there are three separate ligamentous bands fanning out over the broader aspect of the talus. The lateral collateral ligament consists of the anterior and posterior talofibular ligament and the calcaneofibular ligament. When the ankle joint is in plantar flexion the anterior talofibular ligament is in line with the fibula and is under tension, thereby providing the joint with support, as opposed to when the ankle is in dorsiflexion when the calcaneofibular ligament is in line with the fibula and therefore is providing the majority of the support (Fig. 3.6).

The motion that occurs at the ankle joint is that of dorsiflexion and plantar flexion. At the time of initial ground contact, rapid plantar flexion occurs in the ankle joint, which is controlled by an eccentric (lengthening) contraction of the anterior compartment muscles. This rapid plantar flexion helps to absorb the impact of initial ground contact. After plantar flexion has reached a maximum at approximately 12% of the cycle, progressive dorsiflexion occurs at the ankle until

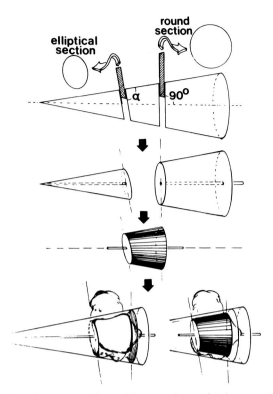

FIG. 3.5. Curvature of trochlear surface of talus creates a cone whose apex is based medially. From this configuration one can observe that the deltoid ligament is well suited to function along the medial side of the ankle joint, whereas laterally, where more rotation is occurring, three separate ligaments are necessary. (From ref. 6, with permission.)

approximately 40% when plantar flexion once again begins and lasts until the time of toe-off. The dorsiflexion of the ankle is controlled by an eccentric contraction (lengthening) of the posterior calf muscles

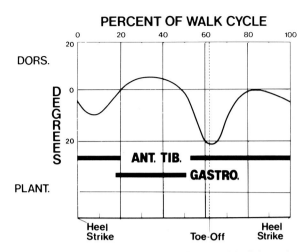

FIG. 3.7. The range of motion of the ankle joint, along with the phasic activity of the muscles of the anterior compartment of the calf, represented by the anterior tibialis (*ANT. TIB.*) and those of the posterior compartment muscles represented by the gastrocnemius-soleus group (*GASTRO*).

until 40% of the cycle when plantar flexion begins and continues until the time of toe-off. The plantar flexion is brought about by a concentric (shortening) contraction of the posterior calf musculature. Following toe-off, dorsiflexion once again occurs, which permits the foot to clear the ground during swing phase. This dorsiflexion is brought about by a concentric contraction of the anterior compartment (Fig. 3.7).

SUBTALAR JOINT

The subtalar joint creates an oblique hinge between the talus and calcaneus that functions to translate mo-

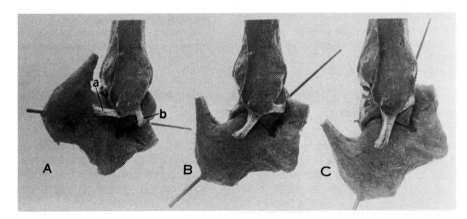

FIG. 3.6. Calcaneofibular ligament (*a*) and anterior talofibular ligament (*b*) are shown. **A:** In plantar flexion, anterior talofibular ligament is in line with the fibula and is providing most of the support to the lateral aspect of the ankle joint. **B:** In neutral position of the ankle joint both anterior talofibular and calcaneofibular ligaments provide support to the joint. Relationship of the calcaneofibular ligament to subtalar joint axis, which is depicted in the background, is noted. Note that this ligament and axis are parallel to each other. **C:** In dorsiflexion, calcaneofibular ligament is in line with the fibula and provides support to the lateral aspect of the ankle joint. (From ref. 6, with permission.)

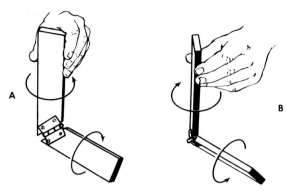

FIG. 3.8. Simple mechanical mechanism demonstrating functional relationships between the tibia above and calcaneus below. The subtalar joint between the talus and calcaneus acts as a mitered hinge, translating motion in the calcaneus to the tibia at the time of heel strike, and translation of tibial movement to the calcaneus at the time of toe-off.

tion that occurs in the lower extremity above to the calcaneus, and conversely functions to translate motion from the calcaneus below into the lower extremity above (Fig. 3.8). Through its mechanism of rotation it also influences the function of the foot through the transverse tarsal joint.

The movement that occurs at the subtalar joint is that of inversion and eversion. At the time of heel strike, eversion occurs, which reaches a maximum at 15% of the walking cycle, following which progressive inversion begins until the time of toe-off (Fig. 3.9). A person with a flat foot has more motion in their subtalar joint than an individual with a normal foot (4). The rapid eversion that occurs at heel strike is a mechanism that helps to absorb the impact of initial ground contract. This motion is not under the control of any specific muscle group. The inversion of the subtalar joint,

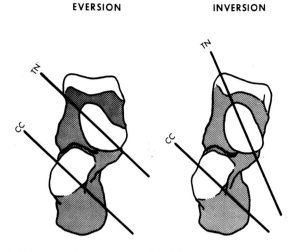

FIG. 3.10. The transverse tarsal joint depicting the head of the talus and head of the calcaneus with its composite axis of motion, *TN* and *CC*. When the calcaneus is in eversion the axis system is parallel to one another, permitting flexibility in the joint. When the calcaneus is inverted, the axes are nonparallel, creating a more stable situation.

however, is under the control of the tibialis posterior and the gastrocsoleus muscles, but the mechanism of the plantar aponeurosis, the external rotation of the lower extremity, and metatarsal break also contribute to the inversion of the subtalar joint.

THE TRANSVERSE TARSAL JOINT

The next joint distal to the subtalar joint is the transverse tarsal joint. It consists of the talonavicular and calcaneocuboid joints. The motion of the subtalar joint controls the stability of the transverse tarsal joint. When the subtalar joint is everted the axes of the trans-

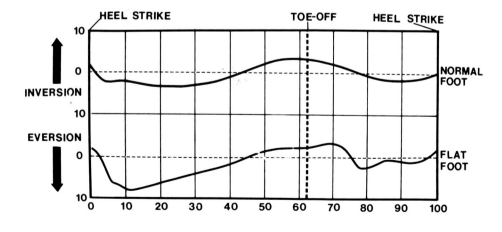

FIG. 3.9. Rotation of the subtalar joint. The rotation of the subtalar joint demonstrates eversion at the time of heel strike, after which there is progressive inversion until the time of toe-off. In a normal foot there is 8 to 10° of motion, and in a flat foot, 12 to 14° of motion.

verse tarsal joint are parallel to one another, which permits the forefoot to be flexible (5). This is the position of the joint at the time of initial ground contact when absorption of the impact occurs. When the calcaneus is inverted, however, the axes are nonparallel, and this results in a rigid forefoot (Fig. 3.10). This is the position that the joint assumes at the time of toe-off when the foot is converted into a rigid lever-arm. Again, this function of the transverse tarsal joint does not stand alone in the creation of a flexible or rigid foot, but is associated with the other joint functions that have been described previously.

DESCRIPTION OF A COMPLETE WALKING CYCLE

In this chapter an isolated series of events have been presented that when taken together constitute a step. A step is a finely coordinated series of events that occurs with a minimal expenditure of energy. If one of these mechanisms fails to function properly, it may impair the function not only of the foot but of the lower extremity.

A step begins with heel strike, which absorbs the impact of the body against the ground. The shape of the articular surfaces of the foot and their supporting ligamentous structures permit the foot to ''bend down'' without the use of muscle force per se. As the foot strikes the ground the heel pad helps to absorb the impact, the ankle joint rapidly plantar flexes, the calcaneus everts, and the knee joint flexes. All these mechanisms help to soften the impact of the body against the ground. One becomes acutely aware of this mechanism if they hold the lower extremity stiff, and strike the ground, and observe the acute jarring of the whole body rather than the almost imperceptible heel strike that occurs normally.

In response to the eversion of the calcaneus and subtalar joint, maximum internal rotation of the lower limb occurs and the transverse tarsal joint is unlocked. This results in a flexible forefoot.

Following opposite toe-off at 12% of the cycle the swing leg starts to move forward and the center of gravity passes over the fixed foot at 34% of the cycle. As this occurs, external rotation of the lower extremity along with subsequent inversion of the subtalar joint begins. As the heel rises, the windlass mechanism of the plantar aponeurosis becomes functional, and along

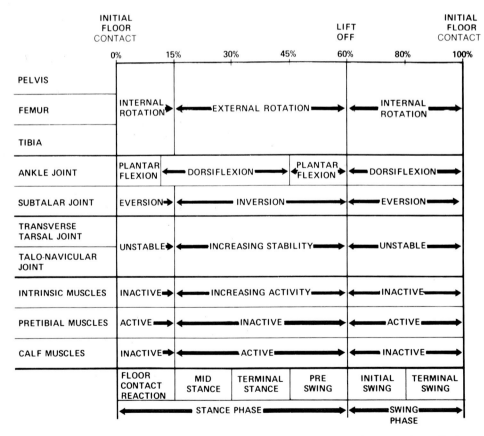

FIG. 3.11. Schematic diagram of the complete walking cycle, showing rotations that occur in the various segments and joints, as well as the activity in the foot and leg musculature. (From ref. 8, with permission.)

with the metatarsal break and the obliquely placed ankle axis, maximum external rotation of the lower extremity is achieved at the time of toe-off. This in turn locks the transverse tarsal joint, creating a rigid lever-arm at the time of toe-off. Following toe-off the foot once again becomes flexible (Fig. 3.11).

REFERENCES

1. Levens AS, Inman VT, and Blosser JA, *Transverse rotation of the segments of the lower extremity in locomotion.* J Bone Joint Surg. 1948, **30A**: p. 859.

2. Isman RE and Inman VT, *Anthropometric studies of the human foot and ankle.* Bull Prosthet Res. 1969, **10–11**: p. 97.

3. Hicks JH, *The mechanics of the foot. II. The plantar aponeurosis and the arch.* J Anat. 1954, **88**: p. 25.

4. Wright DG, Desai ME, and Henderson BS, *Action of the subtalar and ankle-joint complex during the stance phase of walking.* J Bone Joint Surg. 1964, **46A**: p. 361.

5. Elftman H, *The transverse tarsal joint and its control.* Clin Orthop 1960. **16**: p. 41.

6. Inman VT, *The Joints of the Ankle.* 1976, Williams & Wilkins: Baltimore.

7. Mann RA, *Surgery of the Foot.* 1986, CV Mosby: St. Louis.

8. Mann RA, *Biomechanics of the Foot,* in *American Academy of Orthopaedic Surgeons: Atlas of Orthotics.* 1975, CV Mosby: St. Louis.

MRI of the Foot and Ankle,
edited by A.L. Deutsch, J.H. Mink, and R. Kerr,
Raven Press, Ltd., New York © 1992

CHAPTER 4

Traumatic Injuries of Bone and Osteonecrosis

Andrew L. Deutsch

The application of magnetic resonance imaging (MRI) for assessment of trauma- and stress-related osseous abnormalities has emerged as a natural extension of the extraordinary capability of this technique to depict pathologic alterations of bone marrow (1–10). Multiple investigations have now attested to the value of MRI imaging in the assessment of a wide spectrum of injuries to bone, ranging from relatively innocuous bone contusions to bone death (osteonecrosis). The value of MRI in recognizing derangements of bone that have previously not been detectable by conventional radiographic techniques and that span the pathological gamut from stress responses to radiographically occult complete fractures is becoming increasingly recognized (11–20). Recent investigations suggest an emerging role for MRI in the assessment of fracture healing and complications thereof, including injuries to the developing growth plate (21). This chapter reviews these applications of MRI with particular reference to their occurrence in the lower extremity and foot and ankle. As part of this discussion, salient aspects of normal marrow germane to an understanding of the rationale behind the production and interpretation of MRI images of traumatic injuries of bone will be considered.

NORMAL BONE MARROW

Normal marrow is composed predominantly of fat and water (2,3,6,10). Fat is characterized by an extremely short T1 relaxation time and a high proton density (2,3) These two features combine to generate signal intensity for fat that is probably higher than that of any other component tissue of the body on T1-weighted sequences. Fat is also characterized by a

relatively short T2 relaxation time; a feature contributing to lower signal intensity on T2-weighted sequences (2). While fat is referred to in this discussion as a homogeneous tissue component, and appears homogeneous on routine spin-echo imaging, it actually contains several spectral components (aliphatic and olefinic protons) (1). As such, fat may potentially demonstrate chemical shift-induced dephasing and signal amplitude modulation depending on whether the components are in or out of phase with each other (10). This effect is most apparent on gradient-echo techniques, in which the chemical shift-related dephasing that occurs during the free induction decay (FID) is not rephased at the echo (10). With these pulse sequences, signal modulations can be demonstrated in subcutaneous fat (10). The potential effect of chemical shift on the signal from fat in the marrow, however, is generally overshadowed by susceptibility-related signal loss in the marrow space (see below) (1,10). On routine spin-echo pulse sequences, the potential modulation of signal from marrow fat is obscured by overall field inhomogeneity effects, which are significantly greater than the chemical shift between the spectral components of adipose tissue (1). The different spectral components of fat may, however, have an effect on various techniques employed for fat suppression (see below).

The water in bone marrow is contained predominantly within the cellular elements and is compartmentalized into different fractions (2). Intracellular water is comprised of superbound, bound, structured, and bulk water fractions (2,22). The concentration of bulk and structured water contributes most significantly to the signal intensity displayed on MRI studies (2). In particular, bulk water, as a consequence of its long T2 relaxation time, contributes to increased signal intensity on T2-weighted sequences (2). Most disease states are characterized by increases in bulk water and thus high signal on T2-weighted sequences (2).

A.L. Deutsch: Tower Musculoskeletal Imaging Center, Los Angeles, California 90048, and Department of Radiology, University of California, San Diego, California.

In addition to the distribution of fat and water, the structural characteristics of bone significantly contribute to the appearance of the marrow on MRIs (1,2). The honeycomb distribution of the trabeculae separates the marrow space into communicating compartments, providing a large surface area of interfaces between regions of differing magnetic susceptibility (e.g., mineral and bone) (1). The effects of magnetic susceptibility on the appearance of bone marrow are particularly evident on gradient-echo images, in which marrow demonstrates a low signal intensity, even on relatively T1-weighted sequences (1) (see Gradient-Echo Imaging).

At the time of birth, the skeleton is virtually entirely composed of "red" or cellular marrow involved in hematopoiesis (23,24). Cellular marrow consists of granulocyte and red blood cell lines in addition to platelet and lymphocyte precursors (25). Following birth, an orderly conversion of the cellular components of red marrow to fatty marrow occurs with centripetal migration of the red marrow (2,3,23,24). This occurs first in the terminal phalanges of the feet and hands. Within the long bones of the appendicular skeleton, conversion of red to yellow marrow progresses from the diaphyses to the metaphyses (23,24). Epiphyses and apophyses are initially composed of cartilage, and controversy exists as to whether they ever contain hematopoietic marrow (2,26). Epiphyseal and apophyseal ossification centers characteristically contain fatty marrow in normal patients (27). The process of marrow conversion is usually complete by the time an individual reaches the age of 25 years (2,3,23,24). In the adult, the hematopoietic marrow is concentrated in the axial skeleton and to a lesser extent proximal appendicular skeleton (e.g., proximal humeri and femora). As individuals age, there is a continued gradual replacement of hematopoietic with fatty marrow (2,3). In older adults, it is common for the spine and pelvis to demonstrate predominantly fatty marrow. Histologically, the fraction of red marrow decreases from 58% in the first decade to 29% in the eighth decade of life (2,26). Variations in this pattern of marrow conversion exist, presumably reflecting differences between individuals and responses to stress (2,3,25). Residual islands of hematopoietic marrow may occupy long bones well past middle age. Patchy areas of residual marrow are commonly observed in the distal femora on MRI examinations of the knee, and should not be misconstrued as representing significant pathologic lesions (28). Changes in marrow distribution have been seen in association with smoking habits and exercise (28). Islands of fat within hematopoietic marrow are also commonly encountered as normal variants on MRIs with focal fatty infiltration of the axial skeleton reported in 60% of patients in one series (6,29). These variations, however, are more commonly encountered within the axial and more proximal appendicular skeleton than within the bones of the hands and feet, which almost invariably demonstrate uniformly fatty marrow on MRIs of adults.

PULSE SEQUENCE CONSIDERATIONS

Spin Echo

Short TR/TE or T1-weighted spin-echo sequences are well suited for depiction of marrow abnormalities, particularly those involving predominantly fatty marrow (2,3,8,10). Pathological processes, as a consequence of prolonged T1 relaxation times, will appear as areas of decreased signal intensity (e.g., appear dark) contrasted against the background of high signal intensity (e.g., bright) fatty marrow. Using T1-weighted sequences, attention must be directed toward the selection of appropriately short repetition times (e.g., TR 400 or less) and echo times (e.g., TE 20 or less) to maximize T1 contrast (2). At higher field strengths, the relative difference between the T1 of normal marrow and pathological processes is less than at lower field strength as a result of prolongation of T1 relaxation times at higher field strengths (2). As a consequence, T1 contrast decreases at higher field strengths (2). This has proven to be more of a theoretical than practical concern at field strengths commonly used in clinical practice (2).

Proton density weighted spin-echo images are sensitive to changes in mobile protons but relatively insensitive to changes in T1 and T2 relaxation times (2). As most pathological processes have relatively small changes in proton density, these images usually have less contrast for depiction of marrow pathology than T1- and T2-weighted spin echo sequences (2). T2-weighted images are usually not as sensitive as T1-weighted sequences in depicting abnormalities of fatty marrow, but may improve specificity and be of greater value in hematopoietic marrow (2,10,25)

Gradient-Echo Imaging

In contrast to spin-echo sequences, normal marrow is depicted as a relatively low signal intensity structure on all gradient-echo sequences (1,2,30). This appearance occurs as a result of the effects of magnetic susceptibility between trabecular bone and surrounding marrow elements (1,2,10,30). These susceptibility effects are particularly evident on gradient-echo sequences in which tissue contrast is dependent on T2* as opposed to T2 relaxation. T2* is shorter than T2 and represents the decay of transverse magnetization without refocusing of static susceptibility. During the performance of a gradient-echo pulse sequence, there is no rephasing of local magnetic field inhomogeneities by a 180° pulse as in conventional spin-echo imaging (2,10,31,32). As gradients are produced in all directions within a voxel, there will be a dephasing of signal in all directions and therefore signal loss and T2* shortening (1,10). The honeycomb distribution of individual trabeculae divides the marrow space into communicating compartments, providing a large surface area of interfaces between regions of differing susceptibility (e.g., mineral and bone) (1). The amount of trabecular bone varies in the three anatomic segments of tubular bone (1,10). The epiphysis and metaphysis contain more trabecular bone than the diaphysis, which is characterized by a thicker cortex and medullary cavity with few trabeculae (1). As a consequence, the segmental distribution of trabecular bone influences signal intensity of marrow on gradient-echo images (1). Low signal intensity on gradient-echo images may represent fatty marrow with a high content of trabecular bone and should not be interpreted only as hematopoietic marrow (1). Ferritin and hemosiderin, as a consequence of superparamagnetic effects, also increase local magnetic susceptibility (1,2). This contributes to shortening of the T2 and particularly T2* relaxation times, resulting in decreased signal intensity on T2- and T2*-weighted (gradient-echo) images. In situations characterized by excessive iron overload, there will be decreased signal intensity even on T1-weighted sequences (2,25).

Inversion Recovery

Standard inversion recovery sequences produce heavily T1-weighted images (10). If the inversion time (TI) is made short such that the TR time is greater than twice the TI, a "null point" is created (10,33,34). This technique is referred to as short tau inversion recovery (STIR), and is particularly effective for assessment of marrow processes (2,4,10). In the author's experience, this sequence has demonstrated higher sensitivity and lesion conspicuity than any of the other sequences commonly in use. The null point represents the T1 value of a species of spins for which the net magnetization vector will be passing through the transverse plane at the TI and thus will have no net vector along the z-axis at the time of the 90° flip and thus produce no detectable signal (10). Signal from fat can be effectively suppressed by adjusting the TI to the null crossing point of the longitudinal magnetization of fat (2,10). With STIR imaging, for tissues with T1 greater than the null point, the effects of T1 and T2 relaxation are additive, contributing to increased lesion conspicuity (4). The signal-to-noise ratio for STIR sequences is lower than that for T1 and proton density-weighted images (2). While highly sensitive to the depiction of marrow abnormalities, STIR sequences do not contribute to specificity except in settings in which the question arises as to whether a suspected abnormality is fatty or not (10).

Chemical Shift Imaging

Several techniques have been developed in an attempt to exploit the resonant frequency differences between fat and water, the two principal constituents of marrow (5,10). The efforts have been directed toward using these frequency differences in an attempt to depict early abnormalities of marrow more sensitively. Two principal approaches, phase contrast and selective presaturation, have been investigated for purposes of chemical shift imaging (10).

Phase Contrast

The most widely known phase contrast technique is that described by Dixon, which incorporates two separate imaging sequences (2,10,35). Two identical spin-echo sequences are performed with the 180° refocusing pulse of the second sequence applied at a short-time interval earlier than that of the first sequence, producing an out-of-phase or opposed echo (10,35). Adding the initial images (in-phase) and opposed images produces an image of the predominant spectral component, while subtracting the opposed from the in-phase image produces an image of the minor component (10,35). As a consequence, while the image achieved is based on spectral components, the Dixon method does not produce a fat or water image per se (phase ambiguity) (10). The Dixon method is also vulnerable to misregistration errors resulting from motion between the in-phase and opposed images, as well as phase errors resulting from static field inhomogeneities or susceptibility effects (10).

Modifications of the Dixon method incorporating phase correction have been devised in an attempt to overcome some of the previously mentioned limitations (10,36). These methods are capable of producing true fat and water images and are accomplished by applying image processing techniques to the phase information in the opposed image (10,36). Chopper averaging, a technique employed for combining data from multiple acquisitions, can also be used to enhance the Dixon method and eliminate misregistration artifact between acquisitions (10,37). Phase information is preserved as the data from the opposed and in-phase acquisitions are combined before reconstruction. True fat and water images are generated for each acquisition.

Selective Presaturation

The other principal method for accomplishing chemical shift imaging is selective presaturation (10). With this technique, a frequency selective presaturation pulse is applied to water or fat immediately before the excitation pulse. This presaturation pulse effectively destroys the longitudinal magnetization of the water or fat and when the excitation pulse is applied, there will have been insufficient time for longitudinal recovery (10). As such, the "presaturated" component does not contribute to the final image. With presaturation techniques (CHESS, ChemSat) section coverage is decreased, although imaging times are not necessarily increased. While ideal spectral selectivity may not be accomplished, separate fat and water images are available with this method (10).

Combined Chemical Shift and Phase Selective Imaging

As previously discussed, fat is actually composed of two different resonant frequencies related to aliphatic and olefinic hydrogens (10,38). The aliphatic hydrogens represent the predominant signal from fat, are attached to singly bonded carbons, and account for approximately 95% of the total fat protons (38). The olefinic hydrogens (5% of total fat protons) are attached to doubly bonded carbons found in unsaturated fats and resonate close to water hydrogens (38). As a consequence, the previously described techniques that are directed at elimination of the predominant aliphatic fat signal result in incomplete fat suppression (38). In addition, the aliphatic component is not completely suppressed with the CHESS technique as a consequence of steady state effects (38). Combining CHESS fat suppression with the Dixon opposed imaging technique has recently been reported to accomplish superior fat suppression [opposed-fat saturation (OP-FS) sequence] (38). The reported effectiveness of OP-FS relates to saturation of most of the aliphatic component combined with cancellation of the residual signal by the olefinic fat component (38).

TRAUMATIC INJURIES OF BONE

By virtue of its unparalleled ability to depict changes in bone marrow and cancellous bone, MRI has emerged as a powerful technique for the evaluation of traumatic injuries to bone (16–21,39). This has occurred despite the relative insensitivity of MRI to the detection of abnormalities involving the bony cortex. Many of the injuries depicted by MRI have proved to be occult to conventional radiographic detection, and before the development of MRI may have gone undetected. MRI is capable of detecting the full spectrum of injuries to bone, ranging from the relatively innocuous contusions or "bruises" to complete fractures. Additionally, a potential role for MRI in the assessment of fracture complications including the development of osteonecrosis and nonunion is emerging.

Contusion

Contusional injuries of bone, also referred to as "bruises," were first described using MRI in association with major injuries to the collateral ligaments of the knee. These lesions were among the first of the radiographically occult injuries of bone to be depicted by MRI (14,16,40). In the initial reports, the lesions resulted from increased compressive forces, most commonly on the side of the knee opposite a collateral ligament injury (e.g., increased valgus stress secondary to a medial collateral ligament tear) (16). Subsequent experience has resulted in reports of similar injuries secondary to direct bony contusion (41).

On MRI, bone contusions or bruises are manifest as poorly defined, reticulated, inhomogeneous, low signal intensity lesions confined to the medullary space of cancellous bone on T1-weighted images (14,16,17,40) (Fig. 4.1). In the acute stages, the lesions typically demonstrate increased signal intensity on T2-weighted and STIR sequences (Fig. 4.1). While no histological correlation has been available, it has been suggested that these lesions reflect trabecular microfracture with edema and hemorrhage (14,16). This apparent appearance of acute hemorrhage within cancellous bone (e.g., increased signal intensity on T2-weighted images) differs from that classically described with intracerebral hematomas, which may be acutely isointense or hypointense with the surrounding tissue due to the magnetic susceptibility effects of intracellular hemoglobin (16,42,43). It has been suggested that this different appearance of hemorrhage within bone and soft tissue results from the separation of serum from the cellular components of blood in soft tissue (16). As a consequence, the serum proton spins are not as efficiently dephased by cellular magnetic susceptibility effects as in a confined hematoma. This allows the serum water to maintain long T1 and T2 relaxation times and may account for the increased signal intensity observed acutely in these injuries on T2-weighted sequences (16) (see chapter by Crues and Shellock).

On follow-up examinations, persistent signal abnormalities have been present within bruises at 6 weeks postinjury (16). By 3 months, the appearance of the underlying bone has in most instances returned to normal (14,16,40). Cases in which radionuclide bone scan correlation has been available have demonstrated slightly more extensive changes on scintigraphy than

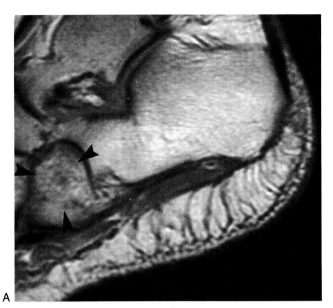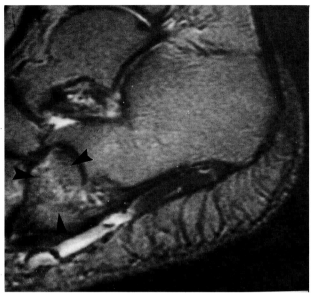

A   B

FIG. 4.1. Bone bruise. **A:** Sagittal TR 2000 TE 20. An ill-defined area of decreased signal intensity is seen within the cuboid (*arrowheads*). The patient had received a direct blow to the area. There is no discrete linear component to indicate a fracture. **B:** Sagittal TR 2000 TE 80. There is mildly increased signal intensity on the T2-weighted image consistent with edema within the cancellous bone (*arrowheads*). The imaging findings are not specific and need to be correlated with the clinical history.

on MRI, a phenomenon that may be similar to the "extended pattern" of uptake described in the context of other skeletal lesions and that has been previously attributed to regional hyperemia (14). Conventional radiographs have been normal in the overwhelming majority of cases of bone bruises (16,40). While the clinical significance of bone bruises remains incompletely known, it has been suggested that a delay in the resumption of normal sports activities be considered in the presence of such lesions to avoid the progression of any weakening of the mechanical properties of bone related to the presumed trabecular disruption (16).

Stress Fracture and Stress Response

Background

The term "stress fracture" refers to the failure of the skeleton to withstand submaximal forces acting over time. Two types of stress fractures have been identified: (a) fatigue fractures such as have been classically described in military recruits and runners in which normal bone is subjected to repeated abnormal stresses, and (b) insufficiency fractures in which normal stresses are applied to a bone whose skeletal composition reflects deficient elastic resistance (i.e., Paget's disease) (40,44–47). Fatigue fractures are particularly common in the lower extremities in athletes, joggers, and dancers. The activity precipitating

the fracture is typically new or different for the patient, is strenuous, and is repeated with a frequency that ultimately results in failure of the bone and the production of symptoms (44). Fatigue and insufficiency fractures are also not uncommon following certain surgical procedures that result in altered stress or an imbalance of muscular forces on normal or insufficient bone (44). A typical example in the foot occurs in the metatarsal bones following bunion surgery (43).

Among the tarsal bones, fatigue and insufficiency fractures most commonly involve the calcaneus (44,47). Fatigue fractures are not uncommonly reported in military recruits, and insufficiency fractures at this site may accompany rheumatoid arthritis, neurological disorders, and other diseases (44,48). The failure of the bone has been attributed to the antagonistic action of the Achilles and plantar tendons. Stress fractures in other tarsal bones are less common. In the tarsal navicular, stress fractures have been reported in active individuals, especially basketball players and runners (44,49,50). Characteristically, this fracture is oriented in the sagittal plane and is located in the central one-third of the bone. It may extend through the navicular for a variable depth, and is typically difficult to image on conventional radiographs. Scintigraphy and computed tomography in the anatomic anteroposterior plane have been advocated for detection of these injuries (49).

The metatarsals are frequent sites of stress fractures. The middle and distal aspects of the shafts of the second and third metatarsals are most commonly affected (44,47). Stress fractures of the first metatarsal are less common and when they occur frequently involve the base. Stress fractures of the base of the second metatarsal have also been reported (44).

A stress fracture should be considered as the final chapter in a series of events (44,46,48). Preceding actual fracture are a number of pathological alterations that are associated with pain, are clearly abnormal, and that place the patient "at risk" for the development of a fracture. The term "stress response" refers to those prefailure events at the cellular level that result in structural weakening (44,46).

When a bone is stressed, gradual and progressive resorption of circumferential lamellar bone and its subsequent replacement by dense osteonal bone are identified (44,46,51). This period is characterized by local hyperemia, edema, and osteoclastic activity with the stressed bone undergoing remodeling. Because of this process, a vulnerable period exists following a stressful occurrence in which the cortical bone is less capable of withstanding further stress and in which foci of osseous resorption may be transformed into sites of microfracture (44,46). Stress events in bone are more likely to occur when there has been an increase in the strength of the acting muscle over a relatively short time as the concomitant increase in strength of bone lags behind that of muscle (46).

The stress fracture begins as a small cortical crack that can progress as the stress continues (44,47). This progression is characterized by the appearance of subcortical infraction in front of the main crack in the bone. Understanding of the above sequence of events provides the basis for the development of conditioning programs for athletes. If the stress is eliminated, the sequence is interrupted or slowed so that new bone formation can "catch up" with the increased demand and a state of increased bone strength is achieved (46). Increasing physical activity under controlled circumstances can result in osseous hypertrophy without microfracture (44). Training programs of professional athletes are designed to allow the bone to compensate for the exaggerated muscular stresses and examples of osseous hypertrophy in athletes are common (e.g, lower extremities of long distance runners) (44).

Imaging of Stress Fractures and Stress Responses

While individuals with stress fractures may demonstrate findings on conventional radiographs, it has become well recognized that many significant injuries to bone may be initially and in many cases forever radiographically occult (16,17,19). In recent years, the radionuclide bone scan has been the principal method

employed for the early detection of stress fractures (48,51–55). Stressed bone undergoing active remodeling, images with poorly defined increased activity on radionuclide bone scans (51). This can clearly occur in the absence of findings on plain radiographs. With appropriate modification of activity, the abnormal scintigraphic activity can resolve without the development of a radiographically evident cortical infraction (44). With unabated continuance of the stressful activity, the bone scan activity develops into a more focal fusiform pattern of sharply marginated activity (44,51). This generally correlates with radiographically evident areas of cortical lucency and periosteal and endosteal activity, findings reflective of frank stress fracture (44).

MRI, by virtue of its enhanced soft tissue contrast resolution, may also permit early (preradiographic) detection of stress injuries of bone (14,17,40,45,46,56). Prefracture stress responses, as previously discussed, are most readily demonstrated on MRI in areas in which bone marrow is overwhelmingly fatty (57,58). This is a distinct advantage for MRI in imaging of the foot and lower extremity, which is overwhelmingly composed of fatty marrow except in the youngest of individuals. On MRI, stress responses appear as globular foci of decreased signal on T1-weighted sequences that are graphically demonstrated against a background of fatty (bright) marrow (Fig. 4.2). The signal variably increases in intensity on T2-weighted sequences. Stress responses are exceedingly well demonstrated on STIR sequences, in which they are depicted as areas of high signal intensity against the suppressed background of fatty marrow (Fig. 4.2). While the detection of stress responses in fatty marrow is relatively straightforward, demonstrating the abnormalities in hematopoietic marrow can be more difficult. We have found STIR sequences to be of considerable value in this setting. This concern, however, represents less of a problem in the foot and ankle than elsewhere in the skeleton.

In the recent MRI literature, lesions that might best have been termed "stress responses" have been referred to as amorphous-type stress fractures (19,40, 41,46,57,59). Stress responses are differentiated from bone bruises (see above) predominantly by the clinical history, as the appearance on MRI may be quite similar. We recently reviewed 11 instances of stress response in bone, diagnosed by (a) history, and (b) resolution by both clinical and MRI criteria (46). Five lesions occurred in the femoral neck, two at the knee, two involving the ankle, and two involving the foot. All lesions had identical MRI findings: inhomogeneous, poorly defined signal decreases on T1-weighted (Fig. 4.3A) sequences that became minimally and inhomogeneously brighter on T2-weighted sequences. All lesions demonstrated dramatically increased signal

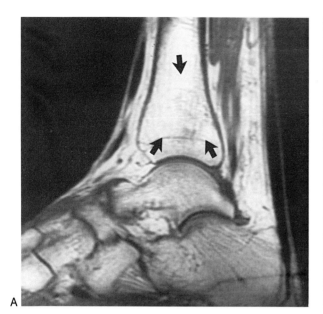
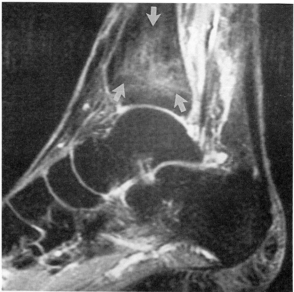

FIG. 4.2. Stress response. **A:** Sagittal TR 500 TE 15. Amorphous areas of decreased signal are identified within the distal tibia metaphysis (arrows). The patient, a ballet dancer, complained of poorly defined pain in the area of several months duration. No acute injury had occurred. **B:** Sagittal STIR TR 2200 TE 35 TI 160. The extent of poorly defined increased signal presumably reflecting edema is better depicted on the STIR sequence (*arrows*). The lack of a clearly defined linear component distinguishes stress response from stress fracture.

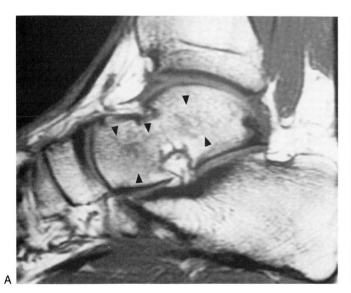
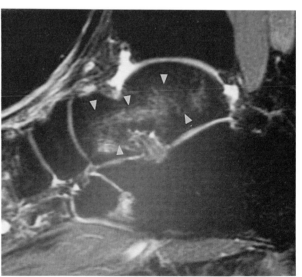

FIG. 4.3. Stress response. **A:** Sagittal TR 300 TE 15. Poorly defined signal is seen within the neck of the talus of another patient who was an active recreational athlete (*arrowheads*). The patient complained of ill-defined pain. No acute injury had occurred. **B:** Sagittal STIR TR 2200 TE 35 TI 160. The STIR sequence is again valuable for depiction of the extent of presumed edema within the bone (*arrowheads*). The patient was treated conservatively with limited weightbearing and the symptoms resolved over a period of 1 month.

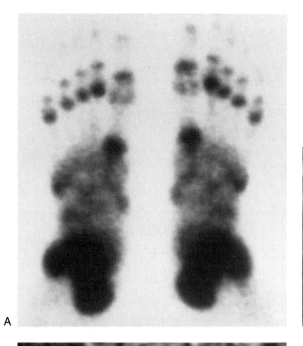

A

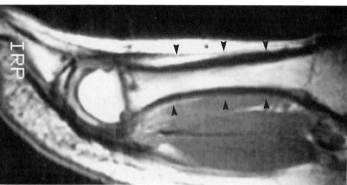

B

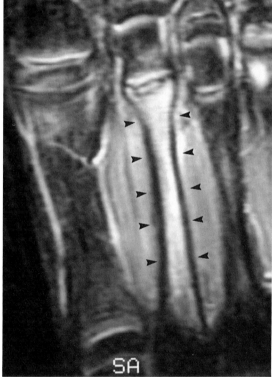

C

FIG. 4.4. Stress response. Value of STIR imaging. **A:** Bone scan. An 11-year-old girl complained of pain in the region of the second metatarsal. Plain radiographs were normal. A ^{99m}Tc MDP radionuclide bone examination demonstrated no significant localized augmented uptake of the isotope. **B:** Sagittal TR 300 TE 15. As a consequence of persistent symptoms, a high-resolution MRI examination was performed 2 weeks following the bone scan. No significant signal changes are noted within the second metatarsal head or shaft on this sequence (*arrowheads*). No fracture line is identified. **C:** Coronal TR 2200 TE 35 TI 160. There is extensive high signal intensity demonstrated throughout the metatarsal shaft most consistent with "marrow edema" (*arrowheads*). As is commonly encountered, lesion conspicuity is often greatest on the STIR sequence. The disparity between the MRI and radionuclide examinations in this case is striking.

intensity on STIR sequences (Fig. 4.3B). In none of the patients were the initial or follow-up conventional radiographs abnormal. Bone scans obtained in 7 patients were positive in 5 and negative in 2 (Fig. 4.4).

The classic appearance of a stress fracture on MRI is a linear zone of decreased signal intensity on T1-weighted sequences that is surrounded by a broad and more poorly defined area that is of lower signal intensity than the linear component (Figs. 4.5 and 4.6). Typically, the linear component remains dark on T2-

weighted sequences, but the surrounding zone of presumed hemorrhagic and nonhemorrhagic edema becomes inhomogeneously brighter. The linear components may be short and straight or long and serpiginous and are typically perpendicular to the adjacent cortex (14,40,41,53,57). Most stress fractures are metaphyseal or epiphyseal in location. It is the linear component that distinguishes a fracture from a stress response. The linear component of the fracture demonstrable on MRI also provides increased speci-

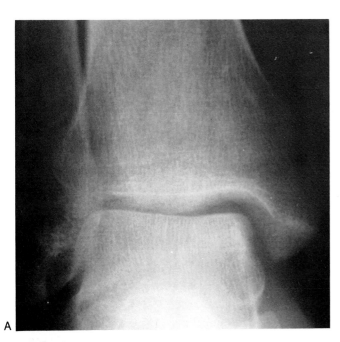

A

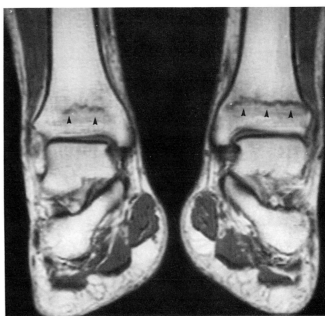

B

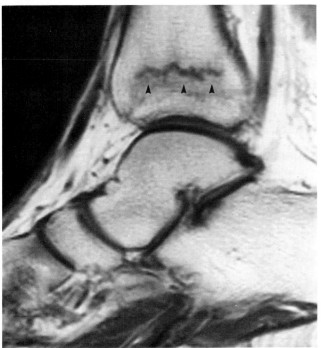

C

FIG. 4.5. Stress fracture (radiographically occult). **A:** An AP radiograph of the distal right tibia demonstrates no evidence of a fracture. The patient complained of excruciating pain in both lower extremities. **B:** Coronal TR 500 TE 30. The classic MRI appearance of stress fractures is evident in both distal tibias. Serpiginous lines of low signal intensity oriented roughly perpendicular to the long axis of the bone are present (*arrowheads*). **C:** Sagittal TR 500 TE 30. Magnified view of the right distal tibia again demonstrates the serpiginous low signal intensity line representing the fracture. The line is surrounded by a zone of less intense signal diminution representing edema.

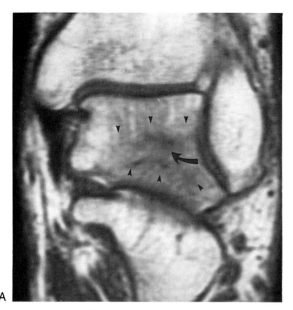

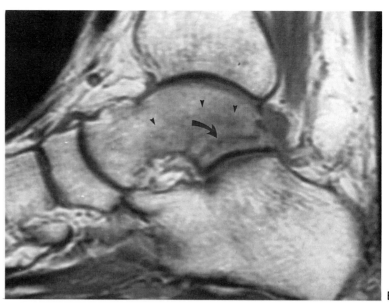

FIG. 4.6. Talar stress fracture **A:** Coronal TR 500 TE 30. Extensive low signal intensity representing edema within cancellous bone is seen abutting the superior margin of the subtalar joint (*arrowheads*). The linear fracture is seen en face (*curved arrow*). **B:** Sagittal TR 500 TE 30. The fracture line is evident as a slightly serpiginous line of low signal paralleling the posterior facet contrasted against the surrounding edema (*curved arrow*). The extensive bone edema is again seen (*arrowheads*).

ficity in diagnosis as compared with radionuclide bone scans. Stress fractures in varying stages of healing may be encountered (Fig. 4.7). Callous may be seen bridging the fracture and appears as intermediate signal intensity material (Fig. 4.7). Furthermore, while initial reports emphasized the changes of bone stress and fracture within cancellous bone, with increasing experience and high resolution images changes in cortical bone and the periosteum can be demonstrated (60). Simple periosteal reaction is most evident as a linear low signal intensity stripe paralleling the cortical margin of the underlying bone (60). The elevated periosteum may be separated from the cortex by material that increases in signal intensity on T2-weighted and STIR sequences and likely reflects reactive edema.

The relative sensitivity of MRI as compared to scintigraphy for detection of stress fracture has not been the subject of a critical study. We have had experience with both MRI positive radionuclide bone scan negative (Fig. 4.4) as well as scintigraphic positive MR negative cases of stress injury, although the latter situation has been rare in our experience. Recent critical studies of MRI versus scintigraphy for the detection of other marrow replacement processes such as metastases have demonstrated an increased sensitivity for MRI. The greater specificity of MRI as compared with scintigraphy would suggest that MRI will be the preferred method of evaluation.

Fractures

The role of MRI in the detection and characterization of radiographically occult injuries to the foot continues to expand. Most of these injuries, as has been discussed, fall in the spectrum short of acute complete fracture. The overwhelming majority of acute fractures of the foot and ankle are demonstrable on conventional radiographs. It has become increasingly apparent, however, from experience with MRI in the setting of acute injury (particularly in the knee) that even complete fractures may be occult on initial radiographic evaluation (14,16,19). In this setting, MRI may be used to advantage for the detection of such injuries. In addition to detection, MRI may be used for further characterization of fractures involving the foot and ankle, and in the assessment of fracture complications including growth plate disturbances, the development of osteonecrosis, and potentially for evaluation of fracture non-union (21,61). In the following section, the potential role of MRI in the detection and assessment of complete fractures at different sites in the foot and ankle will be considered.

Ankle Fractures

Conventional radiographs have provided the benchmark for diagnosis of fractures around the ankle and

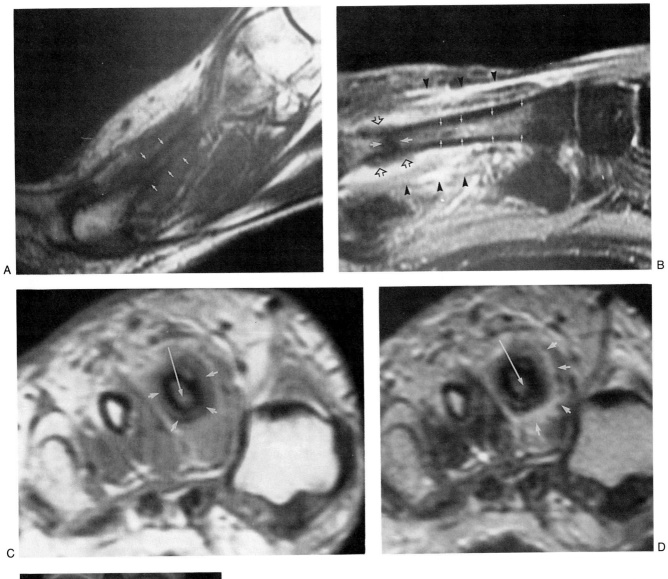

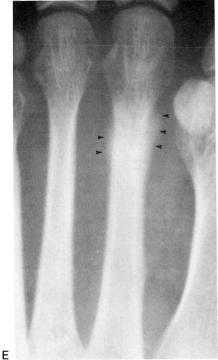

FIG. 4.7. Healing stress fracture. **A:** Sagittal TR 300 TE 15. Diffuse signal diminution reflecting marrow edema is seen throughout the shaft of the second metatarsal (*small arrows*). **B:** Sagittal STIR TR 2200 TE 35 TI 160. High signal intensity throughout the diaphysis of the second metatarsal corresponds to the changes seen on the T1-weighted image (*small vertical arrows*). Additionally, the fracture itself is seen as a zone of low signal intensity within the metaphysis (*horizontal arrows*) and periosteal reaction is noted as a zone of relatively well-marginated intermediate signal intensity along the dorsal and plantar surface of the bone (*black open arrows*). The extent of surrounding soft tissue edema is well depicted (*arrowheads*). **C:** Axial TR 2000 TE 20. Low signal intensity within the medullary bone of the second metatarsal is present (*long arrow*). The zone of periosteal reaction is seen encircling the metatarsal (*small arrows*). **D:** Axial TR 2000 TE 80. On the T2-weighted image, there is mild increase in signal intensity within the medullary bone (*arrow*) and periosteal changes. The surrounding soft tissue edema is again well depicted (*small arrows*). **E:** AP radiograph demonstrates the periosteal changes surrounding the metaphysis of the second metatarsal (*arrowheads*).

85

generally suffice for diagnosis of the osseous component of the injury (62). The stability of the ankle joint, however, is dependent on the integrity of a ring formed by the tibia, fibula, and talus, as well as surrounding supporting ligaments (61). Analysis of ligamentous integrity has principally been accomplished by physical examination, stress radiography, and conventional arthrography (44,62). Increasingly, MRI has been applied toward characterization of severe ankle sprains, and has demonstrated a high accuracy in the direct depiction of the soft tissue components of these injuries (see chapter by Mink on Ligaments of the Ankle). Radiographically occult osseous injuries seen in association with ligamentous injuries may be depicted. The significance of these findings awaits further longitudinal study. There have been no reports to date on the use of MRI for characterization of radiographically evident ankle fractures, with the exception of its use in the further assessment of growth plate injuries (see below).

Ankle fractures may be described on an anatomic basis (e.g., bimalleolar, trimalleolar), or more preferably using a classification system that incorporates the mechanism of injury as well as associated ligamentous abnormalities. Such a comprehensive classification was developed by Lauge-Hansen, who on the basis of experimental studies in cadavers, described five major predictable fracture complexes (63). While a brief description of the system is offered, the interested reader is referred to one of several excellent references for a more comprehensive discussion of this classification schema (44,47,63). Each complex is described by two terms that are modified by progressive increases in stage (force) of injury indicated by Roman numerals. The first term refers to the position of the foot at the time of injury and is designated as either supination or pronation. The second term refers to the direction that the talus is displaced or rotated relative to the mortise and is assigned one of five designations: external rotation, internal rotation, abduction, adduction, or dorsiflexion (44,63). Of the five groups, the supination–external rotation fractures (SER stages I, II, III, IV) account for nearly 60% of all ankle fractures, with supination adduction fractures (SAD stages I, II) and the combined group of pronation–external rotation fractures (PER stages I, II, III, IV,) and pronation–abduction fractures (PAB stages I,II,III) accounting for approximately 20% of ankle fractures each (44). The initial stages of injury are typically ligamentous and thus often not radiographically evident. Additionally, certain groups, such as PER stages I and II and PAB stages I and II, cannot be distinguished on the basis of conventional radiographic findings alone (44). The ability of MRI to directly depict both the osseous and ligamentous components of these injuries represents a significant advantage of this technique and affords a unique opportunity for the further study of these injuries and their commonly proposed pathoanatomic mechanisms and resulting derangements.

Tarsal Fractures

Fractures of the calcaneus are the most common site of tarsal fracture (47). The fractures may be intra- or extraarticular, with the majority (approximately 75%) involving the subtalar articulation and associated with a poorer prognosis (44). Intraarticular fractures most often occur as a result of a fall from a vertical height with the talus driven into the cancellous bone of the calcaneus (44,47). In general, conventional radiography is sufficient for detection of calcaneal fractures. Rarely, acute fractures may be radiographically occult and MRI can be used for their detection (Fig. 4.8). In the more common situation, however, supplemental imaging is often required not for the detection but rather for the complete characterization of the fracture related to the complex anatomy of the calcaneus. Fracture comminution and displacement are common in fractures of the calcaneus and the relationships of the multiple fragments are difficult to appreciate from conventional radiographs (Fig. 4.9).

No studies have been reported in the literature on the value of MRI for characterization of complex calcaneal fractures. MRI has been used elsewhere (principally the knee) for further assessment of complex fractures, and could be applied toward assessment of the calcaneus (41) (Fig. 4.9). It is unclear, however, whether MRI would provide any distinct advantages over CT as a bone tomographic technique. The difficulty for MRI in detection of small intraarticular fragments would likely present a significant limitation for its routine use as compared to CT. MRI, however, could be used effectively in the assessment of the common sequelae of calcaneal fractures including assessment of congruity and arthritis of the subtalar joint and peroneal tendon entrapment between the calcaneus and fibula (see chapter by Mink on Tendons). A recent MRI investigation of heel pain in patients with fractures of the calcaneus provided no evidence for the hypothesis that gross structural changes in the fat pad contribute to the chronic pain often associated with these injuries (64).

Avulsive injuries of the calcaneus, particularly involving the tuberosity, are readily demonstrated on plain radiographs (47). Others including one that arises at the origin of the extensor digitorum brevis along the lateral aspect of the bone may be more subtle (44). Fractures of the anterior process of the calcaneus may also escape detection on conventional radiographs and

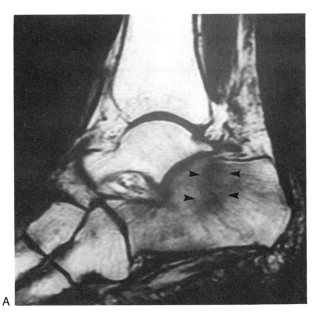 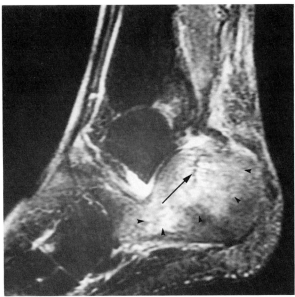

FIG. 4.8. Calcaneal fracture. **A:** Sagittal TR 500 TE 20. Extensive low signal intensity is seen within the body of the calcaneus with a vertically oriented low signal intensity band behind the posterior facet of the subtalar joint (*arrowheads*). The patient had sustained a recent fall. Conventional radiographs were normal. **B:** Sagittal STIR TR 2200 TE 35 TI 160. There is striking increased signal most consistent with hemorrhagic and nonhemorrhagic edema throughout much of the body of the calcaneus. The fracture (*arrow*) is well demonstrated on this pulse sequence contrasted against the diffuse high signal intensity edema (*arrowheads*).

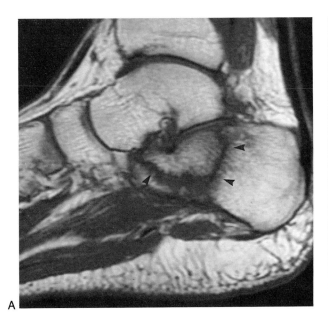 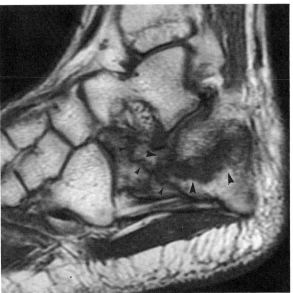

FIG. 4.9. Comminuted calcaneal fracture. **A:** Sagittal TR 500 TE 20. The fracture line is well depicted on this T1-weighted sequence and can be seen to extend into the posterior facet of the subtalar joint (*arrowheads*). **B:** Sagittal TR 500 TE 20. On this section through the most lateral aspect of the subtalar joint, the degree of comminution of the fracture is well demonstrated.

MRI may be useful in the detection of such injuries (Fig. 4.10). Additionally, such injuries may be encountered unexpectedly when performing examinations for unexplained pain and disability.

The talus is second only to the calcaneus as a site of fracture of the tarsal bones (47). It has unique anatomic characteristics including no muscular or tendinous attachments and a tenuous blood supply that increases its susceptibility to posttraumatic osteonecrosis (44). Avulsion fractures predominate and most are produced by a twisting or rotational force combined with flexion or extension stresses and are seen along the superior surface of the neck and lateral, medial, and posterior surfaces of the body (44).

The neck of the talus is particularly prone to fracture, and is the most common site of fracture second only to avulsion injuries of the talus (44). Fractures of the neck usually occur as the result of dorsiflexion of the foot in which the anterior margin of the tibia acts as a wedge on the neck of the talus (44,47). Continued dorsiflexion can cause subtalar dislocation or even extrusion of the body of the talus posteriorly. Talar neck fractures can be classified into three types. The classification scheme has implications for management and

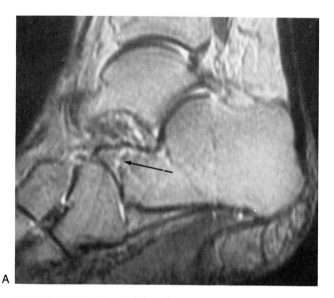

A

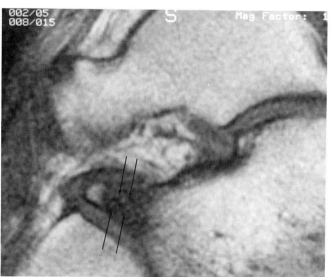

B

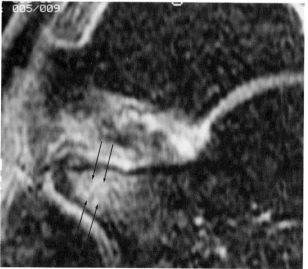

C

FIG. 4.10. Anterior process fracture. **A:** Sagittal TR 2000 TE 80. The patient experienced pain following a twisting injury and fall. Conventional radiographs were normal. A line of high signal intensity is seen crossing the anterior process of the calcaneus consistent with a nondisplaced fracture (*long arrow*). **B:** Sagittal TR 500 TE 20. A striking low signal intensity stripe is seen extending across the anterior process of the calcaneus in a different patient (*arrows*). The patient was referred for foot pain and the diagnosis was clinically unsuspected. **C:** Sagittal TR 2200 TE 35 TI 160. On the STIR sequence, extensive high signal intensity presumably representing edema is seen in the region of the previous low signal intensity stripe (*arrows*).

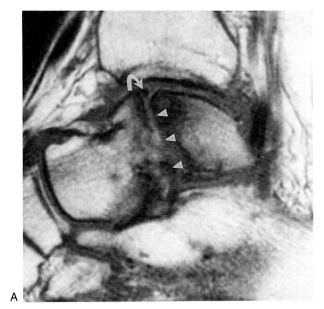

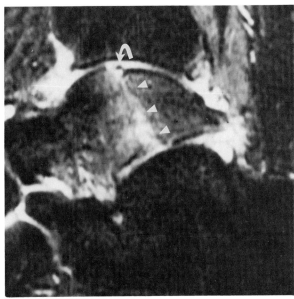

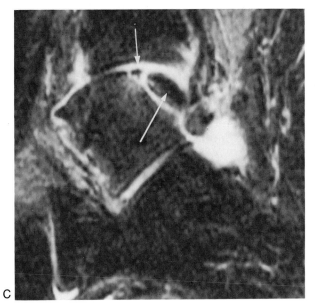

FIG. 4.11. Talar body fracture with articular extension. **A:** Sagittal TR 300 TE 15. A complete comminuted fracture is seen extending vertically through the body of the talus. The fracture extends into both talocrural as well as the posterior facet of the subtalar joint. A small circular low signal intensity osteochondral fragment is seen at the level of the talar dome (*curved arrow*). **B:** Sagittal STIR TR 2200 TE 35 TI 160. On this sequence fluid within the fracture line is well demonstrated and the degree of displacement and incongruity of the posterior facet is well appreciated (*arrowheads*). The loose osteochondral fragment is seen entirely surrounded by joint fluid (*curved arrow*). **C:** Sagittal STIR TR 2200 TE 35 TI 160. On a contiguous section the degree of comminution of the talar dome is well demonstrated. There are two large osteochondral fragments (*arrows*).

for the likelihood of complications. Type 1 are vertical nondisplaced neck fractures, Type 2 are vertical neck fractures with subtalar dislocation, and Type 3 are vertical neck fractures with complete dislocation of the body (47). Osteonecrosis of the body is considered invariable with Type 3 fractures (see Osteonecrosis).

Fractures of the body of the talus are uncommon and may involve the posterior or lateral processes, the articular surface, or all regions in cases of comminution (44). MRI is particularly useful for detection and assessment of congruity of the articular surfaces (e.g., talar dome and posterior facet) (Fig. 4.11). Osteo-

chondral fractures of the talar dome are particularly common and important injuries and are discussed in detail elsewhere in this text (see chapter by Deutsch on Osteochondral Injuries of the Talar Dome).

Metatarsal Bones and Phalanges

Fractures of the metatarsal bones and phalanges are common injuries and usually create few diagnostic problems. Metatarsal fractures may result from a direct blow, chronic stress (see previous discussion), or as a consequence of neuroarthropathy (Fig. 4.12) (44). Fractures of the shaft and metatarsal neck commonly occur as a result of a direct blow. Fractures of the base of the fifth metatarsal have received considerable attention and are of two types: (a) an avulsion injury of the tuberosity, and (b) transverse fracture of the base (Jones fracture). This latter injury is associated with a high incidence of delayed or nonunion (47).

"Turf toe" represents a sprain of the plantar capsule-ligament complex of the great toe metatarsophalangeal (MP) joint. It is most commonly encountered among athletes, particularly football players, playing on artificial surfaces (65,66). The injury is believed to be most commonly produced by forced hyperextension of the MP joint and is contributed to by the use of overly flexible shoes on unforgiving surfaces (65). The injury ranges in severity from stretching of the capsuloligamentous complex to a complete tear of the complex. It has been suggested that with severe Grade 3 injuries, in addition to tearing of the capsuloligamentous complex, there is a compression injury to the articular cartilage and underlying bone of the metatarsal head (65). Clinically, marked point tenderness is noted on the plantar surface especially over the metatarsal head with accompanying soft tissue swelling and ecchymosis. The injury can result in significant functional disability depending on the grade. Athletes may miss 3 to 6 weeks with this injury. Pushoff in particular, which is critically important in football, is markedly impaired.

Conventional x-rays have most commonly demonstrated only generalized soft tissue swelling without evidence of fracture. In some cases, small flecks of bone about the MP joint, possibly representing capsuloligamentous avulsions or osteochondral fragments, have been identified (65). We have had experience with one case of "turf-toe" in a professional football player. On MRI, slight flattening of the articular cartilage overlying the first metatarsal head was evident, accompanied by striking signal alterations with the subchondral and cancellous bone of the metatarsal head most consistent with a "bruise" from direct impaction (Fig. 4.13). The findings corroborate the previously mentioned suspicion that in severe injuries, findings are not limited to the ligamentous complex itself, but extend to include articular cartilage and bone. MRI may be of value in staging and thus assisting in establishing a prognosis in these injuries, as well as in studying their natural history.

Sesamoids

The hallucal sesamoids serve as points of insertion for the flexor hallucis brevis, medial and lateral ses-

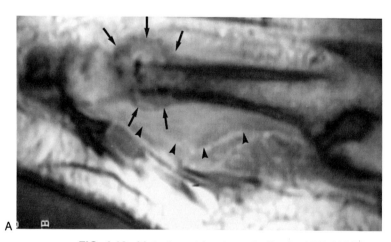
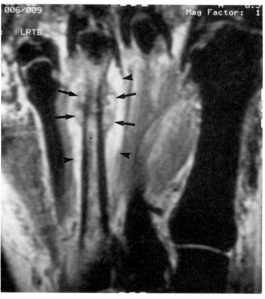

A   B

FIG. 4.12. Metartarsal fracture. **A:** Sagittal TR 300 TE 15. A 50-year-old woman was referred for MRI with the complaint of a 4-month history of ankle and foot pain. There was no history of trauma. A subacute fracture (likely stress related) is depicted with extensive surrounding callous (*arrows*). Extensive soft tissue changes are noted particularly along the plantar aspect of the metatarsal (*arrowheads*). **B:** Coronal STIR TR 2200 TE 35 TI 160. The fracture with reactive edema and bridging callous is again noted (*arrows*). There are extensive signal change in the surrounding soft tissue (*arrowheads*).

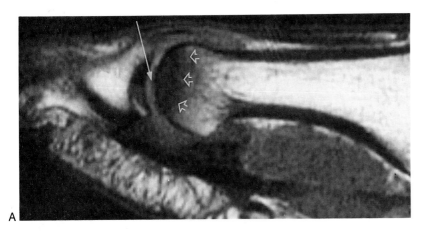

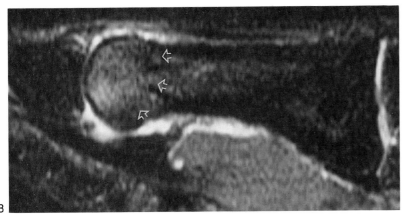

FIG. 4.13. Turf toe. **A:** Sagittal TR 300 TE 15. Professional football player with clinical findings of "turf toe." There is striking decreased signal within the subchondral bone of the first metatarsal head demonstrating an intraosseous contusional component to the injury in addition to the soft tissue changes (*open arrows*). There is subtle flattening of the articular cartilage (*long arrow*). **B:** Sagittal STIR TR 2200 TE 35 TI 160. The area of abnormal signal increases in intensity and is consistent with edema within the subchondral and cancellous bone (*open arrows*). There is a slightly increased amount of joint fluid.

amoid ligaments, and intersesamoid ligaments. There are limited insertions by the adductor hallucis, abductor hallucis, and the fibrous sheath of the flexor hallucis brevis (67,68). Acting as a pulley for the muscle tendon units, they function to increase the power of metatarsal–phalangeal flexion. The sesamoids elevate and protect the metatarsal head and flexor longus tendon. During normal gait, the position of the sesamoids changes. In flexion, the sesamoid lies near the head/ neck metatarsal junction; with extension of the hallux, it is drawn 1 cm distally and tilted dorsally (67). During normal gait, the sesamoids are loaded to three times body weight, with the medial sesamoid transmitting the majority of the force (67,68).

Pain and tenderness over the sesamoids may be associated with one of a number of conditions including fractures, degenerative arthritis in association with hallux valgus, osteochondritis, infection, and parasesamoid lesions including bursitis, conjoined tendon pathology, and sensory neuritis (67). Fractures of the sesamoids are uncommon, generally result from significant trauma, and must be differentiated from partite sesamoids. Acute fractures are associated clinically with significant pain and tenderness, and radi-

ographically with sharp fragmented edges, although the roentgen changes may not be evident initially (67). Partite sesamoids typically demonstrate smooth edges and are enlarged. Sesamoid partition (bipartite, tripartite, or quadripartite) may be seen in 7% to 34% of patients (68). Partite sesamoids may be bilateral in up to 85% of cases and the tibial sesamoid is 10 times more commonly involved than the fibular (68).

Osteochondritis of a sesamoid is a poorly defined pathoanatomic entity that has an inconstant relation to prior injury. The lesion is considered to represent osteonecrosis by many authorities, although histological verification is lacking in many cases. Females are more commonly affected and typically are in the second and third decades of life (68). Both sesamoids are involved with equal frequency. The diagnosis may be initially radiographically occult, with mixed resorptive and sclerotic changes seen later in the condition in association with flattening, elongation, and fragmentation that may mimic fracture (68). Preradiographic diagnosis has frequently been accomplished with scintigraphic methods (68). On MRI, bony sclerosis is manifest as peripheral decreased signal intensity on all pulse sequences and as a consequence, the affected sesamoid may appear "smaller" (Fig. 4.14). Localized increased signal intensity on heavily T2-weighted spin-echo images may be seen (Fig. 4.14). In addition to changes within the sesamoids, associated abnormalities of soft tissue may be seen and exclusion of metatarsal and articular lesions can be accomplished (Fig. 4.15). We have also encountered one case of osteochondritis involving a bipartite tibial sesamoid in which MRI was helpful in establishing the diagnosis (Fig. 4.16). While conservative methods of treatment are often unsuccessful, necessitating surgical extirpation of the affected sesamoid, we have not had the opportunity to obtain pathological correlation of the MRI findings in any of the cases that we have studied to date. As such, the precise diagnosis in these cases remains uncertain, although it is clear that MRI can be useful in precisely detecting the pathoanatomic abnormalities affecting this region.

Growth Plate Fractures

The distal tibia is a common site of growth plate injuries. Salter-Harris type II fractures are the most frequently observed followed by types III, IV, and I injuries (44). Growth disturbances are seen in 10% to 12% of all tibial growth plate injuries (44). The triplane fracture, which accounts for up to 10% of all injuries in this location, has received considerable attention

(44). This injury is classically seen in adolescents around the time of physeal closure. The fracture has transverse, coronal, and sagittal components and represents a variant of a Salter-Harris type IV injury (44). Given the complexity of these fractures, additional imaging is often performed for their complete characterization. This is most commonly accomplished with computed tomography (CT) and to date no reports on the use of MRI in triplane fractures have appeared, although it certainly could be reasonably used.

MRI can be of value in the detection, staging, and assessment of complications of fractures involving the growth plate (21). The normal growth plate on MRI is seen as a relatively high signal intensity band on long TR/TE or T2*-weighted gradient echo pulse sequences (Fig. 4.17). Areas of interruption of the growth plate are manifest as zones of decreased signal intensity within the otherwise bright epiphyseal cartilage on T2- and T2*-weighted sequences (21) (Fig. 4.17). The path of involvement of the injury within the growth plate can be characterized by MRI and may have prognostic significance (21). In a preliminary study, vertical fractures involving the endplate were associated with subsequent growth abnormalities, whereas horizontal fractures were not (65).

The enhanced depiction of the adjacent metaphyseal and epiphyseal components of the growth plate injury using MRI can allow more accurate staging of the fracture than that afforded by conventional radiographic

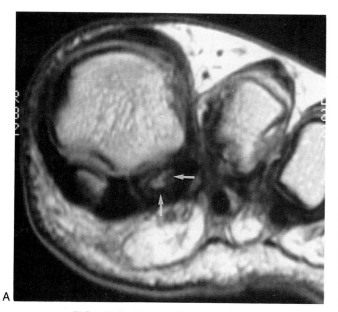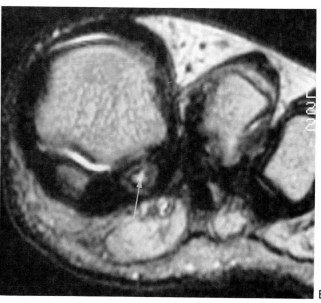

FIG. 4.14. Sesamoid osteochondritis. A: Axial TR 2000 TE 20. The fibular sesamoid appears "smaller" as a consequence of a peripheral rim of low signal intensity presumably relating to bony sclerosis (*arrows*). **B:** Axial TR 2000 TE 80. The central component of the fibular sesamoid demonstrates striking increased signal intensity (*long arrow*). The patient, a 20-year-old female student, had no history of antecedent trauma and a 2-year history of pain localized in the region of the fibular sesamoid. No histological correlation is available.

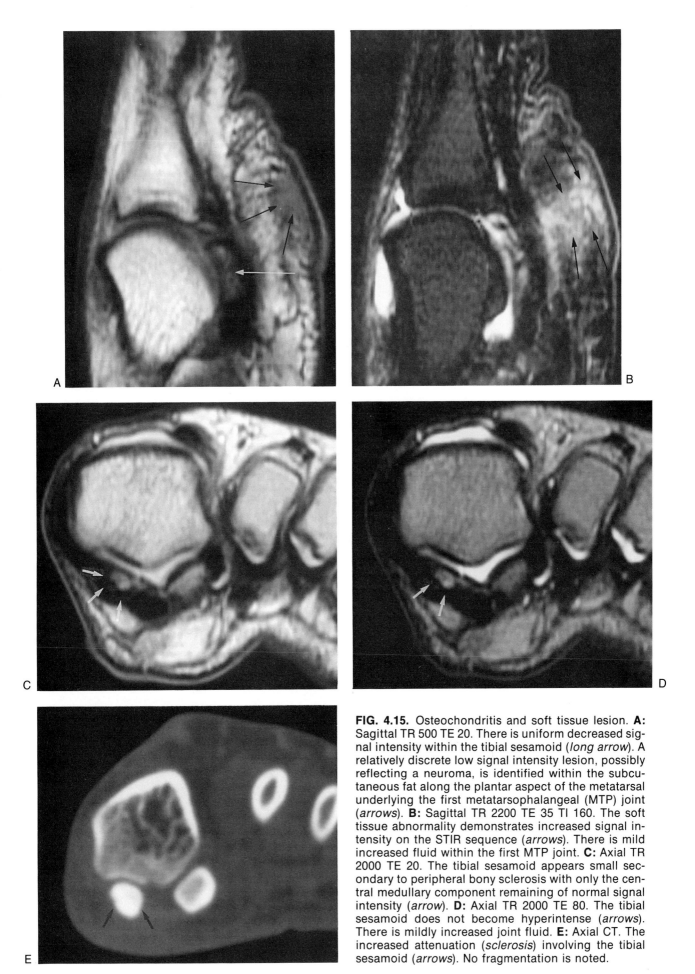

FIG. 4.15. Osteochondritis and soft tissue lesion. **A:** Sagittal TR 500 TE 20. There is uniform decreased signal intensity within the tibial sesamoid (*long arrow*). A relatively discrete low signal intensity lesion, possibly reflecting a neuroma, is identified within the subcutaneous fat along the plantar aspect of the metatarsal underlying the first metatarsophalangeal (MTP) joint (*arrows*). **B:** Sagittal TR 2200 TE 35 TI 160. The soft tissue abnormality demonstrates increased signal intensity on the STIR sequence (*arrows*). There is mild increased fluid within the first MTP joint. **C:** Axial TR 2000 TE 20. The tibial sesamoid appears small secondary to peripheral bony sclerosis with only the central medullary component remaining of normal signal intensity (*arrow*). **D:** Axial TR 2000 TE 80. The tibial sesamoid does not become hyperintense (*arrows*). There is mildly increased joint fluid. **E:** Axial CT. The increased attenuation (*sclerosis*) involving the tibial sesamoid (*arrows*). No fragmentation is noted.

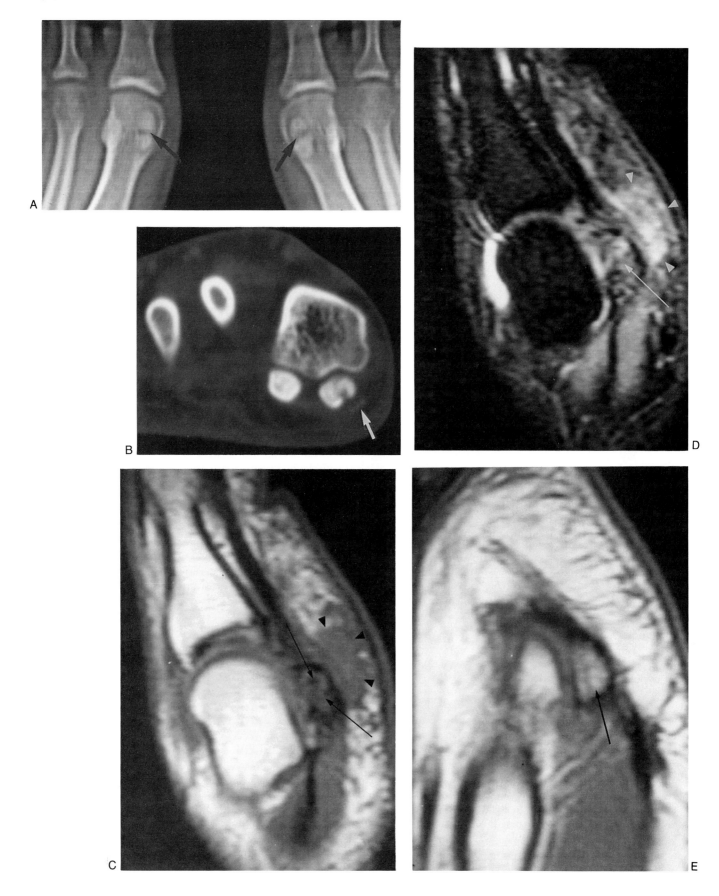

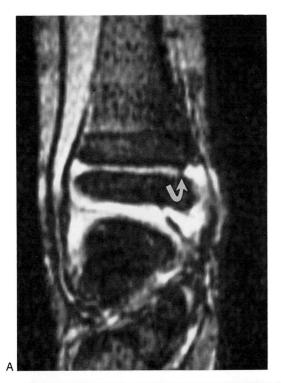

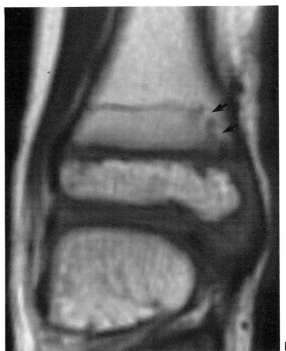

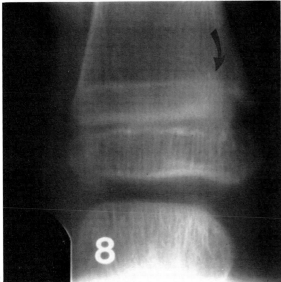

FIG. 4.17. Growth plate injury. **A:** Coronal gradient echo/10 TR 100 TE 25. A 5-year-old girl sustained a Salter IV fracture of the distal tibia. This scan was performed 15 months after the initial injury. There is focal interruption of the medial growth plate manifested by a low signal intensity focus (*arrow*). At surgery, a fibrous bridge was found in the region of interruption. **B:** Coronal TR 500 TE 20. There is focal curving of a growth recovery line medially (*arrows*). More lateral growth recovery line is not affected. **C:** Anteroposterior tomogram obtained near to the time of the MRI examination. The localized curving of the growth recovery line is less apparent than on the MRI (*arrow*). The fibrous bridge is not detectable. (Courtesy of Diego Jaramillo, M.D. Boston, MA.) (From Jaramillo et al., ref. 21, with permission).

FIG. 4.16. Presumed osteochondritis of a bipartite tibial sesamoid. **A:** Digitized image. An AP "scout" image from a CT examination demonstrates bipartite tibial sesamoids bilaterally (*arrows*). **B:** CT scan. Axial section through the right first metatarsal–phalangeal joint demonstrates a mildly fragmented bipartite sesamoid with a small osseous fragment displaced medially within the soft tissues. **C:** Sagittal TR 500 TE 20. High resolution MRI examination demonstrating abnormally decreased signal intensity throughout the tibial sesamoid (*arrow*). An area of abnormally decreased signal is seen within the subcutaneous fat along the volar aspect of the sesamoid (*arrowheads*). **D:** Sagittal TR 2200 TE 35 TI 160. On the STIR sequence, there is again striking increased signal intensity within the abnormal tibial sesamoid (*arrow*). Additionally the soft tissue focus demonstrates high signal on this sequence (*arrowheads*). **E:** Sagittal TR 500 TE 20. The fibular sesmoid (*arrow*) demonstrates normal signal intensity.

analysis (Fig. 4.18). MRI has been particularly valuable in distinguishing between Salter-Harris II and IV injuries when the distal epiphysis has been nonossified and in detecting metaphyseal extension of apparent Salter-Harris III fractures (21). Growth plate fractures may be central or peripheral, with shortening more associated with central fractures, and angular deformity with peripheral lesions (21).

Growth plate injuries may result in the development of a fibrous or osseous bridge across the growth plate with subsequent deformity and or bony shortening. MRI has the potential to depict fibrous bridges that by their nature (i.e., fibrous) are not demonstrable on conventional x-rays or tomography. Osseous bridges crossing the growth plate may demonstrate high signal

related to marrow fat on T1-weighted sequences (21). Small osseous bridges may be difficult to differentiate from fibrous bridges as both may demonstrate low signal intensity. Both fibrous and osseous bridges may require resection, although the physeal cartilage may be able to compensate for small bridges without the development of significant shortening or deformity.

Growth recovery lines are depicted on MRI as low signal intensity linear structures contrasted against high signal intensity marrow (21). Abnormalities of growth recovery lines, ranging from tilting and curving to complete absence, have been described on MRI (21). Extension of physeal cartilage into the metaphysis can also be seen on MRI, and apparently does not cause growth abnormality (21).

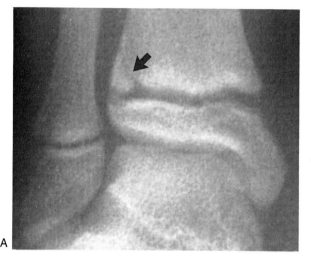

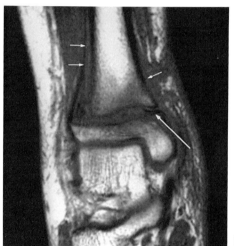

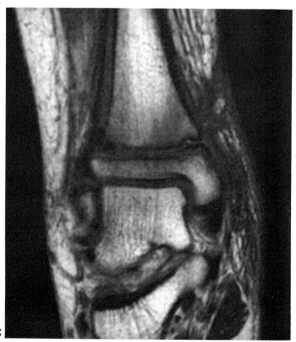

FIG. 4.18. Growth plate injury. A: Anteroposterior radiograph. An 11-year-old girl had what appeared to represent a nondisplaced Salter II fracture of the distal tibia. The radiograph was obtained at the time of reduction. B: Coronal TR 500 TE 20. The MRI study was obtained 2 weeks following the injury. The fracture line extends horizontally to the medial aspect of the physis (*long arrow*). There is persistent physeal widening and evidence of marked periosteal elevation (*arrows*). Decreased signal consistent with marrow edema is seen within the distal tibial metaphysis. C: Coronal TR 500 TE 20. The extent of the fracture line, widening of the physis, and periosteal reaction are well demonstrated. The patient went on to develop a bony bridge.(Courtesy of Diego Jaramillo, M.D. Boston, MA.)

Fracture Complications

MRI may potentially be used in the assessment of fracture complications, although its role in this setting has not been clearly established. The most common indication for MRI in assessment of fracture complications has been in the determination of the presence of osteonecrosis in fractures associated with a high risk for its development (see Talar Fractures). The use of MRI for the detection of osteonecrosis is well established (15,20,39,69,70). Another potential indication for MRI is in the detection of pseudoarthrosis. In patients with delayed fracture healing and nonunion, it is useful for patient management to make a distinction between a fibrous and synovial nonunion (pseudoarthrosis). In cases in which it can be established that a pseudoarthrosis has developed, further conservative management is unlikely to be of value and this synovial-like membrane must be resected to allow union to occur. In a preliminary study, Pathria and colleagues reported on the use of MRI for differentiation of synovial from fibrous nonunion (61). Using T1- and T2-weighted spin-echo sequences, the presence of high signal intensity at the fracture site on long T2-weighted sequences reflected evidence of a pseudoarthrosis (Fig. 4.19). Longer-term studies will be required to substantiate the value of this innovative use of MRI.

MRI may also be used for the assessment of chondral injuries associated with fractures as well as in the detection of degenerative arthritis following intraarticular fractures. Injuries to the growth plate with early epiphyseal closure can be detected (see Growth Plate Injuries). The effect of ankle fractures on surrounding ligaments can be directly evaluated using MRI (see chapter by Mink on Ligaments of the Ankle). In the foot and ankle, fractures may result in injury and entrapment of tendons. In particular, calcaneal fractures are associated with a high incidence of entrapment of the lateral (peroneal) tendons between the widened calcaneus and lateral malleolus. This common complication can be directly evaluated with MRI (see chapter by Mink on Tendons).

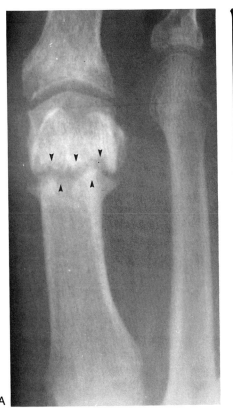 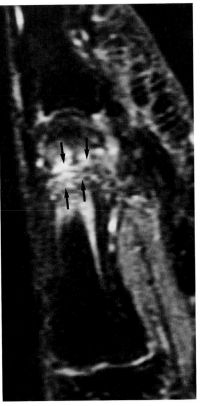

A   B

FIG. 4.19. Pseudoarthrosis. **A:** AP radiograph demonstrating nonunion of a transverse fracture through the distal metaphysis of the first toe. The fracture line remains evident and there is slight bony sclerosis on both sides of the fracture (*arrowheads*). The orthopedist was concerned about the viability of the metatarsal head as well as the possibility of a pseudoarthrosis. **B:** Sagittal STIR TR 2200 TE 35 TI 160. Marked increased band-like signal intensity is seen at the fracture site; MRI findings suggestive of pseudoarthrosis formation (*arrows*). Additionally, there is no evidence of osteonecrosis of the first metatarsal head.

Neuroarthropathy

Neuroarthropathy involving the foot today is most commonly seen as a complication secondary to diabetes mellitus (71). Repetitive microtrauma and macrotrauma in the setting of diminished pain and proprioceptive sensation are considered the principal pathogenetic mechanisms (44,71). Diabetic neuroarthropathy is most commonly seen in the setting of long-standing disease with patients typically in the fifth to seventh decades (44). Pain is often a presenting feature, but is typically less marked than the degree of involvement would suggest. The joints of the forefoot and midfoot are most commonly involved.

At the tarsometatarsal articulation, osseous fragmentation, subluxation, and sclerosis are characteristic findings and complete disintegration of one or more tarsal bones may occur (44, 71–73). Dorsolateral displacement of the metatarsals in relation to the cuneiforms and cuboid may simulate the findings of a traumatic Lisfranc fracture-dislocation (44). Osseous resorption involving the metatarsals is frequent and

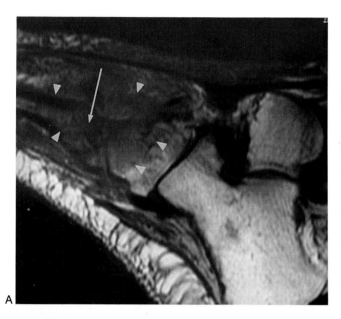

A

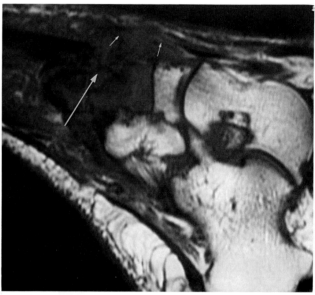

B

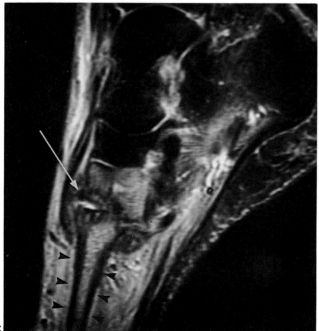

C

FIG. 4.20 Diabetic neuroarthropathy. **A:** Sagittal TR 500 TE 20. A 55-year-old man with a long history of diabetes mellitus presenting with increasing midfoot deformity. On this sagittal section through the lateral aspect of the midfoot, abnormal signal is seen within the cuboid and metatarsal bases (*arrowheads*). Fragmentation consistent with fracture comminution is seen involving the fourth metatarsal base (*long arrow*). The talus and calcaneus are normal. **B:** Sagittal TR 500 TE 20. On a more medial section, extensive deformity and decreased signal intensity is seen within the cuneiforms and metatarsal bases and there is fragmentation at the tarsometatarsal joint (*arrow*). Callous formation displaces an overlying extensor tendon (*small arrows*). The navicular as well as the talus and calcaneus demonstrate normal signal intensity. **C:** Sagittal STIR TR 2200 TE 35 TI 160. There is diffuse increased signal intensity confined principally to the medullary bone of the cuneiforms and metatarsals. Note in particular that the cortex of the metatarsal can be well visualized and is intact and without signal change (*arrowheads*). Deformity at the tarsometatarsal joint space is characteristic of diabetic neuroarthropathy (*arrow*). The signal changes were considered most likely on the basis of neuroarthropathy and the patient received no antibiotic therapy. Fourteen-month clinical follow-up on this patient has revealed no evidence of the development of osteomyelitis.

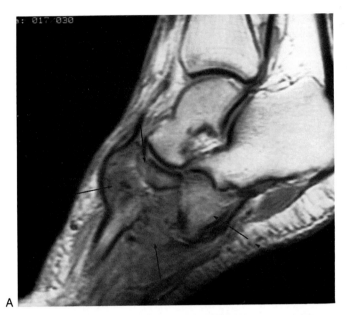

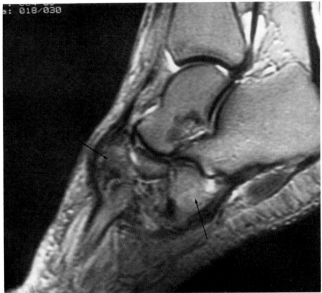

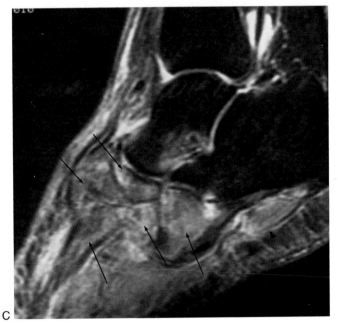

FIG. 4.21. Diabetic neuroarthropathy. **A:** Sagittal TR 2000 TE 20. A 62-year-old woman with long-standing diabetes mellitus and evidence of early cellulitis. There is abnormally decreased signal intensity within the navicular and throughout the cuneiforms and tarsometatarsal articulations (*arrows*). The deformity and distribution are characteristic of diabetic neuroarthropathy. **B:** Sagittal TR 2000 TE 80. The signal changes minimally increase in signal intensity on the T2-weighted image (*arrows*). This lack of significant increase in intensity on this sequence has been suggested as representing a differential feature in distinguishing between changes of osteomyelitis and those on the basis of trauma. **C:** Sagittal STIR TR 2200 TE 35 TI 160. There is markedly increased signal intensity throughout the midfoot depicted on the STIR sequence (*arrows*). The patient was treated with a short course of antibiotics for cellulitis. On clinical follow-up, there has been no evidence of the development of superimposed osteomyelitis.

may lead to complete resorption of a metatarsal head and proximal phalanx. Kraft et al. have classified the changes in diabetic neuroarthropathy as either predominantly destructive (occurring mainly in the tarsal bones and ankle) or resorptive (observed chiefly in the forefoot) (73). Cofield et al. classified the changes of pedal neuroarthropathy into three basic patterns of osteoarticular destruction (72). The most common type occurred at the level of the phalanges and metatarsophalangeal joints and consisted of resorptive changes seen in association with cutaneous ulceration and superimposed infection. The second major pattern occurred at the tarsometatarsal joints and simulated

Lisfranc fracture-dislocations. The third pattern included osseous changes in the navicular, cuneiforms, and head or neck of the talus.

As the diagnosis of neuroarthropathy is readily accomplished on conventional radiographs, the role of the more sophisticated imaging tests, including MRI, is most commonly reserved for evaluation of concurrent complications such as infection. In our experience, extensive signal changes are present within the affected articulations, even in the absence of associated complications such as infection (Figs. 4.20 and 4.21). These changes are most characteristically manifest as marked decrease signal within the medullary and cancellous bone on T1-weighted sequences, with little or relatively mild increases in signal on T2-weighted sequences, and marked increased signal on STIR sequences. The degree of bony fragmentation and articular disruption is generally well characterized by the tomographic and multiplanar capability of MRI.

The differentiation of neuropathic from associated suppurative changes may be difficult, but is best accomplished in our experience by an analysis of associated soft tissue, periosteal, and cortical bone changes. Infection of bone in the diabetic foot most commonly represents the culmination of events resulting from a progression of involvement from the soft tissues to the periosteum (suppurative periostitis) and subsequently the bony cortex (infective osteitis) until the process extends finally to the marrow cavity with the development of osteomyelitis (see chapter by Deutsch on Bone and Soft Tissue Infection). As such, marrow signal changes alone (particularly on STIR sequences), in the absence of definite involvement of the periosteum and cortex, are not necessarily indicative of concurrent osteomyelitis in the setting of neuroarthropathy. Such changes may be seen in neuropathic disease itself, presumably reflecting a manifestation of stress response and microtrauma.

OSTEONECROSIS

Osteonecrosis may develop spontaneously (i.e., idiopathic) or secondary to a number of predisposing factors including trauma, medications (corticosteroids), and marrow infiltrative processes. The hallmark of uncomplicated infarction of medullary bone on MRI is the appearance of the reactive interface (13). This entity represents a distinctive layer of inflammatory fibromesenchymal tissue that develops at the margin between viable and infarcted medullary bone in osteonecrosis (13,74). On MRI, the reactive interface is demonstrated as a well-defined low signal intensity line or arc demarcating the margin of the necrotic segment from viable bone on T1-weighted sequences (13). This line represents replacement of fat by granulation tissue (69). On long T2-weighted sequences, the arc or line demonstrates a bilaminar appearance characterized by an inner margin of increased signal intensity surrounded by an outer border of low signal intensity; a finding termed the "double-line" sign by Mitchell and Kressel (13) (Fig. 4.22). The physical basis for the "double-line" sign has been a subject of some controversy. Mitchell originally ascribed its presence to the combination of granulation tissue (high signal intensity inner margin) and mineralization (low signal intensity outer margin) (13).

Ehman et al. have explained its physical basis on the presence of chemical shift artifact with the high signal intensity component (water image of reactive interface) displaced relative to the low intensity component (fat component of the reactive interface) (69). Whatever its physical basis, the "double-line" sign, when present, should increase the confidence with which osteonecrosis can be diagnosed. A classic "double-line" may, however, not always be present in cases of osteonecrosis.

An MRI staging system for osteonecrosis based on changes in the signal intensity of the osteonecrotic segment has been proposed (13). Described for lesions of the femoral head, the system can potentially be adapted to lesions of the talar dome. While a simplified representation of the pathophysiological events that actually occur, this classification system can assist in understanding the pathologic alterations occurring in the necrotic segment. In MRI class A, the osteonecrotic segment demonstrates signal characteristics similar to fat; high signal on T1-weighted sequences and intermediate signal on T2-weighted images (Fig. 4.23). Class B segments reflect subacute hemorrhage with characteristics of blood: increased signal on both T1- and T2-weighted sequences. As increasing fluid develops within the necrotic segment, a characteristic pattern of decreased signal on T1-weighted and increased signal on T2-weighted images is seen (Class C) (Fig. 4.23). During the later stages of the disease, fibrosis and sclerosis predominate, and the osteonecrotic segment demonstrates decreased signal intensity on both T1- and T2-weighted sequences.

Tarsal Bones

Talus

The talus is unique among the tarsal bones having no muscular or tendinous attachment. As more than 70% of the surface of the bone is covered with articular cartilage, most fractures involving the talus become intraarticular. Since all of the articulations of the talus are weightbearing (62,75), precise anatomic reduction is required to prevent degenerative arthritis. Osteonecrosis develops as a complication of fractures through the talar neck with a varying incidence ranging from a minority of cases in which the fracture is nondisplaced to as many as 80% to 100% of cases in which the fracture is displaced and talar dislocation has occurred (74). It is the proximal portion of the bone (body) that is affected with rare exception (74).

The radiographic diagnosis of osteonecrosis of the talus can be difficult, and is often delayed until relative

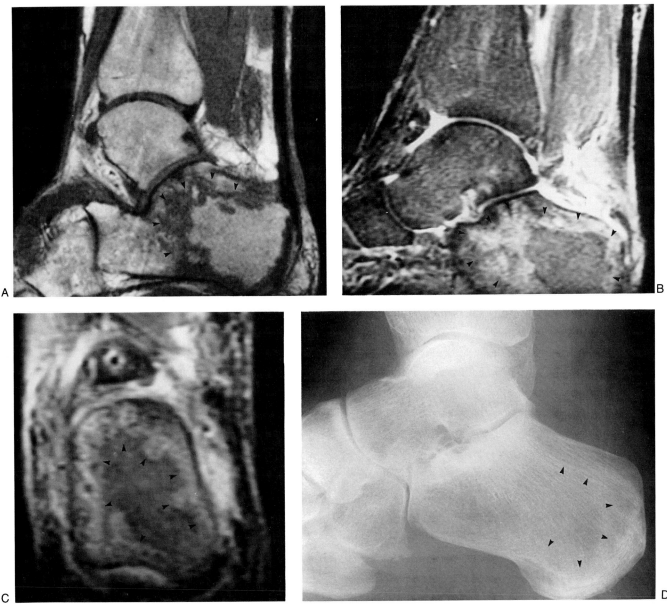

FIG. 4.22. Osteonecrosis. **A:** Sagittal TR 500 TE 20. A 35-year-old patient with Gaucher's disease and multiple bone infarctions. There is a large osteonecrotic segment involving the tuberosity of the calcaneus. A well-defined low signal intensity rim separates the osteonecrotic segment from the remainder of the calcaneus (*arrowheads*). The signal from the osteonecrotic segment is isointense with the remainder of cancellous bone. **B:** Sagittal TR 2000 TE 80. The surrounding rim demonstrates strikingly high signal intensity (*arrowheads*). There is partial demonstration of the classic "double-line" sign. The central segment remains isointense with remaining bone. **C:** Axial TR 2000 TE 80. The large central osteonecrotic segment with surrounding high signal intensity rim (*arrowheads*) is well illustrated in this short axis projection. **D:** Lateral radiograph. There is a subtle peripheral sclerosis correlating with the rim seen on MRI (*arrowheads*). The extent of infarction is difficult to appreciate on the conventional radiographs.

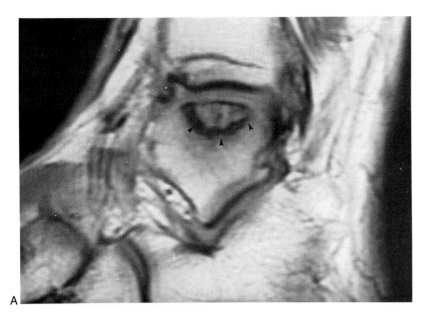

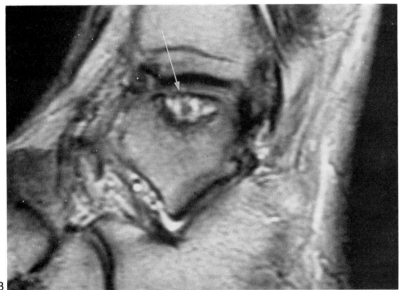

FIGURE 4.23. Talar osteonecrosis. **A:** Sagittal TR 2000 TE 20. A well-defined segment of osteonecrosis is noted within the talar dome (*arrowheads*). The central fragment is of slightly decreased signal intensity compared to the surrounding bone. **B:** Sagittal TR 2000 TE 80. The central fragment becomes hyperintense on this pulse sequence. The findings correlate with MR Class 3 . There is a suggestion of early subarticular collapse (*arrow*).

osteopenia of the surrounding viable bone creates increased density of the talar body (74) (Fig. 4.24). This finding may become apparent within 1 to 3 months following the vascular insult. Generalized osteopenia of the entire talus related to immobilization following injury is a favorable prognostic sign reflecting an adequate blood supply. In a similar manner, Hawkins' sign, characterized by a subchondral radiolucent band in the proximal talus representing subchondral resorption, is also a good prognostic sign reflecting an intact blood supply (74). Revascularization occurs from the medial to the lateral side, emphasizing the importance of the medial blood supply.

MRI can be used both for detection of talar fractures as well as in the assessment of their principal complication (i.e., osteonecrosis). In the acute setting, marrow edema related to the fracture may be present in an extended pattern and does not necessarily imply osteonecrosis. The situation is analogous to fractures of the neck of the femur, where prediction of the viability of the femoral head with MRI may not be possible in the acute setting (58). In the subacute and chronic setting, establishment of the presence or absence of osteonecrosis is readily accomplished with MRI (Fig. 4.25). In addition, the tomographic and multiplanar capability of MRI is valuable in assessment of the talar dome for areas of collapse of the articular surface.

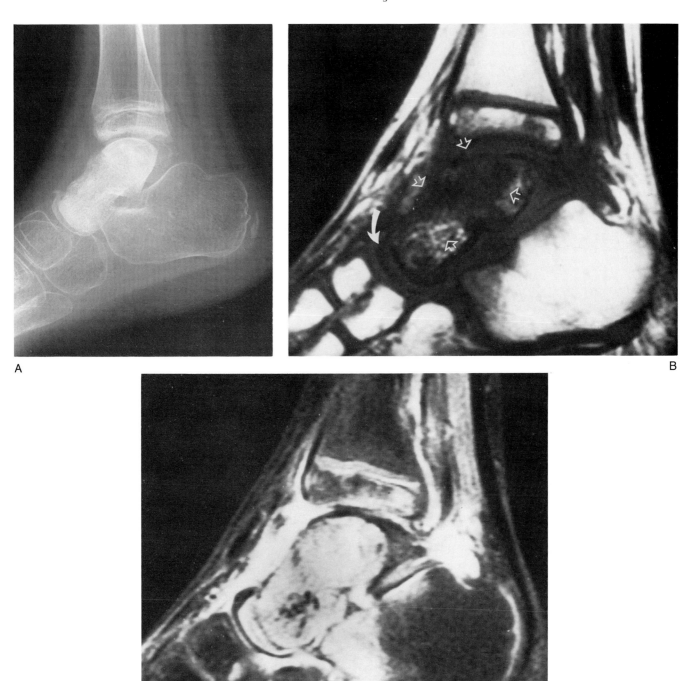

FIG. 4.24. Talar osteonecrosis. **A:** Lateral radiograph demonstrates marked increased density to the talus in comparison to surrounding osseous structures. The patient presented with pain and history of incompletely treated infection. **B:** Sagittal TR 500 TE 15. There is markedly decreased signal intensity within the talus (*open arrows*). The navicular is partially collapsed (*curved arrow*). **C:** Sagittal STIR TR 2200 TE 35 TI 160. There is strikingly increased signal intensity within the talus. Additional signal abnormalities are noted within the anterior aspect of the calcaneus, navicular, and distal tibia epiphysis. There is a large joint effusion; a finding that might contribute to increased intracapsular pressure. Aspiration of the joint revealed no microorganisms. Talar biopsy revealed osteonecrosis.

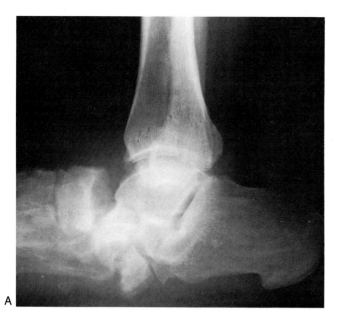

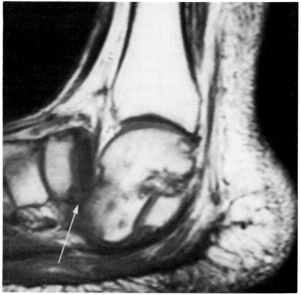

A   B

FIG. 4.25. Exclusion of talar osteonecrosis. **A:** Lateral radiograph demonstrates evidence of a subacute fracture dislocation of the talus. This injury has a high association with the development of osteonecrosis. MRI was obtained before planned surgical reduction to exclude the presence of radiographically occult osteonecrosis. **B:** Sagittal TR 500 TE 20. The talonavicular dislocation is again well demonstrated (*arrows*). There is no evidence of osteonecrosis, the development of which would have changed patient management.

Navicular

Osteonecrosis of the tarsal navicular may be primary or secondary to a number of conditions frequently associated with osteonecrosis including trauma, rheumatoid arthritis, systemic lupus erythematosus, and renal failure (74). Differentiation of primary from secondary osteonecrosis is generally not possible on the basis of imaging characteristics alone, although bilateral distribution, particularly in women, favors the diagnosis of spontaneous disease (76).

Spontaneous osteonecrosis of the tarsal navicular is to be differentiated from the osteochondrosis of the tarsal navicular observed in children (Koehler's disease). Spontaneous osteonecrosis is seen in adults, is most common in women, is symptomatic, and is typically bilateral. Patients with this condition may demonstrate a chronic course with severe pain and disability, and progressive deformity (76). Koehler's disease, in contrast, is seen in children and often is asymptomatic or accompanied by only minor signs and symptoms.

Initial radiographic abnormalities include a loss of volume in the lateral aspect of the tarsal navicular accompanied by increased radiodensity of this segment of the bone (76). As the condition progresses, the navicular assumes a commalike shape because of lateral compression. Eventually, dorsal protusion and fragmentation of the bone may become evident (76). On MRI, the bone demonstrates characteristic decreased signal intensity on short TR/TE sequences (Fig. 4.26). The changes on other pulse sequences have been reported to be more variable and often less obvious, and have most commonly been observed in the lateral, potentially more stressed portion of the bone (76). In our experience, the changes are consistently well demonstrated on STIR sequences. In addition, we have observed striking signal changes with the subchondral and cancellous bone of the talar head and neck in both cases of spontaneous osteonecrosis of the navicular that we have imaged (Fig. 4.26). The precise etiology and significance of the talar signal remains unknown, although it may represent "stress" changes secondary to the altered mechanics across the talonavicular joint. Differential diagnostic considerations include reactive changes secondary to insufficiency fractures, healing of acute traumatic fractures, and stress adaptive sclerosis. A discrepancy between the degree of sclerosis present on radiographs and CT, and the degree of marrow signal changes demonstrated on MRI, favors the diagnosis of spontaneous osteonecrosis (76).

Metatarsals

Osteonecrosis involving the metatarsal heads is most common on an idiopathic basis and referred as Freiberg's infraction, after the investigator who first described a series of patients with metatarsalgia and collapse (hence infraction) of the metatarsal head (74).

The second metatarsal head is most commonly involved, although the third and fourth metatarsal heads may be affected (74). The condition predominates in women (3–4:1) and is most commonly seen in adolescents between the ages of 13 and 18 years (74). Clinical features include pain, swelling, and limitation of motion and the symptoms may be disabling (74). Pathologically, evidence of necrosis may be evident before any radiographic manifestation (74). Collapse of the articular surface may be associated with comminution of subchondral trabeculae (74). Complete healing is not usually seen. It is considered most likely that a single

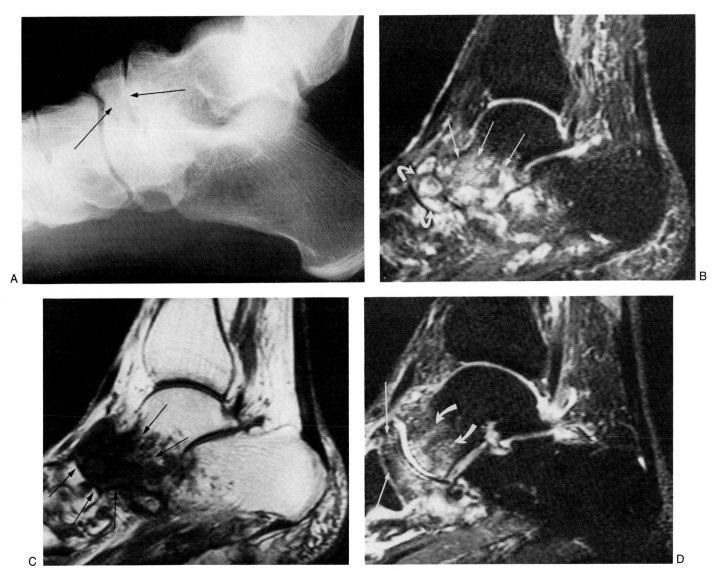

A

B

C

D

FIG. 4.26. Osteonecrosis of the navicular. **A:** Conventional radiograph demonstrates the characteristic loss of volume and dorsal protusion of the navicular; findings consistent with spontaneous osteonecrosis in this 50-year-old woman. **B:** Sagittal STIR TR 2200 TE 35 TI 160. There is striking signal alteration within both the osteonecrotic navicular (*curved arrows*) as well as in the subchondral and cancellous bone of the neighboring talar head and neck (*arrows*). Changes within the talus have not been previously described in this entity and may represent reactive changes secondary to altered stresses across the talonavicular joint. **C:** Sagittal TR 500 TE 35. Sagittal image from another patient with spontaneous osteonecrosis of the navicular demonstrating marked decreased signal intensity within the partially collapsed navicular (*arrows*) as well as characteristic dorsal subluxation. **D:** Sagittal STIR TR 2200 TE 35 TI 160. In addition to the diffuse changes seen within the navicular (*arrows*), this patient also demonstrates signal alteration within the talar head and neck (*curved arrows*).

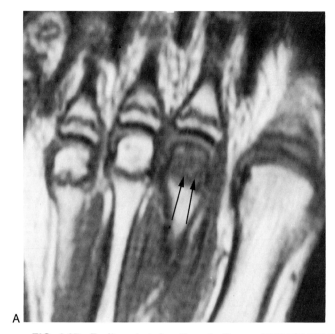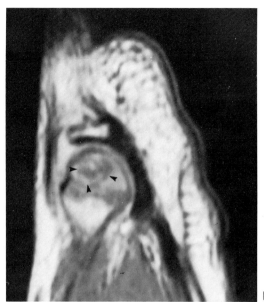

FIG. 4.27. Freiberg's Infraction. **A:** Coronal TR 500 TE 20. A 14-year-old girl presented with metatarsalgia. There is striking low signal intensity within the second metatarsal head (*arrows*). **B:** Sagittal TR 2000 TE 20. A more discrete circular to ovoid focus of osteonecrosis is seen involving the dorsal two-thirds of the metatarsal head (*arrowheads*).

episode or repetitive microtrauma represent the primary pathogenetic event.

The radiographic features are virtually pathognomonic of Freiberg's infraction. Increased density of the metatarsal head is seen in association with variable flattening of the articular surface (74). In the more advanced stages, osteochondral fragments with progressive deformity and enlargement of the metatarsal head may be seen (74). Premature closure of the growth plate may accompany the condition. MRI may be of value in the early setting before the development of the characteristic radiographic features (Fig. 4.27). Additionally, a mild degree of flattening of the articular surface of the metatarsal head (particularly the second) may be encountered as a normal variant (74) and MRI could be used to exclude the diagnosis by demonstrating a normal appearance to the bone marrow.

The differential diagnosis of Freiberg's infraction includes osteonecrosis related to other causes such as systemic lupus erythematosus, which may affect this region (74). Additionally, fragmentation of the metatarsal heads with articular changes may be seen with rheumatoid arthritis, calcium pyrophosphate deposition disease, gout, and diabetes mellitus (74). These entities can usually be distinguished on a clinical basis as well as associated radiographic abnormalities.

TRANSIENT MARROW EDEMA

Transient marrow edema syndrome represents a generic term coined to encompass and account for cases of presumed regional bone marrow edema identified on MRI that have an uncertain relationship to osteonecrosis (77,78). The entity was first described in the hip. Patients present with pain that subsequently resolves with conservative management. On MRI, a regional and typically circumscribed periarticular area of decreased signal intensity is depicted on T1-weighted images that often strikingly increase in intensity on T2-weighted and STIR sequence (Fig. 4.28). Bone scintigraphy typically demonstrates focally augmented activity. Plain radiographs may or may not demonstrate localized osteoporosis. A possible relationship of this entity to the process of transient regional osteoporosis and/or reflex sympathetic dystrophy syndrome has been suggested (77,78).

In the absence of trauma, transient marrow edema represents the principal differential diagnosis to early osteonecrosis in patients presenting with pain and findings of localized "marrow edema" on MRI. The MRI findings typically completely resolve in concert with the patients clinical symptoms. We have encountered one case of apparent regional migratory marrow edema

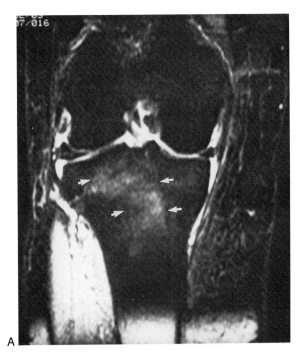

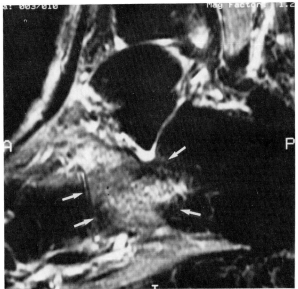

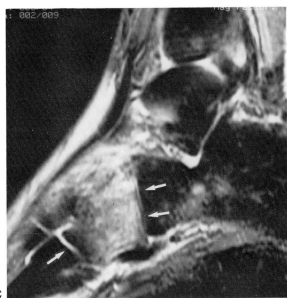

FIG. 4.28. Migratory transient marrow edema. **A:** Coronal "STIR" TR 2200/TE 35/TI 160. A 70-year-old woman presented with pain in the knee. On MRI, a circumscribed area of increased signal intensity was noted within the proximal tibial metaphysis (*arrows*). The patient's symptoms and MRI findings subsequently resolved with conservative management. **B:** Sagittal "STIR" TR 2200/TE 35/TI 160. Approximately one year later, the patient returned with pain in the foot. On MRI, a striking area of signal abnormality manifest as striking increased signal intensity is seen within the calcaneus (*arrows*). The patient's symptoms resolved over the next two months. **C:** Sagittal "STIR" TR 2200/TE 35/TI 160. The patient returned six months later with the onset of recurrent pain in the same foot. On MRI, marked resolution of the findings within the calcaneus is noted. A striking area of increased signal is now noted to have developed within the previously uninvolved cuboid (*arrows*).

involving the lower extremity (Fig. 4.28). Differentiation of transient marrow edema from early osteonecrosis may only be possible by clinical and appropriate imaging follow-up. Conservative management is presently advocated (77).

CONCLUSION

This chapter has reviewed both the current and likely emerging applications for MRI with regard to traumatic osseous abnormalities of the foot and ankle as well as for the detection and staging of osteonecrosis involving the foot. While conventional radiography will continue to serve as the primary and in most instances only imaging examination necessary for assessment of trauma-related abnormalities of the foot and ankle, it is becoming increasingly evident that many potentially important injuries may be initially and in some cases remain forever radiographically occult. It is in this spectrum of musculoskeletal trauma that MRI has had it greatest impact to date. The increasing application of MRI as an investigative method will likely increase our knowledge and understanding of the pathoanatomic mechanisms underlying injuries to the foot and ankle as well as increase our understanding as to their sequelae. This knowledge will undoubtedly affect the approach to management of many of these injuries, although long-term longitudinal studies will be required to learn the natural history of many of the lesions presently depicted by MRI, but previously underappreciated clinically and by other diagnostic methods.

REFERENCES

1. Sebag, GH and Moore, SG, *Effect of trabecular bone on the appearance of marrow in gradient-echo imaging of the appendicular skeleton.* Radiology, 1990. **174**: p. 855–859.
2. Unger, EC and Summers, TB, *Bone marrow.* Top Magn Reson Imaging, 1989. **1**(4): p. 31–52.
3. Vogler, JB and Murphy, WA, *Bone marrow imaging.* Radiology, 1988. **168**: p. 679–693.
4. Porter, BA, Shields, AF, and Olson, DO, *Magnetic resonance imaging of bone marrow disorders.* Radiol Clin North Am, 1986. **24**: p. 269–289.
5. Wismer, GL, Rosen, BR, Buxton, R, et al., *Chemical shift imaging of bone marrow: Preliminary experience.* AJR, 1985. **145**: p. 1031–1037.
6. Dooms, GC, Fisher, MR, Hricak, H, et al., *Bone marrow imaging: Magnetic resonance studies related to age and sex.* Radiology, 1985. **155**: p. 429–432.
7. Lanir, A, Hadar, H, Cohen, I, et al., *Gaucher's disease: Assessment with MR imaging.* Radiology, 1986. **161**: p. 239–244.
8. Sugimura, K, Yamasaki, K, Kitagaki, H, et al., *Bone marrow disease of the spine: Differentiation with T1 and T2 relaxation times in MR imaging.* Radiology, 1987. **165**: p. 541–544.
9. Daffner, RH, Lupetin, AR, Dash, N, et al., *MRI in the detection of malignant infiltration of bone marrow.* AJR, 1986. **146**: p. 353–358.
10. Yao, L and Seeger, LL, *MR effective at detecting pathology of marrow space.* Diagn Imaging, 1991. p. 116.
11. Genez, BM, Wilson, MR, Houk, RW, et al., *Early osteonecrosis of the femoral head: Detection in high-risk patients with MR imaging.* Radiology, 1988. **168**: p. 521–524.
12. Munk, PL, Helms, CA, and Holt, RG, *Immature bone infarcts: Findings on plain radiographs and MR scans.* AJR, 1989. **152**: p. 547–550.
13. Mitchell, DG and Kressel, HY, *MR imaging of early avascular necrosis.* Radiology, 1988. **169**: p. 281–282.
14. Yao, L and Lee, JK, *Occult intraosseous fracture: Detection with MR imaging.* Radiology, 1988. **167**: p. 749–751.
15. Gillespy, TI, Genant, HK, and Helms, CA, *Magnetic resonance imaging of osteonecrosis.* Radiol Clin North Am, 1986. **24**: p. 193.
16. Lynch, TCP, Crues, JV, Morgan, FW, et al., *Bone abnormalities of the knee: Prevelence and significance at MR imaging.* Radiology, 1989. **171**: p. 761–766.
17. Berger, PE, Ofstein, RA, Jackson, DW, et al., *MRI demonstration of radiographically occult fractures: What have we been missing?* Radiographics, 1989. **9**: p. 407.
18. Lee, JK and Yao, L, *Occult intraosseous fracture: detection with MR imaging.* Radiology, 1988. **168**: p. 749–750.
19. Deutsch, AL, Mink, JH, and Waxman, AD, *Occult fractures of the proximal femur: MR imaging.* Radiology, 1989. **170**: p. 113–116.
20. Coleman, BG, Kressel, HY, Dalinka, MK, et al., *Radiographically negative avascular necrosis: Detection with MR imaging.* Radiology, 1988. **168**: p. 525–528.
21. Jaramillo, D, Hoffer, FA, Shapiro, F, et al., *MR imaging of fractures of the growth plate.* AJR, 1990. **155**: p. 1261–1265.
22. Beall, P, *States of water in biological systems.* Cryobiology, 1983. **20**: p. 324–334.
23. Piney, A, *The anatomy of the bone marrow.* Br Med J, 1922. **2**: p. 792–795.
24. Hashimoto, M, *The distribution of active marrow in the bones of normal adult.* Kyushu J Med Sci, 1960. **11**: p. 103–111.
25. Steiner, RM, Mitchell, DG, Rao, VM, et al., *Magnetic resonance imaging of bone marrow: Diagnostic value in diffuse hematologic disorders.* Magn Reson Q, 1990. **6**: p. 17–34.
26. Dunnill, MS, Anderson, JA, and Whitehead, R, *Quantitative histological studies on age changes in bone.* J Pathol Bacteriol, 1967. **94**: p. 275–291.
27. Mitchell, DG, Rao, VM, Dalinka, M, et al., *Hematopoiesis and fatty bone marrow distribution in the normal and ischemic hip: New observations with 1.5T MR imaging.* Radiology, 1986. **161**: p. 199–202.
28. Deutsch, AL, Mink, JH, Rosenfelt, FP, et al., *Incidental detection of hematopoietic hyperplasia on routine knee MR.* AJR, 1989. **152**: p. 333–337.
29. Hajek, PC, Baker, LL, Goobar, JE, et al., *Focal fat deposition in axial bone marrow: MR characteristics.* Radiology, 1987. **162**: p. 245–249.
30. Wehrli, FW, *Fast Scan Magnetic Resonance: Principles and Applications.* 1991, Raven Press: New York. p. 105–109.
31. Haase, A, Frahm, J, Matthaei, D, et al., *FLASH imaging: Rapid NMR imaging using low flip-angle pulses.* J Magn Reson, 1986. **67**: p. 258–266.
32. Haacke, EM and Track, JA, *Fast MR imaging; technique and clinical applications.* AJR, 1990. **155**: p. 951–964.
33. Bydder, GM, Pennock, JM, Steiner, RE, et al., *The short T1 inversion recovery sequence–An approach to MR imaging of the abdomen.* Magn Reson Imaging, 1985. **3**(3): p. 521–254.
34. Bydder, GM and Young, IR, *MR Imaging: Clinical use of the inversion recovery sequence.* J Comput Assist Tomogr, 1985. **9**: p. 659–675.
35. Dixon, WT, *Simple proton spectroscopic imaging.* Radiology, 1984. **153**: p. 189–194.
36. Borrello, JA, Chenevert, TL, and Meyer, CR, *Chemical shift-based true water and fat images: Regional phase correction of modified spin-echo MR images.* Radiology, 1987. **164**: p. 531–537.
37. Szumowwski, J and Plewes, DB, *Separation of lipid and water MR imaging signals by chopper averaging in the time domain.* Radiology, 1987. **1987**(165): p. 274–250.
38. Chan TW, Listerud J, Kressel HY, *Combined chemical-shift and phase selective imaging for fat suppression: Theory and initial clincial experience.* Radiology 1991 **181**: 41–47
39. Ehman, RL, *MR imaging of medullary bone.* Radiology, 1988. **167**: p. 867–868.
40. Mink, JH and Deutsch, AL, *Occult cartilage and bone injuries of the knee: Detection, classification, and assessment with MR imaging.* Radiology, 1989. **170**: p. 823–829.
41. Mink, JH and Deutsch, AL, *MRI of the Musculoskeletal System. A Teaching File*, JH Mink and JH Deutsch, Editors. 1990, Raven Press; New York, p. 251–391.
42. Gomori, JM and Grossman, RI, *Mechanisms responsible for the MR appearance and evolution of intracranial hemorrhage.* Radiographics, 1988. **8**: p. 427–440.
43. Unger, EC, Cohen, MS, and Brown, TR, *Gradient-echo imaging of hemorrhage at 1.5 tesla.* J Magn Reson Imaging, 1989. **7**: p. 163–172.
44. Resnick, D, Goergen, TG, and Niwayama, G, *Physical injury,* in *Diagnosis of Bone and Joint Disorders.*, D. Resnick and G. Niwayama, Editors. 1988, W.B. Saunders: Philadelphia. p. 2756–3009.
45. Stafford, SA, Rosenthal, DI, Gebhardt, MC, et al., *MRI in stress fracture.* AJR, 1986. **147**: p. 553–556.
46. Mink, JH and Rosenfeld, RT, *MR views sports-related bony, muscular injuries.* Diagn Imaging, 1991. Feb: p. 108–114.
47. Rogers, LF, *The foot,* in *Radiology of Skeletal Trauma*, L.F. Rogers, Editor. 1982, Churchill Livingstone: New York. p. 861–920.
48. Greaney, RB, Gerber, FH, and Laughlin, RL, *Distribution and natural history of stress fractures in US Marines.* Radiology, 1983. **146**: p. 339–346.
49. Pavlov, H, Torg, JS, and Freiberger, RH, *Tarsal navicular stress*

fractures: Radiographic evaluation. Radiology, 1983. **148**: p. 641–645.

50. Torg, JS, Pavlov, H, Cooley, LH, *et al.*, *Stress fractures of the tarsal navicular. A retrospective review of twenty-one cases.* J Bone Joint Surg, 1982. **63A**: p. 700–712.

51. Roub, LW, Gummerman, LW, and Hanley, ENJ, *Bone stress: Radionuclide imaging perspective.* Radiology, 1979. p. 132–141.

52. Martin, P, *Basic principles of nuclear medicine techniques for detection and evaluation of trauma and sports medicine injuries.* Semin Nucl Med, 1988. **18**: p. 90–112.

53. Stafford, SA, *MRI in stress fracture.* AJR, 1986. **147**: p. 533–556.

54. Holder, LE, *Clinical radionuclide bone imaging.* Radiology, 1990. **176**: p. 607–614.

55. Rupani, HD, Holder, LE, Espinola, DA, *et al.*, *Three phase radionuclide bone imaging in sports medicine.* Radiology, 1985. **156**: p. 187–196.

56. Lee, JK and Yao, L, *Stress fractures; MR imaging.* Radiology, 1988. **169**: p. 217–220.

57. Deutsch, AD and Mink, JH, *Magnetic resonance imaging of musculoskeletal injuries.* Radiol Clin North Am, 1989. **27**: p. 983–1002.

58. Deutsch, AD, Mink, JH, and Waxman, A, *Occult fractures of the proximal femur: MR imaging.* Radiology, 1989. **170**: p. 113–116.

59. Simon, JH and Szumowski, J, *Chemical shift imaging with paramagnetic contrast material enhancement for improved lesion depiction.* Radiology, 1989. **171**: p. 538–543.

60. Greenfield, GB, Warren, DL, and Clark, RA, *MR imaging of periosteal and cortical changes of bone.* Radiographics, 1991. **11**: p. 611–623.

61. Pathria, M, Wilber, JH, and Yulish, BS, *MR imaging of fracture nonunion,* in *74th Scientific Assembly and Annual Meeting of the Radiological Society of North America.* 1988. Chicago.

62. Rogers, LF, *The ankle,* in *Radiology of Skeletal Trauma,* L.F. Rogers, Editor. 1982, Churchill Livingstone: New York. p. 791–860.

63. Lauge-Hansen, N, *Genetic roentgenologic diagnosis of fractures of the ankle.* Am J Roentgenol, 1954. **71**: p. 456–461.

64. Levy, AS, Berkowitz, R, Corbett, M, *et al.*, *Magnetic resonance imaging evaluation of the calcaneal fat pad in patients with os calcis fractures.* Am Roentgenol Ray Soc, Annual Meeting. 1991.

65. Clanton, TO, Butler, JE, and Eggert, A, *Injuries to the metatarsophalangeal joints in athletes.* Foot Ankle, 1986. **7**(3): p. 162–176.

66. Bowers, KD and Martin, RB, *Turf-toe: A shoe-surface related football injury.* Med Sci Sports Exerc, 1976. **8**(2): p. 81–83.

67. Weiss, JS, *Fracture of the medial sesamoid bone of the great toe: Controversies in therapy.* Orthopedics, 1991. **14**: p. 1003–1007.

68. Jahss, MH, *Disorders of the hallux and the first ray,* in *Disorders of the Foot and Ankle,* MH Jahss, Editor. 1991, W.B. Saunders: Philadelphia. p. 943–1174.

69. Ehman, RL, Berquist, TH, and McLeod, RA, *MR imaging of early vascular necrosis: Reply.* Radiology, 1988. **169**: p. 282–283.

70. Bjorkengren, AG, AlRowaih, A, Lindstrand, A, *et al.*, *Spontaneous osteonecrosis of the knee: Value of MR imaging in determining prognosis.* AJR, 1990. **154**: p. 331–337.

71. Zlatkin, MB, Pathria, M, Sartoris, DJ, *et al.*, *The diabetic foot.* Radiol Clin North Am, 1987. **25**: p. 1095–1105.

72. Cofield, RH, Morrison, MJ, and Beabout, JW, *Diabetic neuroarthropathy in the foot: Patient characteristics and patterns of radiographic change.* Foot Ankle, 1983. **4**: p. 15–22.

73. Kraft, I, Spyropoulos, E, and Finby, N, *Neurogenic disorders of the foot in diabetes mellitus.* AJR, 1975. **124**: p. 17–24.

74. Resnick, D and Niwayama, G, *Osteonecrosis: Diagnostic techniques, specific situations, and complications,* in *Diagnosis of Bone and Joint Disorders,* D Resnick and G Niwayama, Editors. 1988, W.B. Saunders: Philadelphia. p. 3238–3288.

75. Shelton, ML and Pedowitz, WJ, *Injuries to the talar dome, subtalar joint, and mid foot,* in *Disorders of the Foot and Ankle. Medical and Surgical Management.*, MH Jahss, Editor. 1991, W.B. Saunders: Philadelphia. p. 2274–2292.

76. Haller, J, Sartoris, DJ, Resnick, D, *et al.*, *Spontaneous osteonecrosis of the tarsal navicular in adults: Imaging findings.* AJR, 1988. **151**: p. 355.

77. Bloem, JL. *Transient osteoporosis of the hip: MR imaging.* Radiology, 1988. **167**: 753–757.

78. Wilson, AJ, Murphy, WA, and Hardy, DC. *Transient osteoporosis: Transient bone marrow edema?* Radiology, 1988. 167–760.

MRI of the Foot and Ankle,
edited by A.L. Deutsch, J.H. Mink, and R. Kerr,
Raven Press, Ltd., New York © 1992

CHAPTER 5

Osteochondral Injuries of the Talar Dome

Andrew L. Deutsch

Acute and subacute injuries to the articular cartilage and underlying subchondral bone of the talar dome represent common and important injuries for which patients seek medical attention (1–6). Critical to the prognostication and management of these lesions is their accurate detection as well as characterization regarding such features as fragment stability and overlying articular cartilage integrity (2,4,7,8). In this chapter the terminology used to describe these lesions will be reviewed as will the pertinent clinical, biomechanical, pathogenetic, and imaging aspects of these common and important ankle injuries.

Critical to the ability of magnetic resonance imaging (MRI) to detect and characterize osteochondral injuries of the talar dome is the ability of the technique to image both subchondral bone as well as articular cartilage. The basis for imaging bone and marrow, an area at which magnetic resonance has demonstrated considerable strength, is reviewed elsewhere in this text (see chapter by Deutsch on Traumatic Injuries of Bone and Osteonecrosis). To date, the optimal technique for imaging articular cartilage with MRI has remained elusive but remains the subject of active and continuing investigation (9–14). Compounding this difficulty in the talar dome is the thinness of the articular cartilage layer. To provide the interested reader with the requisite background for understanding the currently existing approaches toward articular cartilage depiction and the rationale for future developments in this area, this chapter will also include a review of the salient aspects of the basic composition, organization, and biomechanics of articular cartilage.

ARTICULAR CARTILAGE

Basic Composition, Organization, and Biomechanical Considerations

Articular cartilage consists of cells (e.g., chondrocytes) embedded in an abundant extracellular matrix (15). In contrast to other parenchymal tissues, the cellular component of cartilage contributes relatively little to the total volume (10% or less) (16). The important biomechanical properties of cartilage, including load-bearing, resilience, and durability, depend principally on the chemical nature and complex spatial arrangement of the constituent components of the extracelluar matrix (15–17).

Water constitutes the largest component of the extracellular matrix with tissue fluid accounting for 60% to 80% of the wet weight of cartilage (15–18). This high water content distinguishes articular cartilage from most other connective tissues (15). Approximately 90% of the water is extracellular. The water content of articular cartilage is generally highest next to the articular surface, although its variation in successive layers is not large (15,18). Structural macromolecules including collagens, proteoglycans, and noncollagenous proteins or glycoproteins, comprise 20% to 40% of the weight of cartilage and function to maintain and organize the tissue fluid and impede its flow through the matrix, accounting for the biomechanical properties of cartilage (17,19).

Collagens form the fibrillar meshwork that gives cartilage its tensile strength and form (15–18, 20). Proteoglycans, which form the major macromolecules of cartilage ground substance, bind to the collagen meshwork or become mechanically trapped within it (15,18). The proteoglycans are highly viscous, hydrophillic macromolecules capable of entraining an amount of water 50 times their weight in free solution (17). When

A.L. Deutsch: Tower Musculoskeletal Imaging Center, Los Angeles, California 90048, and Department of Radiology, University of California, San Diego, California.

immobilized as in cartilage by a meshwork of strong collagen fibrils, they can resist very large compressive loads (17). Proteoglycans are composed of a protein core with attached chains of sulfated polysaccharides that radiate out from the core (15,16) (Fig. 5.1). Within the cartilage matrix, the proteoglycans form aggregates that help to immobilize them within the collagen fibrillar meshwork (17). These aggregates are comprised of 100 to 200 proteoglycan monomers attached to a single backbone of hyaluronic acid (15,17). Link proteins stabilize the association between proteoglycan monomers and the hyaluronic acid backbone (15,16).

The physical and chemical properties of the proteoglycans are important to the resiliency of the articular cartilage, the mechanical properties of which are governed by both the composition of the tissue and the movement of interstitial fluid within the tissue (15,17,19). The proteoglycans, which are compressed to only a fraction of their natural aqueous volume by the surrounding meshwork of collagen fibrils, contribute to the turgor of articular cartilage and its ability to resist compressive loads (17). This resistance to compression in large part relates to electrostatic properties of the proteoglycans (15,17). The glycosaminoglycan chains, which comprise up to 95% of the proteoglycan molecules (15), are characterized by a large number of negative charges. As a consequence, they exert an enormous electronegative effect, causing the monomers to remain extended in space and to resist compression into a smaller volume (15,17). With the application of a compressive force, the negatively charged glycosaminoglycan chains are driven closer together (Fig. 5.2). Interstitial fluid is extruded and flows through the interstices of the matrix along the pressure gradient created by the load (19). The compressed negatively charged proteoglycan macromolecules exert a resistive force because of electrostatic charge repulsion, ultimately resulting in a state of equi-

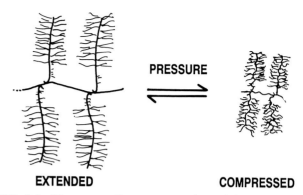

PRESSURE

EXTENDED **COMPRESSED**

FIG. 5.2. Diagrammatic representation of the reversible compressibility of proteoglycan monomers in solution. The negative charges of the glycosaminoglycan chain repel each other, expanding the domain of the proteoglycans. There is decreased charge density and decreased density of chondroitin sulfate chains in the expanded state as depicted on the left. With the application of compression, the negatively charged chains are driven closer together. With release of compression, the molecules are again allowed to expand. In tissue as opposed to in solution, the collagen framework limits the expansion of the proteoglycan monomers. (Adapted from ref. 16.)

librium whereby the matrix-resistive force caused by tissue consolidation balances the applied compressive forces (15,17,19). The movement of fluid through the tissue, which is dependent on the frictional interactions between the fluid and the "branches" of the proteoglycan macromolecules, governs both the rate and absolute amount of deformation (15). With release of the load, the molecules are allowed to expand again (15) (Fig. 5.2).

In tissue, the collagen meshwork limits the expansion of proteoglycans which could, if fully extended, fill a volume many times larger than the tissue that contains them (15). If the collagen fibril meshwork is disrupted, as may occur with chondral injuries, the matrix swells as proteoglycans expand, increasing the concentration of water and decreasing the proteoglycan concentration (15,17). The ability of MRI to detect regional differences in bulk water may form the basis for noninvasive imaging of such structural alterations. In compression and fluid expression experiments, a higher permeability for fluid flow has been found in the superficial cartilaginous zone than in the deep zone; a finding likely reflecting the lower concentration of proteoglycans in the former (19). Thus, as a consequence of its higher hydraulic permeability and fluid flow to nonweightbearing areas, the superficial layer appears to act as a cushion, initially absorbing and distributing the impact of a compressive force (19). Only with higher or prolonged strain is the compressive force also translated to the deeper cartilage zones. In contrast, surface fibrillated cartilage demonstrates far greater deformation as a consequence of perme-

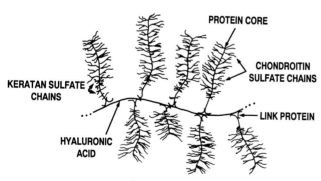

PROTEIN CORE

CHONDROITIN SULFATE CHAINS

KERATAN SULFATE CHAINS

LINK PROTEIN

HYALURONIC ACID

FIG. 5.1. Schematic drawing of a proteoglycan aggregate. Multiple proteoglycan monomers noncovalently associate with a central hyaluronic acid filament via link proteins to form an aggregate. The monomers consist of a central protein core with multiple covalently bound chondroitin and keratan sulfate chains. (Adapted from ref. 47.)

ability increases secondary to cartilage disruption with resulting decreased resistance to fluid motion (19).

One of the unique features of articular cartilage in distinction to other hyaline cartilages is the highly ordered structure that changes from joint surface to subchondral bone (15–18). Cell shape and size, collagen fibril diameter, collagen fibril orientation relative to the articular surface, and matrix water and proteoglycan content all change with increasing depth from the articular surface (15–18). The arrangement of the collagen fibril ultrastructure, in particular, reflects the functional requirements of articular cartilage (17). Four distinct layers or zones have been described and are referred to as the superficial or tangential zone, the middle or transitional zone, the deep or radial zone, and the zone of calcified cartilage (15–17) (Fig. 5.3). Within these zones, distinct matrix regions or compartments can be identified, including the pericellular matrix, the territorial matrix, and the dominant interterritorial matrix, which accounts for many of the biomechanical properties of cartilage (15,16).

The lamina splendens (LS) represents a thin cell-free layer of matrix that grossly corresponds to a fine clear film that can be mechanically stripped from the articular cartilage (15,16,18). It is comprised of a tightly

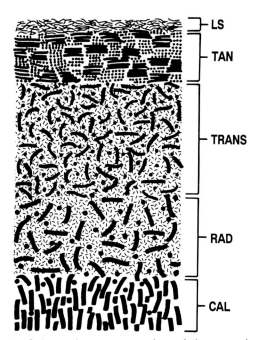

FIG. 5.3. Schematic representation of the organization of articular cartilage. The lamina splendens (*LS*) is a layer of fine fibrils several micra thick that covers the articular surface. The tangential zone (*TAN*) consists of closely arranged bundles of collagen fibers arranged parallel to the articular surface. The collagen fibers in the transitional zone (*TRANS*) are randomly arranged. Collagen fibers of the radial zone (*RAD*) are larger in diameter but also randomly arranged. The collagen fibers of the calcified zone (*CAL*) are arranged perpendicular to the articular surface. (Adapted from ref. 48.)

packed tangentially arrayed layer of fine fibrils and may function in the boundary lubrication mode of synovial joints (15,16). Deep to the LS, the elongated chondrocytes arrange themselves so that their long axis lies parallel to the articular surface (15,18,20). This zone is referred to as the superficial or tangential zone (TAN) (Fig. 5.3). Within this zone the collagen fibers of the dominant interterritorial matrix are arranged in tight bundles oriented parallel to the articular surface (15,17,18). This orientation of the collagen fibrils reflects the functional requirements of the tissue (17). The principal mechanical properties of the collagen fibrils are their tensile stiffness and strength. As such, they make their greatest contribution when oriented in line with the axis of tensile load (17). The spatial arrangement of the collagen in this zone reflects the large tensile stresses that develop parallel to the articular surface with compressive loading.

The transitional zone (TRANS) lies directly beneath the superficial zone and comprises approximately 40% to 60% of the tissue's thickness (15,17,18) (Fig. 5.3). The collagen fibers are larger than in the superficial zone, loosely packed, randomly oriented, and homogeneously distributed (15,20). The deep or radial zone (RAD) usually forms the largest component of articular cartilage (Fig. 5.3). Collagen fibers of the radial zone are also randomly arranged, but are of larger diameter. This zone contains the largest collagen fibrils of articular cartilage and the highest proteoglycan content (15). The water content, which progressively decreases from the superficial to deep zones, is lowest in this layer (21). This distribution of water in part reflects a counterbalance between the osmotic effect of the proteoglycans and the tension effect of the collagen fiber scaffold (15,17).

In the calcified zone and in the deepest area of the radial zone the orientation of the collagen fibers is perpendicular to the subchondral bone (15). Collagen fibrils of the radial zone penetrate directly into the calcified cartilage. The "tidemark" represents a histologically demonstrable line dividing the radial and calcified zones and may function as an anchor for the collagen fibrils (15,17). No structural continuity between hyaline cartilage and subchondral bone is present and the collagen fibers of the calcified zone are not anchored to bone (18). The attachment of hyaline cartilage to subchondral bone has been likened to that of a jigsaw puzzle, whereby the interlocking of the irregular surfaces of the calcified zone and underlying bone provide the necessary attachment (18).

MRI of Articular Cartilage

The reported appearance of articular cartilage and the ability of MRI to depict chondral defects and bio-

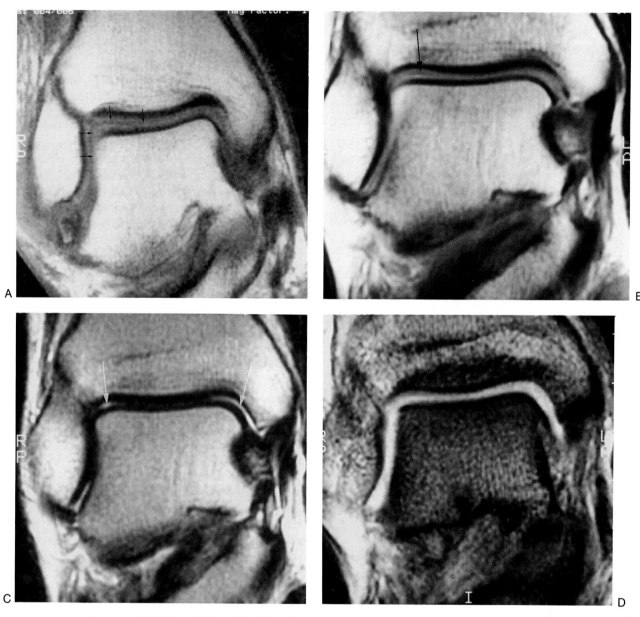

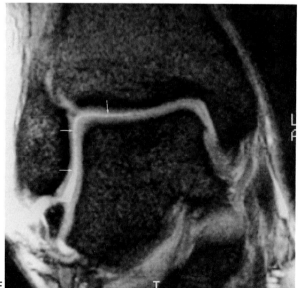

FIG. 5.4. Articular cartilage: appearance with different pulse sequences. **A:** Coronal TR 300 TE 15. High resolution T1-weighted image of the talar dome photographed to optimize depiction of articular cartilage. The articular cartilage along both sides of the joint space is depicted as an intermediate signal intensity structure separated by a thin low signal intensity line presumably reflecting joint fluid (*small arrows*). **B:** Coronal TR 3000 TE 20. The articular cartilage demonstrates intermediate signal intensity and is not clearly distinguished from joint fluid. A small linear low signal intensity line is noted (*arrow*). This should not be misinterpreted as representing a loose body within the joint. **C:** Coronal TR 3000 TE 100. On this high resolution (256 × 256 matrix) "fast" spin-echo image, the articular cartilage demonstrates decreased signal intensity and is difficult to distinguish from subchondral bone. The synovial fluid demonstrates high signal intensity and provides contrast along the articular surface (*arrows*). **D:** Coronal TR 54 TE 13 flip angle 75. Single slice gradient-echo acquisition under steady state condition (*GRASS*). The articular cartilage is of uniform increased signal intensity, although less than that of synovial fluid. **E:** Coronal TR 250 TE 15 flip angle 15. Multiplanar gradient-echo acquisition. The articular cartilage demonstrates intermediate signal intensity on this sequence and is well contrasted against the synovial fluid, which appears as a high signal intensity stripe separating the two articular surfaces (*small arrows*).

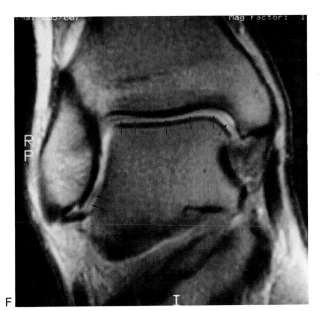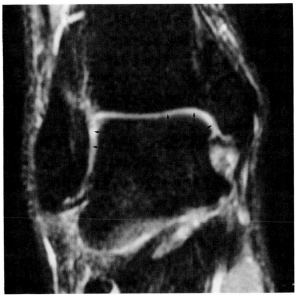

FIG. 5.4. (*Continued*) **F:** Coronal TR 500 TE 20 "Fat Sat." A frequency selective presaturation pulse has been applied to fat immediately before the excitation pulse, destroying the longitudinal magnetization of fat. The hyaline articular cartilage demonstrates uniform increased signal intensity (*arrows*) that is higher than subchondral bone but lower than that of joint fluid. **G:** Coronal TR 2200 TE 35 TI 160. The articular cartilage demonstrates high signal intensity (*arrows*). While well contrasted against subchondral bone, the distinction between cartilage and synovial fluid is not optimal.

mechanical changes has differed significantly between the various approaches adopted by different investigators. These methods have included T1-weighted (short TR/TE); T2-weighted (long TR/TE), various gradient-echo, fat suppression, and inversion recovery pulse sequences as well as T1-weighted sequences in association with gadolinium-enhanced MRI arthrographic techniques (10–14, 19, 21–26). No method to date has proven clearly superior. The challenge has been to depict both the early changes contained within the cartilage, as well as the later changes manifest at the articular surface and at the underlying subchondral bone interface. The patella, which has the thickest articular cartilage in the body, has served as the model for many of the investigations of articular cartilage. As a consequence, several of these studies will be cited in this chapter. Due to the disparity in thickness between the patella and talar dome articular surfaces, however, effective strategies for evaluation of one articular surface may not be directly applicable to the other.

Using conventional T1-weighted sequences, normal articular cartilage most commonly demonstrates a homogeneous intermediate signal intensity (Fig. 5.4A). A subtle bilaminar appearance, with the signal intensity from the basal two-thirds of the cartilage being lower than that of the superficial level, has been reported (24), although this has been more apparent *in vitro* (disarticulated patella cadaver specimens) than *in vivo* and has not been consistently substantiated in other studies (19,24). No zonal differences in the appearance of articular cartilage are routinely evident in our experience on T1-weighted sequences in high-resolution clinical imaging of the talar dome or patella. On proton density (Fig. 5.4B) and T2-weighted sequences (Fig. 5.4C), articular cartilage has also most consistently demonstrated a homogeneous appearance without reflection of the zonal architecture and differential water distribution of the cartilage (14). In an experimental study using bovine patella, however, a bilaminar appearance to the cartilage was described using T2-weighted spin-echo and heavily T1-weighted inversion recovery sequences (19). The bilaminar appearance consisted of a superficial zone, characterized by longer T1 and T2 values, correlating with the tangential and transitional zones of normal articular cartilage, and a second MRI zone, with shorter T1 and T2 values, corresponding to the deeper layers of the articular cartilage. This zonal signal intensity pattern was inverted on heavily T2-weighted spin-echo sequences and the findings correlated with differences between the better hydrated superficial zone and lower water content of the deeper zone (19). This zonal pattern could not be demonstrated with T1-weighted and

T2*-weighted sequences in this study and again has not been routinely demonstrable in the author's experience (21).

In a more recent high-resolution MR study of human articular cartilage, a trilaminar appearance to the cartilage was identified using T1- and T2-weighted spin-echo images (26a). The major difference between this and previous studies related to the depiction in this study of a superficial low signal intensity zone that corresponded in location, although not exactly in thickness, to the superficial zone in correlative histological sections. The depiction of this superficial zone appears dependent on high spatial resolution, and was more consistently depicted on experimental imaging of core cylinders of cartilage in which partial volume effects were minimized (26a). A second zone of intermediate to high signal intensity corresponded approximately to the transitional zone in histological sections. A third zone, which was depicted as a broad band of low signal intensity, corresponded approximately to the deep radial and calcified cartilage zones and the adjacent subchondral bone. The apparent thickness of this latter zone is directly affected by chemical shift effects and thus the direction of the frequency-encoding gradient. The determinants of the signal intensity in the different zones remains unexplained by this study, although the authors suggest that factors other than differences in water concentration (which they believe are insufficient) must be considered, including the possibility that differences in orientation of collagen fibers may affect signal intensity by means of their effect on magnetic susceptibility (26a).

The term ''gradient-echo imaging'' represents a term encompassing a wide number of techniques sharing in common the use of gradient reversal for signal acquisition as well as the application of a radiofrequency (RF) excitation pulse that is generally less than the 90° pulse used in spin-echo imaging (27,28). Image contrast is dependent not only on tissue relaxation times (T1 and T2) and timing parameters (TR and TE), but is additionally affected by pulse flip angle, the presence or absence of steady state conditions, and the mode of acquisition (sequential vs. interleaved) (27,28). A complete discussion of contrast phenomenology for gradient-echo imaging is well beyond the scope of this text and the reader is referred to many excellent sources (27,28). For purposes of articular cartilage and joint assessment, gradient-echo techniques emphasizing T2* contrast, which provide for an arthrogram effect, have been of greatest interest. Under steady state conditions, in which the persistence of the transverse magnetization determines the degree of signal intensity, an arthrogram effect (high signal from long T2 joint fluid) can be produced with short TR times (20–50 ms) and relatively high flip angles (Fig. 5.4D). High

quality T2* images can also be produced in the absence of steady state conditions with relatively longer repetition (TR) (> 200 ms) and echo (TE) times and small flip angles (Fig. 5.4D). In general, regardless of the flip angle chosen, T2* weighting increases with an increase in TE (28). As previously mentioned, the acquisition mode will also affect image contrast with gradient-echo techniques. With sequential acquisition modes that preserve the steady state (e.g., GRASS), joint fluid will demonstrate an arthrogram effect using short TR times (TR less than T2) and moderate to high flip angles (Fig. 5.4E). With slice interleaved (multislice) GRASS (MPGR), the longer TR times required for the multislice mode contribute to spoil the steady state condition (27). With TR times in excess of 200 ms, MPGR sequences with short TE times and small flip angles produce density-weighted images and with large flip angles T1-weighted images result. In a recent study, Konig, using a low flip angle (12°) gradient-echo sequence (FLASH), reported this sequence superior to spin-echo images in depicting early cartilage degeneration. The signal changes seen on MRI (areas of decreased signal within the otherwise high signal intensity cartilage) correlated with a localized reduction of proteoglycan content on histological evaluation of the specimens. We have investigated a number of gradient echo approaches toward assessment of the articular cartilage of the talar dome but have found none to date to be consistently helpful in depiction of articular lesions in this location.

Chemical shift fat suppression techniques have also been applied toward depiction and characterization of articular cartilage. The two principal methods, phase contrast and partial saturation, are discussed in more detail elsewhere in this text (see chapter by Deutsch on Traumatic Injuries of Bone and Osteonecrosis). With short TR/TE partial saturation techniques, the hyaline articular cartilage of the talar dome demonstrates uniform increased signal intensity (Fig. 5.4F). Totterman et al. (12) used chopper fat suppression (CFS), which is a phase-sensitive implementation of the Dixon fat suppression technique, and reported significant improvement in visualization of the hyaline cartilage of the knee in comparison to conventional spin-echo sequences (12). Using a long TR/TE (TR 1500–2000, TE 60–80 ms) CFS sequence, hyaline cartilage appeared as an intermediate signal intensity structure and was well contrasted against high signal intensity joint fluid. Konig compared the use of standard spin-echo (SE) images with ''water'' images obtained using a chemical shift selective sequence (CHESS) for visualization of hyaline articular cartilage (25). With CHESS, hyaline cartilage demonstrated high signal intensity and was well contrasted against low signal intensity subchondral bone, synovial tissues, and ligamentous structures, although contrast between joint fluid and hyaline cartilage was better accomplished in this study with conventional long T2-weighted images. CHESS proved superior to SE sequences in depicting early cartilage degeneration manifest on MRI as localized decreases in cartilage signal intensity and which correlated with a localized reduction of proteoglycan content within the cartilage on histological evaluation of the specimens (25).

Chandnani et al. used a hybrid fat suppression (HFS) pulse sequence for assessment of articular cartilage (26). This technique represents a phase-sensitive variation of chemical shift imaging that involves no postprocessing adjustment or increased actual imaging time, although the necessity for manual pretuning does slightly increase the study time. In their study, Chandnani et al. compared HFS sequences to standard spin echo sequences with and without the intraarticular administration of saline solution and gadopentetate dimeglumine (26). In this investigation, T1-weighted HFS pulse sequences were superior to other sequences for visualization of hyaline cartilage and were the most accurate for depiction of areas of cartilage defects and thinning. Indeed, T1-weighted HFS images performed both with and without intraarticular saline provided greater contrast between hyaline cartilage and surrounding structures than the contrast achieved between hyaline cartilage and intraarticular gadolinium DTPA using standard spin-echo sequences.

The authors have had considerable experience using short tau inversion recovery (STIR) sequences for purposes of accomplishing fat suppression and evaluating articular cartilage. With this pulse sequence, "water" protons are made to dominate the image by using a short inversion time (TI) and adjusting TI to the null crossing point of the longitudinal magnetization of fat (12). With STIR imaging, the effects of T1 and T2 relaxation are additive, contributing to increased lesion conspicuity. This pulse sequence allows sensitive depiction of the subchondral bone, articular cartilage, and the articular surface, which is particularly well delineated when contrasted against high signal intensity synovial fluid. Normal articular cartilage demonstrates a relatively homogeneous intermediate signal intensity appearance using this pulse sequence (Fig. 5.4G). This technique has been quite effective in the author's experience for assessment of the relatively thick articular cartilage of the patella. It has, however, been less successful in consistently characterizing the thinner articular cartilage overlying the talar dome.

The surface features of articular cartilage can also be evaluated using intraarticular contrast. This is most readily accomplished in the presence of sufficient synovial fluid to provide an arthrogram effect on T2- and T2*-weighted sequences. Alternatively, intraarticular saline and/or gadolinium DTPA can be employed for purposes of accomplishing MRI arthrography (see below).

Experimental Chondral Lesions

The ability of MRI to depict experimentally produced cartilage abnormalities has been evaluated in a number of investigations (13,19,22,23). In an early study using relatively limited in plane resolution (0.95 mm/pixel) Wojtys and colleagues were able to depict 15 of 16 experimentally produced chondral lesions of cadaver patellae that were 4 mm or greater in width and all those 3 mm and greater in depth (13). In addition, seven of nine lesions 1 mm in depth were identified in this group. Handleberg et al., using a cadaveric model, detected all experimentally created lesions that ranged from 0.8 to 5 mm in diameter and 1 to 2 mm in depth (23). The images were obtained on a high field strength system (1.5 T) using a T2-weighted spin-echo sequence, and the superficial defects were sharply contrasted against high signal intensity joint fluid. Double contrast CT arthrography, performed after the MRI examination, missed 50% of the 1.5- and 2-mm lesions and detected none of the 0.8-mm holes. In contrast to this favorable experience, Gylys-Morin et al. reported significant limitations for detecting experimentally created defects in the femoral condyles using standard spin-echo imaging and advocated the use of intraarticular gadolinium, in the presence of which all lesions 2 mm or greater could be detected (22). While the results of these investigations are quite impressive with regard to articular cartilage lesion detectability, they may not directly correlate with the ability to detect naturally occurring chondral lesions, as the sharp margins produced by the drill holes of experimentally created chondral defects may enhance their detection as compared to naturally occurring cartilage abnormalities.

MRI has also been used to study the repair characteristics of articular cartilage in experimental models of degenerative arthritis (29). Braunstein et al. demonstrated relative increased thickness of articular cartilage in dogs 3 years following anterior cruciate ligament (ACL) transection (29). This hypertrophic response of articular cartilage is consistent with biochemical observations of increased matrix production manifest by net increased proteoglycan synthesis and concentration in cartilage matrix following ACL transection (29). Using T2*-weighted images, the signal intensity of the hypertrophied cartilage remained similar to that of the contralateral control knee, an observation the investigators attributed to increased proteoglycan concentration rather than merely an increase in bulk water content as contributing to the increased thickness of the repaired cartilage (29).

OSTEOCHONDRAL INJURIES

Terminology

The terminology used to characterize osteochondral lesions of the talar dome has been a source of controversy and confusion for over the past century (2). Konig initially introduced the term "osteochondritis dissecans" to describe the pathological process of loose bodies within the knee joint (30). Konig proposed, without substantiation, that these loose bodies were the result of "spontaneous necrosis" secondary to the occlusion of small end arteries (2,30). Kappis in 1922 described a similar process in the ankle and stated that the loose bodies were the result of "spontaneous necrosis" of the talar dome (31). Rendu (32) followed by Fairbank (33) introduced the concept that these lesions could represent traumatic intraarticular fractures with interruption of the vascular supply and subsequent avascular necrosis (2). The concept that the etiology of osteochondritis dissecans was probably not on the basis of spontaneous necrosis but rather resulted from trauma had become commonly accepted in the orthopedic community by the 1950s (2). In their classic work, Berndt and Harty established the concept of trauma as the principal etiologic factor of osteochondritis dissecans and proposed the term "transchondral fracture" as more appropriate to describe this entity (34). Despite general agreement today that trauma is the principal etiological factor, the term "osteochondritis dissecans" has persisted in the current literature and is believed by some investigators to represent a separate clinical entity with distinct features from that of transchondral fracture (2). In this chapter, the term "osteochondral injury or lesion" will be used to encompass both entities and the entire spectrum of impaction injuries of the talar dome.

Pathogenesis

Oteochondral or transchondral fractures are generally believed to be the result of shearing, rotary, or tangentially aligned impaction forces (34,35). Acute injuries can produce damage to the subchondral bone with preservation of the integrity of the overlying articular cartilage. Alternatively, fragments consisting of cartilage alone (purely chondral fragments) or cartilage and underlying subchondral bone (osteochondral fragments) can result. The depth of the fracture line, which generally parallels the articular surface, determines the cartilaginous and osseous components of the lesions (35).

In their classic pathomechanical study, Berndt and Harty used fresh lower extremity amputation specimens to reproduce medial and lateral talar dome lesions similar to those encountered on a clinical basis (34). Lateral talar dome lesions were reproduced by a strong inversion force to a dorsiflexed foot. As the dorsiflexed foot was inverted, the lateral talar margin impacted and compressed against the medial articular surface of the fibula, creating a shearing and compressing component that if of sufficient strength would displace the fragment (2,34) (Fig. 5.5). Medial talar dome lesions were reproduced by a strong inversion force to a plantar flexed foot with lateral rotation of the tibia on the talus, allowing the posteromedial aspect of the talar dome to impact on the posteromedial lip of the tibia (2,34).

Following the injury, the osteochondral fragment is deprived of its blood supply due to disruption of the subchondral surface (11,35). The overlying articular cartilage may remain viable, receiving sustenance

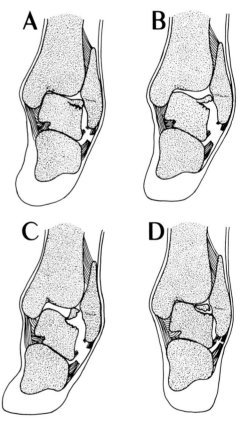

FIG. 5.5. Diagrammatic representation of a lateral talar dome transchondral fracture. **A:** With inversion of the foot, the lateral border of the talar dome is driven against the medial aspect of the fibula. **B:** Initially the ligamentous structures remain intact. With increasing force, ligamentous rupture may be seen in association with the production of an osteochondral fracture. **C, D:** The fate of any fragment produced is variable, it may remain in place or become partially or completely detached. (Modified from ref. 35.)

from the synovial fluid. It is believed that the subsequent healing and revascularization of the osteochondral lesion is dependent on both the stability of the fragment within its bony crater and on the degree of intact overlying articular cartilage (11).

The cartilage overlying the area of the osteochondritic defect may appear normal in the early stages of the condition, or later may variably appear flattened, fissured, discolored, or fibrillated with motion of the fragment and associated with lack of underlying subchondral osseous support (3). Following the injury, the detached portion of the articular surface can remain *in situ*, be slightly displaced, or become loose within the joint. In many cases, the osteocartilaginous fragments attach to the synovial lining at a distant site and become reabsorbed (35). Alternatively, a flap of cartilage or the entire fragment may become loose within the joint and can continue to increase in size, gaining nourishment from synovial fluid. The defect site is typically filled with dense fibrous tissue and underlying eburnated bone (3).

Pathologically, the primary changes occur in the bone with the cartilage affected secondarily (2,3,35). Hemorrhage at the site of the defect develops into a fibrin clot that may eventually be modulated into fibrovascular repair tissue that gradually increases in cellularity and eventually revascularizes the segment deprived of its blood supply. If there is a failure of healing, the interzone between the fragment and the cartilage evolves into a dense fibrous tissue somewhat analogous to the tissue characteristics of a fracture in the stage of delayed union or nonunion (3). The bony bed presents a similar response—the early healing defect demonstrating an active cellular response, early vascularization, and osteogenesis—whereas the nonhealing defect develops dense avascular eburnated bone. This leads to lack of subchondral support, subchondral cyst formation, secondary articular deformity, and subsequent degenerative changes (3).

Clinical Features

Osteochondral injuries of the talar dome are more common in men than women, and the patients are usually in the second to fourth decade of life (3,35). In athletes, the injury is commonly associated with landing on the forefoot in association with a torsional inversion component, as in basketball or football. Medial lesions have also been reported in women having sustained inversion injuries while wearing high heels (35). The middle third of the lateral border of the talar dome and the posterior third of the medial talar border are the most common sites of injury and are involved with approximately equal frequency (medial 57%, lateral 43%) (5,6,35). The medial talar fracture is usually deeper and assumes a more cup-shaped appearance than the lateral, which typically is shallower and more wafer-shaped. Patients typically describe a severe twisting injury to the ankle with a resultant "pop" (6). With lateral injuries, there is marked tenderness over the lateral aspect of the ankle and typically there is a concurrent lateral collateral ligament injury. In anterolateral lesions, pain and tenderness to local palpation often occurs in the area between the talus and the tibiofibular syndesmosis. In the posteromedial lesions, tenderness is most commonly localized behind the medial malleolus. It is important to distinguish a lateral collateral ligament tear from an osteochondral fracture, a task that frequently requires sophisticated imaging as conventional radiographic findings may be quite subtle and frequently are initially occult (6).

Management Considerations

One of the principal orthopedic concerns with regard to talar osteochondral injuries is facilitation of healing and avoidance of intraarticular osteochondral loose body formation. Healing may occur through revascularization of the fragment across the fracture line. The mechanical stability of the fragment and condition of the overlying articular cartilage impact on healing of osteochondral injuries of the dome (6,8,11).

Multiple approaches toward management of osteochondral dome injuries have been advanced, and none has received universal approbation (4, 8, 36–38). If the lesion is mechanically stable and the overlying cartilage intact, conservative measures including a period of nonweightbearing may be sufficient to induce healing (4). Alternatively, the lesions may be percutaneously drilled in an attempt to facilitate revascularization (8,36,38). Larger fragments may also be pinned in an attempt to promote healing. Advances in arthroscopic techniques have allowed a more aggressive approach to these lesions (38). Advanced stage lesions with unstable fragments and articular cartilage violation are commonly approached with curettage and drilling (5). The bony crater is debrided and any loose fragments removed.

Staging Systems

The various treatment options available underscore the need for an accurate lesion staging system. Most work today has used the system initially described by Berndt and Harty based on their cadaver observations and extrapolated to plain radiography (34). This system classifies lesions into four stages (Fig. 5.6). Stage 1 represents a small area of compression of subchondral bone resulting in microscopic damage to bony trabeculae. No lesion may be evident on superficial visual inspection (Fig. 5.6). Stage 2 represents a partially detached osteochondral fragment with fissuring typically evident on plain radiographs. In Stage 3, the fragment is completely displaced from its underlying bed, but remains in anatomic position (Fig. 5.6). In Stage 4, the detached osteochondral fragment has become inverted in the fracture bed or lies displaced elsewhere in the joint (6). A significant limitation of this system, which is based on conventional radiography, is the lack of inclusion of the status of the overlying articular cartilage. In a clinical series, Pritsch et al. classified lesions based on their appearance at arthroscopy (8) (Fig. 5.7). Grade 1 lesions represented a small area of compression of subchondral bone with firm, intact, and shiny articular cartilage evident at arthroscopy. Grade 2 lesions represented partially detached osteochondral fragments with intact but softened cartilage, and Grade 3 lesions represented completely detached osteochondral fragments that remained in the crater and demonstrated significantly frayed cartilage. When the cartilage is intact at arthroscopy, the fragment interface with subchondral bone cannot be evaluated, and in some circumstances, the lesion itself cannot be

demonstrated. Pritsch reported 4 patients with a Grade 1 lesion arthroscopically, but who had a Stage 4 lesion radiographically (8). The ability of MRI to detect the subchondral component as well as to characterize the status of the overlying articular cartilage are significant advantages that contribute to the appeal of applying this diagnostic technique to staging osteochondral lesions.

Imaging of Osteochondral Injuries.

Before the introduction of MRI, both radiographic and scintigraphic methods were applied toward the assessment of naturally occurring osteochondral lesions. The radiographic methods have included plain film radiography, conventional tomography, CT, arthrography, and arthrotomography (5, 35, 39–42). Nonarthrographic methods are limited by their inability to characterize the status of the overlying articular cartilage. The most precise and elegant radiographic technique is that of computed arthrotomography, which may be performed in either the direct coronal plane or with thin overlapping sections and multiplanar reconstruction (39,40). With this technique, the articular cartilage can be defined, and contrast extension between the fragment and underlying bone is considered evidence of cartilage violation and lesion instability. Scintigraphic methods have also been reported of value in the assessment of osteochondritic lesions (41). The presence of focal hyperemia on blood pool phase scintigraphic images has been reported as a strong indicator of loosening (41). Additionally, the likelihood of a loose fragment has been reported to be directly proportional to the extent and degree of radionuclide activity (41). Scintigraphic methods, while apparently sensitive to the detection of osteochondral lesions, are limited by spatial resolution, and provide no direct information regarding articular cartilage. The multiplanar capability of MRI, coupled with its high-contrast resolution and direct capability of depicting both articular cartilage and subchondral bone, represent significant potential advantages of this technique for depiction and characterization of osteochondral injuries compared to existing methods.

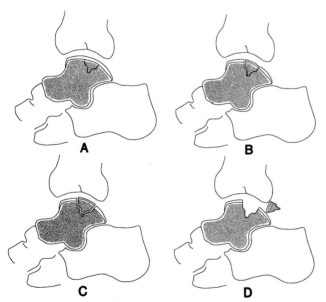

FIG. 5.6. Schematic representation of the different stages of osteochondritis dissecans as described by Berndt and Harty. **A:** The injury is entirely confined to subchondral bone without significant findings at the articular surface. **B:** The fracture has extended through the articular cartilage and the fragment remains largely in place hinged by intact overlying cartilage. **C:** The fragment is unattached and mildly displaced. **D:** The fragment has become completely displaced and lies freely in the joint.

MRI Technique

For evaluation of the talar dome, surface coil imaging is essential. The authors have used several approaches including a standard send-receive extremity coil (GE), dual 3-inch circular coils in a modified Helmholz configuration, and most recently a currently investigational "wrap-around" coil (GE) (see chapter by Crues and Shellock). High spatial resolution is critical to assessment of the articular cartilage of the talar

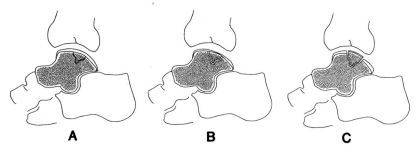

FIG. 5.7. Diagrammatic representation of staging of osteochondritis dissecans after Pritsch **A:** The lesion is entirely subchondral and no surface manifestation will be evident arthroscopically. **B:** A discrete fragment is present but remains covered by intact but attenuated articular cartilage. **C:** The fragment is partially displaced with complete disruption of the overlying articular cartilage.

dome. Small field of view (8–10 cm) imaging is employed. Currently, conventional and fast spin-echo imaging is used to allow T1- and T2-weighted sequences to be obtained at high spatial resolution (256 × 256) and within reasonable examination times. An axial localizer is used to obtain oblique coronal and sagittal images. The location of the lesion will determine whether the coronal or sagittal image will be the most valuable. As a general rule, most lesions are located along the medial and lateral aspects of the dome, and as such are best evaluated in the coronal plane to minimize volume averaging. A STIR and/or partial satu-

ration chemical shift sequence is commonly performed in the plane judged most likely to optimize assessment of the extent of subchondral abnormality and integrity of the overlying articular cartilage. Either T1-or T2-weighted sequences are routinely obtained in one of the three imaging planes.

MRI

Acute osteochondral injuries occur as a result of impaction of the talar dome against either the face of the

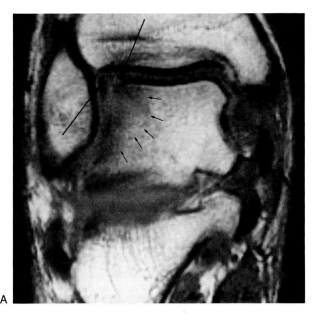
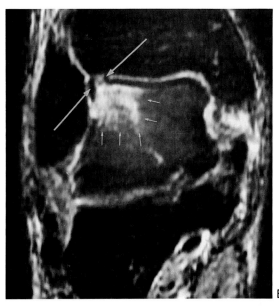

A   B

FIG. 5.8. Acute osteochondral fracture. **A:** Coronal TR/TE 300/15. There is striking decreased signal intensity within the subchondral bone and extending into cancellous bone of the lateral aspect of the talar dome (*small arrows*). Two small loose fragments of bone can be identified within the joint space as low signal intensity structures (*arrows*). The articular cartilage cannot be clearly distinguished from joint fluid using this pulse sequence. **B:** Coronal STIR TR 2200 TE 35 TI 160. There is marked increased signal intensity corresponding to the area of subchondral and cancellous bone contusion identified on the short TR/TE sequence (*small arrows*). The two loose osteochondral bodies within the joint again demonstrate low signal intensity and are well contrasted against high signal intensity joint fluid (*long arrows*). There is complete disruption of the subchondral bone and articular surface along the extreme lateral aspect of the talar dome. (*Figure continues on next page.*)

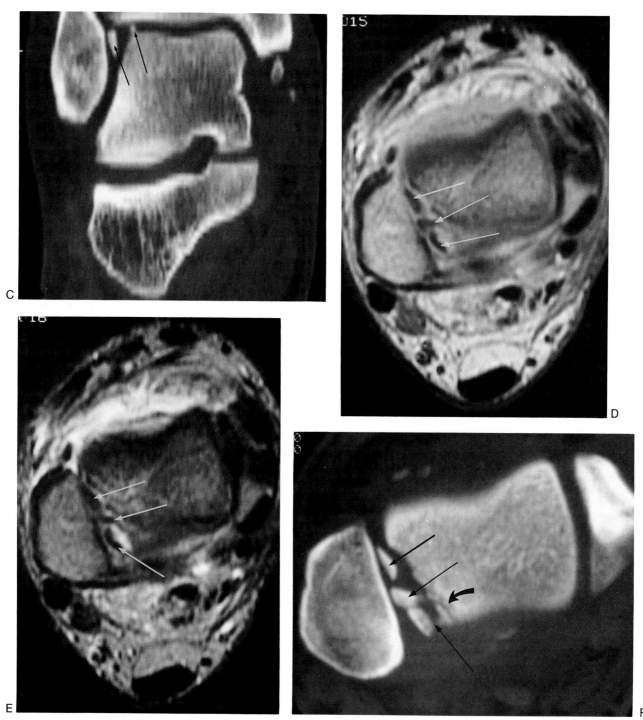

FIG. 5.8. (*Continued*) **C:** CT scan. Coronal reformatted image from a high-resolution CT study demonstrates the two osteochondral fragments within the lateral aspect of the talocrural joint (*arrows*). The contour deformity along the lateral aspect of the talar dome is well demonstrated. There is no evidence of the extension of findings into the underlying cancellous bone. **D:** Axial TR 2000 TE 20. Multiple eliptical shaped low signal intensity fragments are identified between the talus and fibula (*arrows*). **E:** Axial TR 2000 TE 80. The fragments are contrasted against high signal intensity joint fluid (*arrows*). The extent of contusional edema is less evident on this sequence than on the short TR/TE and STIR sequences. **F:** Axial CT. This section directly corresponds to the plane depicted on MR. Multiple eliptical shaped fragments of bone are seen between the talus and fibula (*arrows*). The extent of comminution involving the posterolateral aspect of the talar dome is better demonstrated on CT than MR (*curved arrow*).

lateral malleolus (lateral lesions) or the posteroinferior lip of the tibia (medial dome lesions) (34,35). While findings on conventional radiographs may be occult or quite subtle, the evidence of acute osseous impaction is readily manifest on MRI. On T1-weighted sequences, extensive and poorly defined low signal intensity is seen within the subchondral bone and extending variably into the cancellous bone of the talar dome (Fig. 5.8A). This signal may increase slightly on T2-weighted sequences, and typically demonstrates striking increases in signal intensity on STIR sequences (Fig. 5.8B). These findings are presumed to represent a combination of hemorrhagic and nonhem-

orrhagic edema and resemble other bone contusional injuries (see chapter by Deutsch on Traumatic Injuries of Bone and Osteonecrosis). The overlying articular cartilage may remain intact or be violated, resulting in a transchondral fracture. In the latter situation the elastic properties of the articular cartilage and its resulting capacity to "rebound" from the deforming force allows the injury to be principally transmitted to the underlying subchondral bone. In this setting there will be no obvious surface manifestation of the acute injury (8). These injuries with intact cartilage correspond to Stage 1 lesions in both the previously described systems of Berndt and Harty and Pritsch and associates

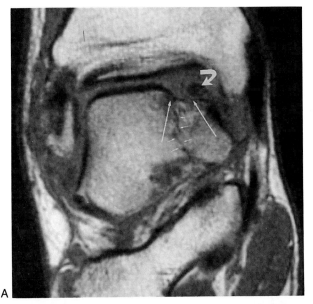

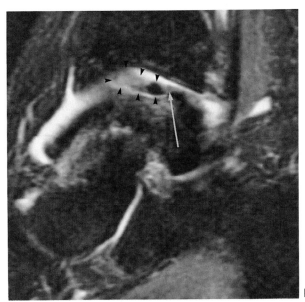

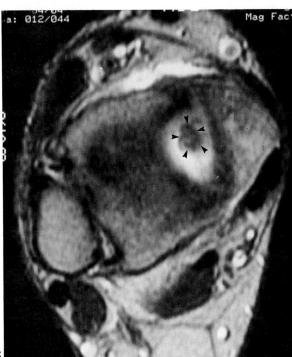

FIG. 5.9. Acute osteochondral fracture. **A:** Coronal TR 500 TE 20. A vertical fracture is seen extending through the medial third of the talar dome (*small arrows*). There is marked depression (11 mm) of the medial fragment; a finding well characterized by the tomographic capability of MR. A circular to ovoid, slightly decreased signal intensity osteochondral fragment is seen within the medial joint space (*curved arrow*). **B:** Sagittal "STIR" TR 2200 TE 35 TI 160. The size of the osteochondral fragment is well delineated on this sagittal scan (*arrowheads*). The cartilaginous component comprises the anterior two-thirds of the fragment and is of intermediate signal intensity. The posterior component comprised of subchondral bone is of low signal intensity. A high signal intensity cleavage plane presumably representing synovial fluid separates the osteochondral fragment from its bony bed throughout its extent except for a small "hinge" of intact articular cartilage posteriorly (*arrow*). The findings correlate with a classic Stage 2 Berndt and Harty lesion. **C:** Axial TR 2000 TE 80. The osteochondral fragment (*arrowheads*) is well contrasted against the high signal intensity joint fluid.

(8,34). The ability of MRI to detect such subchondral injury remains a significant advantage of this method over other techniques including plain film radiography and diagnostic arthroscopy to which the injuries may remain entirely occult. In a recent series evaluating osteochondral fractures of the talar dome, MRI depicted injuries in 14 of 24 patients in whom the fractures remained occult to plain radiographic detection (43). What remains incompletely known at present, however, is the prognostic value of the subchondral signal changes detectable by MRI in the acute setting. The ability to differentiate which lesions will heal conservatively from those that will progress to necrosis and cyst formation would be potentially of great value. It is in this direction that future longitudinal MRI investigations will be of great value.

Extension of the injury to involve the articular cartilage results in the production of classic transchondral injuries that typically have surface manifestations. The transmitted energy of the impaction force determines the extent of the injury. High energy impaction forces may result in comminution of the articular surface with variable degrees of surface depression and production of loose osteochondral fragments (Fig. 5.8). A fracture may be evident extending well beyond the articular surface and subchondral bone into the body of the talus

(Fig. 5.9). On T1-weighted sequences of sufficient resolution, acute osteochondral fragments may be directly recognized as low signal intensity structures within the joint space (Figs. 5.8A, 5.9A). Osteochondral fragments within the joint and purely chondral fragments that would otherwise be occult to detection by conventional radiographic methods can also be depicted contrasted against bright synovial fluid on STIR, T2-, and T2*-weighted sequences (Figs. 5.8C, D,E, 5.9B,C, 5.10A,B). The findings may be quite subtle and must be specifically sought. In this regard, a low signal intensity line normally appearing within the joint space between the opposed articular surfaces of the talus and tibia has been described as a potential pitfall in the detection of loose fragments and should be recognized as such (21) (Fig. 5.4B). In the subacute setting, osteochondral fragments may become ossified and as a consequence demonstrate a more variable appearance on MRI secondary to fat within their central medullary component. Such fragments may actually demonstrate increased signal intensity on T1-weighted sequences that decreases on T2-weighted sequences. In cases in which multiple loose bodies are present, each may have a different composition and thus appearance. Correlation with plain films is particularly valuable in this setting as well as when fragments are

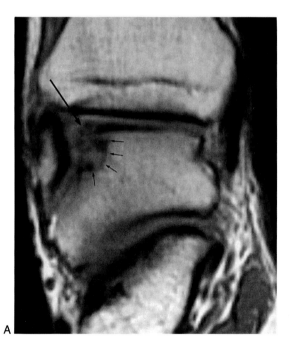 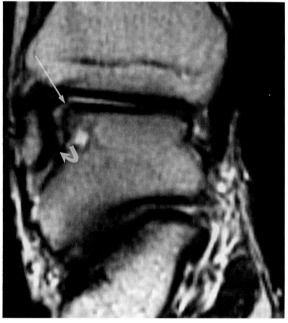

FIG. 5.10. Lateral talar dome lesion. **A:** Coronal TR 2000 TE 20. A subacute transchondral fracture of the lateral dome is present. The low signal intensity subchondral bone plate is focally disrupted (*arrow*). An elliptical shaped subchondral lesion is present (*small arrows*). The articular cartilage cannot be clearly distinguished from synovial fluid utilizing these imaging parameters and no loose body is identified. **B:** Coronal TR 2000 TE 80. The irregularity of the articular surface is better demonstrated highlighted against high signal intensity joint fluid. The site of violation of the articular cartilage and subchondral bone is better seen (*arrow*). A small loose body interposed between the articular surfaces of the lateral gutter is demonstrated as a relative filling defect within the joint fluid (*curved arrow*). (Courtesy of Bert R. Mandelbaum, M.D., Santa Monica, CA.)

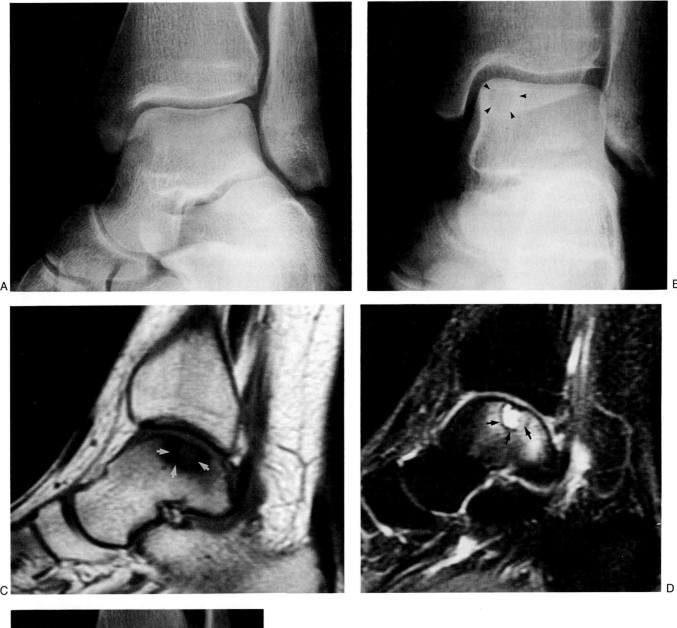

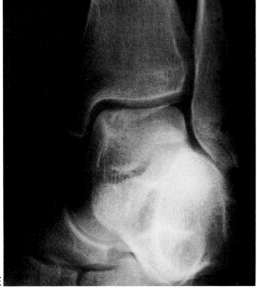

FIG. 5.11. Osteochondritis dissecans. **A:** Conventional radiograph. Mortise view of the ankle taken at the time of the patient's acute ankle injury. No abnormality is evident. **B:** Conventional radiograph. AP radiograph obtained 3 months following the acute injury. An area of cystic rarefaction is seen within the talar dome (*arrowheads*). **C:** Sagittal TR 500 TE 20. The osteochondritic segment is well defined as a roughly circular area of low signal (*arrows*) surrounded by a zone of decreased signal intensity representing edema. The articular cartilage is markedly attenuated over the lesion. **D:** Sagittal STIR TR 2200 TE 35 TI 160. The osteochondritic segment becomes markedly hyperintense (*arrows*). The extent of presumed surrounding edema is more evident on this pulse sequence. At surgery, the articular cartilage was denuded and partially replaced with reparative fibrocartilagelike material. The lesion was percutaneously drilled. **E:** Conventional radiograph. Mortise view obtained 7 months following arthroscopically guided drilling of the osteochondritic lesion. The cystic lesion is smaller and there is surrounding sclerotic bone.

125

nondependent such as when they attach to the synovium. In cases with loose osteochondral fragments, evaluation with CT remains invaluable for their detection and quantification (Figs. 5.8C,F).

Lower impaction force injuries may result in the production of chondral and osteochondral lesions similar to those produced experimentally by Berndt and Harty (34). The articular cartilage in these injuries may be grossly intact or variably disrupted, and the resulting osteochondral fragment may demonstrate a fate ranging from remaining entirely in place to becoming partially or completely detached. Many of these lesions are initially radiographically occult, becoming manifest later following necrosis of the fragment and/or the development of subchondral cyst formation (Fig. 5.11A–E). The term "osteochondritis dissecans" (OCD) is frequently used to refer to such osteochondral injuries that, while considered to be on a posttraumatic basis, are commonly not associated with a single inciting event. In this setting, the extensive areas of bone edema associated with acute injuries are typically not as prominent. The principal role of MRI is in lesion detection and subsequent characterization of the stability of the fragment and subchondral osseous support, as well as in the determination of the status of the overlying articular cartilage.

Osteochondritic lesions may present as variably shaped elliptical or elongate fragments of subchondral bone. The fragment itself may have a signal intensity ranging from decreased (e.g., dark) to increased (bright) in comparison to remaining subchondral bone (Figs. 5.11–5.15). The signal intensity of the fragment has been reported to have no correlation with stability of the fragment (21). In the author's experience, subacute and chronic osteochondritic lesions commonly present as focal, relatively circumscribed areas of significantly decreased signal intensity on T1-weighted images (Figs. 5.11, 5.14, 5.15). Focal areas within the osteochondritic segment may demonstrate significantly increased signal intensity on T2- and T2*-weighted as well as STIR sequences. The focal high signal intensity areas may represent cysts or localized granulation tissue and have been associated with instability of the lesion (3,21). In these latter lesions, the articular surface is frequently markedly attenuated and frayed and often focally replaced by fibrocartilagelike material (see below).

Osteochondral fragments may be defined from the underlying subchondral bone by an interface of low to intermediate signal intensity on T1- and proton density–weighted images. The interface is comprised of either fibrous or fibrovascular tissue along with a variable degree of bordering eburnated subchondral bone (3,21). Partially attached lesions have been reported to demonstrate increased signal intensity at the interface on long T2-weighted pulse sequences (21). Similar

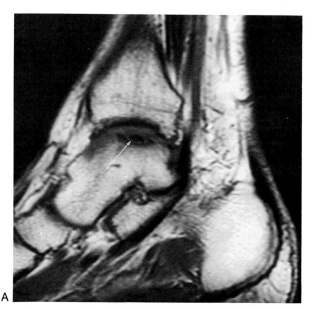 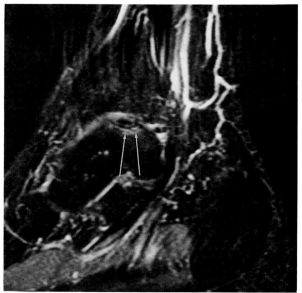

FIG. 5.12. Osteochondritis dissecans. **A:** Sagittal TR 500 TE 20. A discrete ovoid shaped low signal intensity osteochondral fragment is identified along the middle third of the medial aspect of the talar dome (*arrow*). The articular cartilage is not clearly disrupted. **B:** Sagittal STIR TR 2200 TE 35 TI 160. A band of high signal intensity is seen at the interface between the fragment and underlying subchondral bone suggesting a partially attached but unstable fragment (*long arrows*). At surgery, the articular cartilage was intact. On probing, the fragment was readily ballotable.

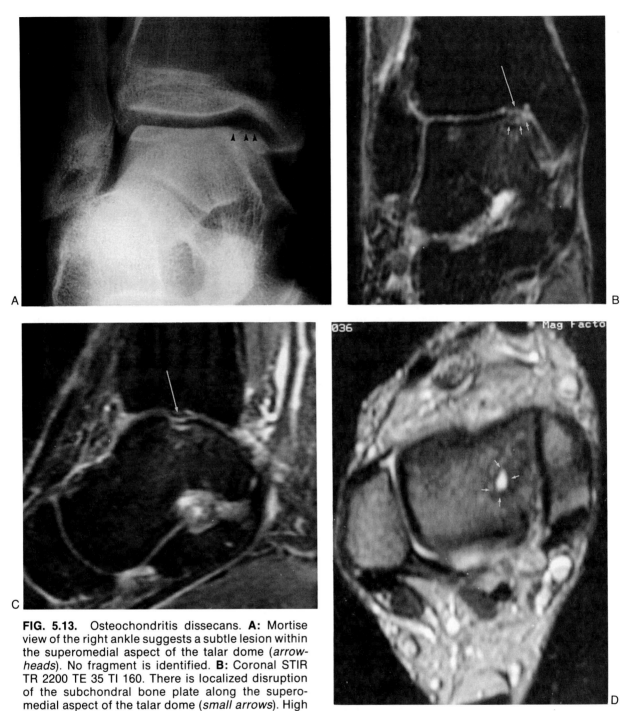

FIG. 5.13. Osteochondritis dissecans. **A:** Mortise view of the right ankle suggests a subtle lesion within the superomedial aspect of the talar dome (*arrowheads*). No fragment is identified. **B:** Coronal STIR TR 2200 TE 35 TI 160. There is localized disruption of the subchondral bone plate along the superomedial aspect of the talar dome (*small arrows*). High signal extends into the subchondral and cancellous bone of the superomedial aspect of the talus. There is a small minimally displaced fragment (*long arrow*). **C:** Sagittal STIR TR 2200 TE 35 TI 160. The radiographically occult chondral fragment is optimally demonstrated on this image minimally displaced from its crater (*arrow*). A circumscribed high signal intensity focus beneath the crater represents a small cyst or localized granulation tissue. **D:** Axial TR 2000 TE 80. On this section obtained just inferior to the subchondral bone plate, the localized high signal intensity cyst is well demonstrated (*small arrows*).

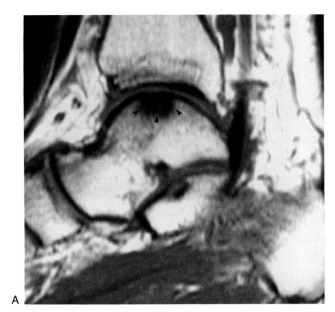

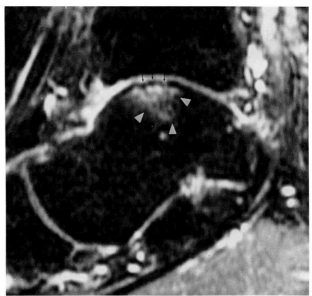

FIG. 5.14. Osteochondritis dissecans. **A:** Sagittal TR 500 TE 30. A well defined circular to ovoid low signal intensity region is seen extending into the subchondral bone of the talar dome. No discrete fragment is identified. There is a subtle suggestion of discontinuity of the subchondral bone plate. **B:** Sagittal STIR TR 2200 TE 35 TI 160. High signal intensity foci are seen within the subchondral component; a finding that has been associated with unstable lesions. There is loss of the normal smooth convexity of the talar dome with slight undulation of the subchondral bone plate (*small arrows*). At surgery, the articular cartilage was frayed and fibrous like component covered the lesion.

findings have also been noted in our experience using STIR and T2*-weighted sequences (Fig. 5.12). These pulse sequences demonstrate granulation tissue as high signal intensity (21) and additionally take advantage of the presence of any fluid tracking between the fragment and underlying bone (11). The presence of a high signal interface between the fragment and underlying subchondral bone has been a reliable but not invariable indicator of fragment instability (21,41). Additionally, whether the signal changes relate to granulation tissue or intrusion of synovial fluid will have direct implications with regard to the integrity of the overlying cartilage (see below). It is clear, however, that a high signal interface between the fragment and underlying subchondral bone can be seen with intact overlying articular cartilage (Fig. 5.12B). The lack of a high signal interface has been considered reflective of a stable or healed lesion, although experience with MRI of a large number of proven stable lesions is limited (21).

The articular cartilage overlying the osteochondritic lesion may be generally intact, intact but attenuated and frayed (Fig. 5.12), partially or completely disrupted (Figs. 5.8–10, 5.13), or variably replaced by fibrocartilagelike material (Fig. 5.11, 5.14, 5.15). On T1-weighted sequences, focal thinning and upward bowing of otherwise intact cartilage may be demon-

strated (21). The integrity of the low signal intensity stripe representing the subchondral bone plate should be specifically sought in evaluation of these lesions. In the presence of sufficient synovial fluid to provide a natural contrast agent, T2, T2*, and STIR sequences, in which the synovial fluid demonstrates high signal intensity, can facilitate evaluation of the cartilage surface (Figs. 5.8B,D, 5.9B,C 5.10A,B 5.14B). The demonstration of extension of synovial fluid beyond the articular surface between the osteochondral fragment and underlying subchondral bone is definitive evidence of cartilage disruption (Figs. 5.9, 5.13). A potential diagnostic pitfall, however, is the previously discussed high signal intensity interface between the fragment and subchondral bone representing granulation tissue and not extension of synovial fluid through a cartilage defect (21) (Fig. 5.12). As such, the mere presence of a high signal intensity band between the fragment and underlying subchondral bone on T2, T2*, and STIR sequences should not be interpreted as necessarily indicative of cartilage violation (Fig. 5.12). In published series, MRI has tended to overestimate cartilage disruption in talar dome lesions (21). It has been suggested that this relates to persistent signal changes related to prior injury within the cartilage that are no longer demonstrable to visual inspection (44).

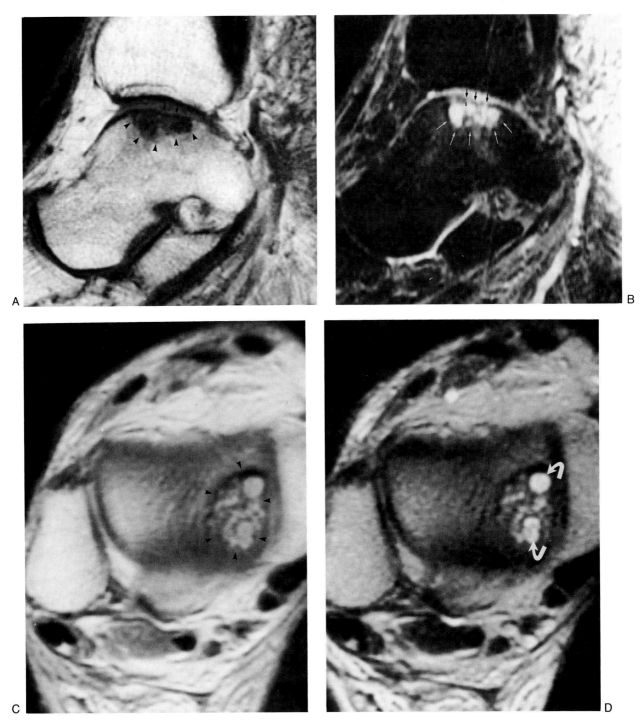

FIG. 5.15. Osteochondritis dissecans. **A:** Sagittal TR 500 TE 30. A 38-year-old man with chronic ankle symptoms. There is a large low signal intensity segment involving subchondral bone along the medial aspect of the talar dome (*arrowheads*). There is flattening and early collapse of the articular surface (*small black arrows*). **B:** Sagittal STIR TR 2200 TE 35 TI 160. The osteochondritic segment becomes markedly hyperintense on this pulse sequence (*small white arrows*). There is slight collapse of the articular surface (*small black arrow*). There is little reactive edema consistent with the chronic nature of the patient's complaints. **C:** Axial TR 2000 TE 20. The size and location of this large lesion is well demonstrated in the axial plane (*arrowheads*). The lesion is composed of several smaller circular to ovoid components. **D:** Axial TR 2000 TE 80. Two discrete subchondral cysts demonstrate markedly increase signal intensity (*curved arrows*). Several smaller cysts and granulation tissue also demonstrate increased signal. At surgery a large necrotic segment was curretted and drilled.

MR Arthrography

As a consequence of the difficulty often experienced in consistently and confidently evaluating the status of the articular cartilage of the talar dome (particularly in the absence of sufficient joint fluid), we have begun to investigate the utility of using intraarticular contrast to assist in this evaluation (Figs. 5.16, 5.17). In much the same manner as CT arthrography, the demonstration of contrast extension from the joint space into the subchondral bone can be considered definitive evidence for cartilage violation. For purposes of MR arthrography, either saline or gadolinium DTPA can be used as the contrast material. When using gadolinium, it is diluted at a ratio of 1 cc of gadolinium to 200 cc of saline. With diluted gadolinium, T1-weighted sequences suffice for assessment of cartilage integrity.

These provide higher signal-to-noise than the T2-weighted images required to provide an arthrogram effect when only saline is injected into the joint. Images are obtained both before and following contrast administration. Before the injection of gadolinium, 1 to 2 cc of iodinated contrast can be injected into the joint and observed fluoroscopically to confirm intraarticular injection. If iodinated contrast is used, it should be limited (1–2 cc) as the presence of iodinated contrast within the joint may change the binding capacity of gadolinium with the DTPA moiety. This may potentially allow for an increase in free gadolinium within the joint, which may become deposited in articular cartilage with potential deleterious effects (45).

The potential role and efficacy of MR arthrography in the assessment of the talar dome has not been the subject to date of any reported critical study. MR ar-

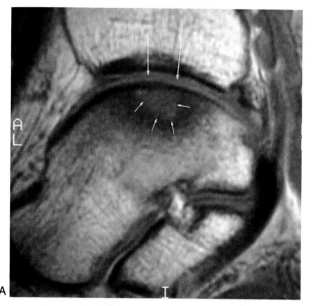

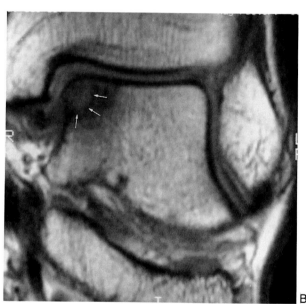

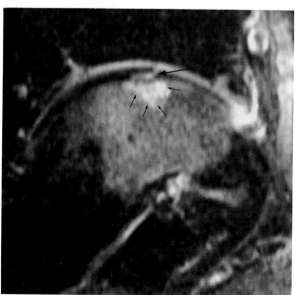

FIG. 5.16. Osteochondritis dissecans: MR arthrography. **A:** Sagittal TR 500 TE 20. A roughly triangular-shaped low signal intensity osteochondritic defect is present (*short arrows*). There is mild surrounding reactive low signal intensity edema. The subchondral bone plate appears intact and there is no evidence of collapse. The articular cartilage appears grossly intact (*long arrows*). **B:** Coronal TR 500 TE 20. The subchondral bone again appears grossly intact. The overlying articular cartilage is more difficult to assess with confidence. The osteochondritic segment is again well visualized (*small arrows*). **C:** Sagittal STIR TR 2200 TE 35 TI 160. The extent of high signal intensity edema throughout much of the body of the talus is far more apparent than on the short TR/TE sequences. The osteochondritic segment demonstrates more localized high signal intensity (*arrows*). An oblique oriented line of high signal crosses the subchondral bone plate suggesting localized disruption (*long arrow*).

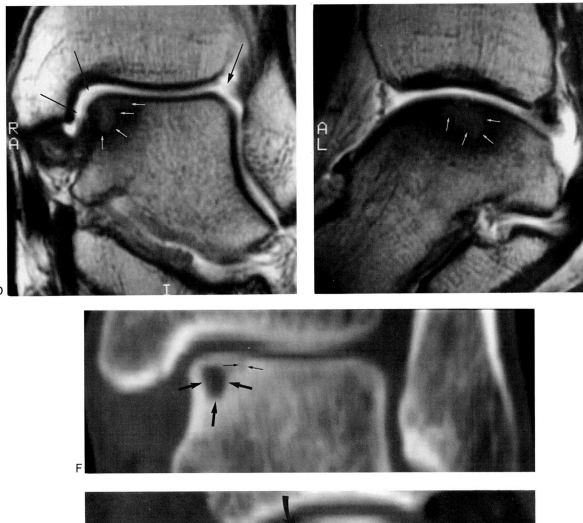

FIG. 5.16. (*Continued*) **D:** Coronal TR 500 TE 20. MR arthrographic image corresponding to the section demonstrated in A. The patient was injected with 10 cc of a diluted solution of gadolinium DTPA. The articular cartilage is well contrasted against the high signal intensity contrast (*arrows*). No contrast material is seen extending into subchondral bone or entering the osteochondritic defect (*arrows*). **E:** Sagittal TR 500 TE 20. The articular cartilage is seen as an intermediate signal intensity layer between the high signal intensity contrast and low signal intensity subchondral bone. No contrast is seen extending beyond the articular surface suggesting cartilage integrity. The osteochondritic defect is again noted. **F:** CT arthrotomogram. Coronal reformatted image. A well-defined circular to ovoid cyst is identified and correlates well with the MR examination (*arrows*). A smaller lesion involving the immediate subchondral bone is also demonstrated and was seen as well on MR (*small arrows*). No contrast could be identified to track into the subchondral lesions. **G:** CT arthrotomogram. Sagittal reformatted image. In addition to the two subchondral cysts (*arrows*), a localized defect in the subchondral bone plate is evident, correlating with the findings on the sagittal STIR image (C) (*curved arrow*). Again, no contrast is seen extending into the subchondral defect to suggest violation of the articular cartilage. At arthroscopy the articular cartilage was attenuated and frayed but grossly intact. The lesion was percutaneously drilled.

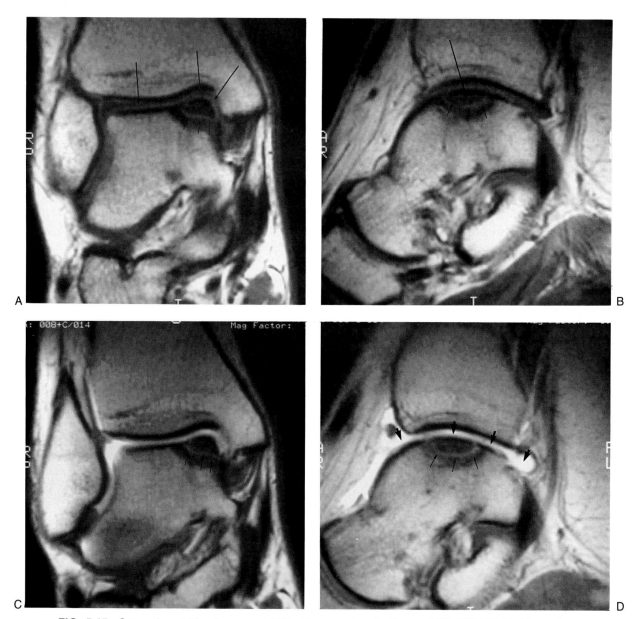

FIG. 5.17. Osteochondritis dissecans. MR arthrography. **A:** Coronal TR 300 TE 20. There is a well-defined osteochondral lesion involving the medial aspect of the talar dome. The fragment is of slightly decreased signal intensity compared to the remainder of the talus. The interface between the fragment and underlying subchondral bone is well delineated and is of slightly increased signal intensity (*small arrows*). The overlying articular cartilage appears grossly intact (*large arrow*). **B:** Sagittal TR 300 TE 20. The well-defined oval-shaped osteochondral lesion is again well depicted. The articular and underlying subchondral interfaces are well defined but not definitively evaluated. **C:** Coronal TR 300 TE 20. Following the intraarticular administration of gadolinium, which appears as high signal intensity, the articular surface can be seen to be intact. No contrast extends into the interface between the fragment and underlying subchondral bone (*small arrows*). **D:** Sagittal TR 300 TE 20. The high signal intensity intraarticular contrast is again well seen and optimally delineates the articular surface (*arrows*). The lack of extension of the contrast between the fragment and underlying subchondral bone further supports the integrity of the overlying articular cartilage (*small arrows*).

thrography appears to be of particular value in cases in which there is a paucity of joint fluid to provide a natural arthrogram effect. In association with high-resolution images and improved signal-to-noise considerations relating to the use of T1- as opposed to T2-weighted images, the surface features of the articular cartilage can be displayed to advantage with intraarticular contrast. It is emphasized, however, that our experience to date remains limited with ankle MR arthrography. Other investigators, using saline and T2-weighted spin-echo imaging, have found the technique quite valuable in assessing talar dome osteochondral injuries (46). There are, however, several obvious arguments against and potential disadvantages to MR arthrography. The principal concern is the changing of a noninvasive examination into an invasive examination with all the risks (e.g., infection) of the procedure. Additionally, the need for fluoroscopy to guide the injection may provide an inconvenience in many scanner settings and complicate scheduling. The use of a contrast agent such as gadolinium may significantly increase the cost of the study as does the need for pre- and postcontrast imaging by increasing the overall examination time. Whether the information acquired using intraarticular contrast will outweigh these other legitimate considerations remains to be determined. Further progress in the noninvasive assessment of articular cartilage may obviate the need for intraarticular contrast.

CONCLUSION

Osteochondral injuries of the talar dome are common problems for which patients seek orthopedic consultation. In the acute setting the injury, if purely chondral, will be entirely radiographically occult, and even if transchondral, in many instances will be subtle, and potentially masked by concern for associated ligamentous and soft tissue injury. MRI, as a result of its ability to image the articular surface directly as well as the underlying subchondral bone, is ideally suited for detection of these injuries. Even in the absence of a single definable acute event, subacute and repetitive microtrauma can result in the development of transchondral fractures—lesions commonly referred to as osteochondritis dissecans. Assessment of the stability of the fracture as well as the integrity of the overlying articular cartilage are important for patient management.

Articular cartilage represents one of the more complex components of the musculoskeletal system and has posed significant challenges for MRI. An understanding of its structure and organization provides a basis for developing rational approaches toward optimizing its depiction and characterization of cartilage abnormalities. Multiple pulse sequence strategies have

been directed toward evaluation of articular cartilage and none has yet received universal approbation. This remains an area of continued and active investigation. Additionally, it is anticipated that with continued improvement in both software and coil technology, higher resolution images, which appear critical for assessment of the talar dome, will be forthcoming, and will likely contribute further to our understanding of osteochondral lesions and our ability to characterize them accurately.

REFERENCES

1. Bauer, M, Jonsson, K, and Linden, B, *Osteochondritis dissecans of the ankle. A 20-year follow-up study.* J Bone Joint Surg, 1987. **69**(1): p. 93–96.
2. Flick, AB and Gould, N, *Osteochondritis dissecans of the talus (transchondral fractures of the talus): Review of the literature and new surgical approach for medial dome lesions.* Foot Ankle, 1985. **5**(4): p. 165–185.
3. Pappas, AM, *Osteochondrosis dissecans.* 1981. **158**: 59–69.
4. Canale, ST and Belding, RH, *Osteochondral lesions of the talus.* J Bone Joint Surg (Am), 1980. **62**: p. 97–102.
5. King, R and Powell, DF, *Injury to the talus*, in *Disorders of the Foot and Ankle. Medical and Surgical Management.*, MH Jahss, Editor. 1991, W.B. Saunders: Philadelphia. p. 2293–2325.
6. Shelton, ML and Pedowitz, WJ, *Injuries to the talar dome, subtalar joint, and mid foot*, in *Disorders of the Foot and Ankle. Medical and Surgical Management.*, MH Jahss, Editor. 1991, WB Saunders: Philadelphia. p. 2274–2292.
7. Lindholm, TS, Osterman, K, and Vankka, E, *Osteochondritis dissecans of elbow, ankle, and hip: A comparison survey.* Clin Orthop, 1980. **148**: p. 245–253.
8. Pritsch, M, Horoshovski, H, and Farine, I, *Arthroscopic treatment of osteochondral lesions of the talus.* J Bone Joint Surg (Am), 1986. **68**: p. 862–865.
9. Lutten, C, Thomas, W, and Dihlmann, W, *Pre- and postoperative magnetic resonance tomography of osteochondrosis dissecans.* ROFO, 1989. **150**(3): p. 290–293.
10. Yulish, BS, Mulopulos, GP, Goodfellow, DB, et al., *MR imaging of osteochondral lesion of talus.* J Comput Assist Tomogr, 1987. **11**(2): p. 296–301.
11. Nelson, DW, DiPaola, J, Colville, M, et al., *Osteochondritis dissecans of the talus and knee: Prospective comparison of MR and arthroscopic classifications.* J Comput Assist Tomogr, 1990. **14**(5): p. 804–808.
12. Totterman, S, Weiss, SL, Szumowski, J, et al., *MR fat suppression technique in the evaluation of normal structures of the knee.* JCAT, 1989. **13**: p. 473–478.
13. Wojtys, E, Wilson, M, Buchwalter, K, et al., *Magnetic resonance imaging of knee hyaline cartilage and intraarticular pathology.* Am J Sports Med, 1987. **15**(5): p. 455–463.
14. Yulish, BS, Montanez, J, Goodfellow, DB, et al., *Chondromalacia patella: Assessment with MR imaging.* Radiology, 1987. **164**: p. 763–766.
15. Buckwalter, JA, Rosenberg, LC, and Hunziker, EB, *Articular cartilage: Composition, structure, response to injury, and methods of facilitating repairs*, in *Articular Cartilage and Knee Joint Function: Basic Science and Arthroscopy*, JW Ewing, Editor. 1990, Raven Press: New York. p. 19–54.
16. Buckwalter, JA, *Articular Cartilage*, in *American Academy of Orthopaedic Surgeons instructional course lectures.* 1983, CV Mosby: St. Louis. p. 349–370.
17. Mow, VC, Fithian, DC, and Kelly, MA, *Fundamentals of articular cartilage and meniscus biomechanics*, in *Articular Cartilage and Knee Joint Function: Basic Science and Arthroscopy*, JW Ewing, Editor. 1990, Raven Press: New York. p. 1–18.
18. Arnoczky, SP. *Articular cartilage injury and repair*, in *Twelfth international seminar on operative arthroscopy.* 1990. Kauai, Hawaii.

19. Lehner, KB, Rechl, HP, Gemeinwieser, JK, *et al.*, *Structure, function, and degeneration of bovine hyaline cartilage: Assessment with MR imaging in vitro.* Radiology, 1989. **170**: p. 495–499.

20. Buckwalter, JA, Hunziker, E, Rosenberg, LC, *et al.*, *Articular cartilage: Composition and Structure*, in *Injury and Repair of the Musculoskeletal Soft Tissues*, S.L. Woo and J.A. Buckwalter, Editors. 1988, American Academy of Orthopaedic Surgeons: Park Ridge, IL. p. 405–425.

21. De Smet, AA, Fisher, DR, Bernstein, MI, *et al.*, *Value of MR imaging in staging osteochondral lesions of the talus (osteochondritis dissecans): Results in 14 patients.* AJR, 1990. **154**: p. 555–558.

22. Gylys-Morin, VM, Hajek, PC, Sartoris, DJ, *et al.*, *Articular cartilage defects: Detectability in cadaver knees with MR.* AJR, 1987. **148**: p. 1153–1157.

23. Handleberg, F, Shahabpour, M, and Casteleyn, PP, *Chondral lesions of the patella evaluated with computed tomography, magnetic resonance imaging, and arthroscopy.* J Arthrosc, 1990. **6**(1): p. 24–29.

24. Hayes, CW, Sawyer, RW, and Conway, WF, *Patellar cartilage lesions: In vitro detection and staging with MR imaging and pathologic correlation.* Radiology, 1990. **176**: p. 479–483.

25. Konig, H, Sauter, R, Deimling, M, *et al.*, *Cartilage disorders: Comparison of spin-echo, CHESS, and FLASH sequence MR images.* Radiology, 1987. **164**: p. 753–758.

26. Chandnani, VP, Ho C, Chu P, *et al.*, *Knee hyaline cartilage evaluated with MR imaging: A cadaveric study involving multiple imaging sequences and intraarticular injection of gadolinium and saline solution.* Radiology, 1991. **178**: p. 557–561.

26a. McCauley, TR, Kier, R, Lynch, KJ, Kohl, P, *Chondromalacia patellae: Diagnosis with MR imaging.* AJR, 1992. **158**: p. 101–105.

27. Wehrli, FW and Atlas, SW, *Fast imaging: Principles, techniques and clinical application*, in *Magnetic Resonance Imaging of the Brain and Spine*, Atlas, SW, Editor. 1991, Raven Press: New York. p. 1013–1078.

28. Prorok, RJ, *Signa Application Guide, Volume II.* GE medical systems.

29. Braunstein, EM, Brandt, KD, and Albrecht, M, *MRI demonstration of hypertrophic articular cartilage repair in osteoarthritis.* Skeletal Radiol, 1990. **19**: p. 335–339.

30. Konig, F, *Veber freie Korper in den Gelenken.* Dtsch Z Chir, 1888. **27**: p. 90–109.

31. Kappis, M, *Weitere Beitrage Zur traumatisch-mechanischen Enstehung der "spontanen" knorpelabiosungen.* Dtsch Z Chir, 1922. **171**: p. 13–29.

32. Rendu, A, *Fracture intra-articular parcellaire de la poulie astraglienne.* 1932. **150**: p. 220–222.

33. Fairbank, HAT, *Osteochondritis dissecans.* J Surg (Br), 1933. **21**: p. 67–82.

34. Berndt, AL and Harty, M, *Transchondral fractures (osteochondritis dissecans) of the talus.* J Bone Joint Surg, 1959. **41A**: p. 988–1020.

35. Resnick, D, Goergen, TG, and Niwayama, G, *Physical injury*, in *Diagnosis of Bone and Joint Disorders*, D Resnick and G Niwayama, Editors. 1988, W.B. Saunders: Philadelphia. p. 2756–3009.

36. Lutten, C, Lorenz, H, and Thomas, W, *Refixation in osteochondrosis dissecans with resorbable material using magnetic resonance tomography in follow-up monitoring.* Sportverletz Sportschaden, 1988. **2**(2): p. 61–68.

37. Convery, FR, Keown, GH, *et al.*, *The repair of large osteochondral defects: An experimental study in horses.* Clin Orthop, 1972. **82**: p. 253.

38. Parisien, JS, *Arthroscopic treatment of osteochondral lesion of the talus.* Am J Sports Med, 1986. **14**(3): p. 211–217.

39. Heare, MM, Gillespy, TI, and Bittar, ES, *Direct coronal computed tomography arthrography of osteochondritis dissecans of the talus.* Skeletal Radiol, 1988. **17**(3): p. 187–189.

40. Zinman, C, Wolfson, N, and Reis, ND, *Osteochondritis dissecans of the dome of the talus. Computed tomography scanning in diagnosis and follow-up.* J Bone Joint Surg, 1988. **70A**(7): p. 1017–1019.

41. Mesgarzadeh, M, Sapega, AA, Bonakdarpour, A, *et al.*, *Osteochondritis dissecans: Analysis of mechanical stability with radiography, scintigraphy, and MR imaging.* Radiology, 1987. **165**: p. 775–780.

42. Bueche, MJ, *Osteochondritis dissecans of the dome of the talus. Computed tomography scanning in the diagnosis and follow-letter [letter-; comment].* J Bone Joint Surg, 1989. **71A**(4): p. 632.

43. Anderson, IF, Chichton, KJ, Grattan-Smith, T, *et al.*, *Osteochondral fractures of the dome of the talus. (ab).* Radiology, 1990. **174**: p. 902.

44. De Smet, AA, Fisher, DR, Graf, BK, *et al.*, *Osteochondritis dissecans of the knee: Value of MR imaging in determining lesion stability and the presence of articular cartilage defects.* AJR, 1990. **155**: p. 549–553.

45. Brahme, S., *MR arthrography of the shoulder*, in *Annual Meeting International Skeletal Society.* 1991. San Diego, California.

46. Pathria, M. Personal communication.

47. Buckwalter, JA, *The fine structure of human intervertebral disc*, in *American Academy of Orthopedic Surgeons Symposium on Idiopathic Low Back Pain*, AA White, III, SL Gordon, Editors. 1982, CV Mosby: St. Louis, p. 108–143.

48. Lane, JM and Weiss, C, *Current comment: Review of articular cartilage collagen research.* Arthritis Rheum, 1975. **18**: p. 558–568.

MRI of the Foot and Ankle,
edited by A.L. Deutsch, J.H. Mink, and R. Kerr,
Raven Press, Ltd., New York © 1992

CHAPTER 6

Tendons

Jerrold H. Mink

Tendon is an inelastic tissue whose primary function is to transmit motion passively from a contracting muscle to a bone or fascia. Tendons are composed primarily of collagen, elastin, and reticulin fibers, materials that give them strength, flexibility, and bulk. The collagen fibers, which dominate the composition of the tendon, are oriented in a parallel wavy pattern that, under tension, straighten along the direction of the load (1). This arrangement accounts for the ability of a tendon to withstand tensile loads more than twice that of its associated muscle (2,3). When the load is released, the elastic fibers facilitate reorientation of the collagen into its resting wavy configuration. Tendons are injured when excessive tensile force is applied, leading to overstretch or a strain. The yield point of collagen occurs when there has been a 6% to 8% increase in length; elastic fibers may increase to twice their length without failure. Collagen, however, is considerably stronger than elastic fibers; collagen can withstand half the tensile stress of cortical bone, whereas elastic fibers tolerate only 10% of such stress.

Tendon injuries that occur in the athlete result from sudden changes in direction, acceleration, or deceleration, and not from forces involved in maintaining static equilibrium (4). Risk factors that predispose to tendon injury include inadequate warm-up, steroid injections, eccentric muscle contractions, prior injury, immobilization, unusual and unaccustomed high levels of activity, and poor conditioning. The dynamic forces that develop in a tendon are a function of the volume of contracting muscle as well as the speed at which it contracts in response to those changes. Rapid contraction of a muscle causes a significant increase in the force within the associated tendon. This may occur with either voluntary maximum push off or an invol-

untary violent reflex contraction in an effort to stabilize the associated joint (4).

Following injury, the tendon and tendon sheath follow a standard sequence of pathologic changes. The first alterations are a disruption of the well-ordered parallel arrangement of collagen fiber (5). With increasing degrees of damage, there is an increase in fibroblasts, endothelial cells, and blood vessel formation. Classical inflammation, consisting of polymorphonuclear leukocytes, is notably absent. The cellular response is usually composed of lymphocytes, monocytes, and a few plasma cells. The final stage of injury and repair is fibrosis; the tendon fibers are twisted and interlaced with new collagen in a haphazard configuration.

Injury to a tendon is termed a strain, which is defined as damage to the musculotendinous unit occasioned by overuse (chronic) or overstretch (acute) (6). A clinical classification system attempting to quantify the degree of acute tendon injury has been established, although it is obvious that precise assessment of the degree of damage is not possible. First degree strains result in very minor amounts of disruption of the structure. Pathologic changes are confined to a low grade inflammatory process. There is swelling, edema, and some discomfort on use of the affected tendon, but there is no loss of strength or restriction of motion. Treatment is directed at relief of symptoms and protection from further damage. Second degree strains are more significant, but still incomplete disruptions. The distinction between first and second degree injuries is the extent to which pathological alteration has occurred. In second degree strains, however, there is enough damage to the unit to result in measurable loss of function. Protection is the primary focus of treatment since by definition, functional damage has occurred. Adequate treatment will result in recovery, but unaltered continuation of activity will result in chronic impairment. Third degree strains imply complete rup-

J.H. Mink: Tower Musculoskeletal Imaging Center, Los Angeles, California 90048.

ture with total or near total discontinuity and major loss of function; surgical reconstitution is essential.

Thirteen tendons cross the ankle joint. They are the peroneus longus and brevis laterally; the Achilles tendon posteriorly; the posterior tibial, flexor hallucis longus, and flexor digitorum medially; the anterior tibial, extensor hallucis longus, extensor digitorum, and peroneus tertius anteriorly. Except for the Achilles tendon, all of the above alter their course from a vertically oriented structure at the distal leg to one oriented horizontally at the foot. They achieve this change in direction by means of a pulley system; in the case of the medial and lateral tendons, the pulley is a bony structure (the malleoli), whereas for the anterior tendons, the soft tissue retinacula provide the fulcrum for direction change.

Two types of tendon investiture can be identified (2,7,8). In locations where the tendons are subjected to high friction forces, as where they must undergo a sudden change in direction, they are invested with a sheath lined by parietal synovium. The necessity of a tendon sheath is evident where two structures move relative to one another, as through a fibro-osseous tunnel (flexor hallucis longus tendon through the talus), under a bony pulley (peroneal tendons under the lateral malleolus), or under a fascial sling (anterior tibial tendon under the extensor retinaculum). The fluid generated by the lining synovial cells facilitates the gliding of the tendon through these high friction regions. The tendon sheath arises from the periosteum and is bordered by the joint complex on its innermost part, forming an osteofibrous groove; ligament and fascia comprise the outer layer of the sheath. In regions where friction forces are minimal, only loose connective tissue, termed the peritenon, surrounds the tendon. The Achilles tendon is the only example of such an arrangement at the ankle.

Tenosynovitis refers to inflammation of the investing soft tissues of the tendon whereas tendonitis refers to an injury or symptomatic degeneration of the tendon itself with secondary inflammation of the synovium or peritenon (9). Tenosynovitis and tendonitis may of course coexist. Inciting factors for tenosynovitis in the lower extremity include direct trauma, late sequelae of fracture, ankle sprains, tendon ruptures, inflammatory arthritis, occupational stress, anatomic anomalies, and increased functional demands caused by static foot deformities (7,8).

The normally avascular synovium reacts to an injury with increased blood supply, generation of inflammatory cells, and oversecretion of synovial fluid with increased fibrin content. This results in adhesions between the tendon and its sheath. The first clinical manifestations of tenosynovitis are crepitation and pain on function. Eventually, the tendon and its sheath become bound together in an inflammatory mass, and the normal gliding motion that occurs between tendon and synovium becomes restricted and ultimately nonexistent. Stenosing, or constrictive tenosynovitis, refers to thickening of the walls of the sheath and narrowing of its lumen (6). This occurs most frequently in those sheaths in which more than one tendon resides (i.e., the peroneal longus and brevis). Peritendonitis refers to pathologic changes identical to those of tenosynovitis, but the former occurs in the loose peritenon about those tendons without a sheath.

IMAGING ASSESSMENT

Until the advent of high-resolution computed tomographic (CT) scanning, the imaging assessment of tendon disorders was limited to those tendons that were surrounded by abundant fat (e.g., the Achilles tendon). The silhouette of the tendon was outlined using low kilovoltage radiographic techniques and xeroradiography (10). Tenography, while an easy procedure to perform and one that does yield important clinical information, achieved rather little popularity as a general diagnostic tool, except in the assessment of the integrity of the calcaneofibular ligament (11–14). Superficial tendons such as the patellar tendon, quadriceps, and Achilles tendons can be examined by ultrasound, but the technique is restricted by overlying structures, limited anatomic detail, and the inability to image bone (8,15–17).

CT has the ability to visualize tendons directly and permits the diagnosis of complete ruptures and limited evaluation of the presence of internal structural lesions (18–22). The contour of the tendon, however, may be obscured by surrounding edema and inflammatory exudate in the tendon sheaths, making evaluation difficult or even erroneous. Additionally, examination of tendons by CT is usually limited to the axial plane since reformatted images generally contain less information than that present in the images generated from a direct scanning plane (15,19,21).

Although magnetic resonance imaging (MRI) assessment of the tendons is a relatively new innovation, early experience suggests that MRI presents significant advantages over CT and ultrasound in assessing traumatic, inflammatory, and infectious tendon abnormalities (9,15,23,24). These advantages include inherently greater soft tissue contrast than any other currently available imaging modality, lack of ionizing radiation, lack of streak artifact, ability to image both bone and soft tissue satisfactorily, and the capability of direct multiplanar imaging (24). The radiologist and clinician can directly image not only the contour abnormalities that occur with many tendinous conditions, but also those aberrations of internal structure that characterize acute and chronic tendonitis, partial tears, and complete tears.

Although every examination should be individualized to answer the clinical question at hand most optimally, certain technical generalizations about MRI assessment of tendons of the foot and ankle may be made (8,25–27). Only the affected limb is examined in a high-resolution send-receive coil (General Electric Medical Systems, Milwaukee, WI). This coil permits the use of a small field of view (12–14 cm), which optimizes image quality and maximizes signal-to-noise. Alternatively, two 3-inch or two 5-inch general purpose coils may be linked together electronically, but the use of a body coil as the receiving instrument has proved unsatisfactory.

We have chosen to divide the foot and ankle into three "examination zones": the hindfoot and ankle, the midfoot, and the forefoot. We have made this anatomic/imaging division for several reasons: (1) the disease processes that affect each zone are often different (osteochondritis dissecans and tendon ruptures occur in the hindfoot; infectious processes occur in the toes and forefoot), (b) the imaging demands for each area are different, and the coils and patient positioning may need to be adjusted for each region. If one chooses a 12- to 14-cm field of view, the hindfoot examination will include the distal tibial metaphysis above, the Achilles tendon posteriorly, the plantar soft tissues inferiorly, and the navicular distally (or the cuneiforms, depending on body size and the precise position of the patient). The midfoot examination will include most of the talus and calcaneus, the cuneiforms, and the metatarsals. The forefoot examination will include the phalanges, the metatarsals, and portions of the tarsals.

For examination of the hindfoot or the midfoot, the patient lies supine and the foot and ankle are positioned within the coil so that the medial malleolus is in the center of the coil. The foot is allowed to lie in a relaxed position; most patients will choose a position that places the foot in 10° to 20° of plantar flexion, and 10° to 30° of external rotation. Permitting the patient to choose a comfortable posture helps insure that motion artifact will be minimized, especially during performance of long repitition (TR) and echo (TE) sequences (28). Specialized positioning, such as purposeful plantar flexion of the foot, may be helpful when performing tailored examinations for detailed problem-solving situations (e.g., assessment of the degree of approximation of the edges of a torn Achilles tendon).

Examination of the forefoot and the toes may be technically challenging. It would be ideal to allow the patient to lie supine (a more comfortable position than the prone position), but one must then have the patient bend the knees so that the toes can be centered within the coil. Alternatively, one can place the patient in a prone position, which makes centering of the foot easier, but often older patients are unable to tolerate the prone position for the relatively long imaging times

used in foot/ankle examinations. Placing one foot in the head coil with the patient in the supine position may be an acceptable alternative. Only rarely in cases in which bilateral disease is suspected is it reasonable to opt for comparison to the opposite side with both feet being placed in a head coil. We have in almost all cases chosen to examine each foot separately rather than compromise the study by increasing the field of view to accommodate both limbs.

Because of their extremely low water content, tendons have very low signal at all pulse sequences (9,15,23,24,28,29). In most situations, T1-weighted images (T1WI) resulting in high contrast between the dark tendon and the bright signal from the surrounding fat yield images of excellent anatomic detail (9). T1WI sequences are most frequently used in the sagittal and occasionally the axial planes. In the axial plane (we define the axial plane as the plane perpendicular to the shafts of the metatarsals, a situation analogous to the hand), long TR studies yield a series of images of good anatomic detail (proton density images), as well as high tissue contrast (long TE) images, maximizing the contrast between a tendon sheath and its contained tendon. In the sagittal plane, long TR/TE, gradient recalled (GRASS), and inversion recovery (STIR) sequences are used to optimize the contrast between the dark tendon and the abnormal increase in water content in the tendon, which characterizes most pathologic processes. In the case of the latter two sequences, there is high conspicuity and contrast that occurs at the expense of resolution of anatomic detail.

For most examinations using the send-receive extremity coil, we choose a 3-mm slice thickness without an interslice gap. A 256 matrix size using one excitation is used when performing a T1WI sequence. The field of view is chosen between 12 and 14 cm. Such an imaging protocol yields an in-plane spatial resolution of 0.47 to 0.62 mm (26). When a T2WI sequence is used, the TR is 2500 to 3000 ms, which allows for the required number of slices; the matrix size is reduced to 128 and two excitations are chosen, while maintaining the slice thickness at 3 to 4 mm without an interslice gap. Most recently, fast spin-echo techniques have been successfully employed to reduce the time necessary to complete long TR/TE sequences while taking advantage of 256 matrix imaging. We have replaced our standard T2 sequences detailed above with the following technique. The TR is chosen between 3000 and 3500, depending on the number of slices necessary to cover the selected area; the double echo TE combination is typically set at 18 to 21/120. A 256 × 256 matrix size and three skip-one spacing with one excitation completes the imaging selections. This sequence can be accomplished in approximately one-half the time of the conventional sequence while achieving a study of higher resolution (256 vs. 128 matrix size).

Two imaging planes with at least two different pulse sequences should be performed in every case to ensure proper assessment of both internal signal and external contour abnormalities, and for the determination of the longitudinal extent of a tendon lesion (26,30). Examination in the axial plane of the affected tendon permits optimal assessment of its contour, the degree of distention of its sheath with fluid, and its relationship to surrounding structures. The axial plane of the tendon is defined as a plane perpendicular to the long axis of the affected tendon at the suspected site of pathology (e.g., the submalleolar region for the posterior tibial tendon). The nonorthogonal axial plane is chosen from a sagittal localizer image demonstrating the longitudinal contour of the tendon. The choice of an unconventional plane reduces the degree of partial volume effect of the tendon with bone and reduces the likelihood of imaging the tendon obliquely at the site of pathology. The full longitudinal extent of a tendinous abnormality is best assessed in the sagittal plane. Rarely is the coronal plane of value for assessment of the tendons of the foot and ankle

THE ACHILLES TENDON

The Achilles tendon is the largest and strongest tendon in the body. It is capable of withstanding forces 5 to 6 times body weight during running or jumping (31,32). The Achilles tendon is the most commonly injured tendon in the foot; in all, Achilles tendon injuries account for 6.5% to 11% of all running injuries (33,34). The tendon is formed by the confluence of the individual tendons of the gastrocnemius and soleus muscles. The gastrocnemius origin is from the lateral and medial femoral condyles, whereas the soleus originates from the posterior aspect of the tibia and fibula. In the most common arrangement, the gastrocnemius contributes two-thirds of the fibers of the Achilles tendon posteriorly and the soleus contributes one-third, but variations on this pattern occur (35). In adults, the tendon is about 10 to 15 cm in length, and has a uniform thickness of 4 to 7 mm (10,36). The Achilles tendon is rather cordlike proximally but fans out just above its insertion so it becomes twice as wide as it is thick (10). Approximately 6 cm from the insertion of the tendon on the posterior aspect of the calcaneus, the fibers of the Achilles tendon take a spiral twist so that the posterior fibers go from a more medial to a more lateral position and the anterior fibers go from lateral to medial (3,35). Unfortunately, this same area has a somewhat tenuous blood supply because the vessels supplying the region are longitudinally oriented and the end vessels are far removed from their origins. The tendon is therefore dependent on short, transversely oriented vessels of the mesotenon for its vascularity (31,34,35,37). Ruptures most commonly occur at this vascular watershed area just above the twist. Ruptures at the musculotendinous junction, so-called tennis leg, are actually ruptures of the medial head of the gastrocnemius.

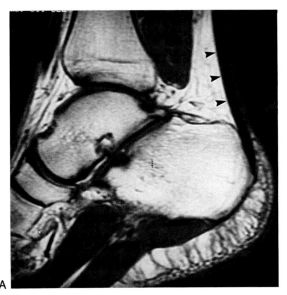
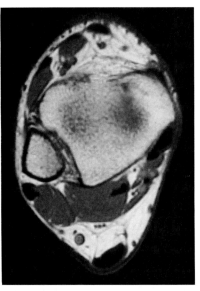

FIG. 6.1. Normal Achilles tendon. **A:** Sagittal MR, TR/TE 500/20. The normal Achilles tendon (*arrowheads*) is sharply demarcated anteriorly by the pre-Achilles fat. From the musculotendinous junction to its insertion, the Achilles tendon has a constant anteroposterior dimension of 4–8 mm. **B:** Axial MR, TR/TE 500/20. This axial sequence is made at the level of the distal tibial epiphysis. The Achilles tendon has a flattened anterior aspect, with rounded sides and posterior margin. Further caudally at the level of the mid-talus.

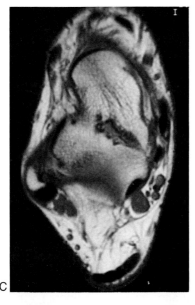

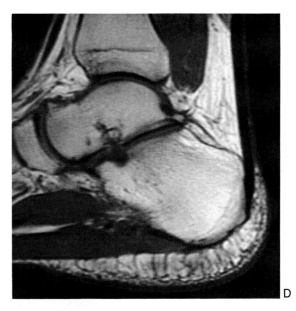

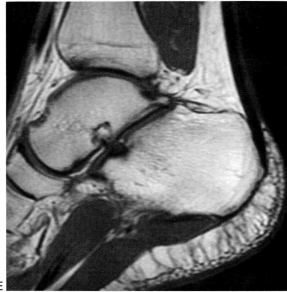

FIG. 6.1. (*Continued*) **C**: Axial MR, TR/TE 500/20. The Achilles widens in its sagittal dimension and assumes a somewhat more ovoid appearance. **D, E**: Sagittal MR, TR/TE 800/20. There is no appreciable change in the shape or the thickness of the Achilles tendon when the foot is in slight dorsi (D) or plantar (E) flexion.

The Achilles tendon is best examined by MRI in both its sagittal and true axial planes (9,36,38,39) (Fig. 6.1). In the axial plane, the normal tendon has a flat to slightly concave anterior margin and rounded medial, posterior, and lateral aspects that give the tendon a crescentic shape. Just above its insertion onto the calcaneus, the tendon assumes a more ovoid and anteriorly flattened configuration. In the sagittal plane, the anterior edge of the tendon is uniformly straight and contrasts sharply with the adjacent fat (T1WI). As with all other tendons, the Achilles tendon demonstrates low signal on all pulse sequences (36).

Achilles tendon injuries are best classified as acute tendonitis and peritendonitis, chronic tendonitis, acute and chronic partial tears, and complete ruptures. Peritendonitis refers to pathological alterations that occur in the peritenon, the tissue in which the earliest changes of Achilles tendon injury occur, whereas the tern tendonitis infers devitalization and disruption of tendon fascicles (32,34,35). Acute tendonitis and peritendonitis may result from a sudden increase in athletic training frequency or intensity, running on hills, tibia vara, tight hamstrings, and cavus feet. Frequently, overpronation of the foot produces a whipping action of the Achilles as the tendon moves from a relatively lateral position at the time of heel strike to a medial position as the foot rolls into pronation; such actions result in an inflammatory response along the medial aspect of the tendon (34). Ischemia may also play a role in the development of Achilles tendonitis. With increased use of the soleus, there is muscular hypertrophy, which increases the intrafascial pres-

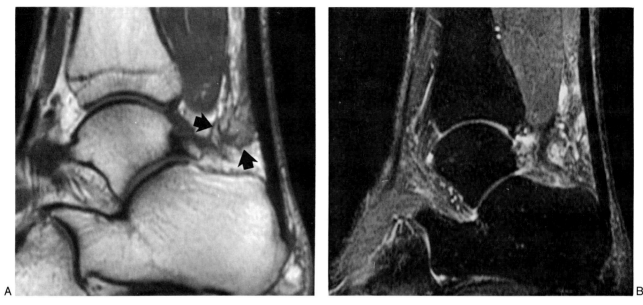

FIG. 6.2. Achilles peritendonitis. **A**: Sagittal MR, TR/TE 500/20. There is an infiltrative "mass" seen in the pre-Achilles fat (*arrows*) that is continuous with the anterior surface of a normally shaped Achilles tendon. **B**: On a STIR sequence (sagittal MR TR/TE/TI 2200/35/160), the mass inhomogeneously brightens. The initial lesion in Achilles tendon disease does not primarily involve the tendon.

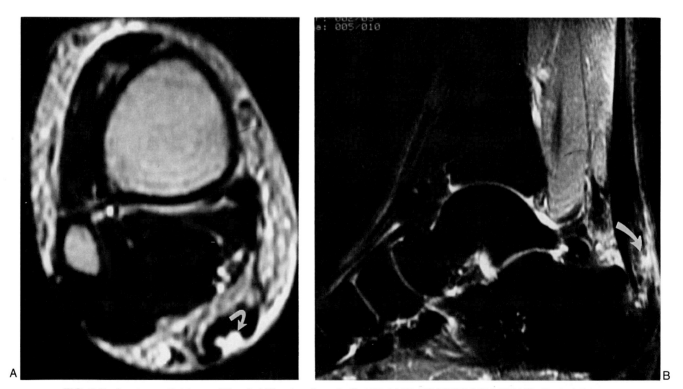

FIG. 6.3. Acute partial tear of the Achilles tendon. **A**: Sagittal MR, TR/TE/TI 2200/35/160. **B**: Axial MR, TR/TE 2000/80. A focus of high signal is seen within the dorsal one-half of the Achilles tendon (*arrows*), and edema is present both within the fat pad and in the subcutaneous tissue.

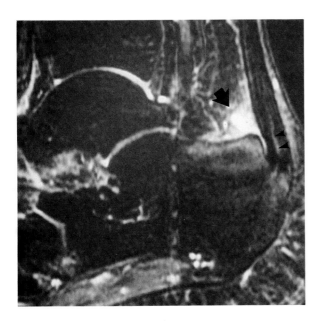

FIG. 6.4. Acute partial Achilles tendon. Sagittal MR, TR/TE/TI 2200/35/160. The distal tendon is widened with longitudinal stripes of high signal (*arrowheads*) in its substance. There is edema of the pre-Achilles fat in the region of the retrocalcaneal bursa (*arrow*). This young male had the sudden onset of pain while playing basketball.

sure, reduces normal blood flow, and results in secondary ischemia of the tendon itself (40). Since the Achilles tendon does not have a true synovial sheath, the primary inflammatory process, termed peritendonitis, occurs in the peritenon (41). Edema, and ultimately thickening and scar formation, manifest themselves by linear and globular foci of decreased signal in the normally bright fat pad (T1WI) immediately adjacent to the anterior margin of the tendon, while the tendon itself maintains a normal contour and internal (dark) signal (Fig. 6.2). Microfractures of the tendon

eventually result in partial tears that are manifest by foci of high intratendinous signal on T2WI, STIR, and GRASS sequences (Figs. 6.3-6.5).

With proper rest, training, and alteration of shoe and running style, most episodes of acute tendonitis will resolve; ''running through'' an episode of acute Achilles tendonitis, however, can result in conversion to a chronic condition (41). When the inflammatory process becomes chronic, longitudinal splits appear within the tendon, and small foci of mucoid degeneration develop (32,36,41); it is this degenerative mate-

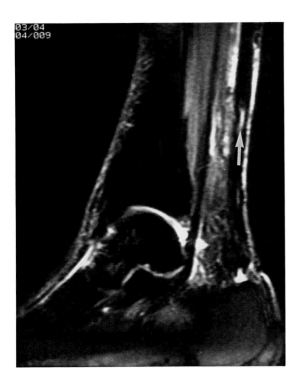

FIG. 6.5. Acute partial tear of the Achilles tendon. Sagittal MR, TR/TE/TI 2200/35/160. The extent of the proximal tear is best appreciated on this STIR sequence. A linear focus of high signal (*arrow*) identifies the site of the tear while T1W sequences did not demonstrate the lesion. Superficial and deep edema surround the proximal tendon.

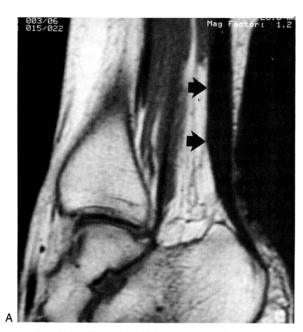
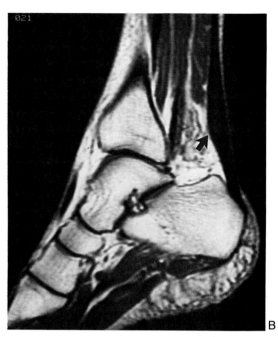

A   B

FIG. 6.6. Chronic Achilles tendonitis. **A**, and **B**: Sagittal MR, TR/TE 800/20. These images are from two different patients and demonstrate the manifestations of chronic Achilles tendonitis. In A, the tendon is thickened throughout its length. In B, there is focal anteroposterior enlargement (*arrow*) of the Achilles tendon.

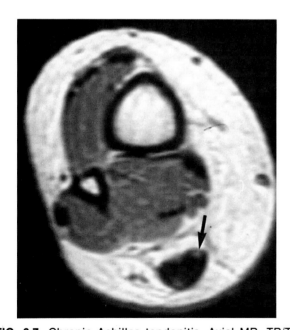

FIG. 6.7. Chronic Achilles tendonitis. Axial MR, TR/TE 500/20. The Achilles tendon has a much more rounded appearance than normal, and its anteroposterior dimension is increased. Multiple small foci of increased signal are seen within the tendon substance on this Tl-weighted image (*arrow*); all became "invisible" on a long TR sequence.

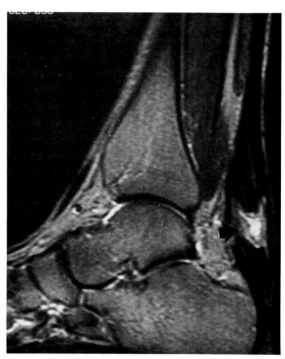

FIG. 6.8. Chronic Achilles tendonitis with an acute partial tear. Sagittal MR, TR/TE 2000/80. Nearly the entire length of the Achilles tendon is markedly widened. A focal area of extremely high signal (*arrow*), indicating the site of the partial tear, is superimposed on an otherwise dark tendon. This aerobic exerciser has had chronic ankle pain, and experienced a pop in the ankle after which he was unable to continue to work out.

rial that is excised if surgical therapy of chronic Achilles tendonitis is deemed necessary (3). On MRI, the hallmark finding of chronic Achilles tendonitis is widening of the tendon contour (Figs. 6.6-6.8). Widening, which may be focal or diffuse, is most readily appreciated along the normally flat to concave anterior surface of the tendon (9,31,36,42–46). Subtle diffuse lesions may go unnoticed unless the examiner remembers that the anteroposterior dimension of the Achilles tendon should not exceed 8 mm. Most commonly, a tendon that is chronically inflamed shows morphologic changes, but no intratendinous signal alteration (31,43); if small foci of increased signal are seen on T1WI images, they may become "invisible" on long TR/TE images (Fig. 6.7). In cases in which a tear is superimposed on a background of chronic tendonitis, the tendon is abnormally widened, and foci of increased signal are found on both T1WI and T2WI (44)

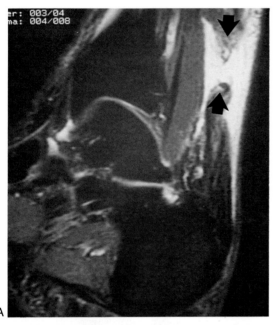

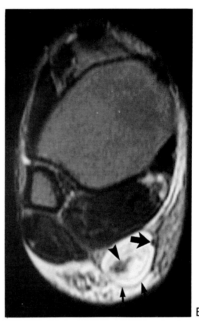

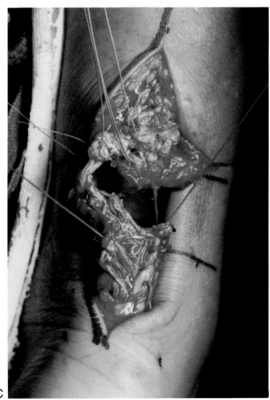

FIG. 6.9. Complete Achilles tendon rupture **A**: Sagittal MR, TR/TE/TI 2200/35/160. The torn ends of the Achilles tendon are separated by 2–3 cm (*arrows*). There is massive edema subcutaneously and deep to the Achilles tendon. In **B**, (axial MR, TR/TE 2200/80), blood and edema are seen to fill the peritenon (*small arrows*). The globular dark foci in the lateral side of the peritenon (*arrowhead*) represent tiny threads of Achilles tendon that were not in continuity at surgery. The small dark focus in the medial side represents the intact plantaris tendon (*arrow*). **C**: This operative photograph demonstrates the wide gap between the torn edges of this completely ruptured Achilles tendon. (Fig. 6.9C courtesy of Frank Shellock, Ph.D.)

(Fig. 6.8). Histological examination of *patellar* tendons afflicted with chronic tears have shown that high signal foci on T2WI represent regions of synovial hyperplasia, fibrinoid necrosis, and inflammatory response (43). This increased signal is consistent with the MRI appearance of necrosis and inflammation elsewhere in the musculoskeletal system. The differentiation of chronic tendonitis with a coexistent tear versus an acute, partial tear may be based solely on history (27).

Complete rupture of the Achilles tendon occurs in unconditioned "weekend athletes" in their third to fifth decades of lie; professional athletes of any age can be affected (3,47). Women uncommonly suffer complete Achilles tendon ruptures except for ballet dancers over the age of 30 (32). In both sexes, the left Achilles tendon is more commonly ruptured than the right, but bilateral rupture has been reported (10,31,48). Systemic and local disorders such as rheumatoid arthritis, gout, hyperparathyroidism, chronic renal failure, diabetes, and steroid injections may weaken the tendon, but most commonly, no predisposing factors can be identified. A perfectly normal Achilles tendon is said not to rupture, and therefore it is assumed that peritendonitis or chronic tendonitis always precedes rupture (32,47). Numerous microfrac-

tures of the collagen fibrils of the tendon occur as a result of recurrent stress; these coalesce over time. Ultimately, tendinous repair is unable to keep pace with degeneration because the vascular supply of the region is tenuous; failure finally occurs (9). Complete rupture typically occurs during push off, jumping with the knee extended, landing with the foot in dorsiflexion, or by direct trauma (42).

The differentiation of a complete tear from a partial tear or from a rupture at the musculotendinous junction may be clinically difficult, and the therapy for each injury is different (49). Therefore, correct preoperative diagnosis is critical. Although complete Achilles tendon rupture is associated with excruciating, unremitting pain, the lesion is misdiagnosed in 25% of patients (4,15,31,40). Neither the Thompson test nor the needle test, both of which are designed to test the flexing capability of the muscle/tendon are infallible (10,49). The marked edema and hemorrhage that accompany the rupture make physical examination difficult, and plantar flexion of the affected ankle is often preserved by action of the posterior tibial tendon, the peroneals, and the flexor hallucis longus.

Rupture of the Achilles tendon is manifest on MRI by gross widening of the tendon contour (often to 3–

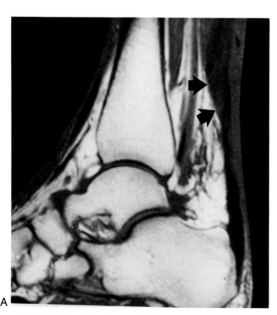

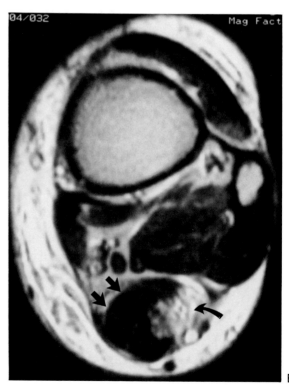

FIG. 6.10. Rupture of the musculotendinous junction of the Achilles ("tennis leg"). **A**: Sagittal MR, TR/TE 500/20. **B**: Axial MR, TR/TE 2000/80. There is marked distortion of the musculotendinous junction of the Achilles tendon. As seen on the axial sequence, the pathologic process in fact is a tear of the distal muscle. In this image, the tendon is somewhat medial (*arrows*) and is essentially intact, while the muscular portion (*curved arrow*) demonstrates disruption and edema of its internal architecture.

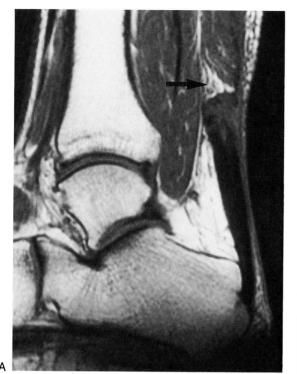 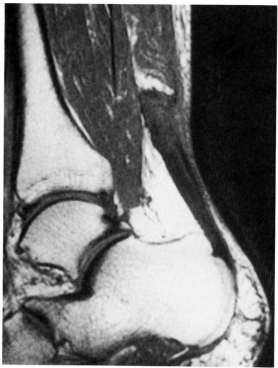

FIG. 6.11. Rupture of the Achilles tendon; effect of plantar flexion on the tear. **A, B**: Sagittal MR, TR/TE 500/20. This patient suffered a tear of the Achilles tendon quite near the musculotendinous junction (*arrow*). The examination in dorsiflexion (A) demonstrates a small gap along the anterior aspect of the muscle/tendon. In B, made in 25° of plantar flexion, there is little reduction in the size of the gap between the torn tendon edges. At exploration, a wide gap in the tendon was found and repaired.

4 times its normal size), partial or complete tendinous discontinuity, and interruption of the normal dark tendon by large areas of signal increase (T2WI), presumably representing edema and hemorrhage that fill the gap (36,38,39,44,45,50,51) (Figs. 6.9-6.11). If the tear is complete, the proximal and distal ends of the tendon retract, the remaining tendon becomes thicker, and the torn tendon edges assume a mop-end appearance (36,51). The sagittal STIR images most graphically depict the size of the gap and the condition and orientation of the torn fiber ends. If the tear occurs at the musculotendinous junction, the muscle usually is the site of the actual tear, while the tendon itself remains intact (Fig. 6.10). Such lesions, since they are largely injuries to muscle and since they remain in continuity, are often treated nonoperatively.

Early data suggest that MRI may be a valuable adjunct to the diagnostic skills of the orthopedic surgeon faced with the patient with a suspected Achilles tendon injury (9,38,46,52). Marcus correlated the MRI findings on 7 patients with clinically suspected Achilles tendon tears to the findings on clinical examination (9). Of the five cases in which a partial or complete tear was identified at MRI, a palpable defect was present in only one, the Thompson test was positive in three,

and plantar flexion weakness was present in only four. In this group of patients, MRI was therefore extremely valuable in making the correct diagnosis. Several studies have semiquantitatively examined the ability of MRI to determine preoperatively the extent of Achilles tendonitis, the degree of rupture and the quality of the torn tendon edges, and all have found MRI to be reliable in such predictions (9,38,46,51,52).

The optimal treatment of complete, acute ruptures of the Achilles tendon remains controversial. Nistor, in a large prospective study, concluded that nonoperative therapy offers advantages over surgical restoration, including lack of anesthetic and surgical complications such as skin slough and infection (53). Inglis critically examined the issue of open versus closed therapy (54). He concluded that those patients treated surgically were more satisfied with the results of the treatment. He found that strength, power, and endurance of the nonoperated group was only 70% of the surgically treated group. No reruptures occurred in the surgical group, whereas the nonsurgical group suffered a nearly 30% rerupture rate (10). Surgical repair most frequently involves reapproximation of the torn ends; the gap may be so large as to necessitate the interposition of a tendon substitute such as the flexor hallucis longus, the fascia lata, or the plantaris (55). Most recently, Achilles tendon substitutes using glutaraldahyde, polylactic acid, or reconstituted type I collagen prostheses have been used (56,57). Although the debate regarding open versus closed therapy continues, most authorities now agree that conservative cast treatment should be reserved for patients who are older than 50 years, sedentary, or debilitated, and all others should undergo percutaneous or open surgical repair (10,58,59).

It is obvious that MRI has inestimable value in confirming the diagnosis of complete Achilles tendon rupture in 25% of patients in whom the diagnosis is uncertain. MRI may find its greatest use in two other situations: selection of patients who should undergo conservative versus operative therapy, and design of rehabilitation programs in those patients who are undergoing either conservative care or open surgical therapy (9,36,38).

Preoperative knowledge of the degree of rupture and separation of the torn tendon edges, and the condition and degree of degeneration of the tendon may help to select those patients who would best benefit from conservative care (3,31,35,38). Proper selection of patients likely to do well with conservative therapy following complete rupture may be very difficult on clinical grounds alone (53). Since plantar flexion of the foot at surgery in a patient with a torn Achilles tendon may bring the edges into apposition, some authors have advocated performing MRI with the ankle in a plantar-flexed position to predict which tears are likely to be apposed if cast therapy were to be chosen (38). In a limited number of cases, however, we have not been able to demonstrate a significant change in the degree of apposition of the torn tendon edges during plantar flexion maneuvers (Fig. 6.11).

If conservative care is chosen, performing MRI at frequent intervals postcasting may permit graphic demonstration of the rate, quality, and degree of restitution of the Achilles mechanism, information critical to rehabilitation (9,36,39,51). Periods of cast immobilization postrupture have been determined largely by trial and error, but just as conventional radiography helps in assessment of fracture healing, MRI may per-

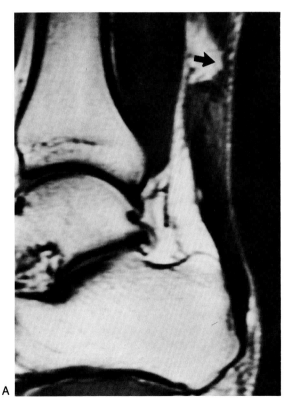 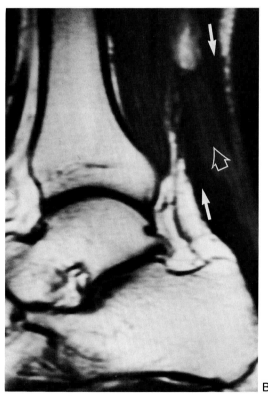

A   B

FIG. 6.12. Healing Achilles tendon rupture. **A**: Sagittal MR, TR/TE 2000/20. This patient suffered an extensive tear of the tendon at the musculotendinous junction; high signal edema is seen to extend caudally within the tendon substance (*arrow*). In spite of marked weakness and advice of his physician to the contrary, the patient opted for equinus cast therapy. After 8 months, the patient was judged to have an excellent clinical result, but a follow-up MR (**B**, sagittal MR, TR/TE 2000/20) revealed intermediate signal (*open arrow*) between the torn edges (*arrows*). The signal of this tissue was felt to be more consistent with scar than regenerated tendon. (Case courtesy of M. Reicher, M.D.) (From ref. 9, with permission.)

mit accurate longitudinal assessment of Achilles tendon healing (9,30,36). In patients treated with cast therapy, MRI may reveal a discontinuous tendon with interposed intermediate intensity tissue, compatible with scar rather than tendon, or areas of mixed signal consistent with incomplete healing (9) (Fig. 6.12).

Achilles tendon ruptures have been evaluated with MRI during the healing phase after either surgical or conservative therapy (Figs. 6.13, 6.14). In one study of ruptured tendons treated either conservatively or open, all tendons had intratendinous fluid spaces on studies performed at 3 and 6 months, but all showed progressive signal decrease over time (T1WI) (60). By 12 months, all tendons demonstrated uniformly low signal, indicative of dense collagen scar, and all ten-

dons had a distinctly widened contour. The widening may be focal at the site of repair, or may be diffuse and dramatic (51,57). In our experience, MRI examinations performed within the first 2 months postoperatively are dramatically abnormal. In fact, the striking degree of edema and apparent tendinous discontinuity suggest that the repair has failed or was improperly performed. We are unable to assess satisfactorily the integrity of the tendon in the immediate postoperative period. Every patient that we have examined more than 6 months postrepair has demonstrated extreme widening of the entire length of the Achilles (up to 15 mm) even though the tear was focal. In patients treated with polylactic acid implants, grafts demonstrate thin streaks of intermediate signal dif-

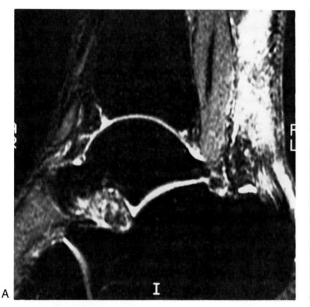

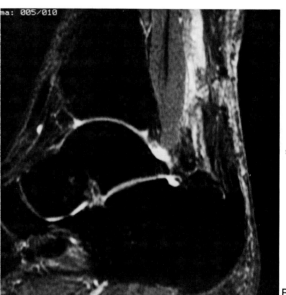

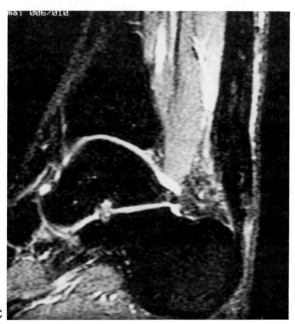

FIG. 6.13. Healing of a surgically treated Achilles rupture. **A–C**: Sagittal MR, TR/TE/TI 2200/36/160. A was performed 1 month following a complete rupture of the Achilles tendon that was surgically repaired. The image demonstrates intra- and peritendinous edema at the site of the rupture (*arrow*). The tendon, in spite of the fact that it was surgically restored, appears remarkably narrow and discontinuous at the site of repair. In B, made 1 month after A, the site of the tear appears thicker, and the degree of intratendinous signal has markedly decreased. By 6 months postoperative, the intratendinous signal has vanished and it is difficult to identify the site of the rupture. The entire Achilles tendon is markedly widened throughout its length.

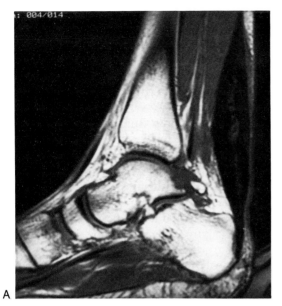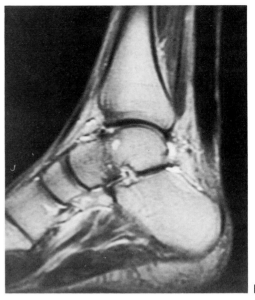

FIG. 6.14. Repaired ruptures of the Achilles tendon. **A**: Sagittal MR, TR/TE 500/20. This patient suffered a complete rupture of the Achilles tendon 12 months prior to this MRI study. There is faint intratendinous signal at the site of repair and the tendon is massively thickened. **B**: Sagittal MR, TR/TE 800/20. This image is made from another patient; the scanning plane is somewhat oblique to the actual plane of the Achilles tendon, so only the proximal portion of the tendon is seen on this image. The Achilles tendon is widened to approximately twice its normal antero-posterior dimension and there is no significant intratendinous abnormality. This appearance might readily be mistaken for chronic Achilles tendonitis. A complete rupture had been repaired 14 months earlier.

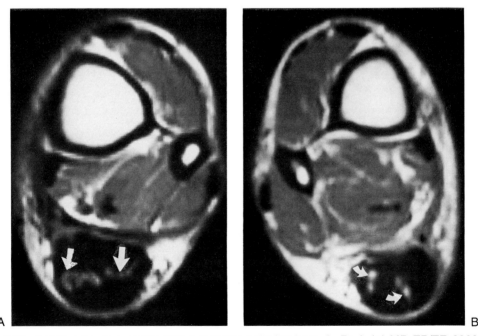

FIG. 6.15. Achilles tendon repair with polylactic acid implant. **A, B**: Axial MR TR/TE 2000/20. These images are from two different patients. In A, made 6 months after surgical repair, there are two well-defined bandlike clusters of high signal foci (*arrows*) corresponding to strands of polylactic acid covered with maturing collagenogenic tissue. In B, made 12 months following implantation, this implant is manifest by a group of sharply defined punctate foci (*arrows*) corresponding to the strands covered by a healed tendon. In both images, the repaired tendon remains markedly thickened. (Case courtesy of M. Liem, M.D.) (From ref. 57, with permission.)

fusely throughout the tendon, and virtually the entire tendon is thickened in a fusiform manner (57) (Fig. 6.15).

While degenerative and traumatic disorders of the Achilles tendon are certainly the most common processes coming to clinical attention, autoimmune and metabolic conditions can lead to inflammation and rupture (Fig. 6.16). Xanthomatous infiltration of the tendons is common in hypercholesterolemic states, especially type II hyperbetalipoproteinemia. MRI assessment of such patients may demonstrate massive thickening of the Achilles tendon (44 mm), pressure erosion of the adjacent bone, intraosseous xanthomata, and affliction of other tendons in the foot (61).

Two other related disorders affecting the heel present with signs or symptoms that are often confused with Achilles tendonitis, rupture, or tumor. There are two bursae at the Achilles insertion that may become irritated, hypertrophied and inflamed, fill with fluid, and become a source of clinical symptoms (35,42,45,50). The retrocalcaneal bursa is situated between the posterior aspect of the calcaneus and the Achilles tendon itself; the superficial bursa is subcutaneous in position, just dorsal to the distal-most

Achilles tendon. Retrocalcaneal bursitis is most commonly seen in athletes who wear boot-type footwear, such as skiers and basketball players. On MRI, a distended retrocalcaneal bursa is a small fluid-filled sac seen just anterior to the Achilles tendon, hugging the posterior aspect of the calcaneus just below its superior margin (Fig. 6.17). Systemic diseases such as rheumatoid arthritis or Reiter's disease may present with a distended retrocalcaneal bursa. In such cases, MRI may be of value in determining the origin and precise etiology of a peri-Achilles mass, and therefore help lead the clinician's search for systemic causes of an Achilles problem. Haglund syndrome is characterized by heel pain and a soft tissue swelling at the level of the Achilles tendon insertion (62). Radiographically, the diagnosis is made by the finding of a prominent calcaneal bursal projection, retrocalcaneal bursitis, thickening of the Achilles tendon, and a "pump bump."

A variety of congenital muscular anomalies in the leg and foot have been described; one of the more common is an accessory soleus muscle (31,63–66) (Fig. 6.18). Persistence of the muscular portion of the soleus distally into the fat pad anterior to the Achilles may

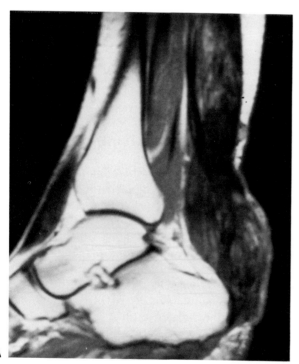
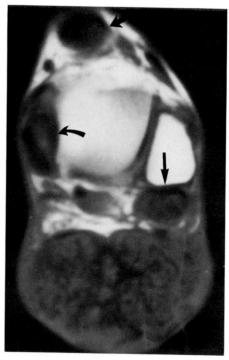

FIG. 6.16. Tendinous xanthomata. **A:** Sagittal MR, TR/TE 500/20. **B:** Axial MR, TR/TE 500/20. The patient is known to suffer from hyperbetalipoproteinemia type II, and she presented to her physician with an Achilles mass. The MRI sequences demonstrate massive enlargement of the Achilles tendon, which is filled with tissue of intermediate signal on the short TR sequences. The axial sequence also demonstrates that the anterior tibial tendon (*arrow*), peroneal tendons (*long arrows*), and posterior tibial tendon (*curved arrow*) are similarly affected by the deposition of this lipid material. (Case courtesy of Scott Kingston, M.D.)

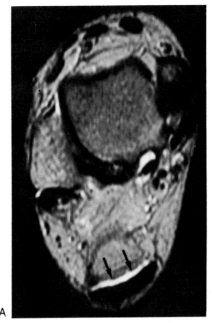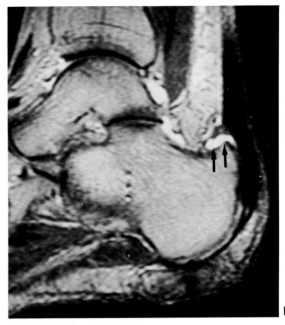

FIG. 6.17. Retrocalcaneal bursitis. **A**: Axial MR, TR/TE 2000/80. **B**: Sagittal MR, TR/TE 2000/80. A fluid-filled bursa (*arrows*) is present immediately anterior to the Achilles tendon just above its insertion onto the calcaneus. Proper diagnosis of this condition is important since intrabursal steroids may afford relief, but intratendinous corticosteroids are contraindicated.

mimic a mass. This "tumor" is most notable after exercise. Patients complain of exercise-induced pain since these muscular anomalies have a tenuous blood supply and therefore exercise may induce ischemia.

FIG. 6.18. Accessory soleus muscle. Sagittal MR, TR/TE 600/20. The large soleus muscle (*arrow*) inserts on the most distal aspect of the Achilles tendon just above the calcaneus. This abnormality is best appreciated when compared to the normal relationship of the soleus muscle and Achilles tendon as seen in Fig. 6.1.

While the differential diagnosis of an accessory soleus muscle must include a soft tissue tumor, an Achilles tendon rupture, or a hematoma, MRI can reliably identify the "lesion" as being continuous with, and having a signal intensity identical to that of the surrounding musculature.

THE POSTERIOR TIBIAL TENDON

The posterior tibial tendon (PTT) is one of the main stabilizers of the hindfoot and is responsible for inversion and plantar flexion. The muscle belly rises from the proximal and middle thirds of the tibia and fibula; the muscle tendon junction is several centimeters above the medial malleolus under which the tendon turns on its course to insert on the navicular, the cuneiforms, and the bases of the second, third, and fourth metatarsals (23,31). Classically, complete rupture of the posterior tibial tendon is a chronic foot disorder of women in their fifth and sixth decades. These women present with a rather marked pain, progressive flat foot deformity, weakness of inversion, and an inability to raise up on their toes. There is lowering of the medial longitudinal arch of the foot, and with full weightbearing, significant flat foot deformity occurs (23,67). The deformity permits the forefoot to drift laterally, allowing the physician, when viewing the patient from behind, to see "too many toes" (28).

A second group of individuals suffering acute posterior tibial tendon injuries have been identified. They are young athletes engaged in sports requiring rapid changes in direction such as soccer, tennis, and ice hockey, or females who point their toes excessively in dance and gymnastics (3,35). We have examined two professional basketball players who suffered PTT injuries as determined by MRI; both were initially misdiagnosed as having sprains of the deltoid ligament.

While on rare occasions the PTT may be acutely avulsed from its insertion, the most common cause of rupture of the PTT is mechanical erosion of the tendon where it passes under the medial malleolus (23,67). While patients with chronic disruption of the posterior tibial tendon have flat arches, it is still not known whether such patients have congenitally flat arches, predisposing to the rupture, or whether rupture results in loss of height of the arch (23). Rheumatoid arthritis and the seronegative spondyloarthropathies, by virtue of the tenosynovitis with which they are associated, can also lead to rupture of the posterior tibial tendon (68). Rarely, closed fractures of the ankle may result

in PTT rupture (69). Posterior tibial tendon injuries are very serious orthopedic problems. The "degenerative" type occurring in older individuals usually progresses relentlessly with severe disability. Orthoses, antiinflammatory medications, casts, and tenovaginotomy may be valuable in lesser degrees of injury, but the severe pain, deformity, and degenerative arthritis that most typically accompanies complete ruptures often necessitate subtalar arthrodesis for stabilization and relief of pain (23,70). One of the two professional basketball players that we examined underwent conservative care for 1 year. Both remained highly symptomatic for 6 months following injury.

Tenography and conventional radiography have played little role in the diagnosis of injury to the PTT, and it was not until the advent of high resolution CT scanning, and more recently MR scanning that accurate preoperative and prerupture diagnosis of PTT injuries could reliably be made (8,21–23,27,71).

The most useful plane in assessing PTT size, shape, and internal signal is a true axial plane of the tendon (27). One can optimize tendon assessment by slightly

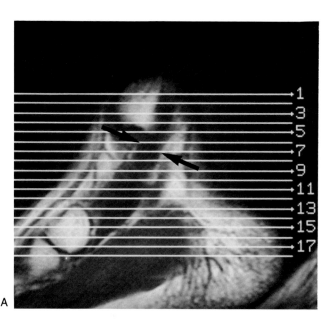

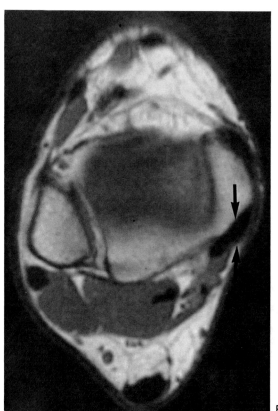

FIG. 6.19. Normal PTT; effect of foot position on PTT visualization. **A:** Sagittal MR, TR/TE 500/20. The sagittal image through the medial aspect of the foot is used to identify the course of the PTT; from this image, the axial plane sequence is proscribed. In this study, the foot is at 90° to the leg, and the axial images will be oblique to the plane of the tendon. **B:** Axial MR, TR/TE 2000/20. This image has been proscribed from A. The PTT (*arrows*) is intimately related to the posterior cortex of the medial malleolus from with which it blends rather imperceptibly. (*Figure continues on next page.*)

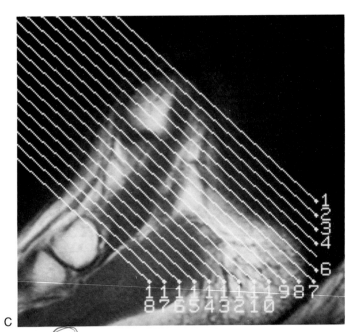

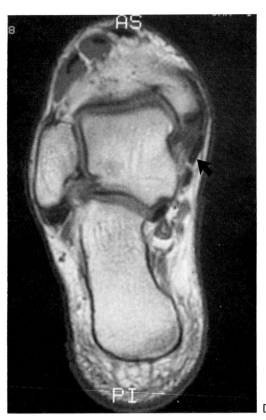

FIG. 6.19. (*Continued*) **C**: Sagittal MRI, TR/TE 500/20. The imaging plane for **D** is selected to be perpendicular to the tendon at the point at which it crosses under the medial malleolus. **D**: Oblique axial MR, TR/TE 2000/20. The PTT is easily distinguished from the medial malleolus. Throughout its course, the PTT is ovoid and has a cross-sectional area 2–3 times that of the flexor digitorum longus.

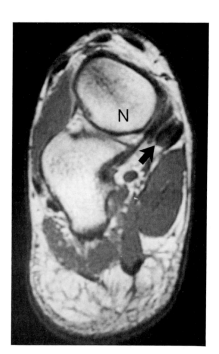

FIG. 6.20. Pseudo-tear of the PTT. Oblique axial, TR/TE 2000/20. Just proximal to its insertion on the medial aspect of the navicular (*N*), the PTT (*arrow*) usually demonstrates increased signal intensity and an increase in its circumference. This appearance must not be mistaken for a type I rupture.

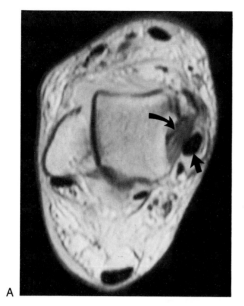 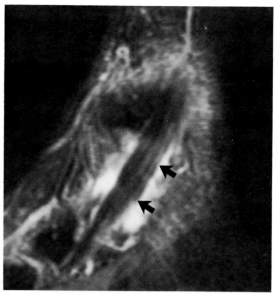

FIG. 6.21. Type I PTT tear. **A**: Oblique axial MR, TR/TE 2000/20. The posterior tibial tendon (*arrows*) is markedly enlarged in its cross-sectional area. It lies immediately superficial to the deltoid ligament (*curved arrow*). **B**: Sagittal MR, TR/TE/TI 2200/35/160. This extreme medial sagittal MRI demonstrates the tendon (*arrows*) to be surrounded by edema. Within its substance, linear signal increases represent longitudinal splits that characterize the type I rupture.

plantar flexing the foot, and by choosing a scanning plane that is perpendicular to the PTT at the point at which it passes under the medial malleolus. By choosing this position, the PTT "moves away" from the groove on the malleolus, and therefore the partial volume effect of the tendon with the malleolus is minimized (Fig. 6.19). The normal PTT can be identified on MRI just above the malleolus under which it curves toward its insertion. The PTT is normally twice as large as the flexor digitorum longus, or the flexor hallucis longus tendons (23,27). The sagittal sequence best demonstrates the longitudinal extent of the injury and

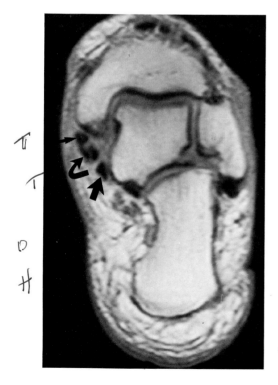

FIG. 6.22. Longitudinal rupture of the PTT. Axial oblique MR, TR/TE 2000/20. The patient has suffered a long, longitudinal split of the PTT that effectively divides the tendon into two tendon fragments. The anterior-most portion of the PTT (*small arrow*) is immediately behind the medial malleolus, and immediately anterior to the posterior fragment of the PTT (*curved arrow*). The flexor digitorum tendon (*large arrow*) and the flexor hallucis longus are seen in normal position. Such longitudinal splitting produces the appearance of four, rather than three medial flexor tendons ("Tom, Tom, Dick, Harry").

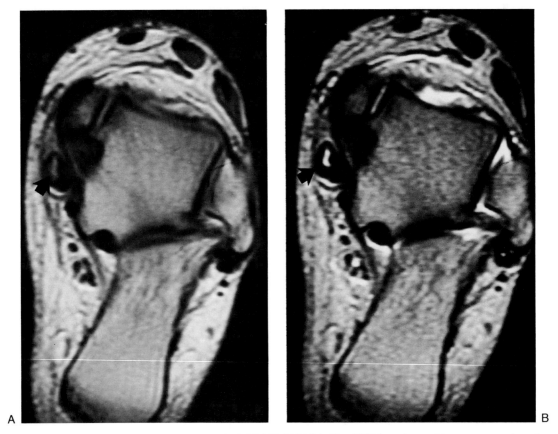

FIG. 6.23. Type I PTT rupture. **A**: Axial MR TR/TE 2000/20. The PTT is enlarged in cross-sectional area and has a focus of increased signal intensity seen within its substance (*arrow*). In **B** (axial MR, TR/TE 2000/80) this signal focus is seen to markedly increase in intensity (*arrow*).

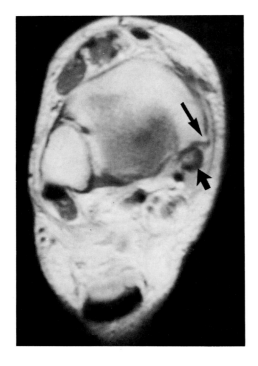

FIG. 6.24. Chronic type I PTT rupture. Oblique axial MR, TR/TE 2000/20. A large globular focus of abnormal signal is seen within the PTT (*arrow*). The spur (*long arrow*) on the posterior aspect of the medial malleolus is consistent with chronic stress in the tendon in this patient with a 2-year history of ankle pain.

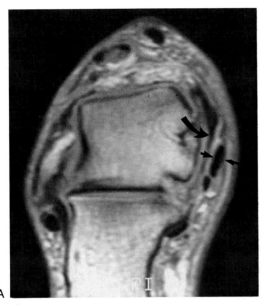 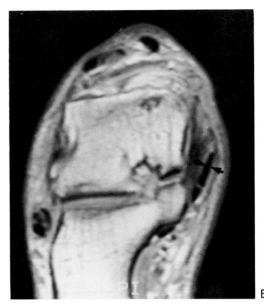

FIG. 6.25. Type II PTT rupture. **A, B**: Oblique axial MR, TR/TE 2000/20. A is 6 mm proximal to B. In A, the PTT (*arrows*) has a normal to somewhat elongated appearance, but would probably be considered normal. It lies just superficial to the tibiocalcaneal (deltoid) ligament (*curved arrow*). In B, however, the sagittal dimension of the PTT has markedly decreased (*arrows*), indicative of a partial rupture pattern. This nonconcentric reduction in size is frequently seen in partial tears of the PTT.

the retraction that accompanies complete rupture (especially on STIR or long TR sequences). The coronal plane is generally not useful in PTT assessment (23).

The PTT is a homogeneously dark, ovoid to rounded structure throughout its course; however, just proximal to its insertion on the navicular, the tendon may "widen" and foci of increased signal on short TR sequences will be seen within it (72) (Fig. 6.20). This normal appearance, thought to be due to a fanlike insertion into the bone, must not be mistaken for a tear (8,23,27,72). This preinsertional contour and signal change is also found in other insertions such as in the deltoid and posterior talofibular ligaments (72). Small amounts of fluid are normally found in the posterior tibial tendon sheath and the presence of fluid is not necessarily indicative of pathology.

There are three patterns of PTT rupture identifiable by both CT and MRI; these patterns correlate well with surgical sub types known to foot and ankle surgeons (8,23,71,73) (Figs. 6.21–6.26). In a type I tear, splits develop within the fiber bundles that compose the tendon. As a result of the splitting, hemorrhage and scar tissue develop and result in increased tendon girth so that the PTT is 4 to 5 times as large as the adjacent flexor digitorum longus (Fig. 6.21). The normally ovoid tendon assumes a much more rounded configuration. On occasion, the splits are extremely long, resulting in division of the tendon into two "subtendons" (Fig. 6.22). In such cases, images in the axial plane may reveal four tendons (the anterior half of the PTT, the

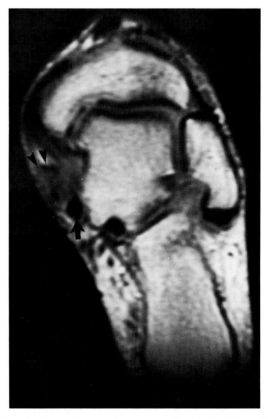

FIG. 6.26. Complete rupture of the PTT. There is no identifiable PTT seen in its expected position (*arrowheads*) over the deltoid ligament. The flexor digitorum longus (*arrow*) and the flexor hallucis longus are in their normal positions.

Type I - hypertrophic
2 - atrophic

posterior half of the PTT, the flexor digitorum, and the flexor hallucis longus) instead of the normal three, along the medial side of the ankle (a similar pattern of rupture may affect the peroneus brevis). Type I rupture patterns may reveal foci of abnormal signal within the tendon best seen on proton density images. Although frequently these foci "disappear" on long TR sequences, they may occasionally become hyperintense, especially on STIR sequences, perhaps indicating a more significant degree of rupture (23) (Fig. 6.23).

While the type I tear may be described as a "hypertrophic" lesion based on increase in tendon size, type II ruptures are atrophic (23,71). Such tears are more severe, but still partial tears in which the tendon undergoes such severe longitudinal splitting that it becomes attenuated to one-half to one-third of its normal size (Fig. 6.25). This reduction in size is not uniformly circumferential; the dominant change in contour is a decrease in width of the tendon with a relative preservation of the anteroposterior dimension. The tendon then assumes a long ovoid configuration, a finding that may best appreciated by careful comparison with images of the tendon just above and below the suspected site of pathology. Both of the professional athletes suffering acute PTT injuries that we have encountered have had type II tears.

Type III tears of the PTT are complete ruptures with retraction of the proximal tendon and development of an obvious gap at the site of rupture, most graphically seen on sagittal STIR images (71) (Fig. 6.26). The proximal and distal edges of the tear may retract and give a pseudowidened appearance. Therefore, the entire length of the tendon must be carefully examined to avoid mistaking the pseudowidened segment of a type III tear for a type I lesion.

In a recent study, MRI had a sensitivity of 95%, a specificity of 100%, and an accuracy of 96% in determining the degree of rupture of a torn PTT. The errors in interpretation generally were ones of underestimation of the severity of the rupture in which partial volume effect of the tendon with the cortical bone of the tibia occurred (23). Type II tears were mistakenly graded as type I. MRI has proved itself to be more accurate that CT in PTT assessment. CT occasionally demonstrated a mild heterogeneity of the tendon that was difficult to differentiate from a normal tendon. Dis-

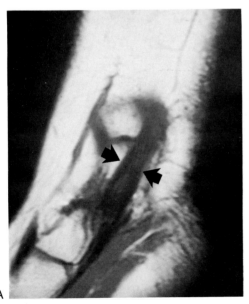
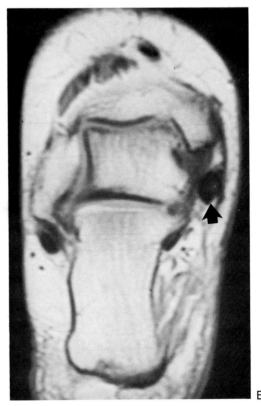

FIG. 6.27. Flexor digitorum longus transfer for a repair of a PTT rupture. This patient is known to have had a complete rupture of the posterior tibial tendon. The flexor digitorum longus tendon was used to repair the rupture. **A**: Sagittal MR, TR/TE 600/20. The PTT appears markedly widened. **B**: Oblique axial MR, TR/TE 2000/20. Just below the medial malleolus, the repaired PTT (*arrow*) is identified. The flexor digitorum longus is "absent" and therefore there are only two tendons along the medial aspect of the foot.

tinction of edema at the site of a recent rupture from an intact but degenerated tendon was difficult by CT. Additionally, CT exaggerated tendon size, particularly in type I ruptures, due to the presence of synovial fluid around the tendon that could not be distinguished from the tendon itself (23).

MRI may prove useful in determining the postoperative outcome of patients undergoing reconstruction of a torn PTT (70). It should be remembered that avulsion, tenosynovitis, and partial and complete rupture may be clinically indistinguishable preoperatively, and the operative therapy is dictated by the precise pathologic stage of disease (67). The MRI findings in patients with PTT tears correlate well with the success of the surgery (70). Tendons with MRI type I tears had satisfactory results after soft tissue reconstruction with flexor digitorum longus tendon transfer (Fig. 6.27). Those patients who had suffered higher grades of tear, as determined on MRI, did poorly with only soft tissue repair. Fusion would best be considered in these groups. Grading of the lesion at the time of surgery did not correlate well with the clinical outcome.

There are variations in the development of the navicular that may cause foot pain and be confused with pathologic changes in the PTT (74,75). One may identify a separate ossicle within the PTT; it is anatomically separate from the navicular, and is uncommonly a source of clinical complaints (type 1) (Fig. 6.28). This sesamoid, the os tibiale externum, is a well-defined round or oval bone, 2 to 6 mm in diameter and within 5 mm medial and posterior to the medial aspect of the navicular. The type 2 variant is a true accessory navicular. A cartilaginous mass that is continuous with the cartilage of the navicular may ossify postnatally as a bone in continuity with the navicular by a synchondrosis (type 2), or the entire mass may ossify and result in a larger, more curvilinear navicular (type 3). The type 2 ossicle is triangular or heart-shaped with its base separated 1 to 2 mm from the posterior aspect of the navicular. The type 2 accessory navicular is the variant most likely to produce symptoms. As noted above, the normal PTT inserts onto the medial and plantar surfaces of the navicular; when it exists, the accessory ossicle may provide the site of attachment of the ten-

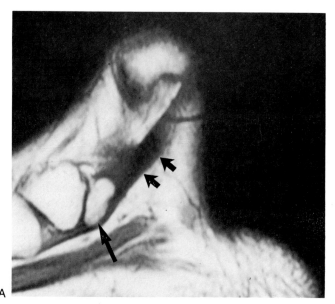

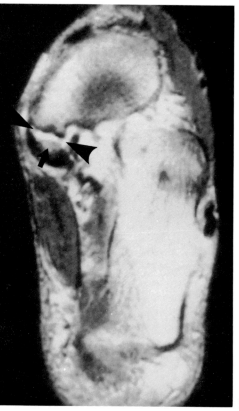

FIG. 6.28. Accessory naviculars. **A:** Os tibiale externum. Sagittal MR, TR/TE 400/20. The PTT (*arrows*) inserts on the os tibiale externum (*long arrow*), a type I accessory navicular. **B:** Symptomatic accessory navicular. Axial MR, TR/TE 2000/80. This 23-year-old dancer has pain on the medial aspect of the foot. This true accessory ossicle (*arrow*) is separated from the navicular by a bandlike area of high signal (*arrowheads*) representing the synchondrosis. (Fig. 6.28B courtesy of R. Fritz, M.D.)

don. This arrangement may alter the leverage of the tendon, interfere with foot mechanics, and lead to painful flat foot (74). Young women may present with signs and symptoms of distal posterior tibial tendon dysfunction. Patients with type 2 variants may have trauma to the bridging synchondrosis between the accessory navicular and the navicular. The injury is analagous to a cartilaginous physeal fracture in a long bone, or to the painful bipartite patella, symptomatic Osgood-Schlatter and Sinding-Larson diseases (74,75). Patients with symptomatic accessory naviculars may require resection of the accessory bone and intervening cartilage, and reattachment of the PTT for relief of pain.

Shin splints, also known as tibial stress syndrome, is the general term applied to vague, exercise-induced pain in the leg, most commonly seen in athletes. Diagnosis should be limited to musculotendinous inflammation, which produces tenderness of medial border of the tibia and is associated with a normal radiographic examination (76–79). The precise site of the lesion remains controversial; radionuclide uptake corresponds to the origin of either/both the tibialis posterior or the soleus muscles (79).

PERONEAL TENDONS

The peroneal muscles pronate and evert the foot; they are primary lateral dynamic stabilizers of the ankle joint and help perform the second stage of walking and push off (3,19). The peroneus longus (PL) arises from the lateral condyle of the tibia, the head of the fibula, and the proximal intermuscular septum; the brevis (PB) arises from the lower two-thirds of the fibula and intermuscular septum, just anterior to the longus (10,35). Behind the malleolus, the tendons, in their common synovial sheath, are retained in position by thick fibrous bands known as the superior and inferior retinacula, which are focal thickenings of the tendon sheaths themselves (4,18–20,80,81). These bands originate from the periosteum of the lateral malleolus, 1 cm posterior and superior to the tip of the malleolus, and insert on the calcaneus. Their function is to prevent the peroneal tendons from bowstringing over the lateral malleolus during muscle contraction. In 80% of patients, there is a groove on the posterior aspect of the lateral malleolus that accommodates the PB (3,31,82). The peroneal tendons, therefore, reside in a fibro-osseous tunnel that is formed by the malleolus in front, the superior peroneal retinaculum posteriorly and laterally, and the posterior talofibular and calcaneofibular ligaments medially (19). Below the malleolus, the tendons diverge from one another and have separate tendon sheaths; the PB inserts on the base of the fifth metatarsal while the longus passes posterior to the peroneal tubercle, curves beneath the calcaneus, and inserts on the base of the first metatarsal and medial cuneiform (31).

Developmental anomalies of the peroneal tendons have been described (66). While several variants exist, the type in which the anomalous muscle arises from the interosseous membrane and peroneus brevis muscle belly and inserts on the calcaneus is the most common. Such anomalies may be symptomatic.

Knowledge of the intimate relationship of the peroneal tendon sheath and the calcaneofibular (CF) ligament is critical to the understanding of the use of arthrography in the diagnosis of lateral ankle sprains. When the CF is torn, the peroneal sheath comes into communication with the ankle joint, a communication that does not normally exist. Peroneal tenography in combination with ankle joint arthrography has a high degree of accuracy in diagnosing lateral ligament tears (13,14).

Until the advent of high resolution CT and MRI, peroneal tenography was the only method whereby one could assess injury to the PB or PL tendons. A peroneal tenogram may demonstrate extrinsic compression, irregularity of the sheath, lateral displacement, or complete obstruction to the normal distal flow of injected contrast material (7,11,13,14).

MRI provides a harmless, noninvasive method of evaluation of all of the components of the peroneal mechanism. The hindfoot protocol is selected for imaging assessment. It should be remembered that the most common site of pathology of the peroneal tendons is where the tendon changes course. Therefore, when specifically examining the peroneal tendons, one should select the axial plane perpendicular to the inframalleolar segment of the PB and PL, rather than the true orthogonal axial plane (39). Selecting the true axial plane of the tendon optimizes image quality at the curve of the malleolus, but above and below that point, the tendons may be viewed obliquely. Partial volume effect with the surrounding fat may produce an appearance in which the tendons are "hazy"; they have a vague increase in signal. One must be careful not to mistake this appearance for pathology.

On MRI, the peroneal tendons are signal-less structures at all imaging sequences (Fig. 6.29). In the axial plane just above the malleolus, the PB is tendinous and lies on the posterior fibula. The PL may still be muscular at this level. The tendons are nearly round and equal in size, although the longus may have a larger tendon sheath (14). The brevis, lying just anterior to the longus, may be difficult to separate from the cortical bone of the malleolus because of partial volume effect. Just behind the malleolus, the superior peroneal retinaculum can nearly always be identified (18) (Fig. 6.30). It is a thin, dark band arising from the lateral aspect of the fibula; its fibers split, engulfing the ten-

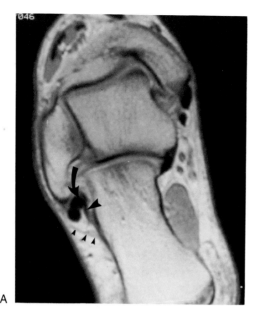

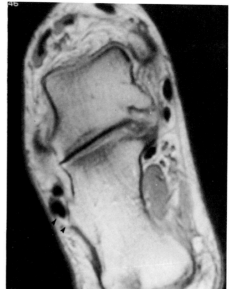

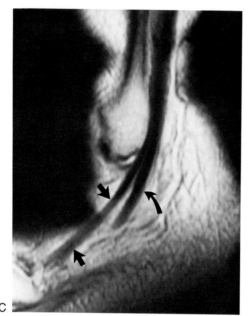

FIG. 6.29. Normal peroneal tendons. **A, B**: Oblique axial MR, TR/TE 2000/20. At the level of the lateral malleolus, the peroneal tendons are approximately the same size, are round, and are signal-less. The peroneus brevis (*curved arrow*), the anterior of the two tendons, is in contact with the fibula. The two tendons lie in a space bounded in front by the fibula, medially by the calcaneofibular ligament (*arrowhead*), and posterolaterally by the peroneal retinaculum (*tiny arrowheads*). Approximately 1 cm more distal (**B**), the tendons are still within the retinaculum but are clearly separable from one another. On the sagittal study (**C**) (sagittal MR, TR/TE 2000/20), the normal tendons lie immediately posterior to the fibula. The peroneus brevis (*arrows*) can be followed from its retrofibular position nearly to its attachment to the base of the fifth metatarsal. The more posterior peroneus longus (*curved arrow*) is apparently "interrupted"; it is at this point that the longus tendon curves under the calcaneus/cuboid and moves out of the imaging plane.

dons, and then reconstitutes on its way to attach to the lateral aspect of the calcaneus. While its course and location are constant, the thickness of the superior peroneal retinaculum is variable, but it can be seen with sufficient confidence to establish its integrity or lack thereof in most instances (18). Because both the peroneal tendons and the retinaculum are dark and may be in contact with one another, separation of one structure from the other may occasionally be difficult. Extreme lateral sagittal images through the ankle invariably demonstrate the two tendons above, and behind the malleolus below which they diverge.

Injuries to the peroneal tendons may be classified

as (a) tenosynovitis, (b) entrapment, (c) dislocation, and (d) rupture (4,7,19,20,31,40,50,80,81,83).

Peroneal tenosynovitis may be idiopathic, but it most commonly occurs as a complication of a comminuted intraarticular calcaneal fracture in which the laterally displaced fragment displaces or impales the tendons, or entraps them against the talus or fibula (19,20,50). Mechanically induced tenosynovitis occurs at the points of direction change such as at the fibular malleolus, the peroneal tubercle, or the cuboid in the case of the peroneus longus (7). Rarely, hypertrophy of the peroneal tubercle, tarsal coalition, inflammatory arthritides, or abnormal foot mechanics leads to ten-

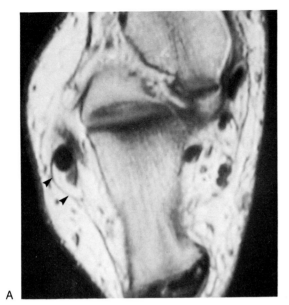

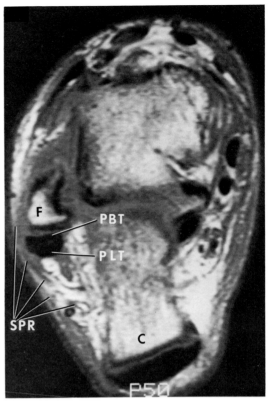

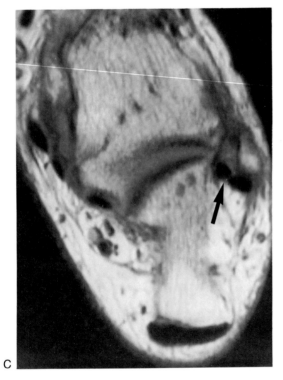

FIG. 6.30. Normal and torn peroneal retinaculum. Axial MR, TR/TE 2000/20. **A:** The thin peroneal retinaculum (*arrowheads*) is seen to surround the peroneals. **B:** The peroneal tendons are slightly subluxed laterally, although they remain behind the fibula. The superior peroneal retinaculum is only vaguely demarcated, and anteriorly is elevated away from the fibular ridge. The retinaculum was found to be torn at surgery. (PBT, peroneus brevis; PLT, peroneus longus; SPR, retinaculum; F, fibula; C, calcaneus) (Case courtesy of J. Zeiss, M.D.) **C:** Medial dislocation of the peroneus brevis. Oblique axial MR, TR/TE 2500/20. This patient gives a history of multiple lateral ankle sprains. The peroneus brevis and longus are both subluxed medially, with the brevis (*arrow*) being displaced into the talofibulocalcaneal articulation. (Fig. 6.30B from ref. 18, with permission.)

osynovitis (7,19). Peroneal tenosynovitis results in pain, swelling, tenderness, and occasionally involuntary inversion of the foot, a situation that results in superimposed ankle sprains (20). Peroneal tenosynovitis is a surgically correctable cause of pain following a calcaneal fracture, and therefore differential diagnosis from subtalar arthritis, loss of plantar soft tissues, and plantar new bone formation is critical (20).

The most common MRI finding in patients with peroneal dysfunction is distension of the synovial sheath with fluid, contrasting with the two dark tendons contained within (Figs. 6.31, 6.32). While a small amount of fluid in the tendon sheath is probably physiologic, significant amounts of fluid must raise the possibility of peroneal tenosynovitis, or in the setting of acute trauma with an ankle joint effusion, a tear of the CF ligament. The tendons have a normal size and contour. With the development of tendonitis, internal splits in the tendon fiber occur, manifest as linear high signal foci, and slight widening of the tendon shape.

Rupture of the peroneal tendons is an uncommon injury (4,81,84,85). It may occur as a result of a calcaneal fracture, or less commonly *de novo*. The mechanical stress on the peroneus brevis where it rides

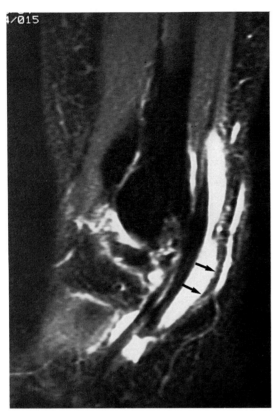

FIG. 6.31. Peroneal tenosynovitis. Sagittal MR, TR/TE/TI 2200/35/160. The peroneal tendon sheath (*arrows*) is markedly distended with fluid, but the contained tendons appear normal.

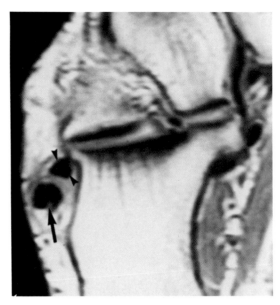

FIG. 6.32. Peroneal tendonitis. Oblique axial MR, TR/TE 2000/20. The peroneus longus is enlarged compared to the peroneus brevis (*arrowheads*) and demonstrates a tiny focus of abnormal signal (*arrow*).

against the malleolus may result in decreased vascularity, longitudinal splitting, and eventually rupture (4,81,85). Rarely, a subcutaneous rupture of the peroneus longus tendon may occur through a fracture of the os peroneum (81,84) (Fig. 6.33). Displacement of the os peroneum, an accessory ossicle that lies within

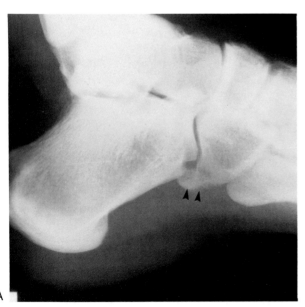

A

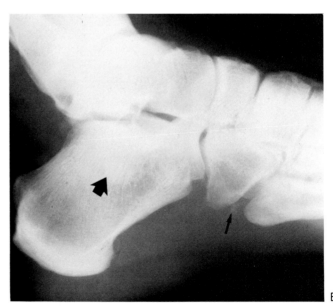

B

FIG. 6.33. Rupture of the peroneus longus, with displacement of the os peroneum. **A**: Preinjury radiographs demonstrate a normal os peroneum situated at the calcaneocuboid junction (*arrowheads*). **B**: Radiographs made following an injury demonstrate that the large proximal fragment has been retracted back to a position nearly under the lateral malleolus (*arrow*), while the small distal fragment has been retracted further distally (*small arrow*). *Case courtesy of J. Tehranzadeh, M.D.)*

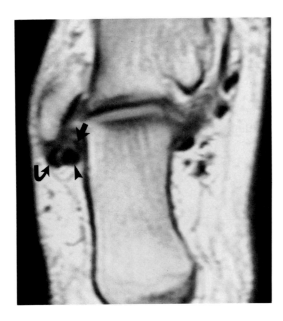

FIG. 6.34. Longitudinal split of the peroneus brevis. Oblique axial MR, TR/TE 2000/20. A long longitudinal split of the peroneus brevis has occurred, dividing it into medial (*arrow*) and lateral (*curved arrow*) halves. The peroneus longus (*arrowhead*) has insinuated itself into the longitudinal split; in fact, traction on the PL may create the split in the PB.

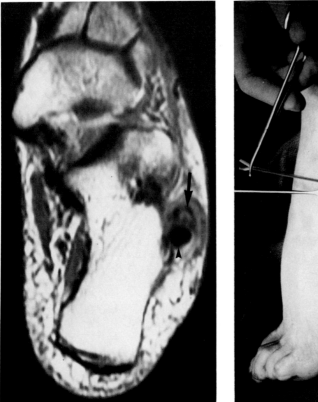

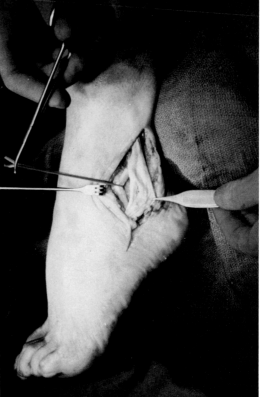

FIG. 6.35. Incomplete rupture of the peroneus brevis. **A, B**: Axial MR, TR/TE 2000/20. This patient suffered a recent ankle sprain, and clinically has weakness of eversion. The peroneus longus (*arrowhead*) is normal, while the brevis (*arrow*) is represented only by a thin irregular linear structure. The tendon sheath is diffusely thickened and distended. **B**: This surgical photograph of the patient demonstrates the torn peroneus brevis being held in the pincers; it is split longitudinally. The intact peroneus longus is held by the tape. (Surgical photograph courtesy of M. Weiss, D.P.M., Irwin Bliss, M.D.)

the peroneus longus quite near the calcaneocuboid joint, may be a helpful conventional radiographic sign of peroneal rupture (86). The rupture occurs just distal to where the tendon slides in the groove of the cuboid (81,84). Therapy for a complete rupture may include tenodesis of the peroneus longus to the peroneus brevis and surgical excision of the os peroneum (84).

The inability of the examiner to identify clearly two signal-less tendons on the lateral side of the ankle in the sagittal plane must raise the question of a partial or complete rupture of one of the peroneal tendons (Figs. 6.34-6.36). A longitudinal split of the peroneus brevis tendon occurs when with forced dorsiflexion, the PL is driven into the posterior aspect of the PB, creating a cleft that never heals (39,85). In such cases, it is critical that the examiner carefully distinguish this unusual type of rupture from a bifurcated insertion of the peroneus brevis; the latter is a normal variant (85). Recently, several cases of partial rupture of the peroneus brevis tendon have been identified; all had marked tenosynovitis in addition to the rupture (8,29). The diagnosis of partial rupture is best made in the axial plane. The PB is difficult to identify; it is attenuated, filled with signal, and/or absent (T1WI or proton density sequences). The tendon sheath is diffusely filled with fluid and edema. In our experience, the per-

oneus brevis does not suffer the retracted type of tear that characterizes complete Achilles tendon ruptures; more frequently, the tears are "interstitial" and some element of continuity of the tendon is maintained.

Peroneal dislocation has been described as congenital, traumatic, and habitual (3,10,83). Following violent contraction of the peroneal muscles, the superior retinaculum may be ruptured or may strip the periosteum from the malleolus, leaving the retinaculum lax and permitting the tendons to sublux lateral to, but rarely anterior to, the lateral malleolus (18,80) (Fig. 6.30). These injuries occur in skiers, ice skaters, and soccer and basketball players (13). We have encountered a single case in which medial subluxation of the tendons occurred following an inversion injury. Such patients present with "sprained ankles" since the mechanism of injury, forced inversion with a plantar flexed foot, can result in both peroneal subluxation and/or lateral ankle ligament sprain (19,31,40). A flake-like fracture on the anteromedial aspect of the distal fibular metaphysis is a characteristic finding seen in patients with torn retinacula and its presence should alert one to an associated peroneal displacement (13,18,80). Congenital laxity of the superior peroneal retinaculum and absence of the fibular groove may predispose patients to peroneal dislocation (19,83). It is

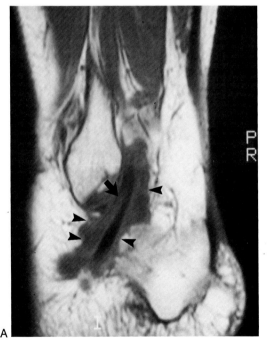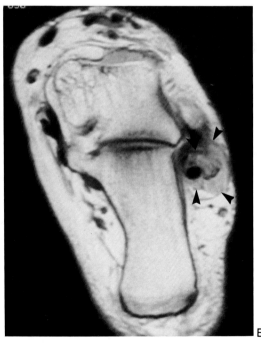

FIG. 6.36. Complete rupture of the peroneus brevis. This patient suffered an injury to the lateral aspect of the ankle after tripping on the carpet 6 months prior. **A:** Sagittal MR. **B:** Axial MR, TR/TE 2000/20. The peroneal tendon sheath is markedly distended with fluid and has a lobulated contour (*arrowheads*). Only a fine thread representing the peroneus brevis (*arrow*) is identified. The peroneus longus is normal.

critical to examine subluxed/dislocated tendons since 50% of patients have been reported to have associated longitudinal splits of the peroneus longus (35). MRI can be useful in the evaluation of superior retinacular injury and spontaneously reduced peroneal tendon dislocation when clinical findings are not definitive. MRI can clearly establish the location of the peroneal tendons, the integrity of the retinaculum, and the contour of the posterior fibula (18).

Following a calcaneal fracture, the peroneal tendons may become displaced secondary to retinacular rupture, or more commonly are entrapped between the talus, fibula, and calcaneus. While entrapment may be suspected clinically, MRI provides graphic representation of the deformity of the lateral wall of the fractured calcaneus, the position of the peroneals, the tear of the retinaculum, and associated peroneal tenosynovitis and/or rupture (Figs. 6.37, 6.38).

MRI has also been of value in preoperatively diagnosing a symptomatic anomalous PB by identification of the muscle itself and by excluding other etiologies for symptoms (66).

A variety of procedures have been advocated for repair of chronic dislocation of the peroneal tendons (3,4,10,35,87–90). The majority opinion supports acute surgical repair of the ruptured superior retinaculum (40). Periosteal reattachment, groove deepening, tenoplasty, and bone block procedures all have their advocates.

FLEXOR HALLUCIS LONGUS

The flexor hallucis longus (FHL) arises from the posterior aspect of the proximal tibia and fibula, and courses posterolateral to the posterior tibial tendon and flexor digitorum longus at the ankle joint. The tendon descends through a fibro-osseous tunnel on the posterior aspect of the talus between the medial and lateral tubercles (35). The FHL then curves under the sustentaculum, courses along the plantar aspect of the foot, passes between the sesamoids at the base of the first metatarsal, and inserts onto the great toe.

Athletes who perform repetitive push-off maneuvers from the forefoot, such as ballet dancers performing en pointe and soccer players, are most likely to injure the FHL (3,32,91). In fact, the FHL has been called the "Achilles tendon of the foot" in ballet dancers (32,35). FHL tenosynovitis and tendonitis may be secondary to inflammatory and degenerative causes such as diabetes, rheumatoid disease, or systemic lupus erythematosus. Rarely, tenosynovitis or even rupture of the FHL may occur at the ankle in association with severely comminuted calcaneal fractures (92). Conservative measures, including orthoses and antiinflammatory medications are usually successful in symptom relief in patients with tenosynovitis and tendonitis. Complete rupture, however, rarely occurs, but in such cases surgical reconstruction is necessary.

Like all other tendons, the normal FHL is a low

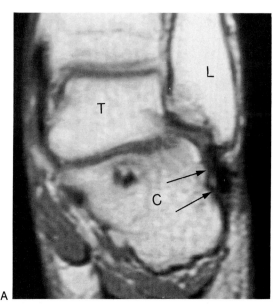 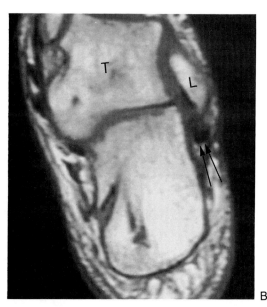

FIG. 6.37. Entrapped peroneal tendons. This patient is known to have suffered a previous calcaneal fracture in which the lateral wall was significantly displaced. In both **A** (coronal MR, TR/TE 2000/20 and **B** (oblique coronal MR, TR/TE 2000/20), the peroneal tendons (*long arrows*) are seen to be entrapped between the fibula (*L*) and the calcaneus (*C*). Entrapment of the peroneal tendons following a displaced calcaneal fracture is common. (T, talus; L, lateral malleolus; C, calcaneus.)

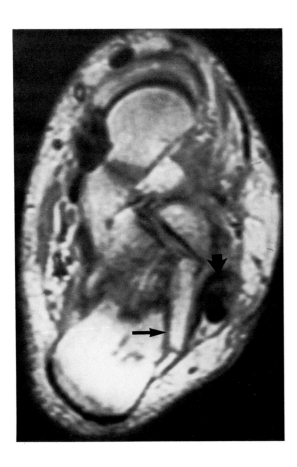

FIG. 6.38. Peroneal rupture following a displaced calcaneal fracture. Axial MR, TR/TE 2000/20. The lateral wall of the calcaneus is displaced (*arrow*). The peroneus brevis (*short arrow*) is difficult to identify; it is morphologically abnormal and is filled with signal. The MRI findings are consistent with a severe tenosynovitis or a rupture.

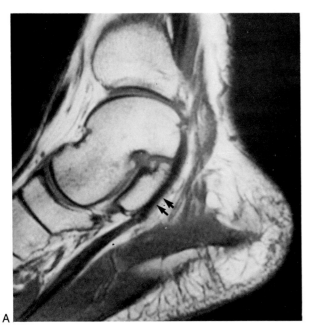
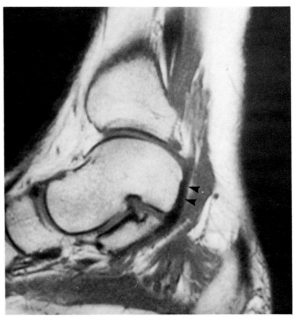

FIG. 6.39. Normal FHL. **A, B**: Sagittal MR, TR/TE 800/20. A is 3 mm medial to B. The normal course and caliber of the FHL can be followed from its position in a groove on the posterior talus (*arrowheads*), under the sustentaculum (*double arrows*), and along the plantar aspect of the foot.

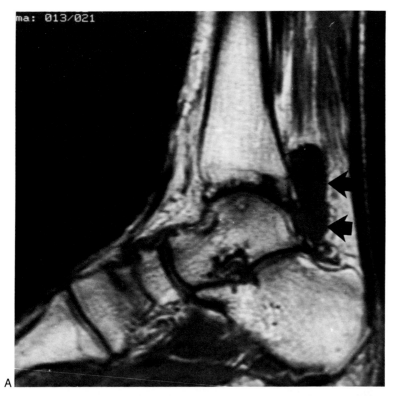

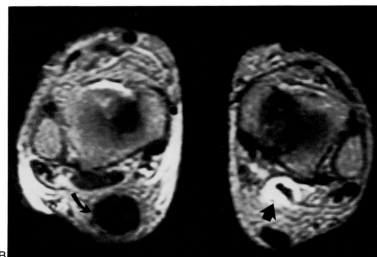

FIG. 6.40. FHL tenosynovitis. This patient is known to have long-standing rheumatoid arthritis. In **A** (sagittal MR, TR/TE 800/20), a tubular "mass" (*arrows*) is seen just posterior to the talus; the mass is in the expected position of the FHL. In **B** (axial MR, TR/TE 2000/80), the FHL tendon sheath (*arrow*) is filled with fluid. Incidentally noted is rheumatoid disease involving the ankle joint in A (joint space narrowing, subchondral cyst formation) and rather marked Achilles tendonitis on the right (*curved arrow*).

signal structure at all imaging parameters (Fig. 6.39). Fluid in the FHL tendon sheath is commonly seen when there is a significant ankle joint effusion since the FHL communicates with the ankle joint in 20% of normal patients. However, a disproportionate amount of fluid in the tendon sheath relative to the joint must be considered diagnostic of tenosynovitis. The FHL is most subject to inflammation, hypertrophy, and rupture either at its position along the posterior talus or between the sesamoids (3,31). Simple inflammatory tenosynovitis may evolve into stenosing tenosynovitis. The patient may be unable to flex the great toe, may

present triggering, or may present with pseudo–hallux rigidus (32,91). Such patients may occasionally require tenolysis for relief. The fluid-filled tubular mass, representing the distended tendon sheath, surrounds the dark tendon (Fig. 6.40). It is best visualized in the sagittal or axial plane using long TR/TE sequences and is best seen above, behind, and just below the tibiotalar joint. Quite similar to the changes that occur in the posterior tibial tendon, the FHL may undergo longitudinal splitting resulting in a fusiform swelling of the tendon, but complete rupture is rare (Figs. 6.41, 6.42).

A much less common form of tenosynovitis may

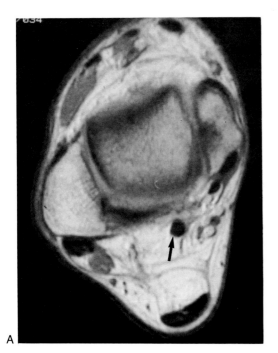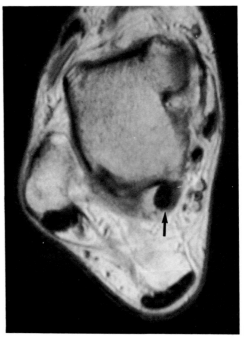

FIG. 6.41. FHL tendonitis. **A, B**: Axial MR, TR/TE 2000/20. A is 6 mm proximal to B. At the level of the ankle joint in A, the FHL (*arrow*) has a normal contour. In B, the tendon markedly enlarges within the groove on the posterior aspect of the talus as it turns to assume a more transverse course. Tendonitis occurs at points of change of direction.

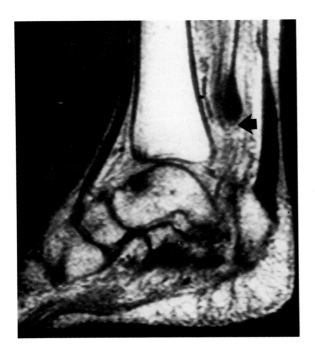

FIG. 6.42. Rupture of the FHL. The patient has sustained a complex calcaneal fracture 8 months prior. (Sagittal MR TR/TE 800/20.) The proximal end of a ruptured FHL (*arrow*) is seen to be retracted cephalad behind the tibia. Rupture of the FHL complicating a calcaneal fracture is uncommon. (Case courtesy of R. Kerr, M.D.)

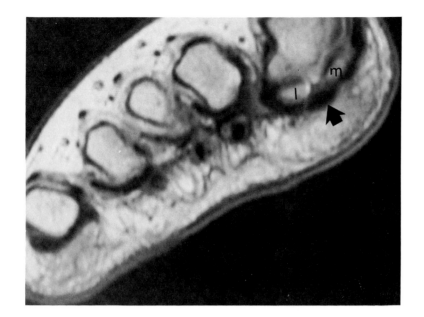

FIG. 6.43. Normal distal FHL. Axial MR, TR/TE 2000/20. The FHL typically becomes inflamed either in its course along the posterior aspect of the talus, or less commonly under the first metatarsophalangeal joint. At this point, the normal FHL (*arrow*) lies in a rather confined space between the medial (*M*) and lateral (*L*) sesamoids.

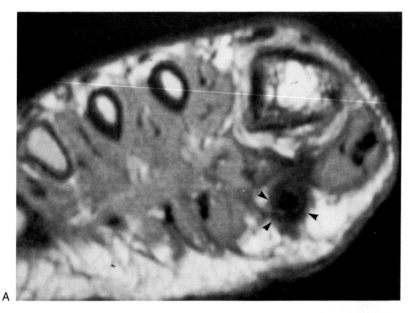

A

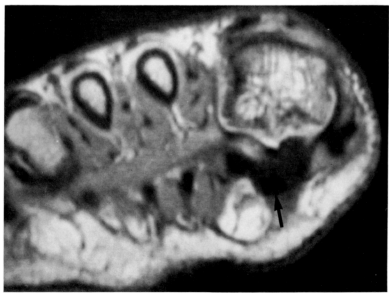

B

FIG. 6.44. Stenosing tenosynovitis of FHL. **A, B**: Axial MR, TR/TE 2000/20. A: On the most proximal image, the FHL tendon sheath is markedly thickened (*arrowheads*). In B at the level of the metatarsal head, 7 mm distal to A, the enlargement of the tendon (*arrow*) and its sheath persists.

develop more distally (Figs. 6.43-6.45). Runners and dancers may develop tenosynovitis at the point at which the flexor digitorum passes beneath the FHL, or where the FHL passes between the sesamoids (3,32,35,42,92). Traumatic lesions of the first metatarsophalangeal joint has been termed "turf toe" because of the frequent occurrence in athletes playing on artificial surfaces with soft-soled shoes. Hyperextension

with varying degrees of valgus is the mechanism of injury. The complex involves osteochondral fractures of the dorsal and medial aspects of the bones, and sprain and rupture of the plantar capsule-ligament complex (93). It is possible that the hyperextension mechanism may result in injury to the FHL tendon. Injuries to the distal FHL may masquerade as primary sesamoid lesions such as fractures (35).

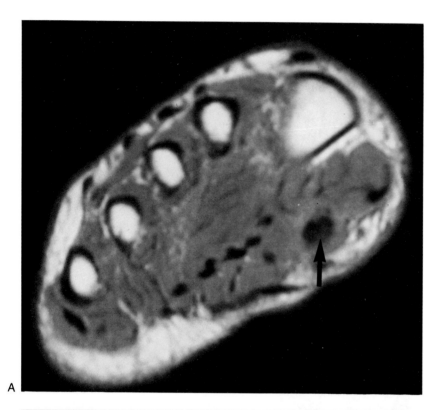

A

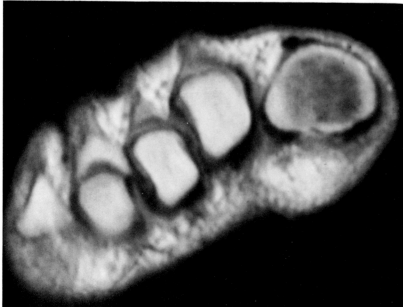

B

FIG. 6.45. Rupture of the distal FHL. **A, B**: Axial MR, TR/TE 2000/20. In A, the FHL tendon (*arrow*) is noted to be enlarged and has a slight increase in signal. In B, just under the first metatarsal head, the tendon is completely absent. It has ruptured and retracted proximally. (Case courtesy of Y. Cheung, M.D.)

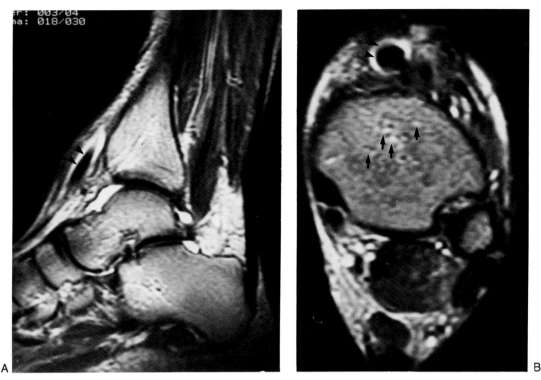

FIG. 6.46. ATT tenosynovitis. (**A**: Axial MR, TR/TE 2000/80. **B**: Axial MR TR/TE 2000/80.) This jogger had anterior pain at the ankle for several months. Just above the ankle joint, the ATT tendon sheath (*arrowheads*) is seen to be filled with fluid, and the contained tendon is focally enlarged in circumference (*arrowheads*). Incidentally noted are poorly defined foci of increased signal in the medullary bone of the tibia (*arrows*); clinically, this edema pattern was a manifestation of a stress response.

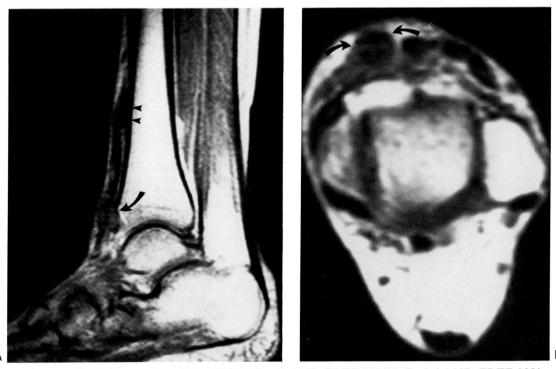

FIG. 6.47. Partial laceration of the ATT. **A**: Sagittal MR, TR/TE 800/20. **B**: Axial MR, TR/TE 800/20. Both images demonstrate widening and increased signal of the distal ATT (*curved arrow*) in this patient who suffered a knife wound and had weakness of dorsiflexion. On the sagittal MRI, several micrometallic artifacts are identified at the point of injury. The proximal tendon (*arrowheads*) is retracted and rolled up.

ANTERIOR TIBIAL TENDON

The tibialis anterior muscle, arising from the proximal two-thirds of the tibia and interosseous membrane, becomes tendinous at the level of the distal tibial metaphysis, and slightly lower, it acquires a synovial sheath. The tendon attaches to the plantar and medial aspects of the first cuneiform and the first metatarsal base. The tendon provides 80% of the dorsiflexion power of the foot and is second only to the Achilles tendon in strength (4,10,35).

The tendon traverses three tough fibrous tunnels that prevent the tendon from displacing away from the subjacent skeletal elements during dorsiflexion; these bands are called retinacula. It is between the superior and inferior retinacula that rupture occurs; in fact, the tough inferior edge of the superior retinaculum may abrade the tendon (10,31). Most tears occur in people over age 50 years, but athletes who might be subject to forced plantar flexion of the foot, such as runners, soccer players, and downhill hikers, can stress and inflame the anterior tibial tendon (31,42) (Fig. 6.46). Since the anterior tibial tendon has a true tendon sheath, the investing synovium may become inflamed primarily and idiopathically, or secondary to rheumatoid disease; spontaneous rupture in these individuals can occur. Inflammation (infection) and penetrating trauma may readily affect the nearly subcutaneous tendon (Fig. 6.47). Patients with ruptures experience a painless drop foot, and differentiation from an L5 nerve root lesion must be made (4,35). Surgical reconstruction of complete ruptures is recommended.

REFERENCES

1. Amiel, D, Harwood, FF, Fronek, J, et al., Tendons and ligaments: A morphological and biochemical comparison. J Orthop Res, 1984. 1: p. 257–265.
2. Frankel, VH and Nordin M, Basic Biomechanics of the Skeletal System. 1980, Lea & Febiger: Philadelphia.
3. Frey, C and Shereff, M, Tendon injuries about the ankle in athletes. Clin Sports Med, 1988. 7: p. 103–117.
4. Scheller, AD, Kasser, JR, and Quigley, TB, Tendon Injuries about the ankle. Orthop Clin North Am, 1980. 11(4): p. 801–811.
5. Trevino, S, Surgical treatment of stenosing tenosynovitis at the ankle. Foot Ankle, 1981. 2(1): p. 37–45.
6. O'Donoghue, DH, Treatment of injuries to athletes. 1984, W.B. Saunders: Philadelphia.
7. Gilula, LA, Oloff, L, Caputi, R, et al., Ankle tenography: A key to unexplained symptomatology Part II: Diagnosis of chronic tendon disabilities. Radiology, 1984. 151: p. 581–587.
8. Rosenberg, ZS and Cheung, Y, Diagnostic imaging of the ankle and foot, in Disorders of the foot and ankle, MH Jahss, Editor. 1991, W.B. Saunders: Philadelphia. p. 109–154.
9. Marcus, DS, Reicher, MA, and Kellerhouse, LE, Achilles tendon injuries: The role of MR imaging. J Comput Assist Tomogr, 1989. 13(3): p. 480–486.
10. Kelikin, H, Disruption and dislocation of some tendons, in Disorders of the Ankle, H Kelikin, Editor. 1985, WB Saunders: Philadelphia. p. 759–791.
11. Szczukowski, M, St Pierre, R, Fleming, L, et al., Computerized tomography in the evaluation of peroneal tendon dislocations: A report of two cases. Am J Sports Med, 1983. 11: p. 444–447.
12. Ala-Ketola, L, Peranen J, Kovivisto, E, et al., Arthrography in the diagnosis of ligament injuries and classification of ankle injuries. Radiology, 1977. 125: p. 63–68.
13. Resnick, D, Arthrography, tenography, and bursography, in Diagnosis of Bone and Joint Disorders, D Resnick and G Niwayama, Editors. 1988, WB Saunders: Philadelphia.
14. Teng, M, Destouet, JM, Resnick D, et al., Ankle tenography: A key to unexplained symptomatology Part 1: Normal tenographic anatomy. Radiology, 1984. 151: p. 575–580.
15. Beltran, J, Noto, AM, Herman, LJ, et al., Tendons: High-field-strength surface coil MR imaging. Radiology, 1987. 162: p. 735–740.
16. Dillehay, G, Deschler, T, Rogers, L, et al. The ultrasonographic characterization of tendons. Invest Radiol, 1984. 19(4): p. 338–341.
17. Fornage, BD, Achilles tendon: Ultrasound examination. Radiology, 1986. 159: p. 759–764.
18. Zeiss, J, Saddemi, SR, and Ebraheim, NA, MR imaging of the peroneal tunnel. J Comput Assist Tomogr, 1989. 13(5): p. 840–844.
19. Rosenberg, Z, Feldman F, and Singson, R, Peroneal tendon injuries: CT analysis. Radiology, 1986. 161: p. 743–748.
20. Rosenberg, ZS, Feldman, F, Singson, RD, et al., Peroneal tendon injury associated calcaneal fractures: CT findings. AJR, 1987. 149: p. 125–129.
21. Rosenberg, Z, Feldman, F, Singson, R, et al., Computed tomography of ankle tendons. Radiology, 1987. 166: p. 221–226.
22. Rosenberg, Z, Cheung, Y, and Jahss, M, Computed tomography scan and magnetic resonance imaging of ankle tendons: An overview. Foot Ankle, 1988. 8: p. 297–307.
23. Rosenberg, Z, Cheung, Y, Jahss, M, et al., Rupture of the posterior tibial tendon: CT and MR imaging with surgical correlation. Radiology, 1988. 169: p. 229–235.
24. Kneeland, JB, Macrander, S, Middleton, WD, et al., MR imaging of the normal ankle: Correlation with anatomic sections. AJR, 1988. 151: p. 117–123.
25. Griffith, JC, Tendon injuries around the ankle. J Bone Joint Surg (Br), 1965. 47: p. 686–689.
26. Beltran, J, Noto, A, Mosure, J, et al., Ankle: Surface coil MR imaging of 1.5T. Radiology, 1986. 161: p. 203–209.
27. Sartoris, D, Mink, J, and Kerr, R, The foot and ankle, in MR of the musculoskeletal system: A teaching file, J Mink and A Deutsch, Editors. 1990, Raven Press: New York.
28. Hajek, P, Baker L, Bjorkengren, A, et al., High-resolution magnetic resonance imaging of the ankle: Normal anatomy. Skeletal Radiol, 1986. 15: p. 536–540.
29. Lance, E, Deutsch, A, and Mink, J, Rupture of the peroneus brevis tendon; MR assessment. (Submitted).
30. Kier, R, Dietz, M, McCarthy, S, et al., MR imaging of the normal ligaments and tendons of the ankle. J Comp Assist Tomogr, 1991. 15: p. 477–482.
31. Berquist, TH and Johnson, KA, Trauma, in Radiology of the foot and ankle, TH Berquist, Editor. 1989, Raven Press: New York: p. 99–113.
32. Hamilton, WG, Foot and ankle injuries in dancers. Clin Sports Med, 1988. 7(1): p. 143–173.
33. James, S, Bates, B, and Ostering, L, Injuries to runners. Am J Sports Med, 1978. 6: p. 40–50.
34. Clement, P, Taunton, J, and Smart, G, Achilles tendinitis and peritendinitis: Etiology and treatment. Am J Sports Med, 1984. 12: p. 179–184.
35. Singer, K and Jones, D, Soft tissue conditions of the ankle and foot, in The lower extremity and spine in sports medicine, J Nicholas, and E Hershman, Editors. 1986, CV Mosby: St Louis. p. 498–525.
36. Quinn, SF, Murray, WT, Clark RA, et al., Achilles tendon: MR imaging at 1.5T. Radiology, 1987. 164: p. 767–770.
37. Lagergren, C and Lindholm, A, Vascular disruption in the achilles tendon and angiographic and microangiographic study. Acta Chir Scand, 1985/59. 116: p. 481–495.
38. Keene, JS, Lash, EG, Fisher, DR, et al., Magnetic resonance imaging of achilles tendon ruptures. Am J Sports Med, 1989. 17(3): p. 333–337.

39. Mitchell, MJ, Sartoris, DJ, and Resnick, D, *The foot and ankle.* Top Magn Reson Imaging, 1989. **1**: p. 57–73.

40. Oden, R, *Tendon injuries about the ankle resulting from skiing.* Clin Orthop, 1987. **216**: p. 63–69.

41. Brody, N, *Running injuries.* CIBA Clin Symp, 1980. **32**: p. 1–64.

42. Forrester, D and Kerr, R, *Trauma to the foot.* Radiol Clin North Am, 1990. **28**. WB Saunders: Philadelphia. p. 423–433.

43. Bodne, D, Quinn, S, Murray, W, et al., *Magnetic resonance imaging of chronic patellar tendonitis.* Skeletal Radiol, 1988. **17**: p. 24–28.

44. Beltran, J, *MRI of the Musculosketal System.* 1990, J.B. Lippincott Co: Philadelphia.

45. Kier, R, McCarthy, S, Dietz, M, et al., *MR appearance of painful conditions of the ankle.* RadioGraphics, 1991. **11**: p. 401–414.

46. Weinstabl, R, Stiskal, M, Neuhold, A, et al., *Classifying calcaneal tendon injury according to MRI findings.* J Bone Joint Surg, 1991. **73 B**: p. 683–685.

47. Fox, JM, Blazina, ME, Jobe, EW, et al., *Degeneration and rupture of the achilles tendon.* Clin Orthop, 1975. **107**: p. 221–224.

48. Price, A, Evanski, P, and Waugh, T, *Bilateral simultaneous Achilles tendon ruptures. A case report and review of the literature.* Clin Orthop, 1986. **213**: p. 249–250.

49. O'Brien, T, *The needle test for complete rupture of the Achilles tendon.* J Bone Joint Surg (Am), 1984. **66**: p. 1099–1101.

50. Pavlov, H, *Athletic injuries.* Radiol Clin North Am, 1990. **28**(2): p. 435–442.

51. Reinig, JW, Dorwart, RH, and Roden, WC, *MR imaging of a ruptured Achilles tendon.* J Comput Assist Tomogr, 1985. **9**(6): p. 1131–1134.

52. Daffner, R, Riemer, BL, Lupetin, AR, et al., *Magnetic resonance imaging in acute tendon ruptures.* Skeletal Radiol, 1986. **15**(8): p. 619–621.

53. Nistor, L, *Nonsurgical treatment of Achilles tendon ruptures.* J Bone Joint Surg (AM), 1981. **63**: p. 394.

54. Inglis, AE, Scott, N, Sculco, TP, et al., *Rupture of the tendon achilles. An objective assessment of surgical and non-surgical treatment.* J Bone Joint Surg (Am), 1976. **58**: p. 990–993.

55. Mann, R, Holmes, GB, Seale, KS, et al., *Chronic rupture of the achilles tendon: A new technique of repair.* J Bone Joint Surg (Am), 1991. **73**: p. 214–219.

56. Kato, YP, Dunn, MG, Zawadsky, JP, et al., *Regeneration of Achilles tendon with a collagen tendon prosthesis.* J Bone Joint Surg, 1991. **73**(4): p. 561–574.

57. Liem, MD, Zegel, HG, Balduini, FC, et al., *Repair of achilles tendon ruptures with a polylactic acid implant: Assessment with MR imaging.* AJR, 1991. **156**: p. 769–773.

58. Bradley, JP, and Tibone, JE, *Percutaneous and open surgical repairs of Achilles tendon ruptures.* Am J Sports Med, 1990. **18**(2): p. 118–196.

59. Ma, GW and Griffith, TG, *Percutaneous repair of acute closed ruptured Achilles tendon.* Clin Orthop, 1977. **128**: p. 247–255.

60. Dillon, E, Pope, C, Barber, V, et al., *Achilles tendon healing: 12-month follow-up with MR imaging.* Radiology, 1990. **177** (P): p. 306.

61. Hertzanu, Y, Berginer, J, and Berginer, VM, *Computed tomography of tendinous xanthomata in cerebrotendinous xanthomatosis.* Skeletal Radiol, 1991. **20**(99–102).

62. Pavlov, H, Heneghan, M, Hersh, A, et al., *Haglund's deformity: Diagnosis and differential diagnosis of posterior heel pain.* Radiology, 1982. **144**: p. 83–90.

63. Dunn, A, *Anomalous muscles simulating soft-tissue tumors in the lower extremities. Report of three cases.* J Bone Joint Surg (Am), 1965. **47**: p. 1397–1400.

64. Nidecker, A, von Hochstetter, A, and Fredenhagen, H, *Accessory muscles of the lower calf.* Radiology, 1984. **151**: p. 47–48.

65. Nichols, GW and Kalenak, A, *The accessory soleus muscle.* Clin Orthop, 1984. **190**: p. 279–280.

66. Sammarco, JD and Brainard, BJ, *A symptomatic anomalous peroneus brevis in a high-jumper.* J Bone Joint Surg (Am), 1991. **73**: p. 131–133.

67. Funk, DA, Cass, JR, and Johnson, KA, *Acquired adult flat foot secondary to posterior tibial tendon pathology.* J Bone Joint Surg (Am), 1986. **68**: p. 95–102.

68. Dezwart, DF and Davidson, JSA, *Rupture of the posterior tibial tendon associated with ankle fractures.* J Bone Joint Surg (Am), 1983. **65A**: p. 260–261.

69. Stein, R, *Rupture of the posterior tibial tendon in closed ankle fractures: Possible prognostic value of a medial bone flake: Report of two cases.* J Bone Joint Surg (Am), 1985. **67**: p. 493–494.

70. Conti, S, *Clinical significance of magnetic resonance imaging in preoperative planning for soft-tissue reconstruction of posterior tibial tendon ruptures,* in *American Academy of Orthopaedic Surgeons Fifty-Eighth Annual Meeting.* 1991. Anaheim, California.

71. Rosenberg, ZS, Cheung, Y, Jahss, M, et al., *Chronic tears of the posterior tibial tendon: A correlative study of CT, MR imaging, and surgical exploration.* Radiology, 1987. **165** (p): p. 149.

72. Noto, A, Cheung, Y, Rosenberg, Z, et al., *MR Imaging of the ankle: Normal variants.* Radiology, 1989. **170**: p. 121–124.

73. Alexander, IJ, Johnson, KA, and Berquist, TH, *Magnetic resonance imaging of the diagnosis of disruption of the posterior tibial tendon.* Foot Ankle, 1987. **8**: p. 144–147.

74. Sella, EJ, Lawson, JP, and Ogden, JA, *The accessory navicular synchondrosis.* Clin Orthop, 1986. **209**: p. 280–285.

75. Lawson, JP, Ogden, JA, Sella E, et al., *The painful accessory navicular.* Skeletal Radiol, 1984. **12**: p. 250–262.

76. Matin, P, *Basic principles of nuclear medicine techniques for detection and evaluation of trauma and sports medicine injuries.* Semin Nucl Med, 1988. **18**: p. 90–112.

77. Michael, RH and Holder, LE, *The soleus syndrome: A cause of medial tibial stress (shin splints).* Am J Sports Med, 1985. **13**: p. 87–94.

78. Rupani, HD, Holder, LE, Espinola, DA, et al., *Three-phase radionuclide bone imaging in sports medicine.* Radiology, 1985. **156**: p. 187–296.

79. Holder, L and Michael, R, *The specific scintigraphic pattern of shin splints in the lower leg: Concise communication.* J Nucl Med, 1984. **25**(8): p. 865–869.

80. Eckert, WR and Davis, EA, *Acute rupture of the peroneal retinaculum.* J Bone Joint Surg (Am), 1976. **58**(5): p. 670–673.

81. Peacock, KC, Resnick, EJ, and Thoder, JJ, *Fracture of the os peroneum with rupture of the peroneus longus tendon.* Clin Orthop, 1984. **202**: p. 223–226.

82. Edwards, M, *The relations of the peroneal tendons to the fibula, calcaneus, and cuboideum.* Am J Anat, 1928. **42**: p. 213–253.

83. Kojima, Y, Kataoka, Y, and Suzuki, S, *Dislocation of the peroneal tendons in neonates and infants.* Clin Orthop Rel Res, 1991. **266**: p. 180–184.

84. Thompson, F and Patterson, A, *Rupture of the peroneus longus tendon. Report of three cases.* J Bone Joint Surg (Am), 1989, **71**: p. 293–295.

85. Munk, RL and Davis, PH, *Longitudinal rupture of the peroneus brevis tendon.* J Trauma, 1976. **16**: p. 803–806.

86. Tehranzadeh, J, Stoll, DA, and Gabriele, OM, *Case report 271: Posterior migration of the os peroneum of the left foot, indicating a tear of the peroneal tendon.* Skeletal Radiol, 1984. **12**: p. 44–47.

87. Micheli, L, Waters, P, and Sanders, D, *Sliding fibular graft repair for chronic dislocation of the peroneal tendons.* Am J Sports Med, 1989. **17**(1): p. 68–71.

88. Kelly, RE, *An operation for the chronic dislocation of the peroneal tendons.* Br J Surg, 1920. **7**: p. 502.

89. Sarmiento, A, *Subluxation of peroneal tendons.* J Bone Joint Surg (Am), 1975. **57**: p. 115–116.

90. Watson-Jones, R, *Fracture and Joint Injuries.* 5th ed. 1976, Williams & Wilkins: Baltimore.

91. Sammarco, GJ, and Miller, ED, *Partial rupture of the flexor hallucis longus tendon in classical ballet dancer.* J Bone Joint Surg (Am), 1979. **61**: p. 149–154.

92. Gould, N, *Stenosing tenosynovitis of the flexor hallucis longus tendon at the great toe.* Foot Ankle, 1981. **2**(1): p. 46–48.

93. Bowers, K and Martin, R, *Turf toe—a shoe surface-related football injury.* Med Sci Sports, 1976. **8**: p. 81–83.

MRI of the Foot and Ankle,
edited by A.L. Deutsch, J.H. Mink, and R. Kerr,
Raven Press, Ltd., New York © 1992

CHAPTER 7

Ligaments of the Ankle

Jerrold H. Mink

CLINICAL CONSIDERATIONS

Ligaments are cords of dense connective tissue that join adjacent bones at their ends, thereby helping to maintain skeletal alignment and body shape. The basic internal structure of a ligament is similar to that of tendon; however, while the collagen fiber bundles of tendon are aligned parallel to one another and are co-linear with the line of pull of the muscle, the fiber bundles of ligament have parallel, oblique, or even spiral arrangements. The precise geometric orientation of the fiber bundles in each ligament represent an adaptation to the specific function of restraining joint displacement (1,2).

Inversion injuries of the ankle are among the most common injuries to the musculoskeletal system. Following inversion, a variety of traumatic lesions may occur singly or in combination, including ligamentous sprain, ankle fractures, osteochondral lesions of the talar dome, and peroneal tendon dislocation (Table 7.1). Because of the frequent difficulty in distinguishing these entities clinically, they have often been lumped together as ankle sprains or turned ankles (3). This chapter will be directed specifically to the anatomy and pathoanatomic changes that occur within the ankle ligaments following trauma.

Ankle Sprains

It has been estimated that there are as many as 23,000 ankle sprains per day in the United States. Such injuries may consititute up to 10% of the visits to emergency rooms in Scandinavia, and 85% of all ankle injuries (4). Inversion injuries occur primarily as a result

of participation in sports; 45% of injuries occurring in basketball and 31% of the injuries occurring in soccer are ankle injuries (4). The majority of ankle injuries occur in people under 35 years, but complete tears of the anterior talofibular ligament occur commonly in patients under 15 years (5). Ankle sprains are not always self-limited. In one study of high school athletes, 50% of those suffering acute lateral ligament tears had residual symptoms from their injuries, and 15% felt that their injury compromised their playing performance (5).

Failure of ligaments is influenced by loading rate of the structure, prior immobilization, exercise, chronic physical activity, age of the patient, and trauma. Age

TABLE 7.1. *Differential diagnosis of ankle sprains*

Fracture
   Lateral malleolus
   Talus
   Anterior process of the calcaneus
   Fifth metatarsal base
   Fifth metatarsal shaft (Dancer's fracture)
   Osteochondral fracture of the talar dome
Dislocations
   Subtalar
   Talonavicular
   Cuboid subluxation
Ligament sprains
   ATIF
   Deltoid
Miscellaneous
   Peroneal subluxation/rupture
   Symptomatic os fibulare
   Impingement syndrome
   Symptomatic os trigonum
   Sinus tarsi syndrome
   Entrapment neuritis (sural and superficial peroneal)
   Rupture of the extensor digitorum brevis
   Retinacular rupture (peroneal and extensor)

J. H. Mink: Tower Musculoskeletal Imaging Center, Los Angeles, California 90048.

and inactivity result in increased stiffness, decreased tensile strength, and less deformation to failure. The administration of even a single dose of steroids directly into collagenous tissue can have a debilitating effect on its strength (2).

Ligamentous sprains are classified as first, second, or third degree injuries, although it is impossible to quantify precisely the true extent of damage (4,6–9). A first degree sprain is a mild injury in which there is local pain, point tenderness, and rather little swelling. There is no instability demonstrable by stress radiography or clinical examination. Microscopically, minor fiber tears may be present. Second degree sprains are more severe injuries in which there is moderate swelling and hemorrhage. This injury must be considered a partial or incomplete tear. The hallmark of the second degree sprain is some loss of function; instability and abnormal motion results. In third degree strains, there is complete loss of ligamentous integrity with abnormal motion and a soft or indistinct end point to stress testing. There is marked edema and tenderness, yet surprisingly the pain may be less than that of a second degree injury. It is thought that with an incomplete tear, tension on partially torn fiber ends produces the pain (6).

During the first week following a ligament tear, a hematoma, fibroblastic proliferation, and a mass of inflammatory tissue form at the site of the disruption. During the third to the sixth week, healing begins by increasing collagenization and reorganization into a more organized ligamentlike histology. The ultimate outcome is dependent on multiple factors including, but not limited to, proximity of the torn tendon edges to each other, local blood supply and local environmental factors (6).

First degree sprains require 5 to 10 days of conservative care. The treatment program includes the immediate institution of conservative care, including rest, ice, compression, and elevation (4). Activity is restricted until there is pain-free motion. Since a second degree sprain implies a more significant injury, treatment is protective. The patient often requires 3 to 6 weeks to recover. First and second degree lateral sprains are treated conservatively with taping or occasionally casting, taping, and crutches. Third degree sprain, if treated conservatively, usually require a short leg cast (6). Occasionally, surgical reconstitution is required (10–12).

MAGNETIC RESONANCE ASSESSMENT

Ankle ligaments, like those elsewhere in the body, are composed of dense fibrous tissue that have rather little free water within their substance. They are dark at virtually every imaging sequence, and inasmuch as they are usually adjacent to fat, they are most graphically depicted on those sequences in which fat is relatively bright (T1 and proton density sequences). Gradient-recalled sequences have been reported to be useful (13), but we have not found this to be true. Because of the general desirability of using the natural arthrographic effect of bright joint fluid contrasted against dark surrounding structures, we choose to use a double-echo, spin-echo sequence (TR/TE 2500/20,80) in examination of the ligaments. The first echo provides an image with a quality comparable to a true T1-weighted image (T1WI), and the second echo image optimizes differences in soft tissue characteristics.

Only the affected ankle is examined in a send-receive extremity coil, allowing for small field-of-view (12–14 cm field of view), high-resolution studies. The patient is allowed to place the foot in the coil in a position that he/she finds most comfortable. Most patients tend to externally rotate, and plantar flex the foot 10° to 20°. By not "forcing" patients to hold their foot in a predetermined position, the examiner is more likely to obtain images without motion artifact. The first images obtained are low-resolution rapidly acquired (localizer) axial images. From this small series of images, the true coronal and sagittal planes can be proscribed. The true coronal plane, equivalent to the mortise view described by conventional radiographic means, is defined by a line drawn between the two malleoli. The true sagittal plane is defined as the plane 90° to the coronal. By standardizing these two planes, one can eliminate the considerable differences in external rotation of the foot among patients. A T1WI sequence in the true coronal plane is obtained, followed by an inversion recovery (STIR) sequence in the sagittal plane. Optionally, STIR coronal and T1W sagittal image sequences may also be obtained. An axial sequence using a double-echo, spin-echo technique is the last sequence performed. If the initial sagittal sequence indicates that the foot is excessively plantar flexed (>15°), the axial plane is deliberately obliqued so that the scanning axial plane is nearly parallel to the plane of the metatarsals. Specialized oblique imaging planes are used if necessary (e.g., examination of the calcaneofibular ligament) (4,14).

Normal ankle ligaments appear either as relatively thin bands connecting adjacent bones, or a series of dark, individual fiber bundles separated by thin layers of fibrofatty tissue (e.g., the deltoid or posterior talofibular ligament). Injured ankle ligaments share a number of common magnetic resonance (MR) features. In acute ligamentous sprains, one finds overlying soft tissue edema and perhaps identifiable hemorrhage, although in our experience, the fluid that accumulates in the deep soft tissues has signal characteristics of water (edema) rather than blood. The contour of the affected ligament is irregular, serpiginous, widened, or discontinuous and the normally dark ligament demonstrates an increase in internal signal (4,15,16). This increase in signal intensity is best seen on T1WI or proton density sequences and may persist on long repitition (TR) time protocols, but uncommonly does the signal within the ligament actually increase in intensity. The combination of periligamentous edema, ligamentous structural damage, thickened and hemorrhagic synovium, and fat plane distortion all lead to the appearance of a poorly defined, lobulated intermediate signal intensity mass replacing the normal structure (4,15). When the affected ligament is capsular (the anterior talofibular ligament, for instance), an effusion in the adjacent joint may be seen to extend directly through the torn ligament into the adjacent soft tissues.

Many of the findings seen in the acutely torn ligament are also found in the ankle that is being assessed for chronic pain syndromes and/or instability, although edema is generally absent. Thickening, contour distortion, and abnormal signal intensity (T1WI or proton density sequences) characterize the chronically torn ligament (4). Evidence of ligamentous damage may also be manifest by marked thinning of the ligament, or its complete absence. The latter sign is a diagnostic sign of a chronic tear only in those instances in which the normal ligament is reliably identified [i.e., 100% for the anterior talofibular ligament (13)].

THE LATERAL COLLATERAL LIGAMENT

The lateral collateral ligament is a complex structure composed of the anterior talofibular (ATAF) ligament, the posterior talofibular (PTAF) ligament, and the calcaneofibular (CF) ligaments (Fig. 7.1). The ATAF is 20 mm long, and 2 to 3 mm thick. It arises from the anterior margin of the lateral malleolus and runs anteriorly and medially toward its attachment to the talus. The ATAF, the weakest and the most vulnerable of all of the ankle ligaments, serves to limit internal rotation and inversion and to prevent the talus from slipping forward from under the tibia (17,18). In its

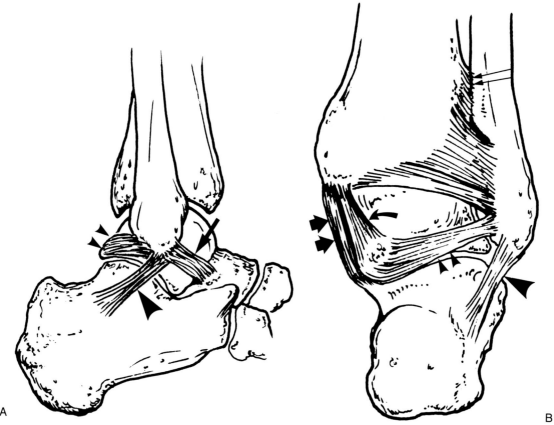

FIG. 7.1. Normal ligamentous anatomy of the ankle. **A–C:** These diagrams demonstrate the normal relationships of the components of the lateral collateral ligament, the medial collateral ligament, and the syndesmotic complex. (ATAF, arrow; PTAF, small arrowheads; CF, large arrowhead; tibiotalar, curved arrow; tibiocalcaneal ligament, double arrow; tibionavicular, double large arrowhead; tibiospring, long arrow; ATIF, double long arrow.) (*Figure continues on next page.*)

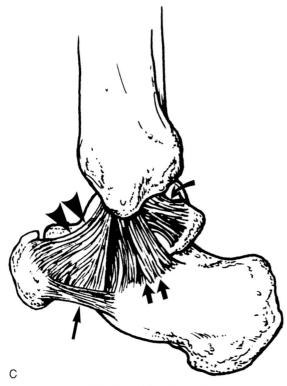

FIG. 7.1. (*Continued*)

course to the talus, the ATAF crosses a ridge of the talar body just behind the neck of the talus. It is this ridge that is in part responsible for a tear of the ATAF. The ATAF tears in its midsubstance 45% of the time, and by talar avulsion 50% of the time (3). A deep branch of the peroneal artery crosses the ATAF, and traumatic aneurysm of the artery has been reported in connection with rupture of the ligament.

The other two components of the lateral collateral ligament are the CF and the PTAF. The CF ligament descends nearly vertically from the lateral malleolus to attach to the lateral calcaneus. The PTAF is generally considered the strongest of the ankle ligaments, and disruption occurs only when the talus is dislocated without an associated fibular fracture (9). It arises from the medial aspect of the distal fibula at approximately the same level as the CF, courses nearly horizontally, and attaches to the posterior lateral talar tubercle, a landmark that defines the lateral margin of the groove for the flexor hallucis longus (the tibiotalar limb of the deltoid ligament attaches to the posterior medial tubercle) (Fig. 7.1). The primary function of the CF ligament is to provide the primary static restraint against inversion of the calcaneus. The CF is situated just lateral to the calcaneus and just medial to the peroneal tendons in their common sheath. Unlike the posterior talofibular ligament and ATAF, the CF ligament is not intimately related to the talocrural joint. Cordlike extracapsular ligaments like the CF have a poorer blood supply than those that are flat and intracapsular. When round ligaments are torn, they tend to retract and often fail to unite even after extended periods of immobilization. Therefore, the arthrographic diagnosis of a CF tear can be made long after the traumatic event, but the opposite is true for the ATAF.

When one speaks of a tear of the lateral ankle ligaments, one is nearly always referring to a tear of the ATAF, with or without a concomitant tear of the CF (17). The combination occurs 40% of the time that the ATAF tears, whereas a tear of the CF without an ATAF tear is quite unusual. Not infrequently, tears of the lateral ligaments will be accompanied by avulsion of the fifth metatarsal base by the tensed peroneus brevis tendon. Lateral ligament injuries occur as a result of inversion motion during which the ATAF is pulled across the ridge along the neck of the talus; the joint capsule, intimately related to the ligament, tears as well. If inversion stresses continue, the CF tears, and ultimately the talocalcaneal interosseous ligament, may also rupture. Ankle ligament tears are characterized by the acute onset of pain, the rapid onset of ecchymosis, and tenderness along the course of the injured ligament.

There is considerable controversy regarding the need for operative repair of acute severe lateral collateral ligament injuries since most patients will have a good to excellent prognosis regardless of therapy (4). In one study, 100 patients with lateral collateral ligament sprains were divided into two groups, one treated operatively and the other conservatively (19). The operative group had a longer delay in return to work, and of course a higher complication rate in the first weeks; however, there was no evidence at 2 years that operative repair offered any symptomatic or functional benefit. Therefore, most grade 3 sprains can be managed nonoperatively, and if late instability occurs, as it may in 10% to 20% of patients, a reconstructive procedure can be performed and the results will be equivalent to that of immediate repair (4,19).

Individuals who suffer extensive recurrent inversion injuries and have documented instability may be candidates for one of the many operative procedures designed to restore lateral ankle stability. While these surgical procedures differ, all are aimed at stabilizing the abnormal inversion of the ankle by the use of static or dynamic stabilizers (4,10–12,20,21).

The diagnosis of lateral collateral ligament sprains has traditionally been made by means of conventional stress radiography, arthrography of the talocrural joint, and peroneal tenography. The inversion and sagittal stress radiographs both take advantage of the fact that the ATAF prevents both inversion of the talus relative to the tibia (talar tilt), and anterior shift of the talus within the ankle joint (Fig. 7.2). To determine the talar tilt, two lines are drawn; the first is a tangent to

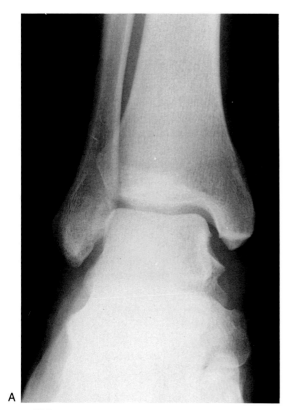
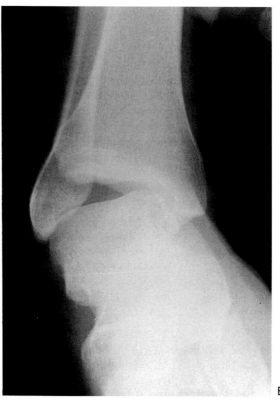

A
B

FIG. 7.2. Talar tilt following an ankle sprain. **A:** The conventional anteroposterior radiograph does not demonstrate any significant abnormalities, but a study performed during varus stress **B:** of the hindfoot demonstrates gross talar tilt, indicating a tear of the ATAF and the CF.

the superiormost surface of the talar dome, and the other is a line drawn along the cortex of the tibial plafond. The degree of divergence of these two lines is defined as the talar tilt, and this angle is usually less than 4° (22). Opinions vary as to the upper limits of normal, but if the angle on the injured side is 10° more than that on the normal side, both the ATAF and CF ligaments are probably torn (7,19,23). Sauser et al. concluded that the inversion stress test was highly specific (99%) when the angle of inversion was greater than 10° but that only 38% of injured ankles with torn ligaments achieved this level of instability (24).

The sagittal stress test, also known as the anterior drawer test, is analogous to a similar test in the knee. The degree of forward shift of the talus relative to the posterior lip of the distal talus is measured (3,22). This measurement does not normally exceed 6 mm, and up to 14 mm of displacement is found when the ATAF is divided alone or in combination with the other ligaments (22,25), but division of the CF alone does not result in any talar displacement. Measurements of both talar tilt and inversion are unfortunately subject to some error; the degree of patient pain/cooperation, the applied force, the amount of plantar flexion of the ankle, and the laxity of the opposite side all affect mensuration. Additionally, the measured values correlate

poorly with symptoms of instability and the extent of the ligamentous disruption (19,23).

Arthrography and tenography have been advocated as relatively painless methods of determining the status of the lateral ligaments of the ankle following trauma (26). In the normal arthrogram, contrast injected into the talocrural joint extends laterally into the space between the lateral malleolus and the talus, but does not extend under the inferior contour of the malleolus (27). As noted above, the ATAF is in intimate relationship with the joint capsule; therefore, a disruption of the former results in a tear of the latter. Contrast injected into an ankle joint in which the ATAF is torn is free to extravasate into the fascial space surrounding the fibular malleolus. The contrast is seen to curve under the fibular malleolus and to extend lateral to it; on lateral radiographs, the contrast dissects anterior to the distal fibula (17,27). Ideally, arthrography should be carried out within 24 h, or at the latest 5 days following trauma, as organization of a soft tissue hematoma may seal the capsular rent and lead to a false negative arthrographic study. The CF ligament is in contact with the anterior aspect of the peroneal tendon sheaths, and an acute rupture of the CF allows contrast injected into the ankle joint to flow into the peroneal sheaths. This communication is unlikely to seal even long after trauma because of the poor vascularity of the ligament, its cordlike structure, and its extracapsular location. There are no distinguishing arthrographic signs of a tear of the PTAF, but isolated injury to this structure is quite unusual (3). The reported accuracy of arthrography in the diagnosis of lateral ligamentous injury to the ankle is 75% to 90%.

Because of the finding of false negative arthrograms in patients with CF ligament tears, Black et al. introduced the concept of performing peroneal tenography to demonstrate the suspected communication with the ankle joint (28). Peroneal tenography is 95% accurate in diagnosing rupture of the CF ligament (29). In the arthrographic assessment of lateral ankle ligament injuries, it is probably best first to perform a stress peroneal tenogram (30), and if it is negative to perform an ankle joint arthrogram (7). The positive predictive value of this regimen approaches 100%, and can reliably distinguish isolated ATAF tears from those combined with CF tears.

On MR examinations, the ATAF is nearly always identified on a single axial section if the foot is in a neutral or slightly plantar flexed position because the ligament has a nearly horizontal course (4,13,15,31 32) (Fig. 7.3). The ligament appears as a 2- to 3-mm thick band running from the anterior lateral malleolus to the anterolateral talus. The ATAF is the most consistently and easily identified ligament at the ankle on MR studies. It has been identified in 100% of normal subjects in the axial plane, but it is uncommon to find this thin structure in any other plane (13,33). In patients who have suffered an acute tear of the ATAF, the proton density images often fail to demonstrate any ligamentous structure at the anterolateral malleolus; the long TR image, however, may reveal a poorly defined mass representing the proximal and/or distal extremities of the torn ligament (Fig. 7.4). A tear of the ATAF is invariably accompanied by a capsular rupture, an event that may permit the natural contrast material joint fluid to escape from the joint space into the soft tissues. This lack of confinement into the joint is the equivalent of the findings on the diagnostic arthrogram. Occasionally, the fibular attachment of the ATAF is "stripped back" along the anterior lateral malleolus, resulting in a ligament that is thickened and redundant. In chronic injuries, ligamentous thickening and a mild diffuse increase in signal predominate (Fig. 7.5). The torn ligament may measure as much as 6 mm in thickness.

The CF arises from the fibula and it courses distally and slightly posteriorly. It is seen on the axial series as a cordlike or linear dark structure, measuring 2 to 3 mm in thickness, situated immediately anteromedial to the peroneal tendons (13,15,32) (Fig. 7.6). The ability to image the CF in the axial plane can be improved by plantar flexing the foot to 25° to 40°, but given its course, it is best to search for the CF on the coronal images (4,15,33). In spite of the use of multiple imaging planes, the normal CF has been identified in only 81% of normal ankles (13). The reasons for this difficulty include the nonorthogonal course of the ligament, the small size of the structure, and the partial volume effect of the dark ligament with the dark peroneal tendons and lateral calcaneal cortex. Therefore, absence of the CF cannot be used as a reliable criterion for CF ligamentous disruption. Tears can be diagnosed when the CF is thickened (up to 5 mm) and assumes a serpiginous character. Findings associated with a CF tear include peroneal retinacular thickening and peroneal tendon abnormalities such as tenosynovitis and subluxation. MR examinations of the ankle must be carefully examined for assessment of these associated disorders.

At approximately the same axial MR level at which one identifies the ATAF, the PTAF can nearly always be visualized as a series of fibers running from the malleolar fossa of the fibula to the posterior lateral talar tubercle (13,15,32–34) (Figs. 7.3, 7.7). The MR image of a parallel arrangement of individual fibers separated by fibrofatty tissue is similar to the appearance of the anterior cruciate ligament of the knee; the appearance must not be mistaken for a pathologic process (15,16). On sagittal images on which it is seen, the PTAF must not be mistaken for a loose body situated just behind the talus (15) (Fig. 7.7). In patients without joint effusion, the PTAF (and the posterior tibiofibular ligament) is closely applied to the posterior aspect of the talus and the joint line where it may simulate a loose body. If the joint is distended, however, the pseudo-loose bodies will be seen to be extracapsular in location.

Posttraumatic Ankle Dysfunction

The long-term consequences of a severe lateral ligament ankle sprain include instability, weakness, pain, osteochondral fracture (osteochondritis dissecans), loose body formation, the sinus tarsi syndrome, and the anterolateral ankle impingement syndrome. It is essential to identify accurately the etiology of posttraumatic ankle pain since the appropriate therapy so critically depends on proper diagnosis.

There is a group of patients who suffer from chronic lateral pain whose etiology remains elusive in spite of the use of stress radiography, high-resolution computed tomography, and single photon emission computed tomography. Affected patients are young and active and 94% have sustained a previous lateral ankle sprain. The term "anterolateral ankle impingement

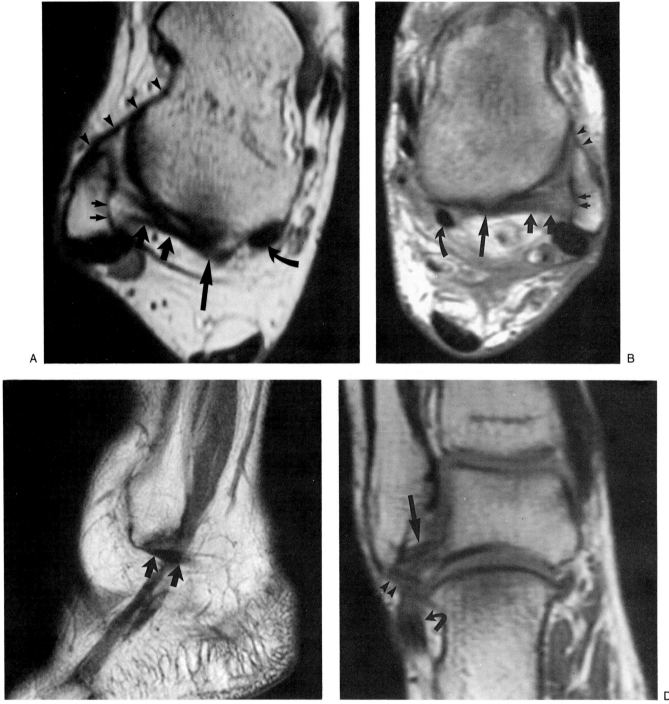

FIG. 7.3. Normal talofibular ligaments. **A, B:** Axial MR, TR/TE 2000/20. The images are from two different patients. In both A and B the ATAF (*arrowheads*) is a thin band that is virtually always identified on a single MRI. The PTAF (*arrows*) has a somewhat fanlike insertion on the fibula, and therefore linear areas of signal within it ought not to be mistaken for pathology. The PTAF originates from the lateral tubercle of the talus (*large arrow*), which forms the lateral wall of the gutter for the FHL (*curved arrow*). The deep malleolar fossa (*tiny arrows*) is the site of origin of the PTAF, and is a reliable landmark in differentiating the position of the talofibular and tibiofibular ligaments. **C:** Sagittal MR TR/TE 2000/20. This fortuitous image demonstrates the PTAF origin (*arrows*) from the fibular malleolus "crossing" the peroneals. **D:** Coronal MR TR/TE 2000/20. This high-resolution image reveals the PTAF (*arrow*) and the CF (*arrowheads*), the latter of which is just medial to the peroneal tendons (*curved arrow*).

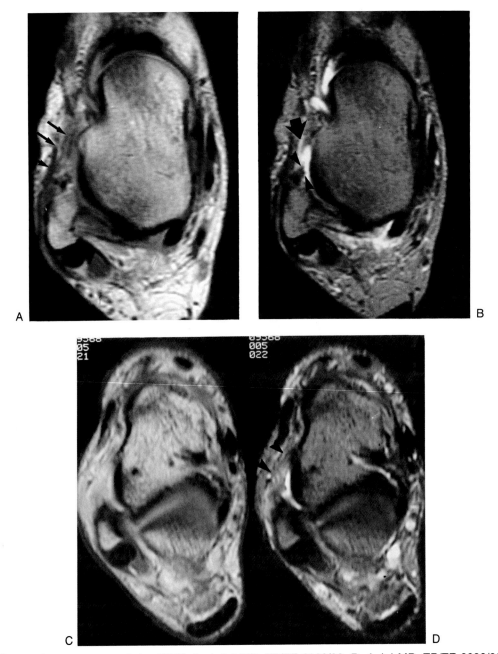

FIG. 7.4. Acute rupture of the ATAF. **A:** Axial MR, TR/TE 2000/20. **B:** Axial MR, TR/TE 2000/80. In neither image is a normal ATAF identified; this alone would markedly raise the index of suspicion of injury. In A, the soft tissues anterolateral to the distal fibula are disorganized (*arrows*). In B, the lateral extremity of the ATAF (*arrowheads*) is discontinuous, and joint fluid (*large arrow*) is seen extravasating through the ligamentous defect. **C:** Axial MR, TR/TE. 2000/20. **D:** Axial MR TR/TE 2000/80. On the proton density image, there is no identifiable ATAF; in D an irregular soft tissue mass representing the torn ligament and capsule (*arrowheads*) is present, but because this injury is 2 weeks old, the joint fluid does not "leak out" of the capsule as in B.

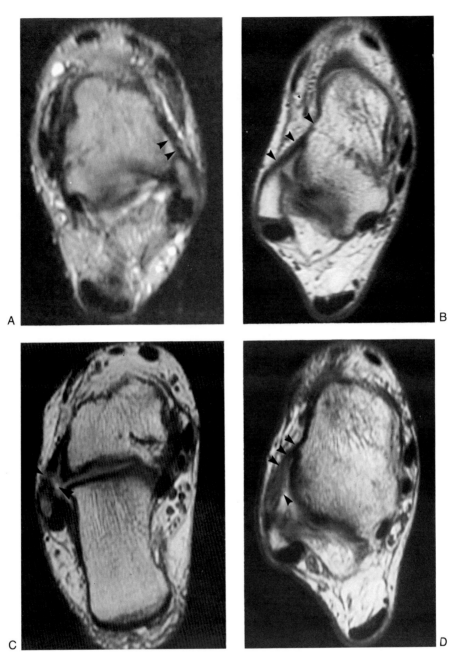

FIG. 7.5. Chronic sprains of the ATAF. Each of the figures are from different patients, all of whom had a remote history of an ankle sprain. These images demonstrate the spectrum of changes in the ATAF following sprain. **A:** Axial MR, TR/TE 2000/80. Two weeks prior, this patient suffered inversion injury. The ATAF (*arrowheads*) is very slightly thickened and irregular, and a thin layer of edema overlies it. The patient in **B** (axial MR, TR/ **E:** 2000/20) has a history of multiple ankle sprains. The ATAF (*arrowheads*) is intact, but is mildly and diffusely thickened. In **C**, the patient had suffered an ankle sprain many months prior. The fibular end of the ATAF is thickened and in fact may be focally discontinuous (*arrowhead*). The patient in **D**, (axial MR, TR/TE 2000/20) had had multiple ankle sprains. The ATAF (*arrowheads*) is represented by a thickened mass that demonstrates diffuse increase in signal intensity throughout its substance. The extreme thickening and masslike character of the ligament in a nonacute situation should suggest the diagnosis of the anterolateral ankle impingement syndrome.

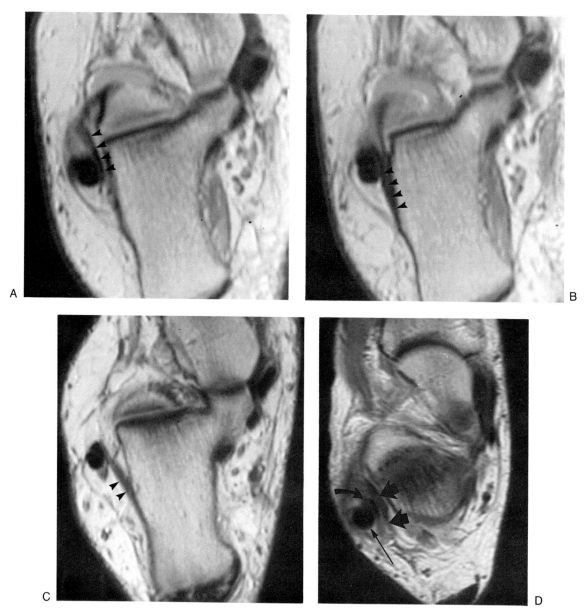

FIG. 7.6. The calcaneofibular ligament. **A, B:** Axial MR, TR/TE 2000/20. A is 3 mm cephalad to B. The calcaneofibular ligament (*arrowheads*) is the most difficult of the collateral ligaments to identify consistently in the axial plane. In these images, the CF is represented by a thin dark band seen anteromedially to the peroneal tendons. The CF blends with the dark peroneal tendons and the lateral calcaneal cortex. **C:** Axial MR, TR/TE 2000/20. In another patient, the CF (*arrowheads*) is more readily discernible and has a more cordlike structure. **D:** Axial MR, TR/TE 2000/20. The CF (*arrows*) is markedly thickened and demonstrates an increase in signal throughout its structure. While the peroneus longus (*long arrow*) is normal, the peroneus brevis (*curved arrow*) has lost its rounded configuration and has increased signal within its substance. Partial tears of the peroneal tendons frequently accompany severe lateral collateral ligament injuries.

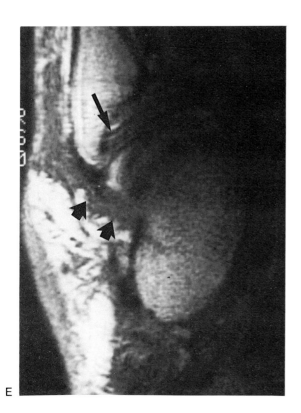

E

FIG. 7.6. (*Continued*) **E:** Coronal MR, TR/TE 2000/20. In another patient, there is marked disorganization of the soft tissues in the expected position of the CF (*arrows*). The normal PTAF is easily identified on this image (*large arrow*). (E courtesy of Javier Beltran, M.D., New York, NY.)

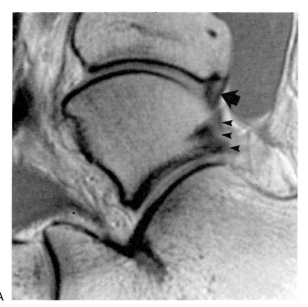

A

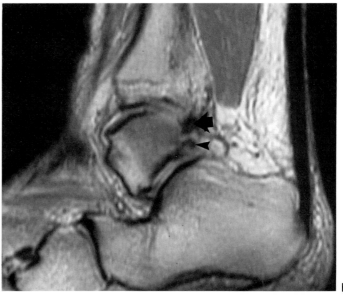

B

FIG. 7.7. Normal PTAF and PTIF: pitfalls in imaging. **A, B:** Sagittal MR, TR/TE 2000/20. The images are from two different patients. Both the PTIF and PTAF can be mistaken for loose bodies within the ankle joint on sagittal MRI. In A, the PTIF (*arrow*) is seen arising from the posterior lip of the tibia and extending obliquely downward and laterally. The fanlike insertion of the PTAF (*arrowheads*) is just below the PTIF. In B the PTIF (*arrow*) and PTAF (*arrowheads*) have more rounded configurations and might easily be mistaken for intraarticular osteochondral fragments.

syndrome" has been applied to the patients suffering from this constellation of symptoms (35,36). Following an inversion injury to the ankle and at least partial tear of the ATAF, an intraarticular hemorrhage may occur. Repetitive motion leads to inflammation of the ligament ends with eventual synovial hyperplasia extending into the lateral talofibular space, also known as the lateral gutter (Figs. 7.8, 7.9). The synovial reaction may extend cephalad to involve the distal anterior tibiofibular joint, and the mass of synovium becomes entrapped between the tibia, talus, and fibula. In some cases, a "meniscoid" lesion of scar tissue forms in the anterolateral aspect of the joint; this mass of tissue is hyalinized connective tissue that assumes a ligamentous contour (37). In extreme cases, the synovium may erode the anterolateral talar dome and produce foci of chondromalacia. Another cause of the anterolateral impingement syndrome is hypertrophy of Bassett's ligament, a structure thought to be a separate inferior fascicle of the anterior tibiofibular ligament (36). All of these pathologic processes may represent a contin-

uum of disease that begins with soft tissue injury and the development of hypertrophic synovitis. At surgery, patients are noted to have hypertrophied, inflamed synovium (38). Pathologically, moderate synovial hyperplasia with subsynovial capillary proliferation is present. Arthroscopic synovectomy and resection of the offending lesion can be expected to improve symptoms in 75% of cases (38,39).

There is only a single documented case in which MR was able to identify preoperatively the cause of the anterolateral ankle joint impingement syndrome (40), although we have subsequently identified a number of other cases (Fig. 7.9). The MR signs of anterolateral ankle impingement syndrome include a thickened and deformed ATAF, with an associated soft tissue mass that is best visualized in either the sagittal or axial planes. This tissue is intermediate in signal on both T1WI and T2WI. The anterior tibiofibular ligament may protrude into the anterior aspect of the joint, and the soft tissue thickening associated with these torn ligaments may preclude uniform distribution of joint

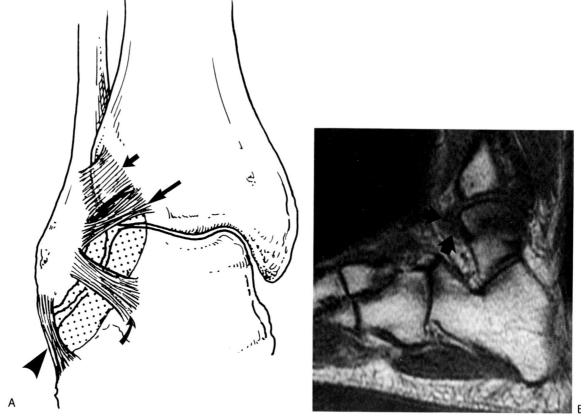

FIG. 7.8. Anterolateral ankle impingement syndrome. **A:** This diagram defines the boundaries of the lateral gutter (*shaded area*), the site at which ligamentous injury and reactive synovitis produce the "meniscoid lesion" typical of the impingement syndrome (ATIF, arrow; Bassett ligament, long arrow; ATAF, curved arrow; CF, large arrowhead). **B:** Sagittal MR, TR/TE 600/20. A soft tissue mass (*arrows*) is seen just anterior to the tibiotalar joint. This mass was most apparent with the foot in dorsiflexion. At surgery, this patient had a mass of synovium resected; the overgrown synovium was thought to be the cause of the patient's lateral ankle pain.

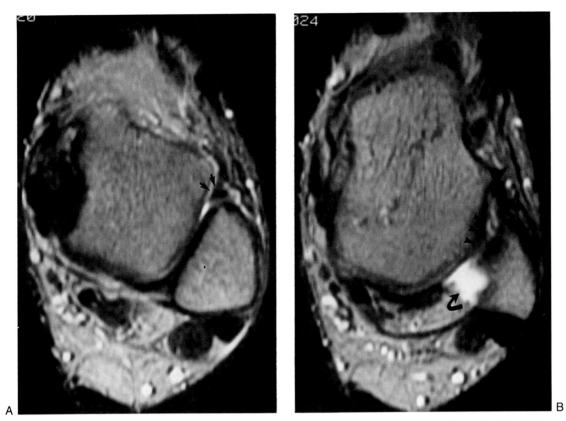

FIG. 7.9. Impingement syndrome. Anterolateral ankle impingement. **A, B:** Axial MR, TR/TE 2000/ 80. The patient has chronic lateral ankle pain years following multiple ankle sprains. The ATIF (A) (*arrows*) is thickened and irregular, and a portion of the ATIF protrudes into the anterior aspect of the talofibular joint (*arrowhead*). At the level of the anterior talofibular ligament (B), a poorly defined soft tissue density (*arrowheads*) is seen in the talofibular joint space; the joint fluid (*curved arrow*) that is present is all posterior. This constellation of findings suggests the diagnosis of the anterolateral ankle joint impingement syndrome.

fluid from front to back within the lateral aspect of the joint. The specificity of this sign is not known. The use of dynamic MRI has been advocated as a means to diagnose this syndrome best (40,41). The foot is placed in a specially designed motion device, and sagittal images are taken with the foot in various degrees of dorsal and plantar flexion. When the foot moves from plantar to dorsiflexion, the synovial mass buckles and thickens and therefore becomes more evident on the sagittal images. More recently, the availability of ultrafast MR has permitted imaging during active motion, closely resembling physiological action (41). The precise and ultimate role of MR and/or intraarticular gadolinium in the diagnosis of this elusive disorder is not known.

THE SYNDESMOTIC COMPLEX

The syndesmosis is composed of the anterior tibiofibular ligament (ATIF), the posterior tibiofibular ligament (PTIF), and the interosseous ligament and membrane (Fig. 7.1). The ATIF is a short bandlike structure. It extends from an origin on the anterola-

terally positioned anterior tibial tubercle and has a caudal, lateral, and slight posterior course to the fibula. The PTIF ligament runs from the posterior malleolus of the tibia, extending slightly downward on its path to insert on the fibula. It is stronger than its anterior counterpart. Some authors consider the lowest fibers of the PTIF ligament to be a separate structure, which is called the transverse tibiofibular ligament (17,42,43). It deepens the ankle joint socket posteriorly. This ligament may withstand torsional forces acting on a distal fibular fracture fragment, and instead may produce an avulsion fracture of the posterior lip of the distal tibia (posterior malleolus).

The interosseous ligament and membrane are a series of short fibers running from a ridge on the tibia in a downward and lateral direction to a similar ridge on the fibula. In some individuals this membrane is thick and strong, whereas it is virtually nonexistent in others (43). This membrane is perforated in two locations. Proximally an oval opening permits passage of the anterior tibial artery, and the caudal opening allows the perforating branch of the peroneal artery to exit onto the anterior aspect of the foot. The syndesmotic complex defines the uppermost extent of the ankle joint and extends 2 to 6 cm above the plafond. Isolated syndesmotic tears are unusual except in the elite skier (44).

There are two predominant mechanisms for tibiofibular diastasis/fractures. The first, referred to as the anterior type, involves lateral rotation of the talus in the mortise so that it impinges on the fibula; the ATIF and the interosseous ligament rupture, and the syndesmosis "books open" with the PTIF as the hinge. Either the medial malleolus fractures or the deltoid ligament ruptures. In the second variety, there is a direct abduction force of the talus against the fibula, producing a fracture and resulting in disruption of the ATIF, the PTIF, and the interosseous ligament; again, either the deltoid ligament is torn or the medial malleolus is fractured. In all significant injuries of the syndesmosis, a fibular fracture is found. The fracture may occur at any point from the top of the inferior tibiofibular joint to the head of the fibula (Maisonneuve fracture) (43).

There is no universal agreement on the proper treatment of syndesmotic tears. Some authors believe that such injuries can be treated by cast immobilization as long as the medial malleolus is not fractured and the deltoid ligament is intact. Diastasis, shortening of the fibular fracture, or displacement of the medial malleolar fracture may mandate operative reduction and fixation (42). Similarly, deltoid ligament tears can also be treated conservatively. Thirty-six patients were followed for 1 year or longer following complete disruption of the deltoid ligament; initial treatment consisted of reduction of the medial joint space and maintenance of the lateral malleolus until bone repair was achieved. None of the patients manifested ligamentous instability (45).

Conventional radiographic assessment of the integrity of the syndesmotic complex is critical as this articulation is most important in maintaining the stability of the ankle joint. Manifestations of rupture of the syndesmosis (ATIF, PTIF, and interosseous membrane) is most simply seen as diastasis of the distal tibiofibular articulation. This diagnosis can be confidently made if the space between the medial malleolus and the medial talus, or between the lateral talar margin and the medial fibula measures greater than 5 mm (42) (Fig. 7.10). It is most important to remember that major syndesmotic disruptions can occur and spontaneously reduce

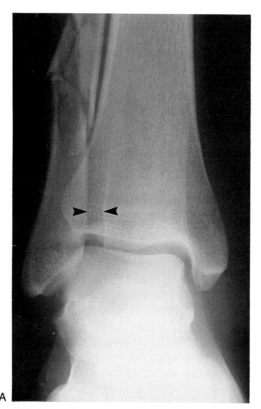
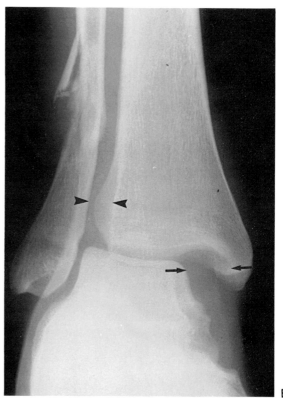

FIG 7.10. Syndesmotic disruption. **A:** The conventional anteroposterior radiograph reveals a fibular fracture approximately 7 cm above the tip of the malleolus. On this nonstressed view, the distal tibiofibular joint space is slightly widened (*arrowheads*). **B:** With valgus stress, gross widening of the medial aspect of the mortise (*arrows*) and the distal tibiofibular joint (*arrowheads*) occurs, indicating disruption of both the syndesmosis and the deltoid ligaments.

before the radiographic examination can be performed. In such cases, the radiographic measurement may be normal, and the examiner must depend on secondary signs such as the combination of a fibular fracture and a medial malleolar fracture to suggest the presence of a severe injury. Stress radiographs are mandatory if a syndesmotic rupture is suspected but not evident on conventional radiographs.

The arthrographic evidence of a tear of the ATIF is manifest by extravasation of the contrast material from the ankle joint out of the joint between the distal tibia and fibula, above the normal syndesmotic recess. This extravasation may occur well up into the interosseous membrane; on the lateral radiograph, the contrast is between the tibia and fibula or just anterior to the fibula (27). Isolated ruptures of the ATIF are rare; most commonly, at least one other ligamentous rupture accom-

panies a syndesmotic disruption (3). There are no specific arthrographic features of a PTIF tear.

On axial MRIs, the shafts of the tibiae and fibulae are seen to be connected to one another by a linear band of dark signal, which represents the interosseous membrane, the caudal extent of which is the interosseous ligament. In some individuals this structure is quite substantial, whereas in others it is virtually absent. The membrane ends at the level of the metaphyseal flare of the tibia. Just above the plafond, a thin dark band representing the ATIF arises from the anterolateral aspect of the tibia (the anterior tubercle) and courses laterally, caudally, and slightly posteriorly (Fig. 7.11). On the next two or three sections, portions of the ATIF are identified, with the lowest section demonstrating the attachment of the ligament to the anterior fibula. The ATIF has a caudal and oblique

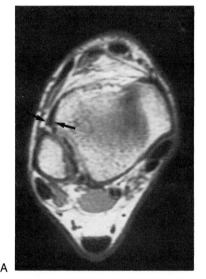
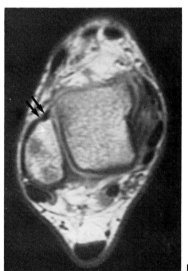
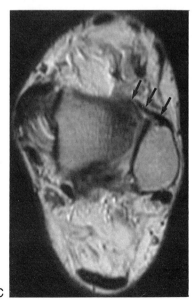

FIG. 7.11. Normal ATIF. **A–C:** Axial MR, TR/TE: 2000/20. Because the ATIF extends from a position superiorly on the tibia to a position inferiorly on the fibula, it is difficult to obtain a single axial image of the ligament completely in-plane. In A, the tibial origin of the ATIF (*arrows*) is identified, but the lateral portion of the ligament is absent. In B, which is 3 mm distal to A, the fibular attachment is identified (*arrows*). In C, which is a slightly oblique image of a different patient, the entire ligament (*arrows*) from tibia to fibula is fortuitously identified.

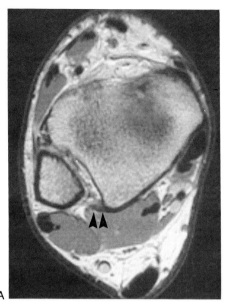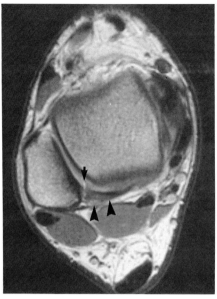

FIG. 7.12. Normal PTIF. **A, B:** Axial MR, TR/TE: 2000/20. Just like the ATIF, the PTIF has a slightly caudal course as it runs from tibia to fibula. In A, the proximalmost tibial origin of the PTIF (*arrowheads*) is seen arising from the posterior tibia/posterior malleolus. B is 5 mm distal to A. The triangular, fan-shaped configuration of the PTIF (*arrowheads*) is best appreciated on this axial image. The PTIF is normally characterized by increased signal "streaks" is arranged in a transverse direction. The small bright streak (*arrow*) seen over the PTIF is an artifact on the film. Inasmuch as most of the PTIF is seen on an image in which the talus is present and the tibia is not, the PTIF has been mistakenly identified as the PTAF.

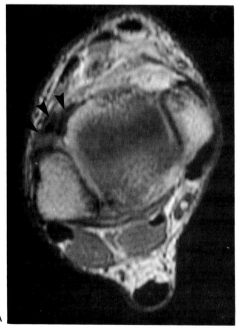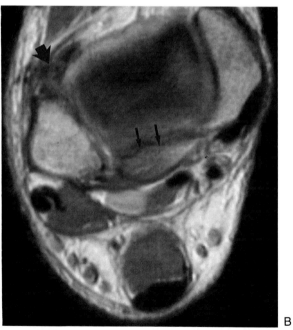

FIG. 7.13. Torn ATIF. **A:** Axial MR, TR/TE 2000/20. One month prior, the patient experienced a severe "sprain" of the ankle with external rotation of the foot. The current study demonstrates thickening and marked deformity of the ATIF (*arrowheads*). There is only a minor degree of subcutaneous edema as this injury is subacute. The masslike appearance of the ATIF should suggest the diagnosis of ankle impingement. **B:** Axial MR, TR/TE 2000/20. This patient stumbled and suffered an eversion injury of the hindfoot. There is marked thickening and distortion of the tissues in the expected position of the ATIF (*large arrow*). The PTIF is intact, but the patient has suffered a nondisplaced posterior malleolar fracture (*arrows*).

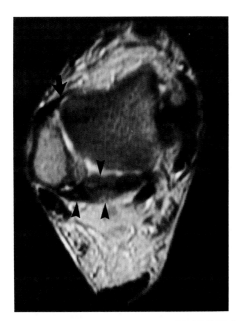

FIG. 7.14. Syndesmotic injury. Axial MR, TR/TE 2000/80. This patient is known to have had a ski injury several months prior, at which time he suffered a severe sprain. The PTIF (*arrowheads*) is markedly thickened in its anteroposterior dimension; it is diffusely filled with signal and has a lobulated anterior margin. The ATIF (*arrow*) is also thickened, but to a lesser degree.

course and is therefore difficult to identify on a single axial image and is also extremely difficult to image coronally (32,46).

At approximately the same axial level at which one images the ATIF, a triangular band, composed of individual fibers (analogous to the anterior cruciate ligament of the knee), is seen with its base on the fibula and its apex on the posterior distal tibia and posterior malleolus; this is the PTIF (and its lowest fascicle, the transverse tibiofibular ligament) (Figs. 7.7, 7.12). It has been noted that the superior margin of the PTIF has a variant appearance. Noto et al., in their review of 30 normal ankles, found that the superior margin of the PTIF was irregular and frayed in 13 (34). This "abnormal" appearance is thought to be due to a fanlike or flared insertion of the ligament, and partial volume effect of the ligament with the surrounding fat. The PTIF is quite frequently seen in all three orthogonal imaging planes. When depicted on the sagittal images, it projects at the posterior margin of the edge of the posterior malleolus. The dark signal, rounded appearance, and proximity to the joint may result in either the PTIF or the PTAF being mistaken for a loose body (Fig. 7.7). Careful medial to lateral examination of adjacent sections will allow one to avoid this potential pitfall (15).

There has been some confusion regarding the identity of the tibiofibular and the talofibular ligaments on

MR examinations (14,15,34,47). Various scientific publications have misidentified these two constant, important groups of ligaments. The most frequent error has been to label the posterior, and occasionally anterior, *tibiofibular* ligament as the *talofibular* ligament. The reason for this confusion is related to the fact that the talus is invariably on the image in which the fibular attachment of the tibiofibular ligament is present. It must be remembered that the anterior tibiofibular ligament has a steeply oblique course from superomedially on the tibia to a more inferolateral attachment onto the fibula; its lateral insertion is more distal than its medial origin. The posterior tibiofibular ligament, while having a more transverse orientation, attaches to the posterior malleolus of the tibia, a structure that dips below the highest point of the talar dome on the axial section; therefore the tibia itself is no longer "in the picture." There are two osseous landmarks, the talus and the fibula, that can be used to identify correctly which group of ligaments one is observing when viewing MR images in the axial plane (Fig. 7.3): (a) at the level of its dome, the talus has a nearly rectangular configuration; this is the level at which the tibiofibular ligaments are observed. The talofibular group is of course identified more distally; the talus has a more elongated shape, and a portion of the sinus tarsi is usually visible; and (b) the most dependable landmark to help distinguish the tibiofibular from the talofibular ligaments is the fibula. The tibiofibular ligaments are identified at the level of the distal fibular shaft; at this level, the fibula has a flattened medial border. The talofibular ligaments are found at the level of the malleolar fossa, a prominent, rather deep indentation along the medial border of the lateral malleolus (15).

In our experience, disruptions of either the ATIF and/or PTIF are most commonly manifest by structural thickening and irregularity (Figs. 7.13-7.15). Since the ATIF is not universally identified on every normal MRI, and given the fact that the ligament has a caudal oblique course, complete absence of this structure cannot be used as a reliable sign of injury. As noted above, rupture of the PTIF is uncommon, and frequently injury to the posterior ankle joint is manifest by an avulsion fracture of the posterior malleolus. Chronic syndesmotic injuries are manifest by heterotopic calcification in the interosseous membrane and at the sites of ligamentous avulsion.

THE MEDIAL COLLATERAL LIGAMENT

The medial collateral ligament, more commonly known as the deltoid ligament, has three main components that, when taken together form a confluent structure that is extremely strong (17) (Fig. 7.1). The proximal attachment is quite confined, but the ligament

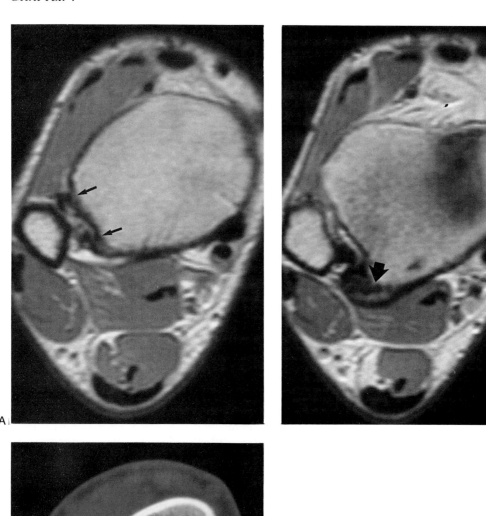

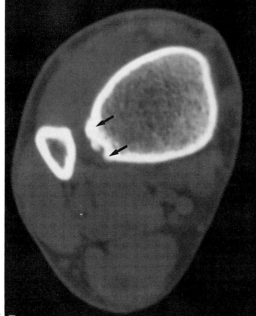

FIG. 7.15. Syndesmotic rupture. The patient gives a history of a severe remote injury to the ankle during skiing. **A, B:** Axial MR, TR/TE 800/ 20. **C:** Axial CT scan at level of syndesmosis. Image A is 6 mm cephalad to B. The dark foci of signal seen in region of the interosseous membrane (*small arrows*) could represent hemosiderin, fibrosis, or calcification in the interosseous membrane. B: There has been an avulsion fracture of the tibial insertion of the PTIF (*thick arrow*). The CT image (C), made at comparable level to A, demonstrates the interosseous membrane ossification.

fans out distally with a very broad insertion. The deltoid ligament is divided into two layers. The superficial layer arises more anteriorly (distally) than the deep. The talonavicular ligament arises from the medial malleolus and extends anteriorly and obliquely plantar to insert into the tuberosity of the tarsal navicular. A separate limb of the deltoid (tibiospring) attaches distally to the plantar calcaneonavicular ligament, also known as the spring ligament. The latter is a specialized fibrocartilaginous structure that bridges the calcaneonavicular gap and supports the medial arch and the head of the talus. If the deltoid ligament is sectioned, the spring ligament sags, the talar head sinks plantar, and the calcaneus slips into valgus, all of which serve to produce a flat foot deformity. The talocalcaneal band of the deltoid ligament descends nearly vertically from the medial margin of the malleolus to insert along the entire length of the sustentaculum of the talus, thereby preventing the calcaneus from assuming a valgus position.

The tibiotalar ligament, also known as the deep layer of the deltoid, extends from the medial malleolus to cover virtually the entire medial, nonarticular portion of the talus. It inserts on the posterior medial talar tubercle and fills the gap left by the short tibial malleolus on the medial side of the mortise (3). The tibiotalar ligament prevents the talus from being displaced laterally against the lateral malleolus. In instances in which a distal fibular fracture is present, displacement of the lateral malleolar fragment by the talus is precluded if the tibiotalar ligament is intact. Isolated rupture of the deltoid ligament is rare (3).

On MR, the tibiotalar ligament is virtually always identified on coronal images, and occasionally on sagittal images as well. It is oriented in a nearly vertical direction and is most readily identified at its origin from the tip of the medial malleolus (Fig. 7.16). This ligament is most optimally visualized if the coronal images are made with the foot in 15° of plantar flexion (16,33,48). The tibiotalar ligament, like the anterior cruciate and posterior talofibular ligaments, is seen to be composed of several fibers that are separated from one another on T1WIs (16). This variant appearance has been identified as a potential source of error in seven of ten normal ankles that have been examined, and is felt to be due to partial volume effect of the dark ligament structure with fibrocartilaginous strands and fatty tissue (34). The posterior tibial and flexor digitorum tendons lie just superficial to the deltoid ligament and can be used as reliable landmarks for identification in both the axial and the coronal planes.

The several components of the superficial deltoid ligament (the tibiocalcaneal and the tibionavicular) are not seen on a single axial or coronal image, but portions can be reliably found on multiple images (Fig. 7.16). The tibionavicular segment is best seen on oblique, axial, or coronal images originating from the medial malleolus and coursing in an anterior direction. The tibionavicular ligament inserts on the medial aspect of the navicular. It is best seen when the foot is held in 40° of plantar flexion (48). The tibiocalcaneal component is best visualized in the coronal plane; it appears as a thin dark band extending from the medial malleolus inferiorly to the sustentaculum. We have not had any experience imaging a disrupted deltoid ligament, but one would expect that thickening, contour distor-

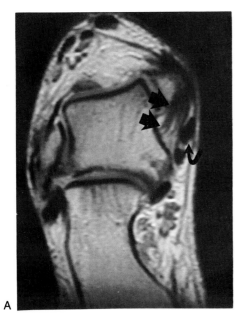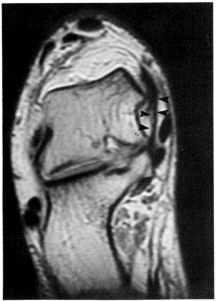

FIG. 7.16. Normal deltoid and spring ligaments. **A, B:** Oblique axial MR, TR/TE 2000/20. A is 3 mm cephalad to B. (*Figure continues on next page.*)

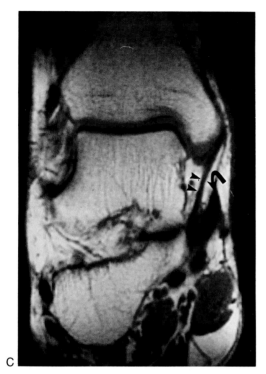

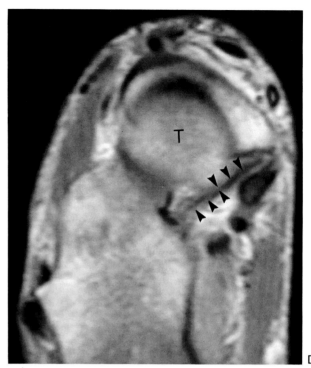

C

D

FIG. 7.16. (*Continued*) **C:** True coronal MR, TR/TE 2000/20. The deltoid is composed of the tibiotalar, tibiocalcaneal, tibiospring, and tibionavicular ligaments. In A, the multiple fibers of the tibiotalar component (*arrows*) can be readily identified situated just deep to the PTT (*curved arrow*). In B and C, the tibiocalcaneal ligament (*arrowheads*) can be identified attaching to the calcaneus at the sustentaculum. **D:** Normal spring ligament. Axial MR, TR/TE 2000/20. The spring or plantar calcaneonavicular ligament (*arrowhead*) supports the head of the talus (*T*). On this fortuitous axial image, the full extent of the ligament from its calcaneal origin to its plantar, medial navicular insertion can be identified.

tion, absence, irregular margins, and increased signal would be present.

THE SUBTALAR LIGAMENTS

The tarsal canal and sinus are the names given to segments of the space between the talus and the calcaneus. This capacious channel extends anterolaterally to posteromedially, opening just behind the sustentaculum. The term "sinus" refers to the larger lateral opening, and the canal is its medial, more narrow continuation (3,13,49,50). Within the sinus tarsi run the artery of the tarsal canal, nerve endings, a small bursa, the cervical (the lateral talocalcaneal) ligament, talocalcaneal interosseous ligament (IOL, also known as the ligament of the tarsal canal), and the medial fibers of the inferior root of the extensor retinaculum. The exact role and significance of these ligaments is somewhat controversial. It appears that the cervical ligament and IOL contribute to the stabilization of the hindfoot, but the fibers of the extensor retinaculum are probably of little import (50,51). This superficial and extracapsular structure serves to limit inversion (52). The cervical ligament lies anterior and lateral to the smaller IOL, the latter which is situated partly in the tarsal canal (13,15,47,50). Both of these ligaments have an oblique course, extending from an inferior and lateral position on the calcaneus to a superior and medial site of attachment to the talus. The IOL attaches just posterior and medial to the sustentaculum. The subtalar ligaments may be injured during forced inversion, or occasionally during hindfoot supination with the foot dorsiflexed (25).

Experimental section of the subtalar ligaments does produce minor instability of the hindfoot, but patients who have clinical injuries to these ligaments rarely have an objective hindfoot abnormality on physical examination (51). The major complaint of such patients, however, is a feeling of instability and weakness, as well as pain over the sinus tarsi. Injection of a local anesthetic relieves the pain. This constellation of symptoms is known as the sinus tarsi syndrome (13). The symptom complex results from an inversion injury to the ankle in 70% of cases, thereby accounting for the frequent association of the sinus tarsi syndrome with tears of the components of the lateral collateral

TABLE 7.2. *Causes of the sinus tarsi syndrome*

Ligamentous disruption
Synovial inflammation (rheumatoid disease)
Osteoarthritis
Peroneal nerve entrapment
Ganglion cyst
Gout
Tarsal tunnel syndrome
Pes cavus/planus

ligament (25,31) (Table 7.2). Treatment of the sinus tarsi syndrome consists of antiinflammatory medications, strengthening exercises for the peroneals, exploration of the sinus, and synovectomy.

While lateral ligamentous instability of the ankle has received considerable attention, there is rather little discussion of the relationship of subtalar instability to chronic ankle pain (3,25,51,53). The problem is compounded by the fact that the mechanisms that produce

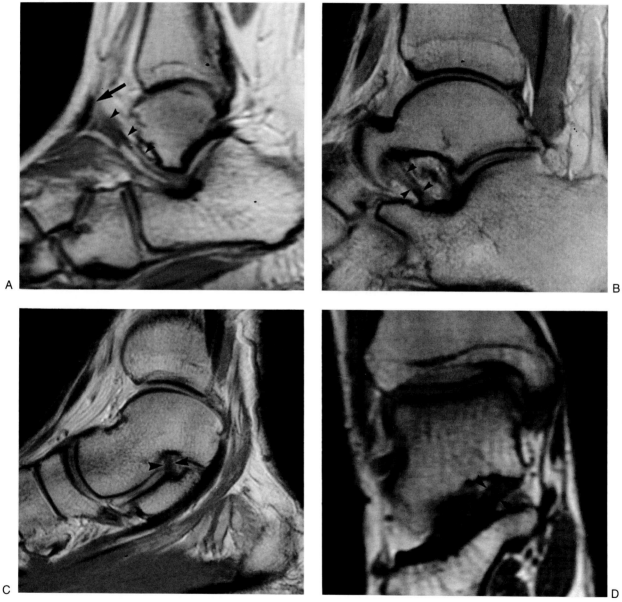

FIG. 7.17. Normal subtalar ligaments. **A–C:** Sagittal MR, TR/TE 2000/20. **D:** Coronal MR, TR/TE 2000/20. The subtalar ligamentous complex is composed of the medial root of the extensor retinaculum, the cervical ligament, and the talocalcaneal interosseous ligament. The extreme lateral sagittal image (A) demonstrates the medial limb of the inferior extensor retinaculum (*arrowheads*) extending from the extensor tendons (*arrow*) to its tarsal sinus insertion. Just medial in B, a well-defined cervical ligament (*arrowheads*) can be seen extending from the talus to calcaneus. Further medially in C and in D, the talocalcaneal interosseous ligament (*arrowheads*), can be readily identified just posterior and medial to the sustentaculum.

ankle joint instability also result in subtalar sprains, and the two injuries may coexist. CF ligament rupture is nearly universal in both ankle and subtalar instabilities. Reconstruction of the lateral ankle ligaments may fail if subtalar instability is overlooked and not simultaneously corrected.

Objective analysis of the integrity of the subtalar ligaments is generally lacking. Stress radiographs and conventional tomography have been employed to determine stability (53). Normal patients have tibiocalcaneal angles of 38° ± 6° and patients with subtalar instability have angles of >50°. In normal patients, the

posterior subtalar articular surfaces of the adjacent talus and calcaneus are always parallel, even under stress. Lack of parallelism must be regarded as indicative of instability.

Arthrography of the subtalar joint can be performed specifically for assessment of the talocalcaneal interosseous ligament (3,25,31). In cases in which the ligament is torn, contrast material injected into the posterior subtalar articulation will extravasate into the sinus tarsi. The normal microrecesses in the synovial membrane abutting the IOL are obliterated in patients suffering from the sinus tarsi syndrome, and the mem-

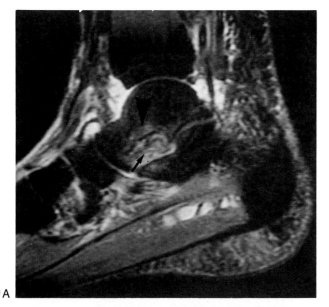

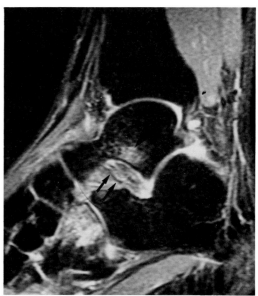

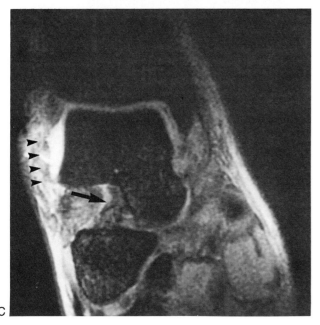

FIG. 7.18. Acute tear of the subtalar ligaments. **A, B:** This patient had suffered a severe inversion sprain of the ankle 4 days prior. Other MRIs had demonstrated a tear of the ATAF and CF. **A, B:** Sagittal MR, TR/TE/TI 2200/30/160. The soft tissues in the sinus tarsi are disorganized (*arrows*) with edema in both the sinus and the adjacent talus (*arrowhead*). Small degrees of intraosseous hemorrhage adjacent to ruptured ligaments is not uncommon. The cuboid in B demonstrates a marked increase in signal intensity; a nondisplaced fracture of the cuboid was evident on other images. **C:** Coronal MR, TR/TE/TI 2200/35/160. In another patient who 1 day prior had suffered an inversion injury of the ankle, the MRI reveals marked lateral subcutaneous soft tissue swelling (*arrowheads*). The interosseous ligament (*large arrow*) is thickened, irregular, and reveals a mild increase in signal intensity.

brane abutting the IOL is flattened. The integrity of the CF and cervical ligaments can also be surmised by the technique.

The ligaments of the normal subtalar articulation are best seen on sagittal MR sequence images, but can, on occasion, be identified in any of the three orthogonal planes (13,33) (Fig. 7.17). On the sagittal images the inferior root of the extensor retinaculum appears as a thin, occasionally fasiculated long band seen on those sections through the extreme lateral aspect of the tarsal sinus. Its entire course from the calcaneus to the extensor tendons can be identified on a single section in 100% of cases (13). The cervical ligament, lying in the anterior portion of the capacious sinus tarsi, can be readily identified in 70% to 90% of normal ankles, depending on the imaging sequence and imaging plane chosen. The coronal and sagittal planes are usually the most fruitful. The cervical ligament is a single band or several identifiable fascicles that appear as discreet structures. The interosseous ligament is the only one of the three subtalar ligaments to lie partially within the tarsal canal. Its calcaneal attachment is lateral, and it courses medially and superiorly to attach to the talus just behind the sustentacular joint. Although it is a broad, bandlike structure, it is the least reliably identified subtalar ligament (13). The IOL can be identified in 80% of high-resolution sagittal and 40% of coronal studies.

Patients with acute subtalar sprains and those suffering from the sinus tarsi syndrome manifest similar MR findings (Figs. 7.18, 7.19). In both groups, images through the sinus tarsi and tarsal canal demonstrate poor definition of the soft tissue anatomy, edema of the sinus tarsi structures (STIR sequences), and lack of visualization of the cervical and talocalcaneal interosseous ligaments (31). These alterations lack specificity. In patients with acute ligament tears, we have occasionally noted bone marrow edema of both/either the talus or calcaneus at the expected insertion sites of the ligaments, and extensive lateral subcutaneous edema.

We have recently attempted to demonstrate subtalar instability by means of an MR compatible device that produces inversion stress to the subtalar joint during performance of sagittal MRI (Fig. 7.20). In normal patients, such maneuvers do not alter the parallelism of the opposing articular surfaces of the talus and calcaneus at the posterior subtalar facet. In a small number of patients with symptoms suggestive of subtalar instability, stress MRI has demonstrated loss of parallelism of the posterior facet. MRI offers advantages over conventional stress radiography in assessment of subtalar instability: MRI is tomographic in nature, it allows direct visualization of the subtalar ligaments in addition to the facet joints and it does not employ ionizing radiation.

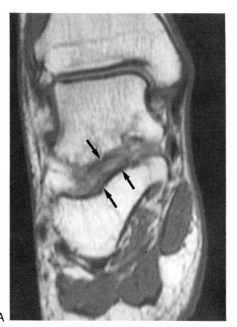 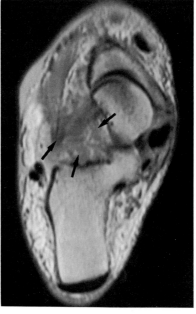

A   B

FIG. 7.19. Sinus tarsi syndrome. This patient has a clinical presentation consistent with the sinus tarsi syndrome. **A:** Coronal MR TR/TE 2000/20. The sinus is diffusely filled with tissue of an intermediate signal (*arrows*), and the definition of the talocalcaneal interosseous ligament is obscured. **B:** Axial MR, TR/TE 2000/20. Again, the wide lateral opening of the sinus tarsi is filled with nondescript soft tissue (*arrows*).

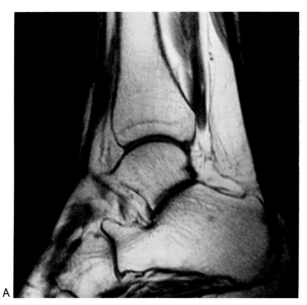
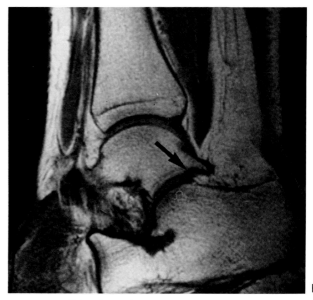

A   B

FIG. 7.20. Subtalar instability. During inversion stress, the tibiotalar calcaneo axis should demonstrate rather little movement. The talocalcaneal relationship should remain unchanged. **A:** Sagittal MR, TR/TE 500/20. The alignment of the posterior talo calcaneal facet is normal during inversion stress. **B:** Sagittal MR, TR/TE 500/20. In another patient, inversion stress results in incongruity (*arrow*) of the posterior subtalar facet, a finding indicative of subtalar instability.

SUMMARY

Currently, MR is rarely used exclusively to image the ligaments at the ankle. It should be remembered, however, that even when the clinical situation suggests that a ligamentous tear is present, a variety of other pathologic states (osteochondritis dissecans, peroneal rupture, etc.) may coexist. While ligamentous tears are nearly always self-limited injuries, the associated disorders may affect prognosis and complicate/alter rehabilitation programs. It is anticipated that MRI will, in the future, be used to a greater degree in assessing foot and ankle injuries.

REFERENCES

1. Amiel, D, Harwood, FF, Fronek, J, *et al.*, *Tendons and ligaments: A morphological and biochemical comparison.* J Orthop Res, 1984. **1**: p. 257–265.
2. Butler, DL, Grood, ES, Noyes, FR, *et al.*, *Biomechanics of ligaments and tendons.* Exerc Sports Sci, 1978. **6**: p. 125–181.
3. Perlman, M, Leveille, D, DeLeonibus, J, *et al.*, *Inversion lateral ankle trauma: Differential diagnosis, review of the literature, and prospective study.* J Foot Surg, 1987. **26**(2): p. 95–133.
4. Kannus, P and Renstrom, P, *Treatment for acute tears of the lateral ligaments of the ankle.* J Bone Joint Surg, 1991. **73-A**: p. 305–312.
5. Smith, R and Reischl, S, *Treatment of ankle sprains in young athletes.* Am J Sports Med, 1986. **14**(6): p. 465–471.
6. Andrish, JT, *Ligament injuries of the knee.* Orthop Clin, 1985. **16**(2): p. 273–284.
7. Berquist, T and Johnson, K, *Trauma,* in *Radiology of the Foot and Ankle,* TH Berquist, Editor. 1989, New York: Raven Press.
8. Hamilton, WG, *Foot and ankle injuries in dancers.* Clin Sports Med, 1988. **7**(1): p. 143–173.
9. Nicholas, JA and Hershman, EB, *The Lower Extremity and Spine in Sports Medicine.* 1986, CV Mosby: St Louis.
10. Sobel, M, Warren, R, and Brourman, S, *Lateral ankle instability associated with dislocation of the peroneal tendons treated by the Chrisman-Snook procedure. A case report and literature review.* Am J Sports Med, 1990. **18**(5): p. 539–543.
11. Korkala, O, Tanskanen, P, Makijarvi, J, *et al.*, *Long-term results of the Evans procedure for lateral instability of the ankle.* J Bone Joint Surg (Br), 1991. **73-B**: p. 96–99.
12. Evans, DL, *Recurrent instability of the ankle joint: A method of surgical treatment.* Proc R Soc Med, 1953. **46**: p. 343–344.
13. Beltran, J, Munchow, AM, Khabiri, H, *et al.*, *Ligaments of the lateral aspect of the ankle and sinus tarsi: An MR imaging study.* Radiology, 1990. **177**: p. 455–458.
14. Mitchell, MJ, Sartoris, DJ, and Resnick, D, *The foot and ankle.* Top Magn Reson Imaging, 1989. **1**: p. 57–73.
15. Erickson, SJ, Smith, JW, Ruiz, ME, *et al.*, *MR imaging of the lateral collateral ligament of the ankle.* AJR, 1991. **156**: p. 131–136.
16. Kier, R, McCarthy, S, Dietz, M, *et al.*, *MR appearance of painful conditions of the ankle.* RadioGraphics, 1991. **11**: p. 401–414.
17. Kelikian, H and Kelikian, A, *Disorders of the Ankle.* 1985, WB Saunders: Philadelphia.
18. Colville, M, Marder, R, Boyle, J, *et al.*, *Strain measurements in lateral ankle ligaments.* Am J Sports Med, 1990. **18**: p. 196–200.
19. Cass, J, Morrey, B, Katoh, Y, *et al.*, *Ankle instability: Comparison of primary repair and delayed reconstruction after long-term follow-up study.* Clin Orthop, 1985. **198**: p. 110–117.
20. Snook, GA, Chrisman, OD, and Wilson, TC, *Long-term results of the Chrisman-Snook operation for reconstruction of the lateral ligaments of the ankle.* J Bone Joint Surg (Am), 1985. **67-A**: p. 1–7.
21. Elmslie, RC, *Recurrent subluxation of ankle-joint.* Ann Surg, 1934. **100**: p. 364–367.
22. Grace, D, *Lateral ankle ligament injuries. Inversion and anterior stress radiography.* Clin Orthop, 1984. **183**: p. 153–159.

23. Cass, J and Morrey, B, *Ankle instability: Current concepts, diagnosis, and treatment.* Mayo Clin Proc, 1984. **59**: p. 165–170.
24. Sauser, D, Nelson, R, Lavine, M, *et al.*, *Acute injuries of the lateral ligaments of the ankle: Comparison of stress radiography and arthrography.* Radiology, 1983. **148**: p. 653–657.
25. Meyer, J, Garcia, J, Hoffmeyer, P, *et al.*, *The subtalar sprain: A roentgenographic study.* Clin Orthop, 1988. **226**: p. 169.
26. Mu Huo Teng, M, Destouet, J, Gilula, L, *et al.*, *Ankle tenography: A key to unexplained symptomatology. Part I: Normal tenography anatomy.* Radiology, 1984. **151**: p. 575–580.
27. Resnick, D, *Arthrography, tenography, and bursography, in Diagnosis of Bone and Joint Disorders,* D Resnick and G Niwayama, Editors. 1988, W.B. Saunders: Philadelphia.
28. Black, H, Brand, R, and Eichelberger, M, *An improved technique for evaluation of ligamentous injury in severe ankle sprains.* Am J Sports Med, 1978. **6**: p. 276–282.
29. Blanchard, K, Finlay, D, Scott, D, *et al.*, *A radiological analysis of lateral ligament injuries of the ankle.* Clin Radiol, 1986. **37**: p. 247–251.
30. Evans, G, Hardcastle, P, and Frenyo, A, *Acute rupture of the lateral ligament of the ankle. To suture or not suture?* J Bone Joint Surg (Br), 1984. **66(2)**: p. 209–212.
31. Beltran, J, *MRI: Musculosketal system.* 1990, J.B. Lippincott: Philadelphia.
32. Kneeland, JB, Macrandar, S, Middleton, WD, *et al.*, *MR imaging of the normal ankle: Correlation with anatomic sections.* AJR, 1988. **151**: p. 117–123.
33. Kier, R, Dietz, M, McCarthy, S, *et al.*, *MR imaging of the normal ligaments and tendons of the ankle.* J Comp Assist Tomogr, 1991. **15**: p. 477–482.
34. Noto, A, Cheung, Y, Rosenberg, Z, *et al.*, *MR imaging of the ankle: Normal variants.* Radiology, 1989. **170**: p. 121–124.
35. Ferkel, R and Fischer, S, *Progress in ankle arthroscopy.* Clin Orthop Rel Res, 1988. **240**: p. 210–220.
36. Bassett, F, Gates, H, Billys, J, *et al.*, *Talar impingement by the anteroinferior tibiofibular ligament.* J Bone Joint Surg, 1990. **72A**: p. 55–59.
37. McCarroll, J, Schrader, J, Shelbourne, K, *et al.*, *Meniscoid lesions of the ankle in soccer players.* Am J Sports Med, 1987. **15**: p. 255–257.
38. Martin, D, Baker, C, Curl, W, *et al.*, *Operative ankle arthroscopy. Long-term follow-up.* Am J Sports Med, 1989. **17(1)**: p. 16–23.
39. Martin, D, Curl, W, and Baker, C, *Arthroscopic treatment of chronic synovitis of the ankle.* Arthroscopy, 1989. **5(2)**: p. 110–114.
40. Sartoris, DJ, Mink, JH, and Kerr, R, *The foot and ankle, in MRI of the musculoskeletal system: A Teaching File,* JH Mink and AL Deutsch, Editors. 1991, Raven Press: New York. p. 389–449.
41. Shellock, F, Foo, T, Deutsch, A, *et al.*, *Patellofemoral joint; evaluation during active flexion with ultrafast spoiled GRASS MR imaging.* Radiology, 1991. **180**: p. 581–585.
42. Sclafani, S, *Ligamentous injury of the lower tibiofibular syndesmosis: Radiographic evidence.* Radiology, 1985. **156**: p. 21–27.
43. Monk, C, *Injuries to the tibio-fibular ligaments.* J Bone Joint Surg, 1969. **51B**: p. 330–337.
44. Fritschy, D, *An unusual ankle injury in top skiers.* Am J Sports Med, 1989. **17(2)**: p. 282.
45. Harper, M, *The deltoid ligament: An evaluation of need for surgical repair.* Clin Orthop, 1988. **226**: p. 156.
46. Beltran, J, Noto, A, Mosure, J, *et al.*, *Ankle: Surface coil MR imaging at 1.5T.* Radiology, 1986. **161**: p. 203–209.
47. Rosenberg, ZS and Cheung, Y, *Diagnostic imaging of the ankle and foot, in Disorders of the foot and ankle,* MH Jahss, Editor. 1991, W.B. Saunders: Philadelphia. p. 109–154.
48. Schneck, J, *Optimization of MR imaging of the most commonly injured structures of the ankle.* Radiology, 1987. **165 (P)**: p. 149.
49. Resnick, D, *Radiology of the talocalcaneal articulations.* Radiology, 1974. **111**: p. 581–586.
50. Cahill, DR, *The anatomy and function of the contents of the human tarsal sinus and canal.* Anat Rec, 1965. **153**: p. 1–18.
51. Kjaersgaard-Anderson, P, Wethelund, JO, Helmig, P, *et al.*, *The stabilizing effect of the ligamentous structures in the sinus and canalis tarsi on movement in the hindfoot.* Am J Sports Med, 1988. **16(5)**: p. 512–516.
52. Reinherz, RP, Sink, CA, and Krell, B, *Exploration into the pathologic sinus tarsi.* J Foot Surg, 198. **28(2)**: p. 137–140.
53. Clanton, T, *Instability of the subtalar joint.* Orthop Clin North Am, 1989. **20**: p. 583–591.

MRI of the Foot and Ankle,
edited by A.L. Deutsch, J.H. Mink, and R. Kerr,
Raven Press, Ltd., New York © 1992

CHAPTER 8

Bone and Soft Tissue Infection

Andrew L. Deutsch

Infections involving the soft tissues and osseous structures of the foot and ankle represent common problems and ones that often provide a significant diagnostic and therapeutic challenge. Early and accurate diagnosis is imperative to allow prompt initiation of appropriate therapy directed at avoiding the development of many of the significant complications associated with infections in this region. In the diabetic patient in whom infection involving the foot is a particularly common clinical problem, coexisting vascular and neurological compromise often further complicate the diagnostic picture (1). Plain radiography, computed tomography (CT), and multiple scintigraphic techniques have been commonly employed in an attempt to detect and accurately characterize the stage of the infectious process (2–20). The high soft tissue contrast and spatial resolution of magnetic resonance (MR) are attributes of this technique well suited toward evaluation of inflammatory conditions of soft tissue and bone. In both experimental studies as well as in initial reported clinical experience, MRI has compared favorably to existing diagnostic methods (21–31). In this chapter the application of MRI to the diagnosis of infection of bone and soft tissue will be reviewed. Integrated into the discussion will be a description of the pathogenesis of soft tissue and bone infection; an understanding of which is critical to the proper interpretation and understanding of the diagnostic studies.

SOFT TISSUE

Background

The detection and characterization of soft tissue infection and its distinction from involvement of bone

represent critical determinants in the management of patients presenting with suspected infections of the foot and ankle. While soft tissue infection may commonly be managed by local wound care, limited antibiotic therapy, and minor surgery, osteomyelitis is more refractory to treatment, frequently necessitating prolonged intravenous antibiotic therapy and in many cases bone debridement (1,32–35). The broad contrast resolution combined with the high spatial resolution of MRI represents a distinct advantage of this method for assessment of soft tissue inflammatory disorders compared to both CT and nuclear medicine techniques (21,29,36).

Soft tissue infection may involve cutaneous, subcutaneous, muscular, fascial, tendinous, ligamentous, or bursal structures. The plantar aspect of the foot is particularly vulnerable to soft tissue infection secondary to a variety of causes including puncture wounds, foreign bodies, and skin ulcerations from weightbearing (37). In diabetics, soft tissue breakdown over certain pressure points (e.g., metatarsal heads, calcaneus) provides the portal of entry for various organisms leading to infection that is often combined with vascular and neurological insufficiencies (38). The initial contamination of the skin and subcutaneous tissues can rapidly progress to infective osteitis, osteomyelitis, and septic arthritis, an occurrence that is particularly frequent about the metatarsophalangeal articulations, calcaneus, and terminal phalanges (21,37,38). Soft tissue dissemination of infection can also occur via the three plantar muscle compartments; medial, lateral, and intermediate (37). The intermediate compartment additionally provides a pathway for spread of infection involving the plantar aspect of the foot to extend into the lower leg via the tendon for the flexor hallucis longus muscle (37). The posterior tibial tendon may also serve as an avenue for spread of infection from the lower leg to the foot. The existence of these avenues for dissemination of infection within the soft tissues of

A. L. Deutsch: Tower Musculoskeletal Imaging Center, Los Angeles, California 90048, and Department of Radiology, University of California, San Diego, California.

the foot underscores the need for early and accurate detection and characterization of the location and extent of soft tissue infection.

Technique

When performing an examination for suspected soft tissue infection versus osteomyelitis, high-resolution, small field-of-view studies are used. At our institution, studies of the entire foot are rarely performed. Examinations are limited to forefoot, midfoot, or hindfoot evaluation, and may be restricted to one or two phalanges in order to obtain sufficiently small fields of view (FOV) for optimal detail. This consideration also argues against the practice of imaging both feet simultaneously for comparison purposes. The FOVs used range from 8 to 14 cm and surface coils are mandatory. We most commonly use a send-receive extremity coil (GE) or dual 3-inch circular coils in a modified Helmholtz configuration. An investigational quadurature coil (GE) has been successfully used for high-resolution studies of the forefoot (see chapter by Crues and Shellock). For examination of the metatarsals and phalanges, sagittal images aligned along the long axis of the metatarsal or phalanx of concern are initially obtained using a short TR/TE (T1-weighted) sequence and 3-mm interleaved sections. A sagittal STIR sequence is then performed along the long axis established on the T1-weighted sequence. An axial long TR/TE (T2-weighted) sequence is obtained with section thickness and gap tailored to cover any area of abnormality depicted on the sagittal sequence. For mid- and hindfoot examinations, initial sagittal T1-weighted sequences at 3-mm section thickness are preferred. Based on the findings on this initial sequence, a STIR sequence is then performed in the plane deemed most appropriate. A T2-weighted sequence is routinely obtained in the axial plane (perpendicular to the long axis of the metatarsals).

MRI

T2-weighted and STIR pulse sequences are preferred for evaluation of soft tissue infection. Inflammatory fluid collections are demonstrated as areas of relatively increased signal intensity on these pulse sequences. Cellulitis typically demonstrates a relatively diffuse, infiltrative pattern, particularly within the subcutaneous tissues. Cellulitis is most typically manifest as diffuse signal alteration replacing and infiltrating the normal high signal intensity subcutaneous fat on T1-weighted sequences. (Fig. 8.1) On long T2-weighted and STIR sequences, areas of cellulitis demonstrate increased signal intensity consistent with edema. The soft tissues are typically thickened. It is common, however, with both STIR and T2-weighted sequences to demonstrate increased signal intensity in the superficial dorsal subcutaneous tissues and/or in the plantar fascia in the absence of infection (21). This pattern may be scattered in the dorsal subcutaneous tissues, and either diffuse or ill-defined in the plantar soft tissues. Its exact nature remains unknown. In diabetic patients, in whom this pattern is particularly prevalent, it has been speculated that it may represent a manifestation of uneven distribution of body weight secondary to peripheral neuropathy with resultant stasis and fluid

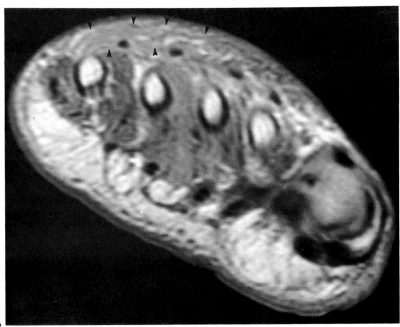

A

FIG. 8.1. Cellulitis. **A:** Axial TR/TE 2000/20. There is diffuse intermediate signal intensity infiltrating the dorsal subcutaneous tissues of the foot (*arrowheads*). The soft tissues are significantly thickened. The findings extend to the dorsal surface of the fifth metatarsal.

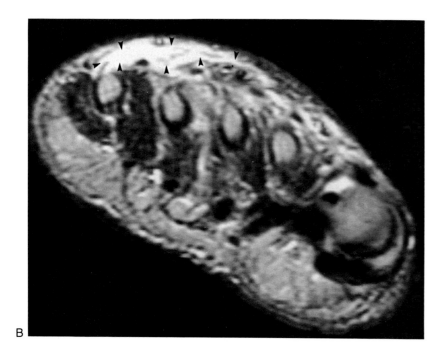

FIG. 8.1. (*Continued*) **B:** Axial TR/TE 2000/80. There is diffuse increased signal intensity without a discrete localized fluid collection (*arrowheads*). While the inflammatory process extends to the dorsal surface of the metatarsals, the underlying signal from bone is normal and the inflammatory process remains confined to soft tissue.

accumulation (21). The presence of this signal complicates the distinction between cellulitis and noninfected edema, and indeed, this differentiation may not be reliably accomplished using MRI (21). Mason et al. have suggested that the presence of distortion of the soft tissues in addition to increased signal intensity may be of value in making the distinction between cellulitis and noninflammatory edema (27).

Despite these limitations with regard to the distinction between cellulitis and noninflammatory edema, a major advantage of MRI has been in the ability of the technique to detect drainable fluid collections and dis-

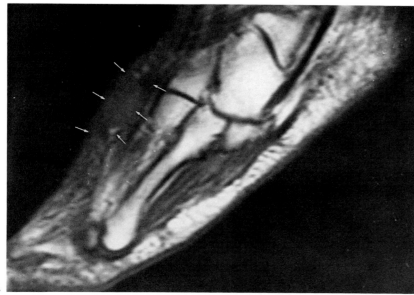

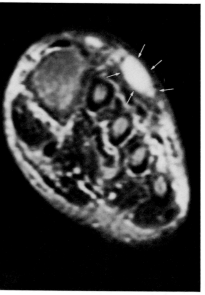

FIG. 8.2. Soft tissue abscess. **A:** Sagittal TR/TE 500/20. The normal high signal intensity of subcutaneous fat along the dorsum of the foot is completely replaced by low signal intensity fluid and edema (*small arrows*). The soft tissues are thickened with a convex outer contour along the dorsal surface of the foot. **B:** Axial TR/TE 2000/20. A circumscribed high signal intensity ovoid-shaped fluid collection is seen dorsal to the second and third metatarsals (*small arrows*). The mass effect and circumscribed nature of the process help in making the distinction between cellulitis and abscess. The MR exam clearly establishes the soft tissue location of the process and complete lack of involvement and separation from underlying bone.

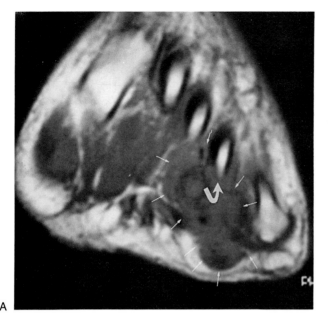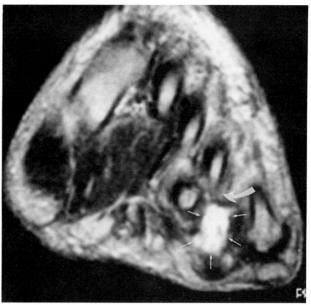

FIG. 8.3. Soft tissue abscess with infective osteitis. **A:** Axial TR 500 TE 20. There is a large "bilobed" inflammatory mass along the plantar aspect of the foot seen most extensively underlying the fourth and fifth metatarsal bones (*small arrows*). The collection is nearly isointense with muscle. The mass effect is seen to displace the plantar subcutaneous fat. A rim of intermediate signal intensity replaces the normal black cortical stripe along the plantar aspect of the fourth metatarsal base (*curved arrow*). **B:** Axial TR 2000 TE 80. The mass demonstrates a complex appearance with the component between the fourth and fifth metatarsals demonstrating more significant increase in signal intensity than the more medial component (*small arrows*). The high signal collection represented readily drainable pus with the more medial collection representing inflammatory but less drainable material. The signal replacing the plantar aspect of the cortex of the fourth metatarsal has slightly increased in intensity (*curved arrow*). The signal from the medullary cavity remains preserved.

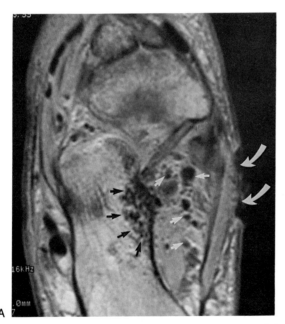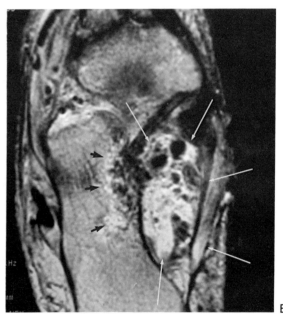

FIG. 8.4. Soft tissue abscess with osteomyelitis. **A:** Axial TR/TE 2000/20. There is an extensive fluid collection within the tarsal tunnel paralleling the medial aspect of the calcaneus. Multiple circumscribed low signal circular to ovoid areas representing gas are noted with the abscess (*small white arrows*). Additionally, evidence of gas and edema are seen within the calcaneus itself (*small black arrows*). A large soft tissue ulcer is present medially (*curved white arrows*). **B:** Axial TR/TE 2000/80. The abscess demonstrates a marked increase in signal intensity. It is relatively well defined and demonstrates characteristic mass effect (*white arrows*). The extensive presence of gas (*circular low signal areas*) is again noted. High signal intensity edema is seen in addition to the gas within the calcaneus (*small black arrows*).

202

crete soft tissue abscess formation. In several studies, MRI has proved superior to conventional radiography, CT, and scintigraphic techniques for the detection of soft tissue abscesses (21,28,29,36,39). T2-weighted, spin-echo, and STIR sequences are preferred for abscess detection to take advantage of the prolonged T2 values of inflammatory fluid collections. On MRI, abscesses appear as localized, relatively well-marginated, and predominantly homogeneous high signal intensity collections on T2-weighted and STIR sequences (Fig. 8.2). The margins are typically convex and the collections may be of higher signal than surrounding background edema (21). The more discrete margination and presence of mass effect distinguish abscesses from areas of cellulitis (Fig. 8.3). A low signal intensity peripheral rim has been reported around abscesses at high field strength but is not a universal finding (24,39). Gas contained within abscesses is depicted on MRI by discrete areas of markedly low signal on all pulse sequences (Fig. 8.4). A recent report has

suggested that the use of intravenous gadopentetate dimeglumine (Gd-DTPA) may be helpful for assisting in the differentiation of abscesses from areas of cellulitis. Areas of cellulitis and walls of abscesses and sinus tracts may demonstrate enhancement while areas of frank pus typically do not (40). The author has no experience with this use of Gd-DTPA in pedal inflammatory disease.

The demarcation between soft tissue involvement and bone is often readily apparent. At times, however, the soft tissue process may appear immediately contiguous with bone, and the distinction is made with more difficulty. The apparent continuity of soft tissue infection and bone does not necessarily indicate involvement of underlying bone. In this setting, longitudinal MRI studies may be of particular value in assessing the adequacy of the treatment protocol and in making the determination of whether extension to bone has occurred (Fig. 8.5).

The value of MRI in detecting soft tissue abscesses

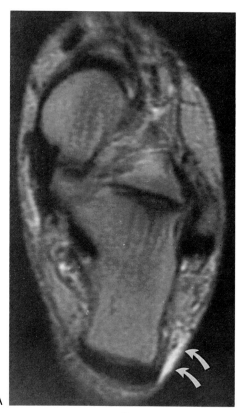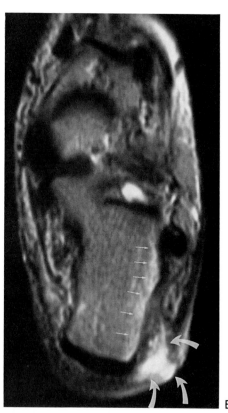

FIG. 8.5. Cellulitis with progressive bone involvement. **A:** Axial TR/TE 2000/80. There is a localized high signal intensity focus confined to the subcutaneous tissues along the posterolateral aspect of the calcaneus (*curved arrows*). No bone involvement is evident. The patient was treated with antibiotics. **B:** Axial TR/TE 2000/80. There has been a progressive increase in size of the fluid collection, which now demonstrates mass effect most consistent with a drainable abscess (*arrows*). Progressive changes within the bone along the lateral aspect of the calcaneus manifest as increased signal intensity on this pulse sequence are evident (*small arrows*). The findings are consistent with the development of infective osteitis. This case demonstrates the value of MRI for monitoring of therapy and for distinguishing between infection involving soft tissue alone as well as soft tissue and underlying bone.

has been studied both experimentally and clinically . Using an animal model, Chandnani et al. demonstrated a higher sensitivity for MRI than CT (97% vs. 52%) in detection of soft tissue abscess (36). These investigators suggested that beam hardening artifact with CT was in part responsible for limiting detection of soft tissue inflammation in the immediate vicinity of small tubular bones. Using the same experimental model, Beltran et al. compared MRI with three-phase bone scans and gallium-67 scintigraphy and found MRI to be significantly more sensitive than radionuclide imaging in the detection of soft tissue infection (29). Additionally, while radionuclide methods did not allow distinction between cellulitis and abscess using existing criteria, MRI demonstrated an overall sensitivity of 85%, specificity of 100%, and accuracy of 92% in differentiating drainable abscess from cellulitis in this experimental model.

The ability of MRI to detect soft tissue infection and distinguish it from bone involvement has also been studied clinically by multiple investigators (21,24, 26,39). In an early study using a low field strength system, Berquist found MRI to be more accurate than radiography and CT in detecting soft tissue infection (26). Beltran found MRI both more sensitive and more specific than bone scintigraphy in the detection of soft tissue infection and attributed the difference to the limited spatial resolution of the scintigraphic methods (39). Both Unger et al. (24) and Yuh et al. (21) corroborated the ability of MRI to distinguish soft tissue from bone infection in clinical series involving foot infections in diabetic patients. In the series reported by Unger et al., the presence of normal signal intensity marrow excluded the presence of osteomyelitis in di-abetic patients with cellulitis and skin ulcerations (24). Yuh et al. successfully differentiated abscesses from edema and cellulitis by the smooth margins and increased signal intensity demonstrated by the infected fluid collections (21). Yuh et al., however, described difficulty in distinguishing small (<1.5 cm) abscesses from background high signal intensity along the plantar aspect of the foot and suggested that T2-weighted sequences were superior to both T1-weighted and STIR sequences in detection of soft tissue abscesses. In a series of 14 diabetic patients with suspected pedal osteomyelitis and/or neuroarthropathic joints, MRI detected seven soft tissues abscesses, five of which were confirmed on the basis of percutaneous aspiration (41). Abscesses were characterized by well-defined areas of high signal intensity in comparison to cellulitis, which was depicted as ill-defined superficial high signal intensity on T2-weighted images. On the basis of these investigations, it is clear that the high spatial resolution of MRI, in conjunction with its broad range of soft tissue contrast resolution, represents the principal advantages of the technique as compared to scintigraphic methods and even CT. These attributes of MRI allow sufficient precision in characterization of soft tissue inflammatory processes required for management considerations and optimal surgical planning when required (42).

Suppurative Tenosynovitis

Infection of a tendon sheath may result from direct puncture or occur secondary to spread from a contiguous source or following trauma (37). Clinically, ex-

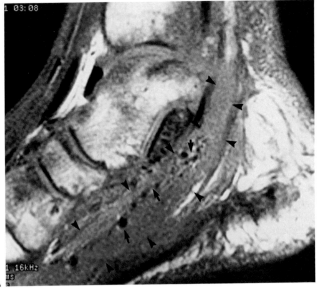

FIG. 8.6. Suppurative tenosynovitis. **A:** Sagittal TR 500 TE 20. The patient was a diabetic man who developed an infection at the site of a distal saphenous vein harvest site following coronary bypass surgery. The infection extended into the sheath of the posterior tibial tendon and via this pathway extended into foot (see Fig. 8.4). Note the increased signal enlarging the posterior tibial tendon sheath (*arrowheads*). Small collections of gas are seen within the fluid collection (*small arrows*).

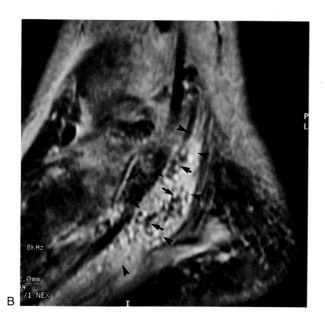

FIG. 8.6. (*Continued*) **B:** Sagittal STIR TR 2200 TE 35 TI 160. The fluid demonstrates marked increased signal intensity (*arrowheads*) and gas is again identified as small circular to ovoid low signal intensity foci (*small arrows*).

quisite tenderness over the course of the sheath can usually be elicited. A tendon sheath infection may perforate into an adjacent bone or joint and ultimately contribute to the development of osteomyelitis or septic arthritis (37). Additionally, an infected tendon sheath may serve as a pathway for spread of infection from one compartment to another. In the foot and lower extremity, the flexor hallucis longus tendon provides a pathway for spread of infection from the intermediate compartment of the foot into the lower leg (37). We have had experience with spread of a soft tissue infection from the lower leg into the medial compartment of the foot along the path of the posterior tibial tendon (Fig. 8.6).

On MRI using T2- and T2*-weighted pulse sequences, a small degree of fluid is commonly detected in all of the major tendon sheaths of the foot and ankle. A significant increase in fluid within a tendon sheath is readily detectable by MRI, but differentiation of septic from noninfective tenosynovitis may not be possible (41). Associated changes within soft tissue and bone may be of value in making this distinction. The presence of gas, manifest as small foci of markedly low signal intensity within the fluid-filled tendon sheath, however, is diagnostic of suppurative tenosynovitis (Fig. 8.6).

BONE INFECTION

Background

The term "osteomyelitis" infers infection of bone and marrow. Precision in diagnosis allowing subse-

quent optimization of therapy makes it desirable to distinguish frank osteomyelitis from other stages of osseous involvement (1,33–35,43). Infective or suppurative osteitis represents infection of the bone cortex (37). This can represent an isolated stage or more commonly be seen as a concomitant to osteomyelitis. Similarly, infective periosteitis infers involvement of the periosteum bordering the bone (37). Subperiosteal accumulation of organisms can lead to infective osteitis and osteomyelitis.

There are four principal routes by which bone may become infected, and accurate interpretation of imaging studies requires an understanding of the potential pathways by which organisms may reach the affected osseous structure. While briefly reviewed here, the interested reader is referred to the elegant treatment of this subject by Resnick and Niwayama (37). In hematogenous spread of infection, organisms reach the bone via the bloodstream and the vulnerability of any specific bone is influenced by and dependent on the anatomy of the adjacent vascular supply (37). Involvement of marrow and medullary bone is early, with later extension toward the cortex and periosteum (37). In the adult foot, spread of infection from a contiguous source overwhelmingly represents the most important mechanism of infection. The direction of infection is opposite to that of the hematogenous route; a critical point in interpreting imaging studies directed at its depiction. Direct implantation of infectious material into the bone or joint as with puncture wounds and penetrating injuries also represents an important route of infection in the foot (37). Postoperative infection is multifactorial and may be contributed to by a combination of direct implantation, spread from a contiguous septic focus, and/or hematogenously (37).

In hematogenous spread of osteomyelitis, the initial involvement is within the medullary canal with subsequent extension outward to involve cortical bone. Cortical penetration is associated with subperiosteal extension and elevation of the periosteal membrane with ultimate subperiosteal bone formation leading to an involucrum or shell of new bone (37). With osteomyelitis resulting from spread from a contiguous source, the direction of contamination is just the opposite, with initial involvement of soft tissue and progressive extension toward the medullary canal (Fig. 8.7). A soft tissue focus of infection can extend to and irritate the periosteum provoking a periosteal reaction without frank invasion of the cortex (37). Actual extension of the infection to the periosteum surrounding the bone is termed "infective periostitis" (37). During this stage, subperiosteal accumulation of organisms and pus leads to the involvement of the cortex, a subsequent stage termed by Resnick as "infective osteitis" (37). Involvement of the cortex may progress to

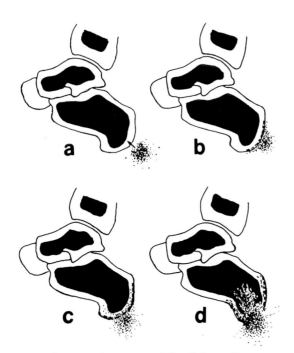

FIG. 8.7. Stages of osteomyelitis. Schematic representation. **A:** A soft tissue focus of infection is depicted (*small black dots*). It is discrete from the underlying bone and there is no evidence of bone involvement. **B:** The soft tissue infection extends to the border of the calcaneus. There is early periosteal reaction depicted (*dashed lines*). Periostitis in this setting may be on an infective or noninfective basis. **C:** The extent of the inflammatory process has extended to involve cortical bone. The findings at this stage can be referred to as infective osteitis. **D:** The infection has extended beyond the cortex to involve the medullary bone. The findings reflect the development of osteomyelitis.(Adapted from ref. 37, with permission.)

spread of the infectious process via haversian and Volkmann's canals (37). Finally, the medullary bone and marrow spaces are involved and frank osteomyelitis is present.

The ability to define the stage of infection reliably underlies the rational choice of therapy (1,33–35,43). Infection limited to the soft tissues or outer cortex responds to therapy that would be insufficient for eradication of frank osteomyelitis (1,43). Plain radiographs, conventional and computed tomography, and scintigraphic methods all have recognized limitations in precise determination of the stage of infection (2,3,5,8,36–38,44,45). In particular, nuclear medicine techniques, while sensitive to the presence of infection, lack spatial resolution to fully define the pathoanatomic sequence (4,6,7,9,10,12–20,46–58). The high contrast and spatial resolution of MRI provides an opportunity for precision in diagnosis that has previously eluded the other available techniques (21–31,42,59–65).

MRI of Acute Osteomyelitis

As has been discussed, MRI can reliably distinguish in most cases between soft tissue infection and extension of the process to involve bone (21,29,60). Initial reports on MRI in the detection of osteomyelitis emphasized the ability of MRI to depict changes in medullary bone consistent with suppurative involvement. With increasing experience, it has become clear that changes within the periosteum and bony cortex can also be reliably detected with MRI and this has significant implications for the diagnosis of pedal osteomyelitis (66). Simple periosteal elevation from the outer cortex may be manifest on MRI as a single linear low signal intensity band paralleling the outer bony cortex (66). Laminated periosteal reaction, as may be seen in some cases of osteomyelitis, may be recognized as concentric low signal intensity lines paralleling the outer cortical margin of the bone (66). Interposed between and beyond the periosteal changes and bony cortex can be high signal intensity changes on STIR, T2-, or T2*-weighted images representing either pus or noninflammatory edema (66). Initial involvement of bone from a contiguous soft tissue focus can be appreciated on high-resolution images using both T1-weighted and T2-weighted or STIR sequences. On T1-weighted sequences, involvement of the bony cortex is appreciated as slight areas of increased signal set against the background of the normally low signal intensity cortex. Care must be taken not to misinterpret findings related to volume averaging from true bone involvement. The stage of infective osteitis is often best diagnosed by increased signal intensity on T2-weighted or STIR sequences, often in a linear or bandlike pattern, confined to the cortex of the involved bone (Fig. 8.8).

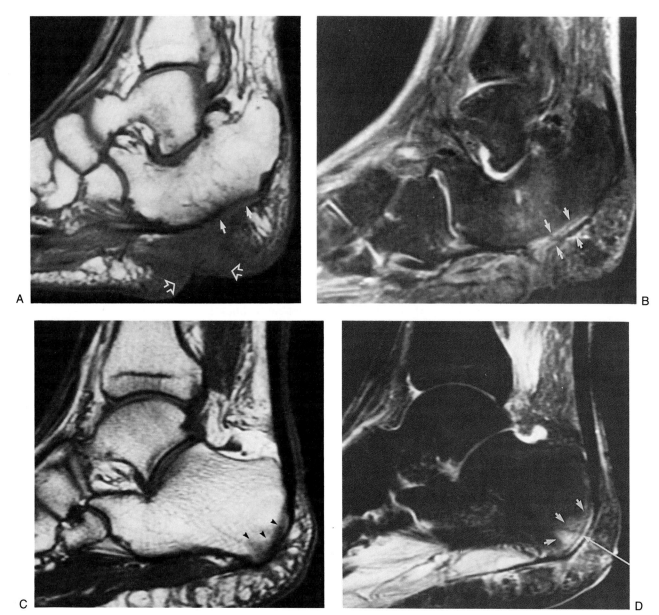

FIG. 8.8. Infective osteitis. **A:** Sagittal TR/TE 2000/20. There is posttraumatic deformity of the calcaneus. A large soft tissue ulcer is noted along the dorsum of the foot (*open arrows*). There is subtle and slightly ill-defined low signal paralleling the cortex and subchondral bone of the plantar aspect of the calcaneus (*small arrows*). **B:** Sagittal STIR TR 2200 TE 35 TI 160. There is a high signal intensity stripe paralleling the periosteal and cortical margin of the plantar aspect of the calcaneus (*arrows*). Minimal and presumably reactive signal changes are seen within the cancellous bone. The findings are most consistent with the stage of infective osteitis bordering on early osteomyelitis. **C:** Sagittal TR 300/15. A low signal intensity band is identified paralleling the posterior/inferior aspect of the calcaneus in another patient with a soft tissue ulcer and suspected early osteomyelitis (*arrowheads*). **D:** Sagittal STIR TR 2200 TE 35 TI 160. A stripe of high signal intensity is again identified paralleling the outer border of the calcaneus (*long arrow*). More discrete and extensive signal alteration is identified extending beyond the subchondral bone plate (*small arrows*). The findings are most consistent with infective osteitis and early osteomyelitis.

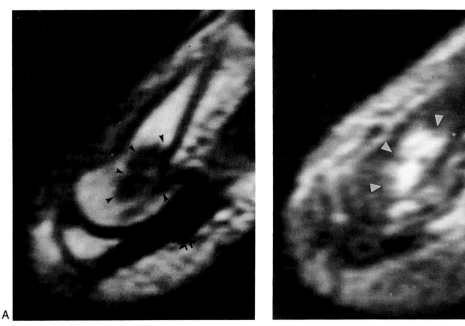

FIG. 8.9. Osteomyelitis. **A:** Sagittal TR 500 TE 20. Magnified view of the second metatarsal head demonstrates irregular focus of low signal intensity contiguous with the volar aspect of the head and extending into cancellous bone (*arrowheads*). Abnormal signal is also seen surrounding the flexor tendon and joint capsule (*open arrow*). **B:** Sagittal TR 2000/80. There is striking increase in signal intensity both within the metatarsal head (*arrowheads*) as well as along the volar soft tissues (*open arrow*). The findings are characteristic of osteomyelitis secondary to direct extension from a soft tissue focus.

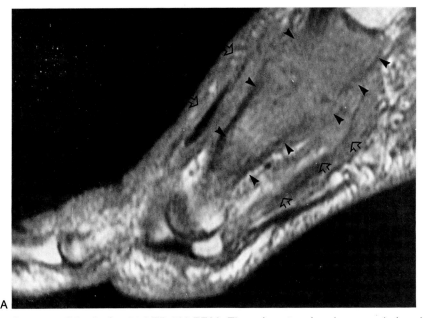

FIG. 8.10. Osteomyelitis. **A:** Sagittal TR 500 TE20. There is extensive decreased signal intensity identified within the proximal first metatarsal shaft and adjacent cuneiform in this diabetic patient (*arrowheads*). The soft tissues, both volar and dorsal, are thickened and normal subcutaneous fat is replaced by low signal intensity edema (*open arrows*).

Extension of signal alteration to the medullary bone, manifest as decreased signal on T1-weighted sequences and increased signal on T2-weighted and STIR sequences is the criterion most commonly used for the diagnosis of osteomyelitis (21,24) (Fig. 8.9). These findings likely reflect a decrease in the normal fat content of the bone marrow and localized increase in the water fraction related to edema and pus (24,42). In bone, in which fatty marrow predominates, T1-weighted sequences generally suffice for detection of osteomyelitis. T2-weighted or STIR sequences are more sensitive for detection of osteomyelitis in regions of hematopoietic marrow, particularly in children (24). In such cases, the red marrow demonstrates lower signal intensity on T1-weighted sequences and there is less contrast between normal bone marrow and that involved by osteomyelitis (24). STIR sequences have been reported to provide the greatest contrast for the detection of osteomyelitis and function well for both fatty and hematopoietic marrow (21,24) (Fig. 8.10). In both experimental studies, as well as in most clinical series in which specimens have been available, there has been excellent correlation between MRI findings and extent of infection (21,27,29). More recently, however, discordance between changes seen on STIR sequences and T2-weighted sequences have been noted in some cases of osteomyelitis and suggests a decreased specificity, albeit extremely high sensitivity,

for STIR imaging in the detection of osteomyelitis (60). The author has also had similar experience with STIR sequences, particularly in the setting of diabetic neuroarthropathy and concurrent foci of osteomyelitis (see below).

The appearance of the cortical bone in acute osteomyelitis will be affected by the route of infection. Cortical bone may appear grossly normal on MRI in cases of acute hematogenous osteomyelitis, although periosteal elevation with subperiosteal pus may be demonstrated (60). In cases in which the bone infection is secondary to preexisting soft tissue infection, as is commonly the situation in the foot, disruption and abnormal signal intensity within the cortex can be demonstrated on high-resolution images. In cases of acute osteomyelitis (even those by the hematogenous route), extensive changes in surrounding muscle and fascial planes, manifest as increased intensity on T2-weighted and STIR sequences, are typically present, and contribute to the specificity of the findings (24). The soft tissue changes most likely reflect a combination of infectious and noninfectious edema. In patients with abscesses, the soft tissue signal changes are commonly more localized with focal disruption of fascial planes and mass effect (60).

The signal changes associated with acute osteomyelitis are nonspecific and can be seen with a number of processes involving bone and marrow. In rare circum-

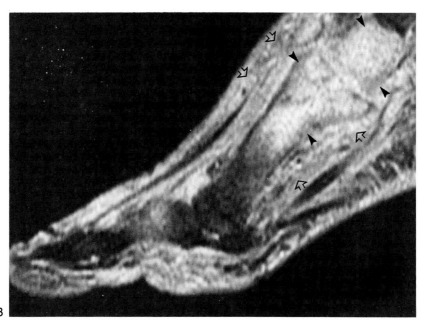

B

FIG. 8.10. (*Continued*) **B:** Sagittal STIR TR 2300 TE 35 TI 160. There is striking increased signal intensity with both bones (*arrowheads*) as well as within the soft tissues (*open arrows*), findings graphically depicted on this pulse sequence. The patient ultimately required amputation and extensive osteomyelitis and soft tissue infection was confirmed.

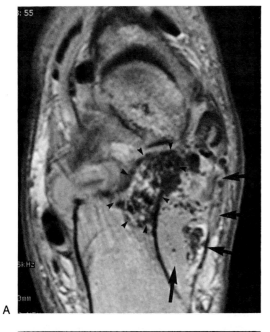

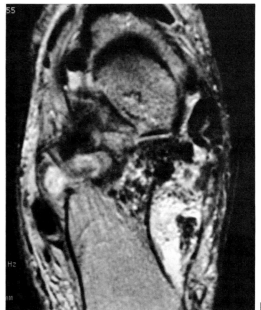

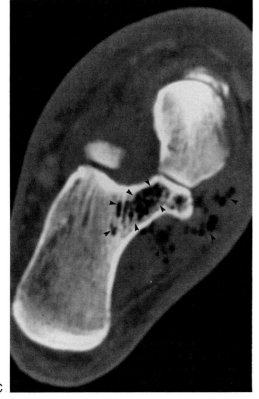

FIG. 8.11. Osteomyelitis. **A:** Axial TR 2000 TE 20. There is a complex appearance to the sustentaculum with intermixed areas of circular to ovoid low and high signal (*arrowheads*). Immediately contiguous with the medial aspect of the calcaneus is a fluid collection containing low signal intensity foci of gas and reflecting an abscess (*arrows*). **B:** Axial TR 2000 TE 80. There is increased signal intensity both within the involved bone as well as within the soft tissue abscess. **C:** Axial CT scan. Corresponding CT section demonstrates the extensive intraosseous gas (*arrowheads*) as well as gas within the soft tissue abscess. Intraosseous gas is an unusual but previously reported manifestation of osteomyelitis.

stances, intraosseous gas may be demonstrated, which in association with the other changes is diagnostic of osteomyelitis (Fig. 8.11). In most other instances, the clinical setting will allow differentiation of the diagnostic possibilities. A potential pitfall, however, in the diagnosis of osteomyelitis using MRI is in distinguishing the signal changes seen in association with recent or subacute trauma from those reflective of osteomyelitis (24). This is a problem of particular concern

in diabetic patients in which subclinical bone injuries are common secondary to altered weightbearing and biomechanics (see below). Acute and subacute fractures may demonstrate similar signal characteristics as osteomyelitis with decreased signal on T1-weighted sequences and increased signal intensity on T2-weighted and STIR sequences. In certain instances, it may be extremely difficult to distinguish confidently between these two possibilities (60).

Diabetic Foot

The challenge of detecting and distinguishing acute osteomyelitis from traumatic-related changes is magnified in patients with diabetes mellitus and particularly so in the presence of diabetic neuroarthropathy, the prototypical setting of bony change related to repetitive microtrauma and macrotrauma. The need for early and accurate diagnosis in the diabetic foot is underscored by the fact that tissue necrosis may necessitate amputation in as many as 40% of patients (32,33,41). Osteomyelitis of the foot is a common complication of diabetes mellitus, occurring in up to 15% of patients (67), and foot disorders account for 20% of all hospital admissions for diabetic patients. It is well recognized that suppurative changes may commonly coexist with neuropathic changes in the diabetic foot (37,38). It is thus of extreme value in patient management to distinguish both between soft tissue infection and involvement of bone, as well as to differentiate in the latter setting between suppurative osseous involvement and nonsuppurative neuropathic changes.

The limitations of plain film radiography with regard to sensitivity in the detection of early osteomyelitis are well recognized and have been previously considered (37,38,45). In the presence of neuroarthropathy, the task of detecting concurrent osteomyelitis is ever the more formidable. Scintigraphic techniques have been widely employed in the assessment of complications of the diabetic foot (16,51–53). The bone scan using ^{99m}Tc-MDP has been the mainstay of diagnosis, and represents a sensitive indicator of altered osteoblastic activity (45,51). While highly sensitive (on the order of 95% in recent series) (51), significant limitations with regard to specificity (particularly in differentiating soft tissue from bone involvement) have led to refinements of the technique of bone scintigraphy with the introduction of three, and more recently four phase scans consisting of dynamic and various delayed static phases (up to 24 hr) (45). Despite these refinements, the continued low specificity of ^{99m}TC bone scintigraphy (45% in recent series) (51) has led to use of adjunctive scintigraphic methods including gallium-67, and more recently indium-111–labeled white blood cells (^{111}In-WBCs) in an attempt to increase specificity. One of the principal disadvantages of gallium-67 imaging is the 48- to 72-hr delay required for sufficient decrease in background activity to allow for diagnostic imaging. While multiple reports of the use of ^{111}In-WBCs for evaluation of suspected osteomyelitis have appeared, experience with large numbers of cases of pedal osteomyelitis in diabetics has been limited (51–58,68). Additionally, the usefulness of ^{111}In-WBC scanning in the setting of diabetic neuroarthropathy has been controversial (51,53,54). In common with other scintigraphic methods, poor spatial resolution

with ^{111}In-WBCs contributes to the difficulty in distinguishing between uptake in bone and adjacent soft tissues, a principal factor contributing to false positive diagnoses (51). In a recent study of 14 patients with Charcot joint, progressive neuroarthropathy of recent onset could not be distinguished from osteomyelitis on ^{111}In-WBC scans (49). Uptake of ^{111}In-WBCs in noninfected stress fractures likely accounted for this difficulty (49). Increased activity of ^{111}In-WBC has also been recently reported in the setting of advanced noninfected diabetic neuroarthropathy (51). In addition to false positive diagnoses, false negative examinations with ^{111}In-WBCs may also result from poor spatial resolution as well as from relative tissue avascularity and tissue necrosis in the diabetic foot (51).

The use of MRI in the assessment of the diabetic foot has been specifically addressed in several clinical series (21,24,41). The markedly increased spatial resolution of the technique appears to represent a significant advantage of MRI over the previously described scintigraphic methods. The utility of MRI in the detection of soft tissue infection has been previously considered (see Soft Tissue Infection). In multiple reports, MRI has reliably depicted suppurative bone involvement. In these reports, the emphasis for the detection of osteomyelitis has been based primarily on observation of signal alteration within the medullary cavity of the involved bone. Acute osteomyelitis in the diabetic foot has been diagnosed on the basis of decreased signal intensity on T1-weighted images and areas of increased signal intensity on T2-weighted and STIR sequences. In several reports, including those of Yuh et al. (21) and Unger et al. (24), areas involved with osteomyelitis have demonstrated greater contrast with STIR sequences than with T2-weighted images, and this pulse sequence has been advocated for lesion detection. In a recent study by Erdman et al. (60), the high sensitivity of STIR images was again corroborated, but discordance between STIR images and T2-weighted images with regard to the presence of osteomyelitis was observed. Areas of increased signal on STIR did not correlate as closely with proved areas of suppurative bone involvement as did areas of increased signal intensity on T2-weighted images. As a consequence of this experience, Erdman et al. suggested that reliance on the findings on T2-weighted images could provide greater specificity for the diagnosis of osteomyelitis without significant sacrifice of sensitivity (60). Beltran et al., in reporting on 14 diabetic patients with suspected pedal infection and/or neuropathic changes, also found increased signal intensity on T2-weighted images a reliable criteria for the detection of osteomyelitis (41). In this series, noninfective neuropathic joints demonstrated relatively low signal intensity on both T1- and T2-weighted images, and MRI could be used reliably to differentiate

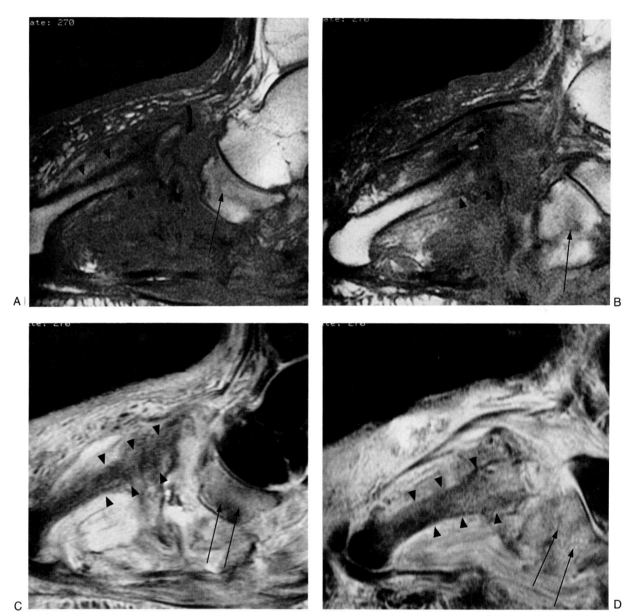

FIG. 8.12. Diabetic neuroarthropathy and soft tissue infection. Anatomic pathologic correlation. **A:** Sagittal TR 500 TE 20. A 70-year-old man with a long history of diabetes mellitus and advanced neuroarthropathy. On this sagittal section through the medial aspect of the foot, extensive soft tissue changes are seen along both the dorsal and plantar aspects. There is slightly decreased signal within the tarsal navicular and more extensive signal diminution involving the fragmented base of the second metatarsal. A fracture dislocation through the Lisfranc joint is evident with dorsal subluxation of the base of the second metatarsal (*curved arrow*). **B:** Sagittal TR 500 TE 20. On a more lateral section there is slight signal decrease within the cuboid (*arrow*) and marked signal decrease within the base of the fourth metatarsal (*arrowheads*). The metatarsal base is dorsally displaced and mildly fragmented. The extensive soft tissue changes are again noted. **C:** Sagittal TR 2200 TE 35 TI 160. Sagittal section approximately corresponding to A. The navicular demonstrates striking increased signal on this STIR sequence, a finding greatly exceeding the changes depicted on the T1-weighted sequence (*long arrow*). Diffuse signal change is also noted also the entire shaft of the second metatarsal (*arrowheads*). On histological analysis, no evidence of osteomyelitis within the navicular or second metatarsal was noted. **D:** Sagittal TR 2200 TE 35 TI 160. Sagittal section approximately corresponding to B. Note the diffuse signal change within the cuboid (*long arrows*) and fourth metatarsal (*arrowheads*), findings again far out of proportion to those depicted on the T1-weighted sequence. On histological analysis, no evidence of osteomyelitis was noted within the cuboid or fourth metatarsal.

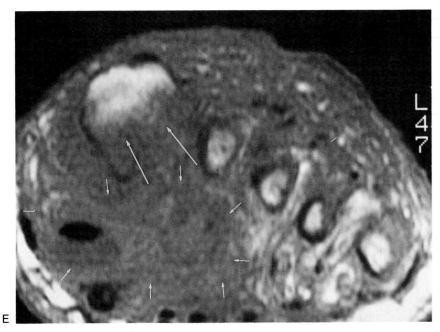

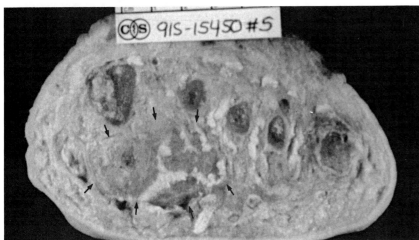

FIG. 8.12. (*Continued*) **E:** Axial TR 500 TE 20. An extensive soft tissue inflammatory process is seen along the volar aspect at the level of the metatarsal bases (*short arrows*). There is diminished signal intensity at the level of the first metatarsal base. **F:** Specimen photograph correlating with E. The extensive soft tissue infection is delineated (*small arrows*) and correlates well with the MRI. No gross or histological evidence of osteomyelitis was detected on analysis of the specimen.

suppurative bone involvement from neuropathic changes in the setting of established diabetic neuroarthropathy. The ability of MRI to differentiate neuropathic change from osteomyelitis has also been reported in others series (21,39,60). Moore and associates, however, have recently reported a case of early pedal neuroarthropathy without evidence of infection that demonstrated striking increased signal on T2-weighted images, a finding that the authors attributed to edema from spontaneous microfractures (40). While neuropathic changes can often be distinguished from areas of osteomyelitis, signal change related to recent trauma, as previously discussed, can create diagnostic difficulty with regard to its differentiation from osteomyelitis in some cases (21,24). This determination, however, has proved less of a problem with MRI, than with scintigraphic methods, but may present a difficult challenge in any individual case (21,24).

In the author's experience, lesion conspicuity has also invariably been greatest using STIR sequences. It is clear, however, particularly in the setting of diabetic neuroarthropathy, that signal changes present in medullary bone, particularly on STIR sequences, may be seen in the absence of suppurative involvement. The author has had both clinical and histological verification of this occurence (see chapter by Deutsch on Traumatic Injuries of Bone and Necrosis, Figs. 19 and 20). In a meticulous MR/pathological correlative study of a surgical amputation specimen obtained from a patient with advanced diabetic neuroarthropathy and concurrent acute soft tissue and bone infection, extensive areas of graphic signal change, particularly on STIR sequences, failed to correlate with areas of either acute or chronic osteomyelitis (Fig. 8.12). As a consequence, medullary signal changes alone (particularly on STIR sequences), in the absence of correlative findings (see below), should be interpreted with caution with regard to establishing the diagnosis of osteomyelitis.

In the author's experience, one of the keys to making the distinction between signal changes reflecting non-infectious bone marrow edema from those representing osteomyelitis is by an analysis of the immediate surrounding soft tissue as well as associated periosteal and cortical bone changes. As has been emphasized, the development of osteomyelitis and septic arthritis within the bones and joints of the foot of diabetic patients occurs in most instances secondary to direct contamination from a soft tissue focus as opposed to hematogenously (33,38). As a consequence, signal changes within the medullary component of bone should be accompanied by appropriate changes in the immediate soft tissues and changes identifiable in the periosteum and bony cortex reflecting the progression of infection (e.g., infective periostitis, infective osteitis) in most cases. Such an analysis, however, requires obtaining high-resolution images of the area of interest. In the author's experience, marrow signal changes alone (particularly on STIR sequences), in the absence of definable involvement of the periosteum and cortex, are commonly seen and are not necessarily suggestive of concurrent osteomyelitis in the setting of neuroarthropathy (see chapter by Deutsch on Traumatic Injuries of Bone and Osteonecrosis, Figs. 19 and 20). Such changes may be seen in neuropathic disease itself, presumably reflecting a manifestation of stress response and microtrauma. Whether T2-weighted sequences can provide significantly greater specificity without sacrifice of sensitivity awaits further investigation. The converse of the previously described situation (i.e., the absence of abnormal signal), however, appears highly reliable in the exclusion of osteomyelitis (24). The role of contrast enhancement with gadopentetate dimeglumine remains to be determined.

Chronic Osteomyelitis

Background

While the clinical stages of osteomyelitis are commonly designated as acute, subacute, and chronic, definitive divisions do not exist between the different stages (37). Resnick and Niwayama have emphasized that patients with apparently acute disease may reveal historical and radiological evidence suggesting long-term indolent infection, and other individuals with documented long-term osteomyelitis may present with acute exacerbations and systemic symptoms (37).

Several descriptive terms have been applied to certain radiographic and pathological features encountered during the course of osteomyelitis. These will be briefly reviewed here and the interested reader is re-

ferred to the discussion by Resnick and Niwayama for a more comprehensive discussion (37). A *sequestrum* represents a necrotic segment of bone isolated from the remaining viable bone by granulation tissue (37). Sequestra may harbor viable organisms capable of evoking an acute exacerbation of the infection (37). An *involucrum* describes a layer of living bone that surrounds the dead bone (37). This may entirely surround and merge with the parent bone, or become perforated by tracts through which pus may escape (37). A *cloaca* represents an opening in the involucrum through which granulation tissue and sequestra may be discharged (37). Sinuses represent tracts leading to the skin surface from the underlying bone.

The principal challenge for diagnostic imaging in assessment of chronic osteomyelitis is in determination of disease activity. The extensive osteolytic and osteosclerotic changes associated with chronic osteomyelitis may obscure the early changes of reactivation and limit the effectiveness of plain radiographic analysis (5). CT has primarily been used in chronic osteomyelitis for detection of sequestra, cloacae, and soft tissue abscesses (2,8,37).

MRI of Chronic Osteomyelitis

The remodeling of the cortex and the medullary cavity of long bones with chronic osteomyelitis is well demonstrated on MR. The cortical changes may often be displayed to best advantage on sagittal and coronal images and appear as a low signal intensity expansion of the cortex (60). In chronic osteomyelitis, the cortical changes may typically be more extensive than the marrow changes (60). The remodeled medullary cavity may demonstrate areas of fat signal intensity presumably related to areas of regenerated or "healed" marrow (24). Areas of active infection are distinguished from regenerative marrow by signal characteristics described for acute infection (42,60,69). T2-weighted and STIR sequences are best used for depiction of foci of active disease, which will demonstrate high signal intensity contrasted against the lower signal intensity of the thickened surrounding bone. In surgical series, these foci of high signal intensity may not necessarily represent frank "pus," but rather regions of infected material that have been described as similar to granulation tissue in consistency (69).

Differentiation of areas of "healed" osteomyelitis from areas of active disease may be difficult with MR (27,60). Unger et al., however, reported the capability of making this distinction on the basis of increased marrow signal on T1-weighted images (24). This increased signal presumably reflects replacement of hematopoietic marrow by fat following resolution of active infection. Bone scintigraphy may demonstrate persistent increased activity while MRI demonstrates high signal intensity marrow on T1-weighted sequences reflective of resolving infection; further enhancing the diagnostic specificity of MRI as compared to scintigraphic techniques in cases of complicated osteomyelitis (24).

Sinus tracts are identified as linear areas of increased signal on T2-weighted sequences that extend from the bone to the skin surface. The site of the disruption of the cortex may be well demonstrated (Figs. 8.13, 8.14). The soft tissue changes in chronic osteomyelitis are typically limited to the area around the sinus tract and are not as diffuse or extensive as the juxtacortical edema seen in cases of acute hematogenous disease (60). In patients with previous surgery or extensive soft tissue deformity secondary to trauma, the differentia-

tion of a sinus tract from a retracted scar may be difficult if continuity with the site of bone infection cannot be clearly depicted. The presence of increased signal intensity within the sinus tract may be a useful sign in distinguishing a sinus tract from a retracted scar (27).

Sequestra are typically sharply marginated bone fragments residing in the medullary aspect of tubular bones surrounded by granulation tissue. They may vary in size from small fragments to long necrotic segments. Radiographically they demonstrate increased density: a finding reflecting the lack of blood supply (37). Tomography has traditionally been employed to identify sequestra within the overall increased bone density associated with chronic osteomyelitis and CT remains an excellent method for detection of sequestra and cloacae (8). On MRI, sequestra appear as areas of

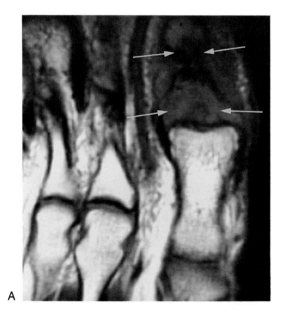

A

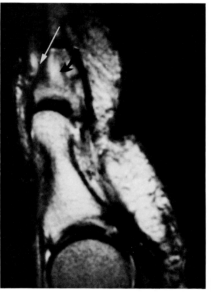

B

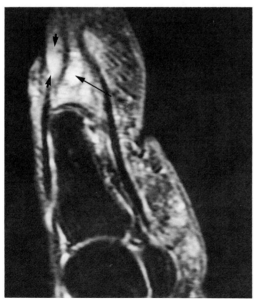

C

FIG. 8.13. Chronic osteomyelitis with sinus tract. **A:** Coronal TR/TE 500/20. There is marked decreased signal intensity within the distal phalanx of the great toe (*arrows*).**B:** Sagittal TR 2000/TE 20. Localized hyperintense signal is seen within the distal phalanx (*curved arrow*). A linear sinus tract extends from the dorsal aspect of the bone to the skin surface (*white arrow*). A micrometallic artifact related to prior surgery is seen within the distal phalanx. **C:** Sagittal STIR TR 2200 TE 35 TI 160. The central hyperintense focus is again demonstrated (*arrow*) but note the enhanced depiction of edema throughout the remainder of the distal phalanx using this pulse sequence as compared to the long TR/TE sequence. The extent of the abnormal soft tissue collection is also better depicted (*small arrows*).

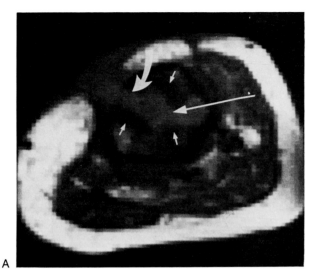
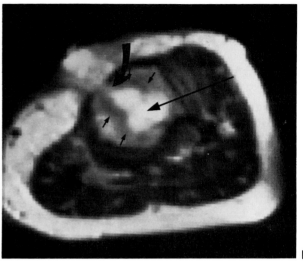

A   B

FIG. 8.14. Chronic osteomyelitis: rim sign and sinus tract. **A:** Axial TR 500 TE 30. A 38-year-old woman with a history of a draining sinus since age 10. A "mulitilobular" focus of abnormal signal is seen within the medullary canal of the tibia. There is a surrounding zone of lower signal intensity presumably representing fibrous tissue (*small arrows*). There is localized disruption of the cortex with demonstration of a sinus tract extending to the skin surface (*curved arrows*). **B:** Axial TR 2000 TE 80. The central focus increases significantly in signal intensity (*long arrow*). The surrounding band remains of low signal intensity consistent with its presumed fibrous nature (*small arrows*). The sinus tract is again well demonstrated (*curved arrow*). (Courtesy of William A. Erdman, M.D. Dallas, TX). (From ref. 60, with permission.)

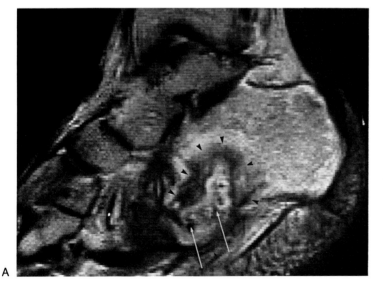
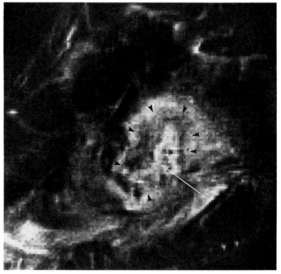

A   B

FIG. 8.15. Chronic osteomyelitis: rim sign. **A:** Sagittal TR 2000 TE 80. This 42-year-old man developed chronic osteomyelitis following a gunshot wound. A central area of surgically proven active infection is surrounded by a low signal intensity (*dark*) band (*arrowheads*). Low signal intensity foci within a sinus tract may represent sequestra of bone but cannot be absolutely distinguished from fracture or bullet fragments (*arrows*). **B:** Sagittal TR 1500 TE 30 TI 160. The low signal intensity band representing the rim sign (*arrowheads*) is again demonstrated surrounding the central area of active infection (*arrow*). The low signal intensity foci within the site of active infection, possibly representing sequestra, are again well demonstrated. (Courtesy of William A. Erdman, M.D. Dallas, TX.) (From ref. 60, with permission.)

diminished signal intensity or areas of intensity similar to cortical bone within and contrasted against the high intensity foci of infection on T2-weighted sequences (25,60) (Fig. 8.15).

Foci of chronic osteomyelitis may demonstrate a "rim sign" consisting of a well-defined rim of low signal intensity surrounding the area of focal active disease on MRI scans (60) (Fig. 8.15). This sign was demonstrated in 14 of 15 patients (93%) with chronic osteomyelitis secondary to trauma in the series reported by Erdman et al. (60). In contrast, the "rim sign" was depicted in only 1 of 38 other cases of either acute, diabetic, or decubitus-related osteomyelitis. The peripheral rim presumably reflects fibrous tissue or reactive bone (60). Tang et al. reported similar findings in subacute osteomyelitis, and Berquist described a dark margin of "fiber bone" surrounding the area of chronic infection (25,26). This appearance may be less evident at high (1.5 T) than at mid-field strength (60).

Mason reported on the use of MRI in the assessment of active infection in patients with extensive deformities of the bones and soft tissues of the lower extremities due to previous trauma, surgery, and chronic infection (27). Using the criteria of increased signal intensity on long T2-weighted sequences, MRI successfully identified active osteomyelitis in all patients subsequently demonstrated by surgery to have active infection. In addition, MRI was true positive for infection in three cases in which scintigraphy performed with ^{111}In-WBCs was negative. The authors attributed the poorer performance of scintigraphy to the chronic course of disease in these patients with extensive scarring and avascularity from prior trauma and surgery (27).

Bone abscesses (Brodie's abscess) reflect sharply delineated foci of infection that are seen most commonly in the subacute and chronic stages of hematogenous osteomyelitis. These lesions are commonly sharply circumscribed and demonstrate a predilection for the ends of tubular bones and are often of staphylococcal origin (37). Brodie's abscesses are particularly common in children with the distal tibia a common location of occurrence. In young children, Brodie's abscesses may occur in the epiphyses and in the carpus and tarsus (37). The walls of typical bone abscesses are lined by granulation tissue and may be surrounded by eburnated reactive bone. The fluid contained within may be purulent or mucoid and bacteriological analysis may not reveal the organism (37). On MRI, a Brodie's abscess will demonstrate low to intermediate signal on T1-weighted sequences that significantly increases in intensity on T2-weighted sequences: findings reflective of the central fluid component and granulation tissue (25). The signal is homogeneous and outlined by a thick rim that is of low

signal intensity on all pulse sequences and corresponds to the eburnated surrounding reactive bone ("rim sign") (25).

Septic Arthritis

Background

Septic arthritis may affect individuals of all ages, although it predominates in the young. The potential pathogenetic sequence for articular infection parallels that already described for osteomyelitis. Thus, contamination of a joint may occur either (a) via hematogenous seeding of the synovial membrane, (b) spread from a contiguous source as in intraarticular extension of osteomyelitis from an epiphyseal, metaphyseal, or from a neighboring soft tissue location, (c) via direct implantation as may occur with a penetrating injury, or (d) postoperatively (37).

In response to infection, the synovial membrane becomes edematous and hypertrophied and increased amounts of joint fluid are produced. After a few days, frank pus accumulates and destruction of articular cartilage begins (37). This may occur centrally or at the margins of the articulation. With further accumulation of hypertrophied synovium, the capsule becomes distended, surrounding soft tissue edema is evident, and osseous abnormalities may develop (37). Involvement of adjacent osseous structures produces typical features of osteomyelitis (37).

MRI

The changes that may be evident on MRI parallel this pathologic sequence and may precede conventional radiographic findings. MRI is quite sensitive to the detection of joint fluid, which demonstrates increased signal intensity on T2-weighted and STIR sequences. The mere depiction of joint fluid does not allow differentiation of septic arthritis from a reactive or noninfectious effusion (41). Increased signal intensity within the surrounding soft tissues reflective of edema, in association with increased joint fluid, is suggestive of infection (39). Evidence of cartilage destruction may be evident on MRI, and its depiction is enhanced in the presence of joint fluid using T2-weighted or STIR sequences. Signal changes may also be evident within the adjacent medullary bone: findings that may reflect reactive edema or extension of the inflammatory process (60) (Figs. 8.16, 8.17). This distinction may be extremely difficult during the early course of the infection (60). Erdman et al. reported

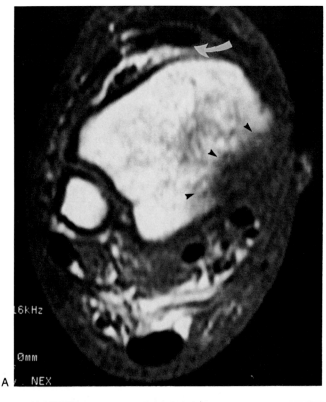

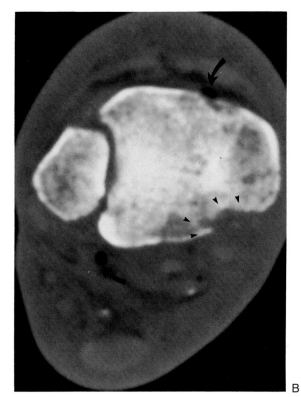

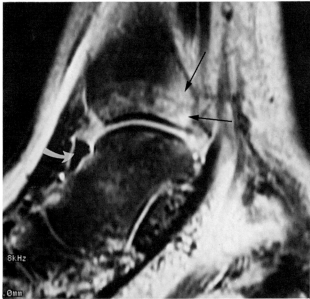

FIG. 8.16. Septic arthritis. **A:** Axial TR 500 TE 20. There is ill-defined low signal replacing the normal fatty marrow of the tibial plafond (*arrowheads*). A low signal intensity crescent, representing gas, is seen with the joint anteriorly (*curved arrow*). **B:** Axial CT. Corresponding CT section of the extent of bone destruction involving the plafond (*arrowheads*) as well as pockets of gas within the joint (*curved arrows*). **C:** Sagittal STIR TR 2200 TE 35 TI 160. High signal intensity fluid is seen within the joint as well as low signal intensity gas in the anterior joint space (*curved arrow*). There is focal high signal intensity within the posterior aspect of the tibial plafond representing extension of infection with concurrent osteomyelitis (*long arrows*).

signal changes within marrow subsequently demonstrated to be noninfectious in nature in 60% of cases of septic arthritis (60). In cases with noninfectious marrow changes, the findings on T1-weighted and STIR sequences far exceeded those on T2-weighted images. As a consequence, Erdman et al. have suggested that the inclusion of increased signal on all three pulse sequences for the diagnosis of osteomyelitis may increase the specificity of the examination for osteo-

myelitis without significantly decreasing sensitivity (60).

When septic arthritis develops secondary to a preexisting osteomyelitis, the changes within bone characteristically exceed those seen in the joint. Reported clinical experience with MRI and detection of septic arthritis remains limited (39,41,60). Erdman et al. reported on 10 cases of septic arthritis, 4 with concurrent osteomyelitis and 6 without (60). In a report by Klein et al., MRI compared favorably to bone scintigraphy, gallium scanning, and CT in the detection and characterization of septic arthritis involving the sacroiliac joint (61).

CONCLUSION

The role of MRI in the detection and characterization of infections of the musculoskeletal system continues to evolve. Multiple studies have now attested to the ability of MRI to depict and differentiate between infection of soft tissue and that of neighboring bone. Additionally, MRI has the unique capability of precisely defining both the pathoanatomic sequence of bone infection as well as the ability to differentiate suppurative involvement of bone from changes related to trauma and other causes. This is a particular advantage in assessment of pedal osteomyelitis and particularly so in the diabetic patient in whom changes related to trauma and ischemia often complicate the diagnostic picture. Multiple scintigraphic methods have been used for assessment of musculoskeletal infection. These methods, while highly sensitive, lack specificity, and share in common low spatial resolution, a feature further limiting their diagnostic utility. In an attempt to increase specificity, scintigraphic methods are often used in combination, a practice contributing to both increased cost and prolongation in the time of work-up. The high spatial resolution of MRI overcomes many of the limitations encountered with the more traditional methods that have been used for characterization of musculoskeletal infections. The high soft tissue contrast resolution and multiplanar capability of MRI is ideally suited for assessment of complicated musculoskeletal infections and as a single examination, MRI can contribute to efficiency in diagnostic work-up and compete on a cost-effective basis with the more traditional diagnostic algorithms. With its now general availability, it is anticipated that MRI will increasingly be used for assessment of complicated musculoskeletal infections and may become the primary diagnostic method employed for this purpose. The use of small field of view, high-resolution

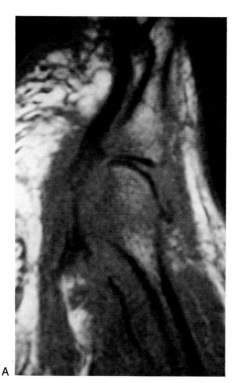 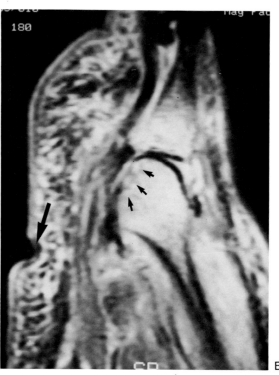

FIG. 8.17. Septic arthritis and osteomyelitis. **A:** Sagittal TR 500 TE 20. A 50-year-old nondiabetic man developed pain and swelling in the region of the first tarsometatarsal joint 4 weeks following a puncture injury related to a nail. There is markedly decreased signal intensity along the volar aspect of the first metatarsal head as well along the base of the first proximal phalanx (*arrows*). **B:** Sagittal TR 2200 TE 35 TI 160. On the STIR sequence the site of the puncture wound is seen along the plantar aspect of the foot (*arrow*). There is striking increased signal within the entire metatasal head and much of the base of the first proximal phalanx. More localized cartilage and subchondral destruction is noted along the plantar aspect of the first metatarsal head (*small arrows*). The findings on the STIR seqence far exceed the area of actual active infection and relate to reactive changes within the marrow. (*Figure continues on next page.*)

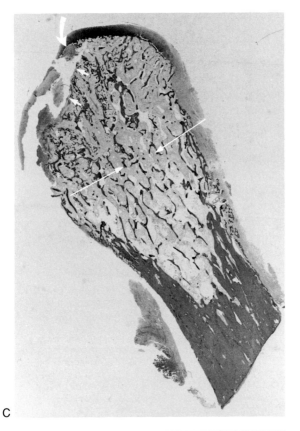

C

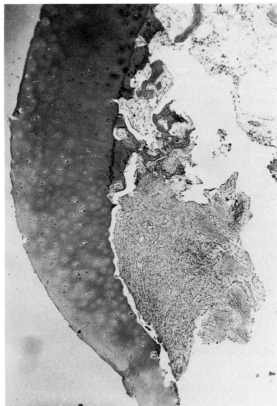

D

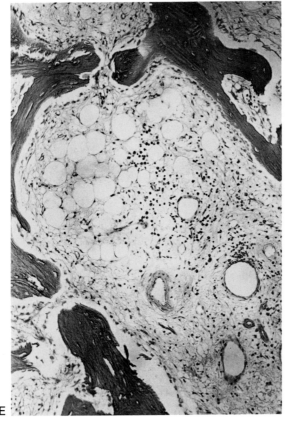

E

FIG. 8.17. (*Continued*) **C:** Whole mount section. There is destruction of articular cartilage extending into subchondral bone (*short arrows*). **D:** Higher power histologic section corresponding to curved arrow in C. There is destruction of subchondral bone with partial replacement by granulation tissue and new bone production. The findings are consistent with resolving osteomyelitis. **E:** Higher power histologic section corresponding to long arrow in C. There is marked reduction in medullary fat and increased medullary fibrosis. There is mild mononuclear cell infiltration but no evidence of active infection.

images is strongly encouraged to maximize the diagnostic capability of MRI.

REFERENCES

1. Bamberger, DM, Daus, GP, and Gerding, DN, *Osteomyelitis in the feet of diabetic patients: Long-term results, prognostic factors, and the role of antimicrobial and surgical therapy.* Radiology, 1988. **167**: p. 295.

2. Seltzer, S, *Value of computed tomography in planning medical and surgical treatment of chronic osteomyelitis.* J Comput Assist Tomogr, 1984. **8(3)**: p. 482–487.

3. Hald, JJ and Sudmann, E, *Acute hematogenous osteomyelitis: Early diagnosis with computed tomography.* Acta Radiol, 1982. **23(1)**: p. 55–58.

4. Hemingway, D and Lieberman, C, *Bone scan findings with radiographic, clinical, and surgical correlation in extensive osteomyelitis: A case report.* Clin Nucl Med, 1980. **5(1)**: p. 29–30.

5. Williamson, B, Teates, C, Phillips, C, et al., *Computed tomography as a diagnostic aid in diabetic and other problem feet.* Clin Imaging, 1989. **13(2)**: p. 159–163.

6. Tumeh, SS, Aliabadi, P, Weissman, BN, et al., *Disease activity in osteomyelitis: Role of radiography.* Radiology, 1987. **165(3)**: p. 781–784.

7. Tumeh, SS, Aliabadi, P, Weissman, BN, et al., *Chronic osteomyelitis: Bone and gallium scan patterns associated with active disease.* Radiology, 1986. **158**: p. 685–688.

8. Hernandez, RJ, *Visualization of small sequestra by computerized tomography. Report of 6 cases.* Pediatric Radiol, 1985. p. 238–241.

9. Esterhai, J, Alavi, A, Mandell, GA, et al., *Sequential technetium-99m/gallium-67 scintigraphic evaluation of subclinical osteomyelitis complicating fracture nonunion.* J Orthop Res, 1985. **3(2)**: p. 219–225.

10. Seldin, DW, Heiken, JP, Feldman, F, et al., *Effect of soft tissue pathology on detection of pedal osteomyelitis in diabetics.* J Nucl Med, 1985. **26(9)**: p. 988–993.

11. Alazraki, N, Dries, D, Datz, F, et al., *Value of a 24-hour image (four phase bone scan) in assessing osteomyelitis in patients with peripheral vascular disease.* J Nucl Med, 1985. **26(7)**: p. 711–717.

12. Herndon, WA, Alexieva, BT, Schwindt, ML, et al., *Nuclear imaging for musculoskeletal infections in children.* J Orthop Pediatr, 1985. **5(3)**: p. 343–347.

13. Hernandez, RJ, Conway, JJ, Pozanski, AK, et al., *The role of computed tomography and radionuclide scintigraphy in the localization of osteomyelitis in flat bones.* J Pediatr Orthop, 1985. **5(2)**: p. 151–154.

14. Schauwecker, DS, Park, HM, Mock, BH, et al., *Evaluation of complicating osteomyelitis with Tc-99m, MDP, In-111 granulocytes, and Ga 67 citrate.* J Nucl Med, 1984. **25(8)**: p. 849–853.

15. Raptopoulos, V, Doherty, PW, Goss, TP, et al., *Acute osteomyelitis: Advantage of white cell scans in early detection.* AJR, 1982. **139(6)**: p. 1077–1082.

16. Park, HM, Wheat, LJ, Siddiqui, AR, et al., *Scintigraphic evaluation of diabetic osteomyelitis: Concise communication.* J Nucl Med, 1982. **23(7)**: p. 569–573.

17. Jones, DC and Cady, RB, *Cold bone scans in acute osteomyelitis.* J Bone Joint Surg, 1981. **63B**: p. 376–378.

18. Leonard, JC, Marks, MI, and Kolyvas, E, *False-normal radionuclide scans for osteomyelitis [Letter].* Am J Dis Child, 1981. **135(4)**: p. 383–384.

19. Scoles, PV, Hilty, MD, and Sfakianakis, GN, *Bone scan patterns in acute osteomyelitis.* Clin Orthop, 1980. **153**: p. 210–217.

20. Sullivan, DC, Rosenfield, NS, Ogden, J, et al., *Problems with the scintigraphic detection of osteomyelitis in children.* Radiology, 1980. **135(3)**: p. 731–736.

21. Yuh, W, Corson, J, Baraniewski, H, et al., *Osteomyelitis of the foot in diabetic patients: Evaluation with plain film, 99mTc-MDP bone scintigraphy, and MR imaging.* AJR, 1989. **152(4)**: p. 795–800.

22. Modic, M, Feiglin, D, Piraino, D, et al., *Vertebral osteomyelitis: Assessment using MR.* Radiology, 1985. **157**: p. 157–166.

23. Fletcher, B, Scoles, P, and Nelson, A, *Osteomyelitis in children: Detection by magnetic resonance. Work in progress.* Radiology, 1984. **150(1)**: p. 57–60.

24. Unger, EC, Moldofsky, PJ, Gatenby, RA, et al., *Diagnosis of osteomyelitis by MR imaging.* AJR, 1988. **150(3)**: p. 605–610.

25. Tang, JS, Gold, RH, Bassett, LW, et al., *Musculoskeletal infection of the extremities: Evaluation with MR imaging.* Radiology, 1988. **166**: p. 205–209.

26. Berquist, TH, Brown, ML, Fitzgerald, RH, et al., *Magnetic resonance imaging: Application in musculoskeletal infection.* Magn Reson Imaging, 1985. **3**: p. 219–230.

27. Mason, MD, Zlatkin, MB, Esterhai, JL, et al., *Chronic complicated osteomyelitis of the lower extremity: Evaluation with MR imaging.* Radiology, 1989. **173**: p. 355–359.

28. Hovi, I, Hekali, P, Korhola, O, et al., *Detection of soft-tissue and skeletal infections with ultra low-field (0.02 T) MR imaging.* Acta Radiol, 1989. **30**: p. 495.

29. Beltran, J, McGhee, RB, Shaffer, PB, et al., *Experimental infections of the musculoskeletal system: Evaluation with MR imaging and Tc-99m MDP and Ga-67 scintigraphy.* Radiology, 1988. **167**: p. 167–172.

30. Cohen, MD, Cory, DA, Kleiman, M, et al., *Magnetic resonance differentiation of acute and chronic osteomyelitis in children.* Clin Radiol, 1990. **41**: p. 53–56.

31. Scott, JA and Palmer, EL, *Musculoskeletal infection of the extremities: Evaluation with MR imaging.* Radiology, 1988. **168**: p. 284–285.

32. Bessman, AN and Wright, W, *Nonclostridial gas gangrene.* JAMA, 1975. **233**: p. 958.

33. Edmons, ME, *The diabetic foot: Pathophysiology and treatment.* Clin Endocrinol Metab, 1986. **15**: p. 889.

34. Kaufman, J, Breeding, L, and Rosenberg, N, *Anatomic location of acute diabetic foot infection. Its influence on the outcome of treatment.* Am Surg, 1987. **53**: p. 109.

35. Robson, MC and Edstrom, LE, *The diabetic foot: An alternative approach to major amputation.* Surg Clin North Am, 1977. **57**: p. 1089–1099.

36. Chandnani, VP, Beltran, J, Morris, CS, et al., *Acute experimental osteomyelitis and abscesses: Detection with MR imaging versus CT.* Radiology, 1990. **174**: p. 233–236.

37. Resnick, D and Niwayama, G, *Osteomyelitis, septic arthritis, and soft tissue infection: The mechanisms and situations,* in *Diagnosis of Bone and Joint Disorders,* D Resnick and G Niwayama, Editors. 1988, W.B. Saunders: Philadelphia. p. 2524–2619.

38. Zlatkin, MB, Pathria, M, Sartoris, DJ, et al., *The diabetic foot.* Radiol Clin North Am, 1987. **25**: p. 1095–1105.

39. Beltran, J, Noto, AM, McGhee, RB, et al., *Infections of the musculoskeletal system: High-field-strength MR imaging.* Radiology, 1987. **164**: p. 449–454.

40. Moore, TE, Yuh, WTC, Kathol, MH, et al., *Pictorial essay abnormalities of the foot in patients with diabetes mellitus: Findings on MR imaging.* AJR, 1991. **157**: p. 813–817.

41. Beltran, J, Campanni, DS, Knight, C, et al., *The diabetic foot: Magnetic resonance imaging evaluation.* Skeletal Radiol, 1990. **19**: p. 37–41.

42. Totty, WG, *Radiographic evaluation of osteomyelitis using magnetic resonance imaging.* Orthop Rev, 1989. **18**: p. 587–592.

43. Benton, G and Kerstein, M, *Cost effectiveness of early digit amputation in the patient with diabetes.* Surg Gynecol Obstet, 1985. **161(6)**: p. 523–524.

44. Ram, PC, Martinez, S, Korobkin, M, et al., *CT detection of intraosseous gas: A new sign of osteomyelitis.* AJR, 1981. **137**: p. 721–723.

45. Gold, RH, Hawkins, RA, and Katz, RD, *Bacterial osteomyelitis: Findings on plain radiography, CT, MR and scintigraphy.* AJR, 1991. **157**: p. 365–370.

46. Segall, G, Nino-Murcia, M, Jacobs, T, et al., *The role of bone scan and radiography in the diagnostic evaluation of suspected pedal osteomyelitis.* Clin Nucl Med (A), 1989. **14(4)**: p. 255–260.

47. Keenan, AM, Tindel, NL, Alavi, A, et al., *Diagnosis of pedal osteomyelitis in diabetic patients using current scintigraphic techniques.* Radiology, 1990. **175**: p. 888.

48. Gupta, NC and Prezio, JA, *Radionuclide imaging in osteomyelitis*. Semin Nucl Med, 1988. **18**: p. 287.
49. Seabold, JE, Flickinger, FW, Kao, SCS, *et al.*, *Indium-111-leukocyte/technetium-99m-MDP bone and magnetic resonance imaging: Difficulty of diagnosing osteomyelitis in patients with neuropathic osteoarthropathy*. J Nucl Med, 1990. **31**: p. 549–556.
50. Lisbona, R and Rosenthal, L, *Observations on the sequential use of 99m Tc-phosphate complex and 67-Ga imaging in osteomyelitis, cellulitis, and septic arthritis*. Radiology, 1977. **123**: p. 123–129.
51. Lartos, G, Brown, ML, and Sutton, RT, *Diagnosis of osteomyelitis of the foot in diabetic patients: Value of 111 In-leukocyte scintigraphy*. AJR, 1991. **157**: p. 527–531.
52. Hartshorne, MF and Peters, V, *Nuclear medicine application for the diabetic foot*. Clin Podiatr Med Surg, 1987. **4**: p. 361–375.
53. Keenan, AM, Tindel, NL, and Alavi, A, *Diagnosis of pedal osteomyelitis in diabetic patients using current scintigraphic techniques*. Arch Intern Med, 1989. **149**: p. 2262–2266.
54. Schauwecker, DS, Park, HM, Burt, RW, *et al.*, *Combined bone scintigraphy and indium-111 leukocyte scans in neuropathic foot disease*. J Nucl Med, 1988. **(q)**: p. 1651–1655.
55. Schauwecker, DS, *Osteomyelitis diagnosis with In-111-labeled leukocytes*. Radiology, 1989. **171**: p. 141–146.
56. McCarthy, K, Velchik, MG, Alavi, A, *et al.*, *Indium-111-labeled white blood cells in the detection of osteomyelitis complicated by a pre-existing condition*. J Nucl Med, 1988. **29**: p. 1015–1021.
57. Splittgerder, GF, Stiegelhoff, DR, and Buggy, BP, *Combined leukocyte and bone imaging used to evaluate diabetic osteoarthropathy and osteomyelitis*. Clin Nuc Med, 1989. **14**: p. 156–160.
58. Merkel, KD, Brown, ML, Dewanjee, MK, *et al.*, *Comparison of indium-labeled-leukocyte imaging with sequential technetium-gallium scanning in diagnosis of low-grade musculoskeletal sepsis*. J Bone Joint Surg (Am), 1985. **67A**: p. 465–476.
59. Sanchez, RB and Quinn, SF, *MRI of inflammatory synovial processes*. Magn Reson Imag, 1989. **7**: p. 529.
60. Erdman, WA, Tamburro, F, Jayson, HT, *et al.*, *Osteomyelitis: Characteristics and pitfalls of diagnosis with MR imaging*. Radiology, 1991. **180**: p. 533–539.
61. Klein, MA, Winalski, CS, Wax, MR, *et al.*, *MR imaging of septic sacroilitis*. J Comput Assist Tomogr, 1991. **15(1)**: p. 126–132.
62. Modic, MT, Pflanze, W, Feiglin, DHI, *et al.*, *Magnetic resonance imaging of musculoskeletal infections*. Radiol Clin North Am, 1986. **24**: p. 247–258.
63. Quinn, SF, W., M, Clark, RA, *et al.*, *MR imaging of chronic osteomyelitis*. J Comput Assist Tomogr, 1988. **12**: p. 113–117.
64. Tehranzadeh, J, Spoliansky, G, and Post, J, *MR imaging in osteomyelitis*. Radiology, 1990. **177 (P)**: p. 367.
65. Post, M, Sze, G, Quencer, R, *et al.*, *Gadolinium-enhanced MR in spinal infection*. J Comput Assist Tomogr, 1990. **14**: p. 721–729.
66. Greenfield, GB, Warren, DL, and Clark, RA, *MR imaging of periosteal and cortical changes of bone*. Radiographics, 1991. **11**: p. 611–623.
67. Wheat, J, *Diagnostic strategies in osteomyelitis*. Am J Med, 1985. **78**: p. 218.
68. Jacobson, AF, Harley, JD, Lipskey, BA, *et al.*, *Diagnosis of osteomyelitis in the presence of soft tissue infection and radiological evidence of osseous abnormalities: Value of leukocyte scintigraphy*. AJR, 1991. **157**: p. 807–813.
69. Quinn, SF, Murray, WT, Clark, RA, *et al.*, *MR imaging of chronic osteomyelitis*. J Comput Assist Tomogr, 1988. **12**: p. 113–117.

MRI of the Foot and Ankle,
edited by A.L. Deutsch, J.H. Mink, and R. Kerr,
Raven Press, Ltd., New York © 1992

CHAPTER 9

Tumors and Tumorlike Lesions of Soft Tissue and Bone

Roger Kerr

IMAGING APPROACH

Soft tissue tumors and tumorlike lesions are common in the foot and ankle and the great majority are benign. Conversely, primary bone tumors and tumorlike lesions rarely arise in the foot and ankle, as this location accounts for only 3% to 4% of all such lesions (1,2). Primary malignant bone tumors are particularly uncommon and skeletal metastases are extremely rare in the foot and ankle.

Tumors and tumorlike lesions of the foot and ankle usually present earlier in their course, compared to other locations, for several reasons: (a) soft tissue masses are more readily palpated through the relatively thin layers of subcutaneous fat and muscle; b) the pressure and mechanical demands of weightbearing tend to elicit symptoms from both soft tissue and bone lesions; c) peritendinous lesions cause pain and discomfort due to interference with tendon function; and d) because of the compact structure of the foot, small lesions may cause focal nerve entrapment and cause pain or paresthesia. The early production of symptoms creates an opportunity to diagnose a lesion while it is small in size and readily amenable to excision. The clinical diagnosis may be unclear, however, as deep lesions may be small and nonpalpable and may produce vague, poorly localized signs and symptoms. Furthermore, the nature and extent of palpable lesions often may not be reliably deduced by physical examination (3). In these cases, the presence and extent of

the offending lesion may be accurately determined with magnetic resonance imaging (MRI).

Conventional radiographs remain the cornerstone for the initial evaluation of bone and soft tissue masses. For a primary bone tumor, a probable histologic diagnosis or a limited differential diagnosis can usually be generated based on the radiographic appearance and consideration of clinical data. The aggressiveness of a bone tumor may also be estimated from the radiograph. In the foot, however, tumors arising within the tarsal bones often have a nonspecific appearance and, unless there is calcified or ossified matrix, or an obvious fatty composition, it may not be possible to generate a narrow differential diagnosis. Radiographic determination of the extent of lesions originating within the bones of the foot may also be difficult. The tarsal bones and the metatarsal bases are irregularly shaped, with many undulating surfaces. Consequently, cortical destruction by a primary bone lesion or bony invasion by a soft tissue lesion may be difficult to identify with conventional radiography (Fig. 9.1).

If a primary bone lesion appears benign and well circumscribed on radiographs, further imaging is probably not necessary. For lesions in which the diagnosis or extent are indeterminate, and for lesions that appear malignant, local staging with MRI is indicated before biopsy. A well-performed MR examination, with attention to anatomic detail, is superior to computed tomography (CT) for determining the intramedullary and extraosseous extent of bone tumors and tumorlike lesions of the extremities (4–9). CT is more sensitive in demonstrating cortical bone destruction and in revealing intralesional calcification or ossification (8,9).

Radiography is somewhat limited in evaluating soft

R. Kerr: Department of Radiology, Musculoskeletal Imaging, Cedars–Sinai Medical Center, Los Angeles, California 90048; USC School of Medicine, Los Angeles, California.

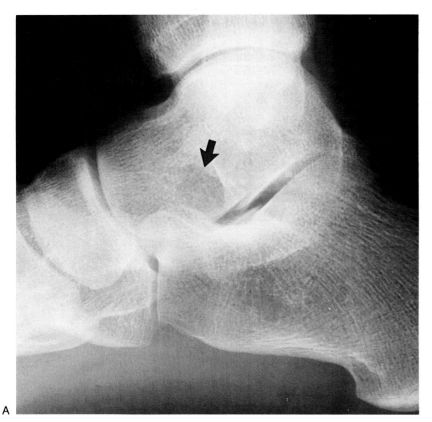
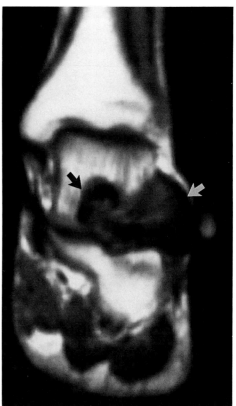

A

B

FIG. 9.1. Pigmented villonodular synovitis arising from the sinus tarsi. **A:** Lateral radiograph reveals a subtle radiolucency (*arrow*) within the talus. **B:** Coronal MR, TR/TE 2100/28 reveals a large low signal intensity mass (*arrows*) eroding the talus and extending into the lateral soft tissues. (B from ref. 59, with permission.)

tissue masses. Many such masses will not be detected and, for others, only a general estimate of lesion extent is possible. Findings that suggest a specific diagnosis, such as phleboliths in a hemangioma, are rarely present. Radiolucent fat suggests a lipoma; however, it may also be a significant component of a hemangioma or liposarcoma. Intralesional calcification may be seen in a variety of lesions ranging from synovial sarcoma to leiomyoma. Secondary invasion of bone indicates an aggressive growth pattern, but may occur with both benign and malignant lesions.

Because of its superior soft tissue contrast, MRI has replaced CT as the imaging modality of choice in evaluating all soft tissue processes (10–14). In the foot and ankle, MRI is useful in distinguishing between bone and soft tissue lesions that may cause similar signs and symptoms. For soft tissue mass lesions, MRI may not establish a specific diagnosis, but is the most sensitive means to detect such lesions and determine their extent (15). The anatomic information provided by MRI facilitates the planning and performance of a biopsy or surgical excision, when warranted.

MRI CHARACTERISTICS OF TUMORS AND TUMORLIKE LESIONS

Most bone tumors reveal low to intermediate signal intensity on T1-weighted images and high signal intensity on T2-weighted images. Lesions with high signal intensity on T1-weighted images contain either fat or blood. Very low signal intensity is seen on T2-weighted images in cellular, densely fibrous lesions and in lesions containing bone, calcification, or hemosiderin. Most mass lesions demonstrate some heterogeneity of signal intensity, reflecting a compound histologic composition, intralesional hemorrhage, necrosis, or cyst formation.

Most soft tissue tumors also demonstrate a pattern of low to intermediate signal intensity on T1-weighted images and high signal intensity on T2-weighted images. Certain benign lesions, such as lipomas, hemangiomas, and ganglion cysts, reveal a characteristic morphology and pattern of signal intensity on MRI. The diagnosis of other benign lesions such as interdigital neuroma, plantar fibroma, and giant cell tumor of tendon sheath may often be correctly deduced by considering their location and signal characteristics. Conversely, the histologic diagnosis of malignant soft tissue lesions is not usually predictable based on the MRI appearance.

Attempts have been made to distinguish benign from malignant soft tissue masses based on the margin definition, intensity and homogeneity of signal, and the involvement of bone or neurovascular structures. Berquist et al. were 90% accurate in predicting the benign or malignant nature of 95 soft tissue masses (16). In their study, benign lesions tended to be well marginated, have homogeneous signal intensity, and not encase neurovascular structures or invade bone. Malignant lesions tended to reveal the converse properties but there was significant overlap between these two categories. In contrast, the studies of Kransdorf et al. and Totty et al. encompassed 145 soft tissue masses and concluded that MRI was not capable of reliably distinguishing between benign and malignant soft tissue tumors (14,17).

MRI may be used to detect recurrent tumor in patients who have had prior surgical excision (18,19). When radiation therapy has been given, however, it is often not possible to distinguish active tumor from radiation-induced inflammation (19). There have been several studies of MRI in assessing the response of bone and soft tissue tumors to chemotherapy (20–23). These studies have not, thus far, yielded reliable criteria to distinguish residual viable tumor from other tissue. Preliminary work indicates that dynamic gadolinium (Gd)-DTPA–enhanced MRI may be useful to distinguish viable or recurrent tumor from regions of inflammation, edema, or necrosis (24,25).

MRI IN STAGING OF MALIGNANT TUMORS

MRI has become an essential component in the surgical staging of musculoskeletal neoplasms (26,27). Musculoskeletal sarcomas are staged according to histologic grade and anatomic extent (28). A low histologic grade is denoted as Stage I and a high grade lesion as Stage II. A lesion associated with metastatic disease is designated Stage III. Lesions are further classified according to anatomic extent as: (a) intracompartmental or (b) extracompartmental. An intracompartmental lesion is confined to an anatomic site such as a bone, joint, or an interfascial soft tissue compartment. In order to be defined as intracompartmental, both the tumor and its reactive zone must be within the compartment. The compartment is bounded by natural barriers to tumor spread, such as cortical bone, joint capsule, articular cartilage, and fascial septae. An extracompartmental lesion violates compartmental

barriers and may readily spread and involve the neurovascular bundle. In the foot, a lesion confined to a ray is intracompartmental. Because of a lack of anatomic boundaries, the midfoot and hindfoot are defined as extracompartmental locations. In patients with sarcomas involving the foot, adequate surgical treatment usually requires some form of amputation. In order to achieve a radical margin lesions in the toe distal to the metatarsophalangeal joint require a ray resection, midfoot lesions distal to the talonavicular or calcaneocuboid joints are managed with a disarticulation of the ankle joint (Syme's amputation), and lesions in the hindfoot and periarticular soft tissues of the ankle require below knee amputation above the musculotendinous junction. The key to effective surgical treatment is resection of the tumor with adequate margins (2).

In patients with sarcomas, recent advances in the use of adjuvant therapy combined with limb salvage surgery have produced enhanced survival with preservation of the involved extremity and improved quality of life. The goal of limb salvage surgery is to excise tumor adequately while preserving useful function. Accurate imaging of tumor extent is essential in deciding if a patient is a candidate for limb salvage surgery, to ensure adequate surgical margins, or to define a radiotherapy field. MRI has been shown to be useful in planning limb salvage surgery of malignant bone and soft tissue tumors primarily because of its ability to delineate the intramedullary and extraosseous extent of tumor accurately (27).

The use of limb salvage surgery in treating malignant tumors of the foot and ankle is controversial (29–31). For limb salvage, the optimal excision includes tumor, surrounding edema and reaction, and a layer of uninvolved tissue. Because of the close anatomic confines of the foot, excisions that are less than radical often do not achieve a margin free of tumor. Consequently, persistent or recurrent disease is more common in the foot than in other locations (2). Although soft tissue sarcomas are enclosed by a fibrous pseudocapsule, microscopic spread of tumor beyond this boundary is common (32). Therefore, "shelling-out" of an apparently encapsulated sarcoma usually leaves tumor cells behind. There has been a hesitancy to use adjuvant radiation therapy, because the weightbearing demands are believed to render the foot more prone to complications (29,30). Encouraging results were recently reported in patients with soft tissue sarcomas of the foot treated with preoperative chemotherapy and irradiation, followed by conservative resection (31). It was concluded that for selected patients, limb salvage therapy resulted in a high probability of local control and useful function without compromising survival. In order to be eligible for this treatment approach, however, nonexpendable osseous, neural, or tendinous structures must not be involved by tumor.

Prognostic factors that affect survival with soft tissue sarcoma of an extremity may be divided into those that relate to the patient, the tumor, and the mode of therapy. A recent study identified several factors as independent predictors of a poor outcome (33). These were an age greater than 53 years, local symptoms, high grade of tumor, proximal location within the extremity, size greater than 10 cm, positive regional lymph nodes, and inadequate surgical margins. Favorable aspects of soft tissue sarcomas arising in the foot or ankle are the distal location and the fact that tumors are usually detected in this location before attaining a large size. In the foot, local control and an improved prognosis is most readily achieved with subcutaneous lesions that involve the dorsum (3).

MRI TECHNIQUE

In evaluating mass lesions of the foot or ankle, a combination of T1-weighted and T2-weighted spin-echo (or fast spin-echo) pulse sequences and a short tau inversion recovery (STIR) acquisition are routinely obtained. The intramedullary extent of tumor is best shown on T1-weighted images (Fig. 9.2), whereas evaluation of cortical bone and soft tissue extent is usually best accomplished with T2-weighted images. The extent of most soft tissue lesions is best shown on T2-weighted images wherein the high signal intensity lesion contrasts sharply with the lower signal intensity of bone, muscle, or fat. Enhanced detection of bone or soft tissue neoplasms may be achieved using STIR imaging. This imaging sequence more sensitively detects abnormal tissue (including tumor and edema), and enhances lesion conspicuity compared to routine spin-echo imaging (15).

For lesions arising in the ankle, a coronal or sagittal scout image with a large field of view is used to exclude proximal skip metastases or to establish the proximal extent of a soft tissue lesion. A dual echo T2-weighted sequence is obtained in the axial plane for definition of anatomic compartments and to evaluate involvement of cortical bone, the neurovascular bundle, or tendons. T1-weighted and STIR sequences are obtained in the coronal or sagittal plane depending if the lesion is predominantly anterior or posterior (use sag-

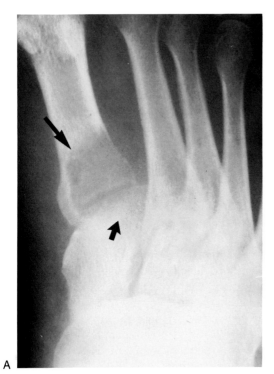

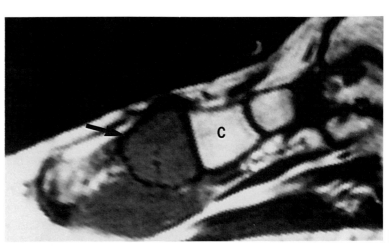

A B

FIG. 9.2. Use of MRI to evaluate the marrow space. **A:** Dorsoplantar radiograph reveals a lytic lesion of the base of the first metatarsal (*long arrow*) and radiolucency within the distal aspect of the medial cuneiform (*short arrow*). Infection or tumor, with involvement of the medial cuneiform, was suspected. **B:** Sagittal MR, TR/TE 500/20 reveals a lesion (giant cell tumor) localized to the first metatarsal (*arrow*) and demonstrates a normal marrow space within the cuneiform (**C**). The radiolucency was presumably due to localized osteopenia related to disuse or local hyperemia. (Courtesy of Mark D. Murphey, M.D., Kansas City, KS.)

ittal) or medial or lateral (use coronal). These images are used to determine the longitudinal extent and the relation to the tibiotalar joint.

In the foot, the coronal imaging plane becomes a cross-sectional imaging plane and the axial image plane is longitudinal, parallel to the sole of the foot. Sagittal images are obtained parallel to the calcaneus. A T1-weighted sagittal scout image, encompassing the foot and ankle, is obtained first to assess the general extent of the lesion (Fig. 9.3). The anatomic extent, relation to cortical bone, neurovascular bundle, and tendons are best shown with a coronal dual echo T2-weighted acquisition. The longitudinal extent is determined with sagittal T1-weighted and STIR images or a combination of sagittal and axial images.

Once the general extent of a lesion is determined, the examination should be performed with the smallest field of view that will include the entire tumor (usually 12–16 cm) in order to optimize anatomic detail. A dedicated, send-receive extremity coil is used. If the examiner is inexperienced, both feet/ankles may be imaged side-by-side in a head coil on axial and coronal images. This may facilitate detection of subtle abnormalities, but the increased field of view required results in loss of spatial resolution. Intravenous Gd-DTPA is not routinely used in imaging mass lesions.

INCIDENCE OF SOFT TISSUE AND BONE LESIONS

Tables 9.1 through 9.4 list the most common tumors and tumorlike lesions encountered in the foot or foot and ankle in a variety of clinical settings. Table 9.1 is a compilation representing all soft tissue biopsies of the foot performed over a 5-year period in a hospital orthopedic department. Table 9.2 is derived from lesions excised in a podiatric office setting, excluding skin lesions. Table 9.3 is a compilation of all bone lesions of the foot diagnosed in a hospital setting over a 40-year period. Table 9.4 lists the most common bone tumors of the foot and ankle diagnosed in a tertiary care hospital (1,34–37).

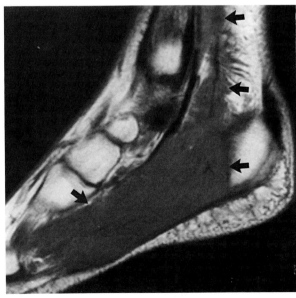
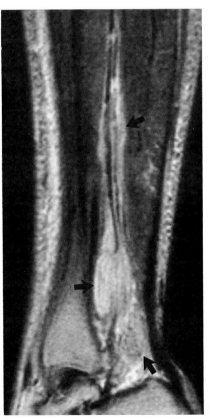

FIG. 9.3. Rhabdomyosarcoma involving foot and leg. **A:** Sagittal MR, TR/TE 500/20 image reveals a large, low signal intensity mass within the medial-plantar soft tissues of the foot, that appears to extend into the ankle (*arrows*). **B:** A sagittal MR, TR/TE 1800/20 image of the leg was added and reveals extensive proximal infiltration of tumor (*arrows*) along the posterior tibial neurovascular bundle.

TABLE 9.1. *Most common soft tissue tumors and tumorlike lesions of the foot, from 83 cases[a]*

	Number of lesions
Ganglion cyst	24
Plantar fibromatosis	11
Epidermal inclusion cyst	7
Lipoma	6
Synovial sarcoma	5
Giant cell tumor of tendon sheath	3
Rheumatoid nodule	3
Leiomyoma	2
Angiomyoma	2
Extraosseous myxoid chondrosarcoma	2
Unspecified fibromatosis	2
Unspecified sarcoma	2
Metaplastic cartilage/bone	2

[a] Representing all biopsies over a 5-year period, orthopedic department, hospital setting.
From ref. 34, with permission.

TABLE 9.2. *Most common mass lesions of the foot[a]*

	Number of lesions
Interdigital neuroma	10,427
Neuroma	5,097
Ganglion cyst	1,800
Exostosis	1,382
Fibroma	582
Digital mucous cyst	277
Plantar fibromatosis	262
Lipoma	196
Hemangioma	147
Leiomyoma	138
Neurofibroma	124
Rheumatoid nodule	111
Gouty tophus	101
Giant cell tumor of tendon sheath	85
Nodular subepidermal fibrosis	83
Osteochondroma	70
Thrombosed varix	66
Neurilemoma	32

[a] Excised in a podiatric office setting (excluding skin lesions).
From ref. 35, with permission.

TABLE 9.3. *Most common bone tumors and tumorlike lesions of the foot, of 554 lesions[a]*

Benign	No. of lesions	Malignant	No. of lesions
Osteochondroma	340	Ewing's sarcoma	16
Enchondroma	48	Chondrosarcoma	10
Simple bone cyst	31	Osteosarcoma	9
Juxtacortical chondroma	13	Malignant giant cell tumor	7
Intraosseous ganglion	10		
Osteoid osteoma	8		
Giant cell reparative granuloma	8		
Brown tumor	7		
Giant cell tumor	6		
Osteoblastoma	5		
Chondromyxoid fibroma	4		
Intraosseous lipoma	3		
Aneurysmal bone cyst	3		

[a] Diagnosed over a 40-year period, hospital setting.
From ref. 36, with permission.

TABLE 9.4. *Most common bone tumors of the foot and ankle: from 8,542 primary bone tumors[a]*

Benign	No. in foot and ankle	Percent in foot and ankle	Malignant	No. in foot and ankle	Percent in foot and ankle
Osteochondroma	34	4.7	Osteosarcoma	38	2.8
Nonossifying fibroma	32	32.3	Ewing's sarcoma	35	8.7
Osteiod osteoma	26	10.6	Chondrosarcoma	23	3.5
Giant cell tumor	26	6.1	Hemangioendothelial sarcoma	10	16.7
Aneurysmal bone cyst	24	11.5	Fibrosarcoma	9	4.4
Simple bone cyst	21	—	Lymphoma	8	1.7
Enchondroma	16	6.5	Adamantinoma	4	17.4
Chondromyxoid fibroma	11	28.2			
Chondroblastoma	6	7.6			
Osteoblastoma	4	6.3			

[a] From the Mayo Clinic.
From ref. 1, with permission.

SOFT TISSUE TUMORS AND TUMORLIKE LESIONS

Vascular Lesions

Hemangioma

The term "hemangioma" is used to refer to a group of vascular lesions that vary in their clinical appearance and histologic features. They include the capillary hemangioma, cavernous hemangioma, arteriovenous malformation, angiolipoma, and hamartoma. Each of these lesions is characterized by an increase in the number of normal or abnormal-appearing blood vessels. Hemangioma is broadly defined because the histologic and clinical distinction between these lesions is often impossible (38).

Hemangiomas are classified as capillary or cavernous, depending on the size of the blood vessels that comprise the majority of the lesion. They are composed of dilated blood vessels that contain stagnant or slow-flowing blood and may have calcified phleboliths. These lesions, especially the cavernous form, often contain fat and other nonvascular components including fibrous tissue, smooth muscle, and bone (39). Most hemangiomas are superficial lesions that do not require any form of imaging in their evaluation. Deep, intramuscular hemangiomas are relatively uncommon and present as a nonspecific soft tissue mass. They tend

to occur in young adults under the age of 30 years and usually involve the muscles of the lower extremity (38). Clinical diagnosis is often not straightforward, for, unlike superficial hemangiomas, deep lesions are not associated with discoloration of skin, visible pulsation, or an audible bruit. Misdiagnosis and delay in diagnosis are common (39). Intramuscular hemangiomas may be diffuse and infiltrative and involve multiple compartments. Rapid enlargement, bony deformity, and bone destruction may occur (40). In the foot, deep hemangiomas tend to involve the medial and plantar aspect (40). They may produce pain, swelling, and paresthesia (41,42). Surgical excision is usually performed because of pain, deformity, or impaired function and is often preceded by ligation or embolization of feeding vessels (43).

Angiomatosis is a congenital process that refers to diffuse, infiltrative involvement of an extremity by a hemangioma or arteriovenous malformation (39). These lesions usually present during infancy or childhood and are prone to local recurrence. They may be seen in association with Klippel-Trenaunay-Weber syndrome (39).

The MRI appearance of hemangiomas is fairly characteristic, reflecting the presence of multiple, dilated vascular spaces with slow-flowing or stagnant blood and variable amounts of nonvascular tissue (44–49) (Fig. 9.4). On T1-weighted images the lesion is usually

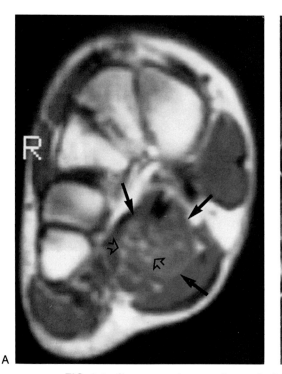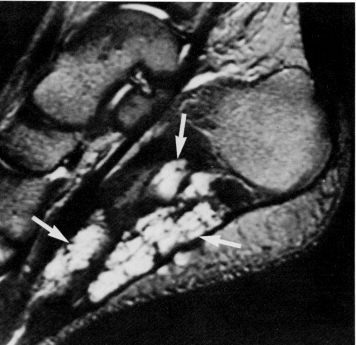

A   B

FIG. 9.4. Cavernous hemangioma. **A:** Coronal MR, TR/TE 500/20 image reveals a soft tissue mass that is isointense with muscle (*arrows*). Punctate regions of high signal intensity represent intralesional fat (*open arrows*). **B:** Sagittal MR, TR/TE 2500/80 image reveals a mass (*arrows*) composed of globular and tubular regions of high signal intensity, separated by fine, low signal intensity septae. These represent dilated vascular channels. (Courtesy of Scott Kingston, M.D., Los Angeles, CA.)

isointense or of slightly increased signal intensity compared to muscle. Punctate, linear, or coarse regions of increased signal intensity are often seen interspersed within the lesion due to the presence of fat (44). Fibrous septae produce a reticular pattern of low signal intensity but are more evident on T2-weighted images. Delineation of the margins of the lesion is usually difficult on T1-weighted images due to the similar signal intensity of adjacent muscle. On T2-weighted images a hemangioma typically reveals globular, tubular, and serpentine regions of high signal intensity, bordered by low signal intensity fibrous septae. These represent vessels with slow-flowing blood. Regions of very low signal intensity or signal void may be produced by vessels with fast-flowing blood, phleboliths, or foci of calcification or ossification (46,47). Phleboliths and small calcifications are best seen on T2-weighted images. The extent and margins of a hemangioma are usually well defined and are best seen on T2-weighted images (47,48). Infiltrating forms of hemangioma (angiomatosis) tend to have poorly defined margins on all pulse sequences and may erode bone (Fig. 9.5). Partial enhancement may be seen following intravenous injection of Gd-DTPA (Fig. 9.5). MRI is superior to CT or angiography in determining the extent of hemangiomas (46,49). If embolization is being considered, angiography or MR angiography are required to identify feeding arteries.

Lesions of Fat Origin

Lipoma

Lipoma is the most common soft tissue tumor and may arise in any part of the body. All age groups are affected, but lipoma is usually diagnosed in the fourth to sixth decades. Lipoma is typically a solitary lesion that presents as an asymptomatic, slow-growing mass. The lesion is often superficial but may also arise deep within muscle. Lipoma usually arises in areas with significant adipose tissue and is uncommon in the foot and ankle (38,50). There is a propensity for lipomas of the distal extremities to occur within tendon sheaths (51). Marginal excision is usually curative.

Two forms of lipoma with a predilection for the distal extremities are congenital lipomatosis and macrodystrophia lipomatosa. Congenital lipomatosis becomes apparent soon after birth and grows in an aggressive, infiltrative manner. It is nonencapsulated, tends to involve large portions of an extremity, and has a strong tendency to recur. It is composed of mature adipose tissue and may be associated with bony hypertrophy (52). Macrodystrophia lipomatosa is a neurofibrolipoma associated with localized overgrowth of the bone and soft tissue of one or more digits. The median nerve

in the hand and the digital plantar nerves in the foot are most often affected (53).

On radiographs, lipoma appears as a radiolucent soft tissue mass. Metaplastic calcification or ossification may develop in long-standing lesions (53). On MRI, a soft tissue lipoma appears as a well-marginated, lobulated mass with signal characteristics identical to those of subcutaneous fat (Fig. 9.6). The mass is often traversed by fine fibrous septae. Calcification or ossification may occur within a lipoma, resulting in regions of very low signal intensity on MRI. In congenital lipomatosis, MRI reveals the extent of fatty infiltration throughout the involved extremity (Fig. 9.7). There are several variants of lipoma that have a significant nonlipomatous component and consequently do not appear purely fatty on MRI. These include lipoblastoma, angiolipoma, spindle cell lipoma, pleomorphic lipoma, and atypical lipoma (53,54). These lesions may appear identical to a liposarcoma in that they consist of a combination of fat and other elements.

Liposarcoma

Liposarcoma is a common tumor that principally affects adults but may occur at any age. It has a predilection to involve the deep soft tissues and, although it commonly involves the extremities, is rare in the foot and ankle. This lesion usually presents as a painless, well-circumscribed mass and often attains a large size. The amount of fat within a liposarcoma varies depending on its histologic type. There is a propensity for local recurrence and survival is most dependent on the histologic type and location (deep vs. superficial) of the tumor (38).

On radiographs a well-differentiated liposarcoma appears as a mass with an obvious fatty content and variable calcification. On MRI, liposarcoma typically appears as a well-marginated mass containing variable amounts of fat and regions characterized by low signal intensity on T1-weighted and high signal intensity on T2-weighted images. Poorly differentiated liposarcomas, however, may not contain any detectable fat and are indistinguishable from other benign and malignant soft tissue masses (53,55). A potentially useful sign of liposarcoma is the presence on T1-weighted images of linear, high signal intensity septae (representing fat) within a low signal intensity mass (55).

Lesions of Fibrous Origin

Fibromatoses

The fibromatoses are a group of benign fibrous tumors characterized by a pattern of growth intermediate

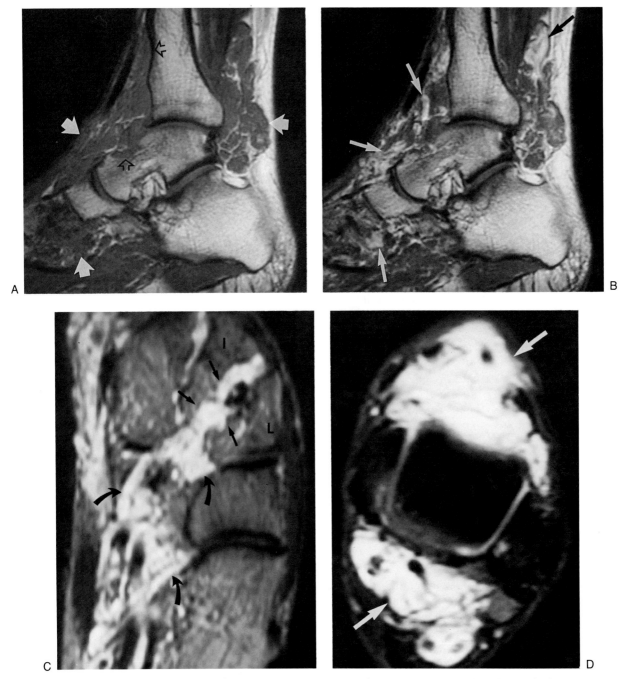

FIG. 9.5. Angiomatosis. **A:** Sagittal MR, TR/TE 500/25 reveals a diffuse, infiltrating soft tissue mass of intermediate signal intensity (*arrows*). There are pressure erosions of the anterior distal tibia and dorsal talus (*open arrows*). **B:** Sagittal MR, TR/TE: 500/25 following intravenous Gd-DTPA demonstrates multiple linear and tubular regions of enhancement (*arrows*). **C:** Axial MR, TR/TE: 2500/80 reveals erosion (*arrows*) of the intermediate (*I*) and lateral (*L*) cuneiforms by an infiltrating high signal intensity mass (*curved arrow*). **D:** Axial MR, STIR (2200/35/160) at the ankle level reveals a globular, septated high signal intensity mass within the anterior and posterior compartments (*arrows*).

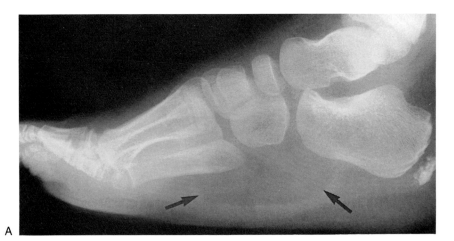

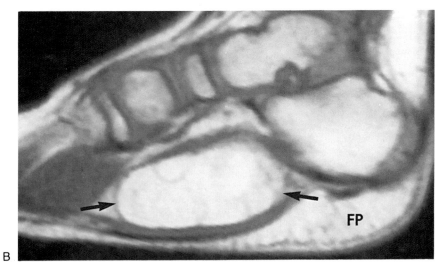

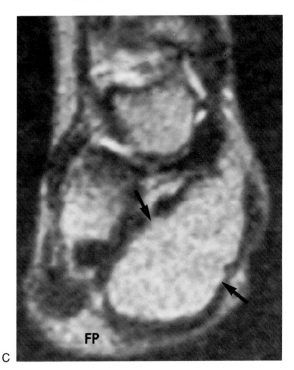

FIG. 9.6. Lipoma. **A:** A lateral radiograph reveals a well-defined, radiolucent mass (*arrows*). **B:** Sagittal MR, TR/TE 500/20 and **C,** Coronal TR/TE 1800/80 images reveal a lobulated, well-demarcated mass (*arrows*) with signal characteristics identical to those of the plantar fat pad (*FP*).

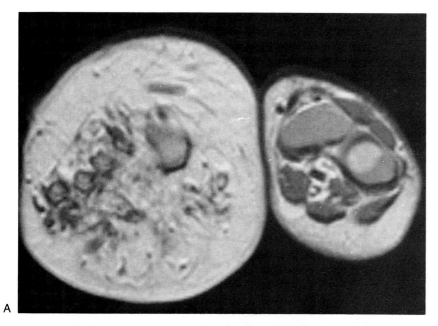

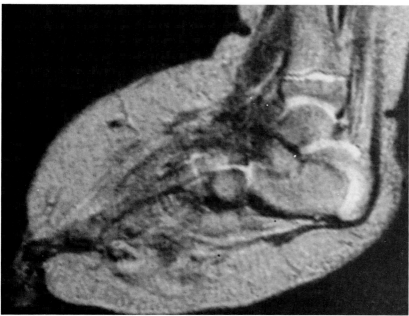

FIG. 9.7. Congenital lipomatosis. A: Coronal MR, TR/TE 800/20 and B, sagittal MR, TR/TE 1800/80 images demonstrate enlargement and diffuse infiltration of the entire foot by a lipomatous mass.

between that of a benign lesion and a fibrosarcoma. These lesions show a strong tendency for local recurrence and may grow in an infiltrative manner, but never metastasize. The fibromatoses are subdivided into superficial and deep forms and have a predilection for certain anatomic sites (38). These lesions are usually seen in adults and may be solitary or multiple. The superficial fibromatoses are small, grow slowly, arise from the fascia or aponeurosis, and rarely involve deeper structures. The deep fibromatoses are often large, grow rapidly, and tend to be more aggressive and infiltrative in their pattern of growth. The deep

fibromatoses rarely occur in the foot or ankle. Superficial lesions occur in the form of plantar fibromatosis.

Plantar Fibromatosis

Plantar fibromatosis is a benign nodular fibrous proliferation arising within the plantar aponeurosis. It is roughly twice as common in men than women, and is bilateral in 10% to 40% of cases (56,57). It has a broad age incidence, occurring in children and young adults as well as the middle-aged and elderly. In general, this lesion appears to increase in incidence with advancing age. Lesions may arise asynchronously in the plantar and palmar fascia, usually separated in time by an interval of 5 to 10 years. Patients typically present with a firm nodule, 2 to 3 cm in diameter, located on the middle and medial aspect of the plantar surface of the foot. Initial presentation with multiple nodules is infrequent, occurring in 10% of patients (56). Multiple lesions are most often seen as a recurrence following the excision of a single nodule. Patients are usually asymptomatic or complain of mild pain after walking or long standing. Involvement of the superficial plantar

nerve may cause paresthesia of the distal sole and undersurface of the toes. In contrast to the high rate of digital contractures seen in palmar fibromatosis, contraction of the toes is rare in plantar fibromatosis (38).

Pathologic examination reveals a single nodule or a conglomerate of multiple small nodules embedded within the plantar fascia. Microscopically, the lesion is composed of fibroblasts, separated by variable amounts of collagen. The early, cellular phase may be mistaken for fibrosarcoma histologically, whereas long-standing lesions are less cellular and predominantly contain dense collagen (38). Due to the infiltra-

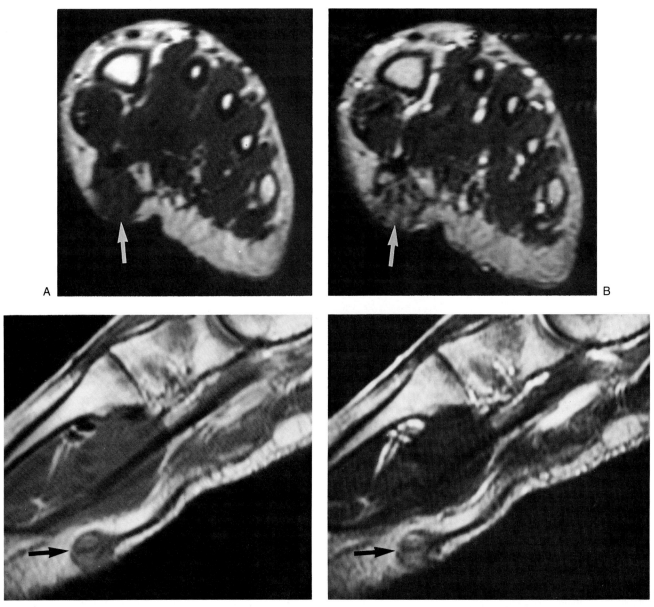

FIG. 9.8. Plantar fibromatosis. **A:** Coronal MR, TR/TE 400/25 image reveals a low signal intensity plantar mass (*arrow*). **B:** *Coronal* MR, TR/TE 2400/80, the lesion (*arrow*) is hypointense to fat and surrounds multiple, very low signal intensity fibers of the plantar aponeurosis. **C:** On sagittal MR, TR/TE 2000/25, and **D,** TR/TE 2000/80 images the plantar aponeurosis appears splayed about a low-to-intermediate signal intensity nodule (*arrow*).

tive and multinodular pattern of growth within the plantar fascia, the limits of the tumor are not always readily discernible with gross inspection. Invasion of the muscles and deeper structures of the foot, however, is not observed. Treatment options include conservative management and surgical removal. In one study, a complete fasciectomy was curative in 92% of patients, whereas local excision resulted in a 57% recurrence rate (57).

On MRI, plantar fibromas appear as single or multiple nodules and are usually less than 3 cm in diameter (58). The lesions are confined to the subcutaneous soft tissue. They reveal low signal intensity on T1-weighted images and low to intermediate signal intensity on T2-weighted images (59) (Fig. 9.8). High signal intensity may be observed on STIR images (Fig. 9.9).

Extraabdominal Fibromatosis

Extraabdominal fibromatosis (also known as aggressive fibromatosis and desmoid tumor) is a histologically benign tumor that arises from the connective tissue of muscle and fascia, and tends to grow in an aggressive, infiltrative manner, similar to that of a sarcoma. It predominantly occurs between the ages of 15 and 40 years, and tends to involve the muscles of the shoulder, chest wall, back, and thigh. Involvement of the foot or ankle is rare (38). Symptoms vary depending on the site and extent of the lesion. Pain, numbness, or weakness tend to occur with neurovascular involvement. The recurrence rate ranges from 25% to 90% and depends primarily on the completeness of local excision (38,60–62). The preferred method of treat-

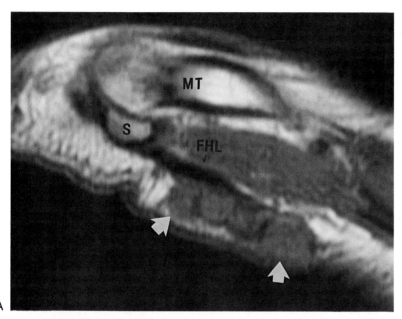

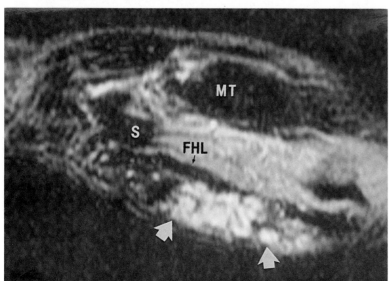

FIG. 9.9. Recurrent plantar fibromatosis. **A:** Sagittal MR, TR/TE 500/20 image shows a low signal intensity, multinodular plantar mass (*arrows*) that on **B** sagittal MR, STIR (2200/35/160) image reveals predominantly high signal intensity (*arrows*) (MT, first metatarsal; S, sesamoid bone; FHL, flexor hallucis longus tendon).

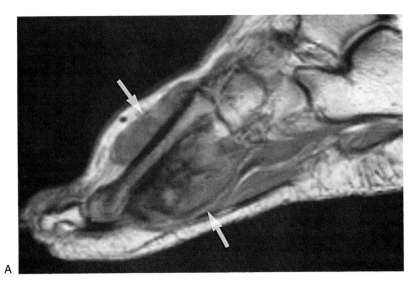

A

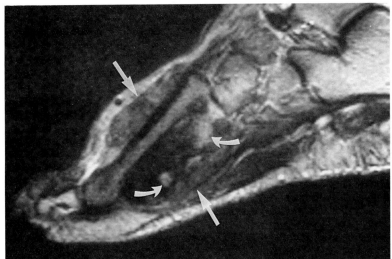

B

FIG. 9.10. Extraabdominal fibromatosis. A: Sagittal MR, TR/TE 1800/20 and B, sagittal MR, TR/TE 1800/80 images reveal a mass (*arrows*) of predominantly low to intermediate signal intensity dorsal and plantar to the second metatarsal. Small foci of intermediate to high signal intensity (*curved arrows*) are noted at the periphery in B.

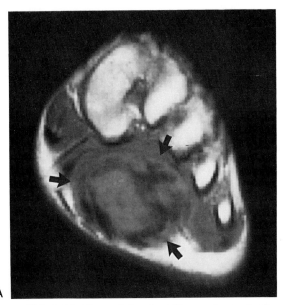

A

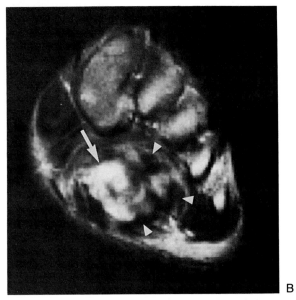

B

FIG. 9.11. Extraabdominal fibromatosis. A: Coronal 500/17 image reveals a plantar mass (*arrows*) with predominant low signal intensity at the periphery and intermediate signal intensity centrally. B: On a coronal MR, TR/TE 2100/90 image there is a heterogeneous pattern of predominant low signal intensity at the periphery (*arrowheads*) and high signal intensity centrally (*arrow*). (From ref. 59, with permission.)

ment is radical excision, including a wide margin of uninvolved tissue (62). The lesion is characteristically poorly circumscribed and, given its fibrous content, it may be particularly difficult to distinguish recurrent tumor from scar on gross inspection (38).

Extraabdominal fibromatosis demonstrates a varied appearance on MRI depending primarily on the degree of cellularity and density of collagen deposition (63). Most lesions are predominantly isointense or hyperintense relative to muscle on T1-weighted images and reveal a mixture of high and low signal intensity on T2-weighted images (64,65). A heterogeneous pattern of varied signal intensities is typical. Some lesions are predominantly very low in signal intensity on both T1-weighted and T2-weighted images (63,65) (Fig. 9.10). The lesions are not surrounded by edema. The low signal intensity regions correspond to densely collagenous, hypocellular portions of tumor. Hypercellular portions of the tumor account for regions of high signal intensity on T2-weighted images. A pattern on T2-weighted images of peripheral low signal intensity and central medium to high signal intensity has also been reported in extraabdominal fibromatosis (66) (Fig. 9.11). Moderate enhancement of the central areas may be observed following intravenous administration of Gd-DTPA (66). The margins of fibromatosis vary on MRI from well defined to infiltrating. Gd-DTPA–enhanced T1-weighted images may be used to clarify the tumor margins (67). This is of limited benefit, however, as microscopic invasion is always present beyond the gross margins of the tumor (65).

Proliferative Fasciitis

Proliferative fasciitis is a common lesion that is believed to represent a posttraumatic, reactive process. Most lesions arise in the extremities, especially in the forearm and thigh. Affected patients are usually between 40 and 70 years of age and present with a rapidly growing subcutaneous nodule. The lesion usually stabilizes in size after 2 to 3 weeks and is usually between 1 and 5 cm in size (38). It is usually not painful. Histologically, proliferative fasciitis consists of immature fibroblasts and varying amounts of mucoid material and collagen (38). It may be multifocal, is often poorly circumscribed, and may extend into underlying muscle (38,67). Proliferative fasciitis shares several clinical and histologic features with two other reactive lesions: proliferative myositis and nodular fasciitis (38). MRI of proliferative fasciitis may reveal a lesion with signal characteristics similar to those of plantar fibroma (Fig. 9.12). Lesions with a large mucoid component may be expected to reveal high signal intensity on T2-weighted images.

Fibroma of Tendon Sheath

Fibroma of tendon sheath is a slowly growing lesion that is found attached to a tendon or tendon sheath. It is not known if this lesion is a reactive process or a neoplasm. It occurs chiefly in adults aged 20 to 50 years and almost always involves an extremity. Patients

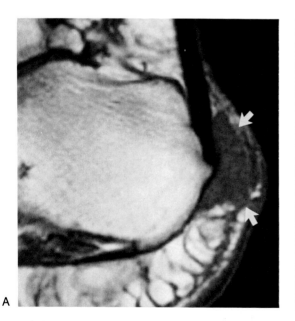
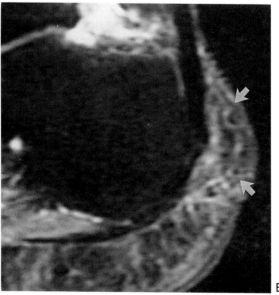

A

B

FIG. 9.12. Proliferative fasciitis. **A:** Sagittal MR, TR/TE 400/20 image reveals a focal mass of intermediate signal intensity (*arrows*) that contacts the posterior aspect of the Achilles tendon and calcaneus. **B:** Sagittal STIR (2200/35/160), the mass (*arrows*) reveals a heterogeneous pattern of low and high signal intensity and is difficult to distinguish from the adjacent fat pad. (*Figure continues on next page.*)

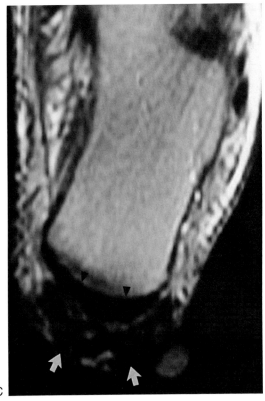

C

FIG. 9.12. (*Continued*) **C:** Axial MR, TR/TE 2300/80 image reveals a predominantly very low signal intensity mass (*arrows*) posterior to the distal Achilles tendon (*arrowheads*).

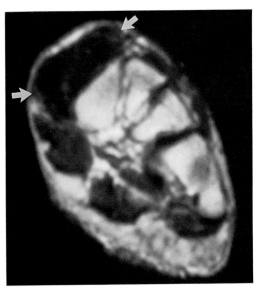

FIG. 9.13. Fibroma of tendon sheath. Coronal MR, TR/TE 1800/80 image reveals a very low signal intensity mass (*arrows*) arising from the tibialis anterior tendon sheath. (Courtesy of D.M. Forrester, M.D., Los Angeles, CA.)

complain of a painless, slowly enlarging mass that may limit motion of an involved digit. The typical lesion is a loculated, densely collagenous mass, between 1 and 2 cm in size (68). It is distinguished from the more common giant cell tumor of tendon sheath by an absence of xanthoma cells or giant cells and is much less cellular (38). It is treated by local excision, although in one study 24% of fibromas recurred (68). On MRI, fibroma of tendon sheath has an appearance identical to that of giant cell tumor of tendon sheath, revealing low signal intensity on both T1-weighted and T2-weighted images (Fig 9.13).

Fibrous Proliferation of Infancy and Childhood

There are a variety of fibrous lesions unique to infancy and childhood. Two such lesions that occur in the feet (and hands) are digital fibromatosis and calcifying aponeurotic fibroma. In the foot, digital fibroma exclusively involves the toes and usually presents before age 2 years. It produces single or multiple nodular lesions up to 2 cm in size. The great toe and the thumb are spared. Surgery is performed to correct contracture or functional impairment; however, about 60% of lesions recur locally (38,69).

Calcifying aponeurotic fibroma occurs between birth and age 16 years and principally involves the hands and feet. The plantar surface of the foot and the ankle region are favored sites of involvement. The lesion is usually painless and less than 3 cm in diameter. Local recurrence is seen in at least half of patients following surgical excision (38). The MRI appearance of both of these lesions has not been reported.

Malignant Fibrous Histiocytoma

Malignant fibrous histiocytoma (MFH) is the most common soft tissue sarcoma in adults and, although it may be seen at any age, is most common between the ages of 50 and 70 years. The lower and upper extremities as well as the retroperitoneum are the most common sites of involvement. The tumor usually presents as a painless, enlarging mass. MFH has a strong tendency to recur and to metastasize. An infiltrative growth pattern is observed and erosion of adjacent bone is not uncommon. Prognosis is improved if the lesion involves the distal rather than proximal extremity and if it is superficial rather than deep-seated (38).

On MRI, MFH may have a variety of appearances. A heterogeneous pattern of low to intermediate signal intensity on T1-weighted images and intermediate to high signal intensity on T2-weighted images may be seen (12,14,70). There may be predominant high signal intensity on T2-weighted images due to intralesional hemorrhage (27,71). The margins may be either well defined or infiltrative (14,27,71).

Fibrosarcoma

Fibrosarcoma is a malignant tumor that chiefly occurs in adults between the ages of 25 and 55 years. It predominantly involves the lower extremity (69). When arising in the foot, fibrosarcoma is usually deep-seated and demonstrates an infiltrative, destructive growth pattern (67,72). Its MRI characteristics are similar to those of malignant fibrous histiocytoma (11).

Lesions of Neural Origin—Peripheral Nerve Sheath Tumors

Neurilemoma

Neurilemoma is a benign peripheral nerve sheath tumor that may occur at any age but is most common between ages 20 and 50 years. This lesion is also known as a schwannoma, neurinoma, and perineural fibroblastoma (38). Neurilemoma is a well-encapsulated tumor that arises eccentrically from a nerve sheath and is usually solitary. It is usually firmly bound to the nerve sheath and varies in size from several millimeters to greater than 20 cm (73). It grows slowly and is usually asymptomatic until it is large enough to cause nerve impingement. It tends to occur in the head and neck and, in one study, 4% involved the ankle region (74). When arising in an extremity, the tumor tends to involve the flexor region (75). Neurilemoma is distinguished histologically from a neurofibroma by the fact that it is encapsulated and is composed of two different types of zones: a cellular zone of compact spindle cells (Antoni A area) and a loose, myxoid zone (Antoni B area) (38). Multiple neurilemomas tend to be associated with neurofibromatosis. The tumor does not recur after simple excision (39). On MRI, neurilemoma usually reveals intermediate signal intensity on T1-weighted images, high signal intensity on T2-weighted images, and has well-defined margins (Fig. 9.14).

Neurofibroma

Neurofibroma may occur as a solitary lesion or as part of neurofibromatosis. Most solitary neurofibromas occur in the third decade of life and arise in the

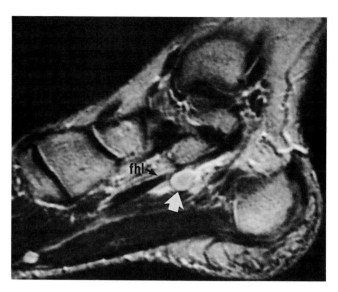

FIG. 9.14. Neurilemoma. Sagittal MR, TR/TE 1800/80 reveals a small, round, high signal intensity lesion (*arrow*) adjacent to the flexor hallucis longus tendon (*fhl*). Also see Fig. 12.10. (From ref. 213, with permission.)

skin or subcutaneous tissue. The lesion grows slowly and is usually asymptomatic. In patients with neurofibromatosis, the lesions may develop at any age but most often appear during childhood or adolescence. They may be found in superficial or deep locations and may involve the viscera, including the heart and gastrointestinal tract. A variety of skeletal abnormalities may occur in patients with neurofibromatosis. Bony erosion may occur due to a contiguous neurofibroma or reflect bone dysplasia (76). Unlike neurilemoma, a neurofibroma is not encapsulated and often breaks through the epineurium and infiltrates the adjacent soft tissue. These tumors are therefore difficult to remove without compromising nerve function (38). Surgical excision is usually reserved for lesions that are large, painful, or in a position to cause compromise of organ function (76). Recurrence is common, due to the inability to excise the tumor completely because of its infiltrative nature. The risk of malignant transformation in patients with neurofibromatosis is estimated to be in the range of 2% to 4% (38).

On MRI, neurofibromas demonstrate low to intermediate signal intensity on T1-weighted images and intermediate to high signal intensity on T2-weighted images (Fig. 9.15). Variable degrees of inhomogeneity are observed on all pulse sequences (77–79). In neurofibromas, the large amount of fluid within the endoneural matrix is believed responsible for the high signal intensity on T2-weighted images (80,81). This matrix spreads apart the residual axons to produce the

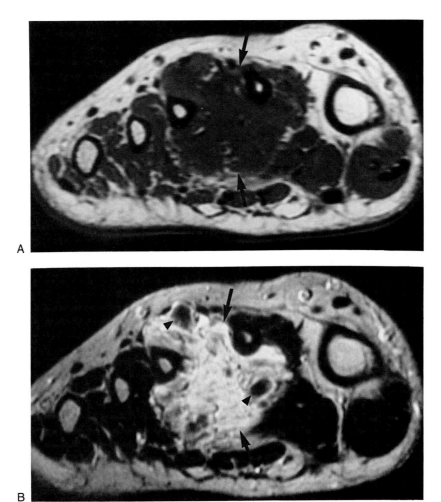

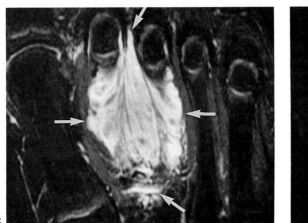

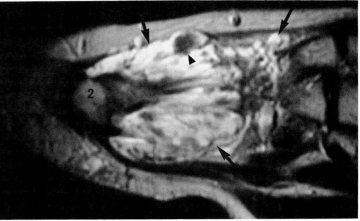

FIG. 9.15. Neurofibroma. **A:** Axial MR, TR/TE 400/20. **B:** Axial MR, TR/TE 3500/100. **C:** Coronal STIR (2200/35/160). **D:** Sagittal MR, TR/TE 3000/120. MR images reveal a mass (*arrows*) that is isointense with muscle in A and of high signal intensity in B, C, and D. Rounded foci of low signal intensity (*arrowheads*) are noted within the mass in B and D. An infiltrative growth pattern is observed as the mass involves the dorsal and plantar soft tissues and has widened the space between the second and third metatarsals ("2" in D, second metatarsal head).

fusiform shape of a neurofibroma (80). Focal areas of low signal intensity on T2-weighted images may be seen in neurofibroma, representing fibrous tissue (80). The margins are typically smooth and well defined; however, irregular, ill-defined margins may rarely

occur (73). Muscle atrophy may be seen in association with any of the peripheral nerve sheath tumors (73). In patients with neurofibromatosis, MRI may be used to distinguish between bone dysplasia and invasion or erosion of bone by tumor (Fig 9.16).

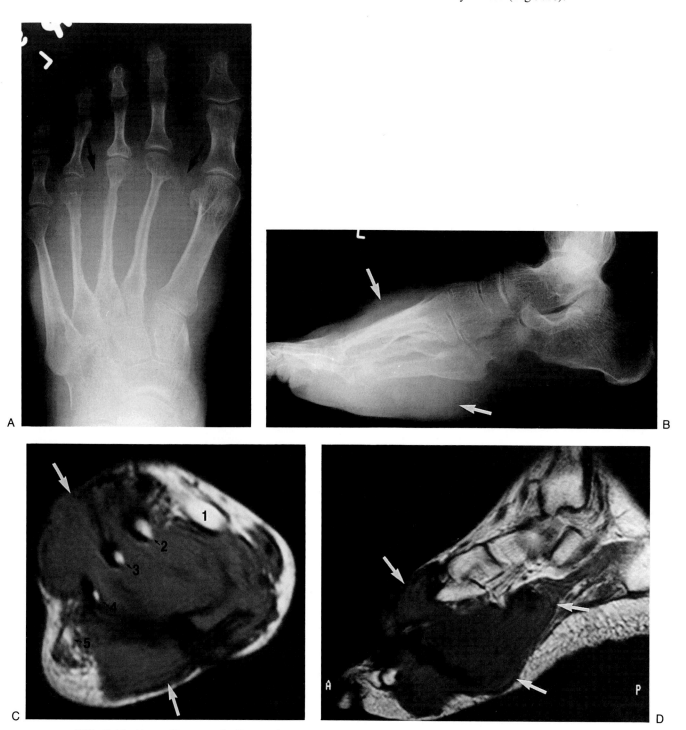

FIG. 9.16. Neurofibroma. **A:** Dorsoplantar and **B,** lateral radiographs demonstrate a large soft tissue mass in the forefoot (*arrows*) and modeling deformities of the second, third, and fourth metatarsals. **C:** Coronal MR, TR/TE 600/20 and **D,** sagittal MR, TR/TE 600/20 images reveal a large, infiltrating, low-to-intermediate signal intensity mass (*arrows*) interposed between the metatarsals and extending proximally into the plantar soft tissue of the midfoot. The coronal images are most useful to confirm the absence of bone invasion (1–5, first through fifth metatarsals).

Malignant Peripheral Nerve Sheath Tumor

The great majority of malignant tumors arising from a peripheral nerve are classified as malignant peripheral nerve sheath tumor (MPNST). This lesion is also known as malignant schwannoma, neurogenic sarcoma, and neurofibrosarcoma. It usually occurs between the ages of 20 and 50 years. Roughly 50% of MPNST occurs in patients with neurofibromatosis (82). Affected patients usually have a 10- to 20-year history of disease. Pain or sudden enlargement of a preexisting neurofibroma are important clinical signs of possible malignant transformation. Patients with MPNST and neurofibromatosis have a poorer survival than patients with MPNST alone (83). Compared to the solitary form, MPNST arising in neurofibromatosis tends to be of higher grade, tends to occur in the trunk and proximal extremities (where early detection and adequate surgical removal are difficult), and may be multiple. The tumor commonly infiltrates along the nerve sheath and treatment is by radical excision or amputation (84).

Benign and malignant peripheral nerve sheath tumors cannot be reliably distinguished with radiographs, CT, or MRI (73,77–79). MPNST shares the MRI characteristics described above for neurofibroma and neurilemoma (Fig. 9.17). One differentiating point is that irregular, ill-defined margins may be seen with MPNST and neurofibroma but not with neurilemoma (73).

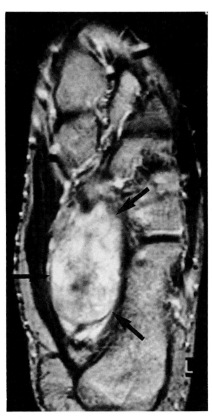

FIG. 9.17. Malignant peripheral nerve sheath tumor. Axial MR, TR/TE 1800/80 image reveals a well-demarcated mass (*arrows*) with a heterogeneous pattern of intermediate and high signal intensity.

Pigmented Villonodular Synovitis

Pigmented villonodular synovitis (PVNS) is a lesion of unknown etiology that arises from the synovium of a joint, bursa, or tendon sheath. A variety of terms is used to describe this lesion, depending on its site of origin and growth pattern. Lesions arising from the synovium of a joint may be solitary and localized (localized nodular synovitis) or diffuse and villous (PVNS). The tendon sheath lesion is typically localized and discrete (giant cell tumor of tendon sheath or nodular tenosynovitis). The diffuse form of tendon sheath lesion is rare and most often involves the ankle, foot, or hand (85,86).

These lesions usually occur between ages 20 and 50 years. The knee is the most commonly affected synovial joint, followed in decreasing order of frequency by the hip, ankle, small joints of the hands and feet, shoulder, and elbow (87). The tenosynovial form most often involves the flexor and extensor tendons of the fingers of the hand. Less commonly, the tendons of the foot, ankle, and knee are involved. All of these lesions tend to grow as a lobulated, partially encapsulated mass. Intraarticular lesions usually cause pain and swelling, although the duration and severity of

symptoms are quite variable. The tendon sheath lesion often presents as a painless or only mildly painful swelling (88). A slowly progressive course is typical for both diffuse and nodular forms, and patients often wait 2 to 3 years before seeking medical care (89). Histologically, these lesions are characterized by acute and chronic synovial inflammation and reveal varying amounts of giant cells, collagen, and lipid-laden macrophages. Hemorrhage results in hemosiderin deposits within the stroma, macrophages, and synovial lining cells. The etiology is unknown. Although a neoplastic process has been proposed (90), most investigators favor a reactive, inflammatory origin (87,91).

In intraarticular PVNS, radiographs typically demonstrate a joint effusion and/or soft tissue mass. Erosive or cystic lesions of bone tend to occur in "tight" articulations without a redundant or capacious joint capsule. One study of intraarticular PVNS revealed erosive bone lesions in 93% of hips, 75% of shoulders, 63% of elbows, 56% of ankles, and 26% of knees (87). Joint space narrowing is uncommon and is usually seen in long-standing lesions with superimposed degenerative joint disease.

The appearance of PVNS on MRI reflects its het-

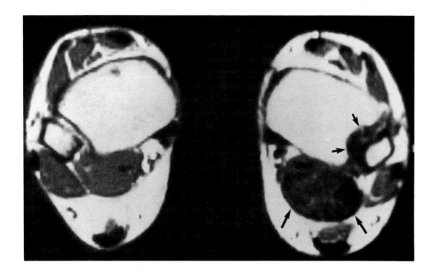

FIG. 9.18. Pigmented villonodular synovitis. Axial MR, TR/TE 2000/40 image reveals a low signal intensity mass (*long arrows*) extending posteriorly from the ankle, filling the tibiofibular joint space, and eroding the lateral aspect of the tibia (*small arrows*).

erogeneous composition (92–94). The typical lesion demonstrates regions of intermediate and low signal intensity on T1-weighted images and a mixture of high and low signal intensity on T2-weighted images. PVNS may be predominantly low in signal intensity on both T1- and T2-weighted images (Fig. 9.18). Low signal intensity regions are produced by chronic synovial proliferation and by hemosiderin. The paramagnetic effects of hemosiderin produce a decreased T2 relaxation time (causing decreased signal intensity) and become more prominent with increasing field strength (i.e., 1.5 T). Lipid-laden macrophages may impart the signal characteristics of fat to the lesion. High signal intensity on T1-weighted images may also result from subacute hemorrhage in the synovium. Synovial inflammation and intraarticular fluid produce intermediate signal intensity on T1-weighted images and high signal intensity on T2-weighted images. A low signal intensity rim may be seen at the periphery of the lesion. A variety of appearances is produced, as the relative proportion of these components varies considerably from lesion to lesion.

Giant cell tumor of tendon sheath is usually evident on radiographs as a soft tissue mass. Erosion of cortical bone is observed in 10% of patients and is seen in a higher proportion of lesions occurring in the foot (95,96). It has been postulated that outward growth of the lesion is prevented in the foot due to its compact structure (95). When this lesion occurs in the foot, it tends to be larger and more irregularly shaped than in the hand (95,97). Following local excision, there is a 10% to 20% rate of recurrence (38).

The diffuse form of giant cell tumor of tendon sheath is a rare synovial lesion that affects the same age group and same anatomic sites as the other forms of PVNS. It is often difficult to define clearly the site of origin of the tumor as being from joint, bursa, or tendon sheath. Most lesions demonstrate joint involvement

and may be considered as a subtype of PVNS characterized by extraarticular extension, rather than a primary tendon sheath lesion (38). In the foot, this lesion has been reported to arise from the peroneal tendon sheath and from a flexor tendon sheath (86). As opposed to the localized form, this form tends to grow outward without a confining fibrous capsule, and may erode bone and widen the joint space (Fig. 9.19). The recurrence rate for this diffuse form has been estimated at 40% to 50% (38).

On MRI, giant cell tumor of tendon sheath is similar to intraarticular PVNS and usually reveals low to intermediate signal intensity on both T1- and T2-weighted images (98–100) (Fig. 9.19). High signal intensity may be observed on T2-weighted or STIR images (100) (Fig. 9.20). MRI accurately delineates the extent of both localized and diffuse forms.

Synovial Chondromatosis

Synovial chondromatosis refers to a process of synovial metaplasia resulting in the formation of multiple cartilaginous nodules that commonly ossify or calcify. It may arise in the synovium of a joint, bursa, or tendon sheath. It usually affects young or middle-aged adults and produces nonspecific symptoms of pain, swelling, and limitation of motion. Synovial chondromatosis is usually monoarticular and most often affects the knee. It has also been reported in the elbow, shoulder, hip, and ankle (101–103). The extraarticular form is rare, most often affects the hands, feet, and wrists, and shows a predilection to originate from flexor tendon sheaths (104).

Synovial chondromatosis has been shown to follow a temporal sequence that may be divided into three phases: (a) active intrasynovial disease with no free loose bodies; (b) transitional lesions with cartilaginous

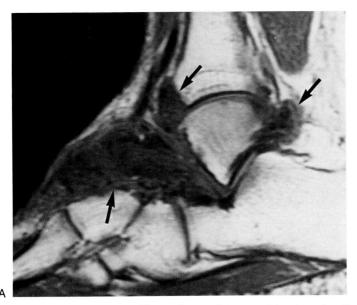
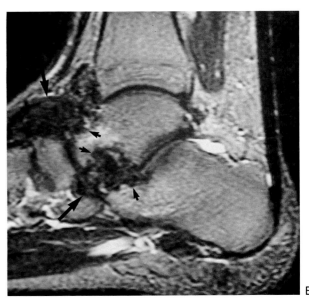

FIG. 9.19. Diffuse giant cell tumor of tendon sheath. **A:** Sagittal MR, TR/TE 2000/20 and **B,** 2000/80 images reveal an infiltrating mass of low to intermediate signal intensity involving the tibiotalar and posterior talocalcaneal joints, the sinus tarsi, and the dorsal soft tissues of the midfoot (*long arrows*). The mass is eroding the talus and calcaneus (*short arrows* in B).

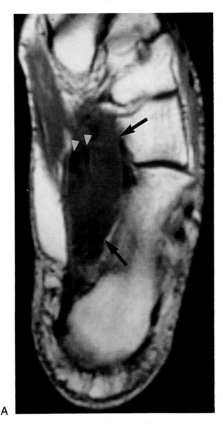
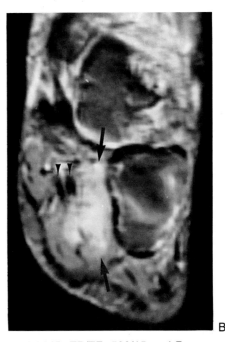

FIG. 9.20. Giant cell tumor of tendon sheath. **A:** Axial MR, TR/TE: 500/15 and **B,** coronal STIR (1900/25/130) images reveal a well-marginated mass (*arrows*) of intermediate signal intensity in A and high signal intensity in B, partially engulfing the flexor digitorum longus and flexor hallucis longus tendons (*arrowheads*). (Courtesy of Allan M. Haggar, M.D., Detroit, MI).

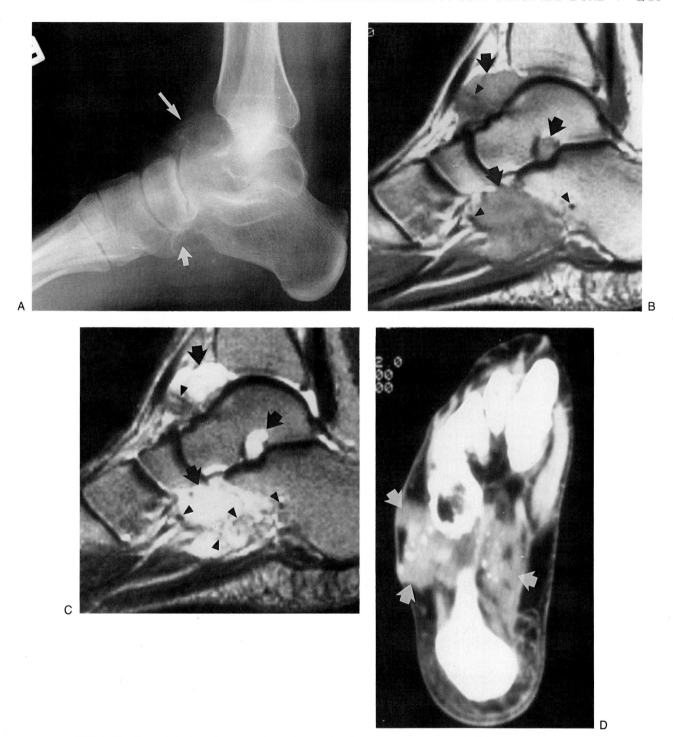

FIG. 9.21. Synovial chondromatosis. **A:** Lateral radiograph reveals a calcified mass (*long arrow*) extending anterior to the ankle and vague calcifications adjacent to the calcaneocuboid joint (*short arrow*). **B:** Sagittal MR, TR/TE 500/20 and **C,** sagittal 2000/80 images: A mass (*arrows*) of intermediate signal intensity in B and high signal intensity in C is noted anterior to the ankle, within the sinus tarsi and within the plantar soft tissues adjacent to the calcaneus. Low signal intensity foci (*arrowheads*), reflecting calcifications, are better seen in C. **D:** Axial CT demonstrates the mass (*arrows*), with punctate calcifications, extending from medial to lateral under the calcaneus. (Courtesy of Mark D. Murphey, M.D., Kansas City, KS.)

nodules in the synovial membrane and loose bodies; and (c) multiple free loose bodies with quiescent synovial disease (102). Primary synovial chondromatosis should be distinguished from the synovial metaplasia that occurs secondarily in traumatic and degenerative joint disorders. Treatment consists of removal of the loose bodies and partial or complete synovectomy.

Synovial chondromatosis is diagnosed radiographically when multiple calcified bodies of variable size and shape are seen within a joint. A noncalcified soft tissue mass may be the only radiographic clue to the diagnosis. It has been estimated that 5% to 33% of lesions are not apparent on radiographs due to lack of calcification or ossification (105). Bone erosion has been reported in association with lesions of the hip and shoulder (105). Rarely, synovial chondromatosis may extend through the joint capsule and continue to proliferate (Fig. 9.21).

Extraarticular tenosynovial chondromatosis commonly involves the foot and may be a locally aggressive process. Although unusual, erosion of the anterior aspect of the distal tibia was reported in a lesion arising from the tendon sheath (106). On radiographs, the tenosynovial form usually appears as a mass with multiple, variable-sized calcified or ossified nodules (106–108).

On MRI, synovial chondromatosis reveals low signal intensity on T1-weighted images. Depending on the histologic composition, these lesions may reveal intermediate or high signal intensity on T2-weighted images (Fig. 9.21). If large enough, calcified nodules are apparent as low signal intensity structures and are usually best seen on T2-weighted images. Lesions that do not contain calcified nodules may simulate a joint effusion. In such cases, the presence of slight inhomogeneity is a clue that a mass lesion, rather than a joint

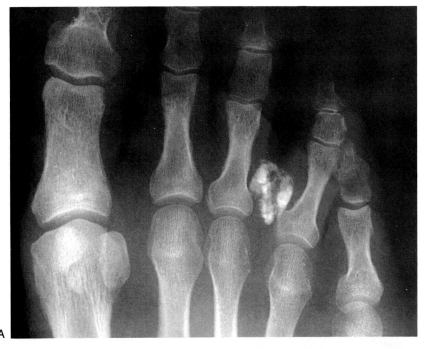

A

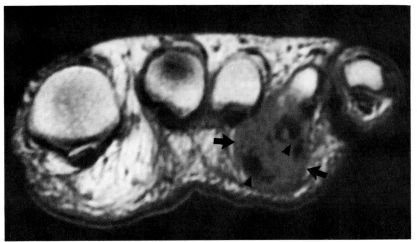

B

FIG. 9.22. Tenosynovial chondromatosis. **A:** Dorsoplantar radiograph reveals a calcified mass between the third and fourth proximal phalanges. **B:** Coronal MR, TR/TE 500/20 image demonstrates an intermediate signal intensity plantar mass (*arrows*) containing calcified foci of low signal intensity (*arrowheads*) arising from the fourth flexor tendon sheath.

effusion, is present. For tenosynovial lesions, MRI may be useful in demonstrating lesion extent and to document a tenosynovial origin (Fig. 9.22).

Soft Tissue Ganglion

Soft tissue ganglion is a common lesion and was described by Hippocrates as a "knot of tissue containing mucoid flesh" (109,110). It is a unilocular or multilocular mucin-filled cystic lesion with a synoviumlike inner lining and a fibrous capsule. Fibrous septae often compartmentalize the lesion into cystic cavities. A ganglion is usually found adjacent to a joint capsule or tendon sheath, but may occur completely separate from such synovial structures. Ganglia most often arise in the wrist, hand, ankle, foot, and knee. A pattern of multiple ganglia of the wrists and ankles may be observed (111). Patients of all ages are affected but this lesion is most common in the second through fourth decades of life (110).

A ganglion may consist of three components: a lobulated main cyst, multiple pseudopodia that extend from the main cyst along fascial planes, and small capsular cysts that extend into the substance of an adjacent joint capsule or tendon sheath (110). Actual communication between a ganglion and an adjacent joint space is controversial and in one study of 80 ganglia, no such communication was identified (110). The pathogenesis of soft tissue ganglia has not been established but it is believed to represent differentiation and proliferation of multipotential mesenchymal cells that exist near joints or tendons (112). If symptoms are persistent, local excision is performed; however, recurrence is likely if the excision is not complete.

Most ganglia are 1 to 4 cm in size and present as a circumscribed soft tissue swelling. The mass may fluctuate in size and may resolve spontaneously. The consistency varies from a soft compressible cyst to a tense hard mass depending on the duration, location, and content of the lesion. Fibrous septae often proliferate over time, causing the lesion to become more firm. Ganglia that form adjacent to joints often produce a dull ache and a feeling of weakness or instability (110,111). Ganglia within or adjacent to tendon sheaths may interfere with tendon motion and produce pain. Nerve palsy is uncommon but has been reported involving the median or ulnar nerve in the palm of the hand and the lateral popliteal nerve at the neck of the fibula (110). The diagnosis may be confirmed by aspiration of the lesion. Definitive treatment requires complete excision, including the outer fibrous capsule.

In the foot, most ganglia arise in the dorsal or dorsolateral soft tissues and are more frequently painful when compared with lesions about the wrist (113) (Fig. 9.23). A ganglion may also arise in the tarsal sinus and produce sinus tarsi syndrome (Fig. 9.24). It may also occur in the subcutaneous soft tissue, unattached to synovial structures (Fig. 9.25).

On radiographs a ganglion may be detected as a soft tissue mass, provided it is of sufficient size. On MRI, a ganglion typically appears as a well-marginated, lobular, septated lesion with a homogeneous pattern of low to intermediate signal intensity on T1-weighted and proton density images and high signal intensity on T2-weighted images. The relationship of the cyst to the adjacent joint capsule is best shown on T2-weighted images (109,114). MRI is an excellent means of determining the extent of the ganglion. Potential sources of recurrence, such as small pseudopodia, capsular cysts, and deep extensions of the ganglion, are well demonstrated (Fig. 9.26).

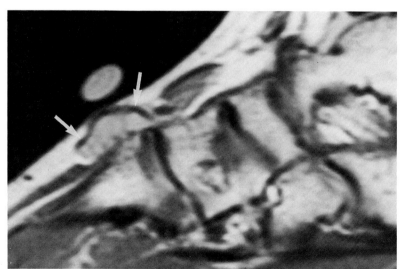

A

FIG. 9.23. Ganglion. **A:** Sagittal MR, TR/TE 2500/25 and **B,** sagittal MR, TR/TE 2500/80 images reveal a lobulated mass (*arrows*) with the signal characteristics of fluid and a low signal intensity fibrous capsule, dorsal to the middle cuneiform–second metatarsal joint space. (*Figure continues on next page.*)

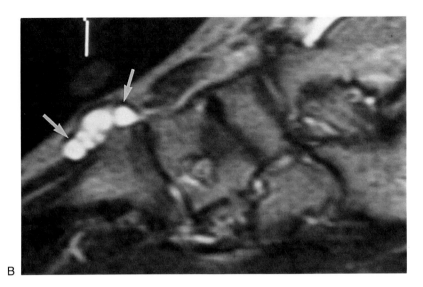

B

FIG. 9.23. (*Continued*)

Synovial Sarcoma

Synovial sarcoma is an uncommon tumor that typically arises adjacent to a joint, tendon, or bursa. Despite its name, this lesion is intraarticular in only 5% of cases (38). It is thought to originate from primitive mesenchymal cells that differentiate in a pattern that resembles synovial membrane. Synovial sarcoma accounts for approximately 10% of all soft tissue sarcomas and most often occurs between the ages of 15 and 40 years. It is rare under the age of 10 years. Patients usually present with a slow-growing mass, with pain or tenderness occurring in 30% to 50% of cases (38,69,115). This tumor has a strong predilection to

arise in the extremities. Approximately two-thirds of lesions involve the lower extremity and one-quarter involve the upper extremity. The most common sites of involvement are the knee region (30%), the foot (13%), and the lower leg or ankle (10%) (38). Synovial sarcoma typically arises in the deep soft tissues and often adheres to tendon or the external surface of a

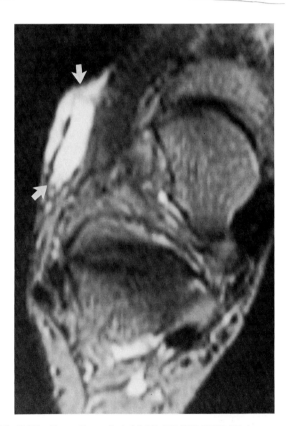

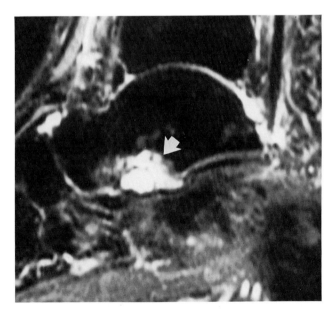

FIG. 9.24. Ganglion.   Sagittal STIR (2200/35/160) image reveals a lobulated, high signal intensity lesion (*arrow*) within the tarsal sinus. (T, talus; C, calcaneus).

FIG. 9.25. Ganglion. Axial MR, TR/TE 2500/80 image reveals a septated, high signal intensity lesion (*arrows*) within the lateral subcutaneous tissue of the foot. This lesion had fluctuated in size for several months.

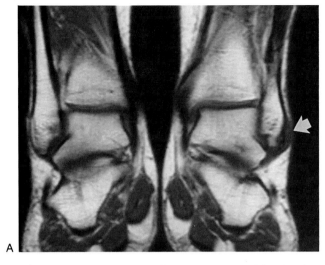

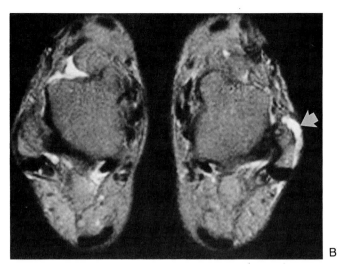

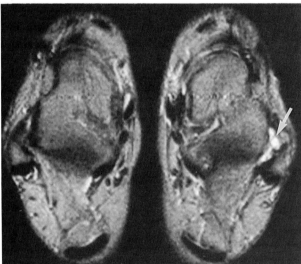

FIG. 9.26. Ganglion. **A:** Coronal MR, TR/TE 600/20 image reveals a subtle low signal intensity mass (*arrow*) overlying the lateral malleolus. Compare to opposite side. **B, C:** Axial 1800/80 images reveal a lobulated, high signal lesion (*arrow*) overlying the lateral malleolus in B and extending into the talofibular joint in C.

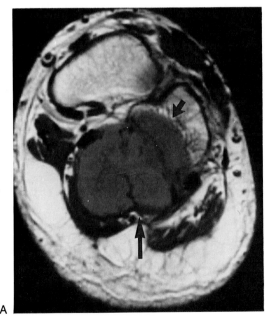

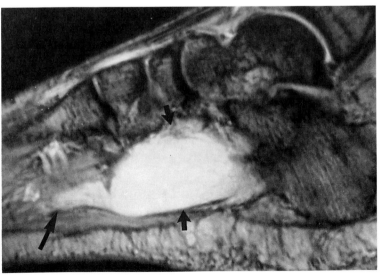

FIG. 9.27. Synovial sarcoma. **A:** Axial MR TR/TE 2000/20 image reveals a low signal intensity plantar mass (*long arrow*) invading the cuboid (*short arrow*). **B:** Sagittal MR gradient echo (400/ 30/30°) image reveals a high signal intensity mass (*short arrows*) infiltrating into the forefoot (*long arrow*). (Courtesy of Lynne S. Steinbach, M.D., San Francisco, CA.)

249

joint capsule. Because of its slow rate of growth, the tumor often is surrounded by a pseudocapsule; however, its microscopic margins are invasive. Histologically, this tumor is typically biphasic, consisting of spindle cell and epithelial components.

Metastatic disease is common, principally involving the lung, lymph nodes, or bone marrow, and may occur several years after diagnosis. The long-term prognosis is poor. An improved prognosis is seen in younger patients, tumors smaller than 5 cm, lesions in the distal extremities, and in heavily calcified lesions (38,69).

On MRI, synovial sarcoma typically reveals a heterogeneous pattern of predominantly low to interme-

diate signal intensity on T1-weighted images and intermediate to high signal intensity on T2-weighted images (100,116–119) (Fig. 9.27). A homogeneous pattern of high signal intensity on T2-weighted images is unusual (119). It often appears as a lobulated mass with internal septae. Regions of necrosis or cyst formation may result in fluid/fluid levels (119) (Fig. 9.28). Synovial sarcoma may appear well demarcated by a pseudocapsule or have infiltrative margins. Neurovascular involvement by tumor is suggested if the tumor is adjacent to or displaces the neurovascular bundle. Extension to adjacent bone is well demonstrated with MRI (120).

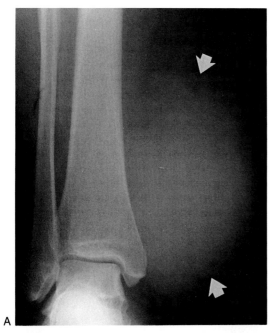

A

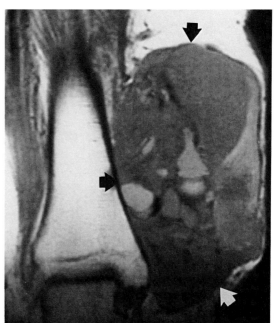

B

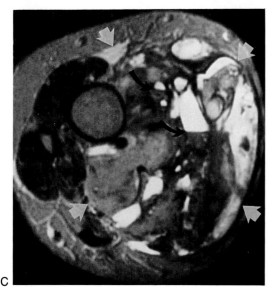

C

FIG. 9.28. Synovial sarcoma. **A:** AP radiograph reveals a large, medial soft tissue mass (*arrows*). **B:** Coronal MR TR/TE 600/20 and **C,** axial MR TR/TE 2000/80 images reveal a large lesion (*arrows*) with a heterogeneous pattern of signal intensity and fluid-fluid levels (*curved arrows* in C). There is no evidence of medullary involvement. (Courtesy of Phoebe Kaplan, M.D., Omaha, NE.)

Lesions of Muscle Origin

Rhabdomyosarcoma

Rhabdomyosarcoma is the most common soft tissue sarcoma of children under 15 years of age, of adolescents, and of young adults. Rhabdomyosarcoma compromises 15% to 20% of all soft tissue sarcomas; however, the majority of lesions involve the head and neck regions and visceral organs in children (38,69). This tumor is classified into four histologic subtypes. The embryonal form accounts for 75% of rhabdomyosarcomas and typically involves the head and neck region in young children but may also affect the extremities. Two of the histologic subtypes have a predilection to involve the extremities: alveolar rhabdomyosarcoma involves the upper and lower extremities of adolescents and young adults, and pleomorphic rhabdomyosarcoma affects the large muscles of the extremities in adults (121). When arising in an extremity, rhabdomyosarcoma usually presents as a rapidly enlarging mass and is often painless. There is an infiltrative pattern of growth and erosion of bone may be observed in lesions of the hands and feet (38) (see Fig. 9.3). Rhabdomyosarcoma has a strong tendency to metastasize to lymph nodes. The combination of radical surgery and chemotherapy has improved the 5-year survival to as high as 70% to 80%; however, an inadequate surgical margin, local recurrence, or metastatic disease diminish survival significantly (69). On MRI, rhabdomyosarcoma has a nonspecific appearance. It often reveals intermediate, rather than high, signal intensity on T2-weighted images. STIR imaging may be the best technique to delineate the lesion (Fig. 9.29).

Lesions of Cartilage Origin

Soft Tissue Chondroma

Soft tissue chondroma is a rare, benign tumor that chiefly arises within the soft tissues of the hands and

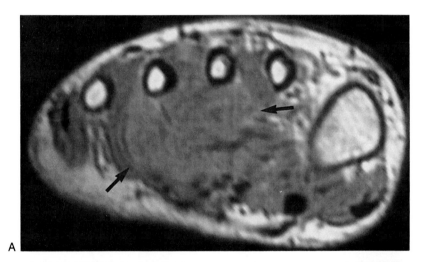

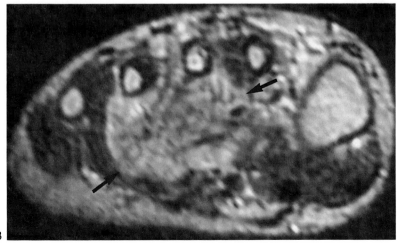

FIG. 9.29. Rhabdomyosarcoma. **A:** Coronal MR TR/TE 2000/18, **B,** coronal MR TR/TE 2000/80. (*Figure continues on next page.*)

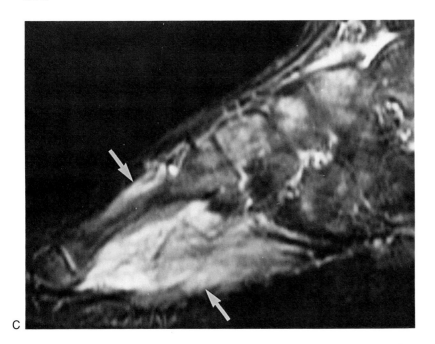

FIG. 9.29. (*Continued*) **C:** sagittal STIR (2000/43/160). An infiltrating soft tissue mass (*arrows* in A, B, and C) is isointense with muscle in A and isointense with fat in B. The lesion reveals high signal intensity and is most conspicuous with STIR imaging in C. (Courtesy of Randall M. Patten, M.D., Kirkland, WA.)

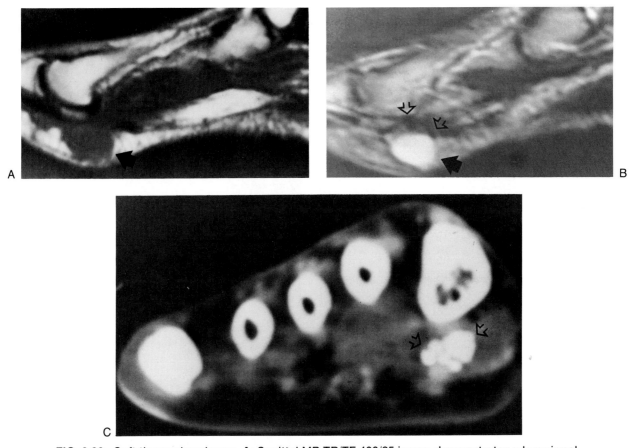

FIG. 9.30. Soft tissue chondroma. **A:** Sagittal MR TR/TE 400/25 image demonstrates a low signal intensity mass in the plantar soft tissue under the first metatarsal head (*arrow*). **B:** Sagittal MR TR/TE 2500/80: the mass (*arrow*) reveals predominant high signal intensity and contains low signal intensity calcifications at its dorsal aspect (*open arrows*). **C:** Axial CT through a different part of the lesion reveals multiple central calcifications (*open arrows*) within the mass. (From ref. 214, with permission.)

feet (122). The lesion presents as a slowly growing mass and is usually not tender or painful. It is usually less than 3 cm in diameter and, on palpation, may be firm or rubbery and is often mobile. The lesion is predominantly composed of hyaline cartilage, although fibrosis, myxoid change, and hemorrhage may be observed (38). A variable degree of focal or diffuse calcification has been reported in 33% to 70% of cases (123). Calcification tends to occur in the center of the lesion. On MRI, purely cartilaginous lesions reveal low signal intensity on T1-weighted images, high signal intensity on T2-weighted images, and variable foci of very low signal intensity, depending on the extent of calcification (Fig. 9.30). A heterogeneous pattern of signal intensity may be observed in lesions with a mixed fibrous and cartilaginous matrix.

Extraskeletal Myxoid Chondrosarcoma

Extraskeletal myxoid chondrosarcoma is a rare, low grade malignant tumor of cartilage that tends to arise within the deep muscles of the extremities. It is an uncommon tumor and its peak incidence is in the fifth decade. Seven of 40 reported cases involved the foot or ankle (124). Patients typically complain of a slowly growing mass that is often not painful or tender. Symptoms may be present for several years before medical attention is sought. Pathologically, the tumor appears as a lobulated, well-circumscribed mass that frequently contains regions of hemorrhage. Intralesional calcification or bone formation is not observed (38). The prognosis for this tumor is strongly dependent upon its histologic composition. Those tumors that are least cellular and most myxoid have the lowest rate of recurrence and metastasis. Extraskeletal myxoid chondrosarcoma is less aggressive than chondrosarcoma of bone or extraskeletal mesenchymal chondrosarcoma. The latter is a rare, highly malignant neoplasm that usually affects young adults and has a propensity to metastasize. It often contains regions of calcification or ossification (125).

On radiographs, extraskeletal myxoid chondrosarcoma appears as a nonspecific, uncalcified soft tissue mass. On MRI it reveals the typical lobular growth pattern of a cartilage lesion and may erode bone (Fig. 9.31).

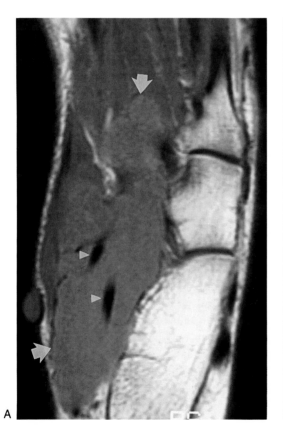
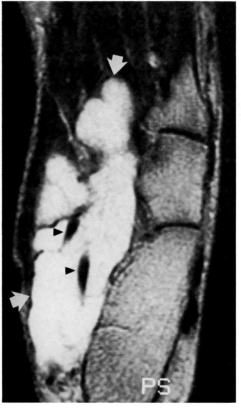

A

B

FIG. 9.31. Extraskeletal myxoid chondrosarcoma. **A:** Axial MR TR/TE 1800/18 and **B,** axial MR TR/TE 1800/80 images reveal a large, lobulated mass (*arrows*) of intermediate signal intensity in A and high signal intensity in B. The flexor tendons (*arrowheads*) are embedded within the mass. (*Figure continues on next page.*)

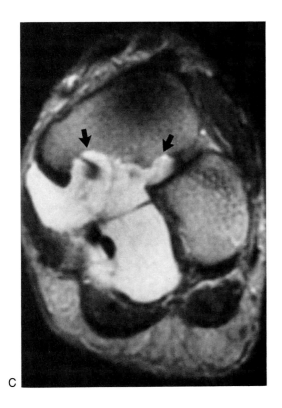

C

FIG. 9.31. (*Continued*) **C:** Coronal MR TR/TE 2000/80 image reveals invasion of the navicular (*arrows*) by the high signal intensity mass. (Courtesy of Randall Patten, M.D., Kirkland, WA).

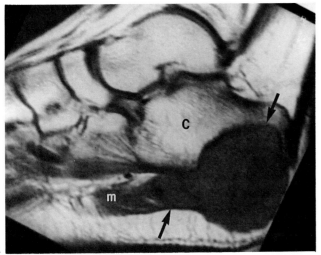

A

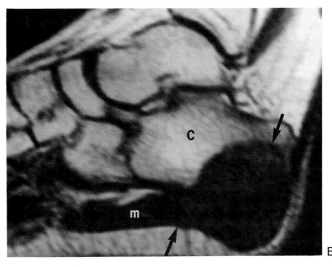

B

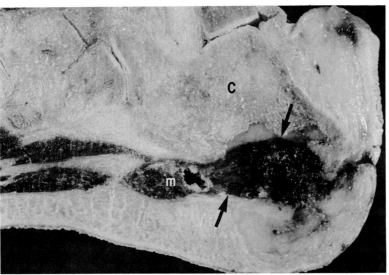

C

FIG. 9.32. Clear cell sarcoma. **A:** Sagittal MR TR/TE 600/25 image reveals a mass (*arrows*), isointense with muscle, arising near the origin of the plantar aponeurosis. The tumor is infiltrating the flexor digitorum brevis muscle (*m*) and invading the calcaneus (*C*). **B:** Sagittal MR TR/TE 2000/90 image. The tumor reveals low signal intensity, reflecting its melanin content. **C:** Gross section just medial to plane of images confirms infiltration of muscle (*m*) and invasion of calcaneus (*C*) by tumor (*arrows*). (From ref. 59, with permission.)

254

Miscellaneous Soft Tissue Lesions

Clear Cell Sarcoma

Clear cell sarcoma is a rare malignant tumor that most often affects young adults between 20 and 40 years of age. This tumor usually produces melanin and has been termed malignant melanoma of soft parts (38). It is usually deep-seated and intimately associated with tendons or aponeuroses. It typically involves the extremities, with the foot and ankle the most common site. This lesion presents as a slow-growing, often painful mass and may be present for several years before diagnosis. Invasion of bone is uncommon (38). Clear cell sarcoma has a poor prognosis and a strong tendency for local recurrence and metastasis (126,127). The appearance of clear cell sarcoma on MRI depends on its melanin content. Melanin causes paramagnetic relaxation enhancement, with shortening of T1 and T2 relaxation times. This acts to increase signal intensity on T1-weighted images and decrease signal intensity on T2-weighted images (59). Lesions that contain a significant amount of melanin reveal intermediate signal intensity on T1-weighted images and low signal intensity on T2-weighted images (59) (Fig. 9.32).

Epidermoid Inclusion Cyst

Epidermoid inclusion cyst is a common tumorlike lesion that arises in the subcutaneous tissue. It usually arises in the plantar soft tissues under the first and second metatarsal heads or medial to the first metatarsal head. The cyst usually contains a thick material and is surrounded by a thick fibrous wall (128). It is most likely a posttraumatic, reactive lesion and is treated by surgical removal (129). Large lesions may be confused with other soft tissue masses. MRI may be used to demonstrate the depth of the lesion (Fig. 9.33).

Accessory Muscle

MRI may be useful in characterizing unusual soft tissue masses that are not neoplastic in origin. An accessory soleus muscle may present as a soft tissue mass in the posteromedial aspect of the distal leg and ankle (130,131). This muscle extends from the deep surface of the soleus to the superior or medial aspect of the calcaneus. Although patients are usually asymptomatic, teenagers or young adults may complain of

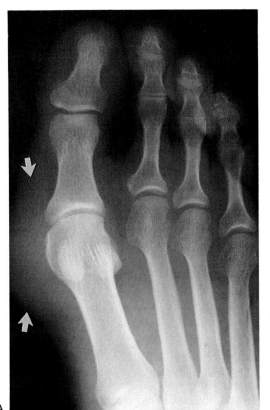

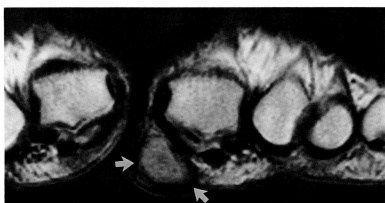

A   B

FIG. 9.33. Epidermoid inclusion cyst. **A:** Dorsoplantar radiograph demonstrates a soft tissue mass medial to the first metatarsal head (*arrows*). **B:** Coronal MR TR/TE 600/20 image reveals a discrete, intermediate signal intensity mass (*arrows*) with a low signal intensity capsule within the plantar subcutaneous fat.

pain and swelling with exercise. This is thought to be due to a closed compartment ischemia. Fasciotomy or excision of the accessory muscle is sometimes performed (130).

On MRI an accessory soleus muscle replaces a portion of the pre-Achilles fat pad and demonstrates the signal characteristics of muscle on all pulse sequences. On axial images at the ankle level, it appears as a mass between the flexor hallucis longus muscle and the Achilles tendon (Fig. 9.34A). It may have a distal insertion on the medial wall of the calcaneus and appear in the hindfoot as an abnormal mass posterior to the posterior tibial neurovascular bundle (Fig. 9.34B).

Foreign Body

MRI may also be used to localize foreign substances within the soft tissues that present as mass lesions (Fig. 9.35). In order to optimize lesion detection, several pulse sequences (such as T1- and T2-weighted images and STIR) should be used.

BONE TUMORS AND TUMORLIKE LESIONS

Simple Bone Cyst

A simple bone cyst is a common lesion that is not a true neoplasm but is believed to represent a devel-

opmental or reactive process (132). It is usually discovered during the first two decades of life. The distribution varies with age. In patients aged 17 years or younger, 81% of cysts arise in the proximal humerus or proximal femur, whereas in patients older than 17 years, 52% arise in the ilium or calcaneus (133). Lesions in tubular bones are usually detected because of pathologic fracture. Cysts in the flat bones, including the bones of the foot, rarely fracture and are usually discovered incidentally.

Most cysts contain serous or serosanguinous fluid and are often bridged by fibrous septae. The fluid often has a high protein content (134). Treatment is usually by curettage or intralesional steroid injection; however, a recurrence rate of 10% to 50% has been reported (132,135).

The typical radiographic appearance of a simple bone cyst arising in a tubular bone is that of a metaphyseal, centrally located radiolucency with cortical thinning and mild expansion of the bony contour. It may appear trabeculated but does not penetrate the cortex or extend into soft tissue. Roughly 3% of simple bone cysts arise in the calcaneus and the lesion is otherwise rare in the bones of the foot or ankle (135–138). In the calcaneus, this lesion characteristically arises anteriorly within the radiolucent triangle between the major trabecular groups, just inferior to the anterior margin of the posterior facet. It usually appears as a well-defined radiolucency with an ovoid or

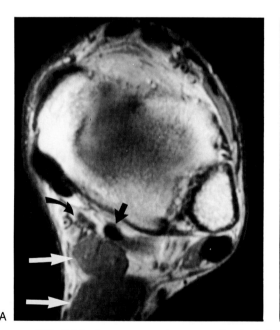
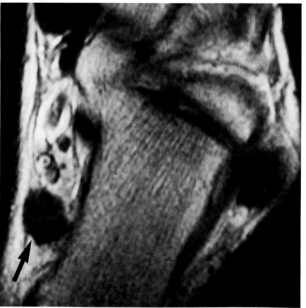

A   B

FIG. 9.34. Accessory soleus muscle. **A:** Axial MR TR/TE 2000/20 image at the level of the ankle reveals an intermediate signal intensity mass (*large arrows*) posterior to the flexor hallucis longus tendon (*short arrow*) and the posterior tibial neurovascular bundle (*curved arrow*). **B:** Axial MR TR/TE 2000/80 image reveals a low signal intensity mass (arrow), posterior to the neurovascular bundle, representing the distal portion of the accessory muscle. This "mass" is isointense with muscle on both pulse sequences.

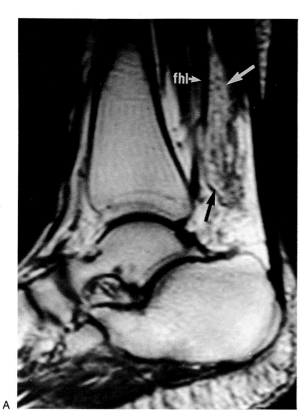 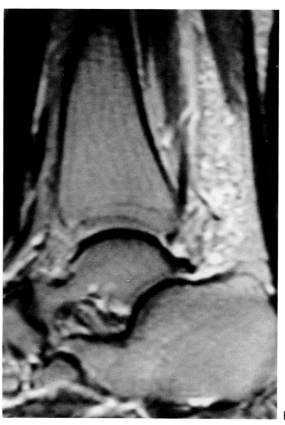

A   B

FIG. 9.35. Distal migration of injected silicone. **A:** Sagittal MR TR/TE 600/20. **B:** Sagittal MR TR/TE 1800/80 images. In A, an intermediate signal intensity "mass" (*arrows*) is noted extending into the pre-Achilles fat pad, adjacent to the flexor hallucis longus tendon (*fhl*). In B, this "mass" cannot be distinguished from fat. Patient had undergone cosmetic injection of silicone into calf and complained of loss of cosmetic effect and increasing pain in ankle region.

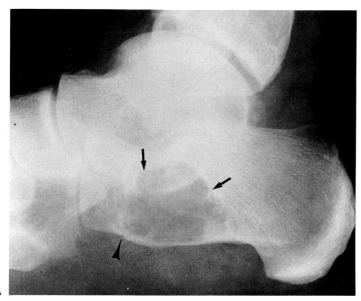

A

FIG. 9.36. Simple bone cyst. **A:** A lateral radiograph reveals a well-defined, quadrangular, lytic lesion (*arrows*) within the anterior calcaneus and a minimally displaced fracture (*arrowhead*). (*Figure continues on next page.*)

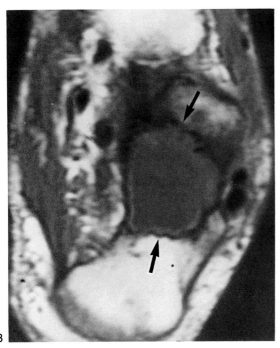

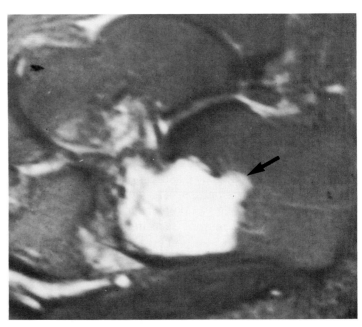

B

C

FIG. 9.36. (*Continued*) **B:** Axial MR TR/TE 600/20 image. **C:** Sagittal MR TR/TE 2500/80 image. The cyst (*arrows*) reveals intermediate signal intensity in B and high signal intensity with internal separations in C. (Courtesy of Morrie Kricun, M.D., Philadelphia, PA.)

quadrangular shape. It typically involves one-third to one-half the length of the calcaneus, one-half to two-thirds of the width, and abuts the lateral cortex (137).

On MRI, most simple cysts reveal homogeneous low to intermediate signal intensity on T1-weighted images, and high signal intensity on T2-weighted images (Fig. 9.36). Linear regions of low signal intensity within the lesion correspond to fibrous septae. Hemorrhage into the lesion will produce a more heterogeneous pattern of signal intensity and may create fluid-fluid levels (139) (Fig. 9.37).

Aneurysmal Bone Cyst

Aneurysmal bone cyst (ABC) is an expansile lesion composed of distended, thin-walled, blood-filled spaces. It is believed to be a reactive rather than a neoplastic process and may occur secondarily in association with other bone lesions. Approximately 80% of affected patients are less than 20 years old and the lesion is rare over the age of 30 years (132). ABC may occur in any bone and is most common in the craniofacial bones, spine, and the metaphyses of long tubular bones. Most ABCs in tubular bones are intramedullary but an intracortical and juxtacortical origin has also been described (140). ABC has been reported in almost all of the bones of the foot and between 11% and 13% of all cases involve the foot or ankle

(1,36,132,141–143). Treatment is usually by resection or curettage with bone graft.

On radiographs, ABC appears as an expansile, lytic lesion with variable trabeculation. Occasionally it has an aggressive appearance, with cortical breakthrough and soft tissue extension. The soft tissue component

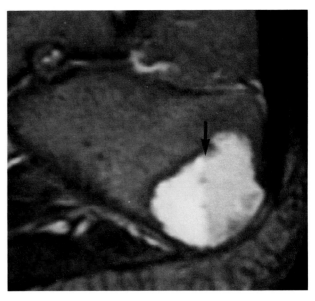

FIG. 9.37. Simple bone cyst. Sagittal MR TR/TE 2000/70 image reveals a well-demarcated lesion within the posteroinferior calcaneus with a fluid-fluid level (*arrow*). (Courtesy of Robert J. Binder, M.D., Oakland, CA.)

is usually at least partially contained by a thin rim of periosteal bone. This rim is a useful sign of benignancy but may only be visible with CT.

On MRI, ABC typically appears as an expansile, lobulated, multicystic lesion (Fig. 9.38). There are multiple internal septations and it is surrounded by a low signal intensity rim (144–147). This peripheral rim may be composed of fibrous tissue or bone. Multiple, variable-sized cysts with fluid-fluid levels of varying signal intensity are characteristic. These fluid-fluid levels are probably due to settling out of the byproducts of hemoglobin degradation (144,146). They are usually most evident on T2-weighted images and may not be identifiable on T1-weighted images. The appearance of multiple fluid-fluid levels is not pathognomonic for ABC, however, as this may be seen in any bone or

soft tissue tumor that undergoes hemorrhage or cystic degeneration (139). Partial or complete erosion of cortical bone and soft tissue extension of the lesion may also be demonstrated with MRI (Fig. 9.38).

Intraosseous Lipoma

Intraosseous lipoma is an uncommon lesion that is probably neoplastic in origin, although a degenerative pathogenesis has also been proposed. It has been observed in patients from age 3 to 85 years but its peak incidence is in the fourth and fifth decades of life (132). Between one-third and two-thirds of patients are symptomatic, complaining of local pain and variable soft tissue swelling (132,148–150). It is usually found in the

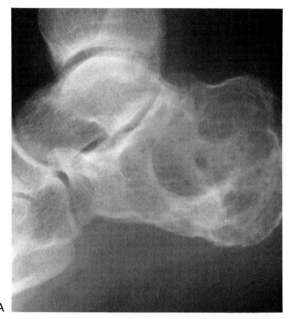

A

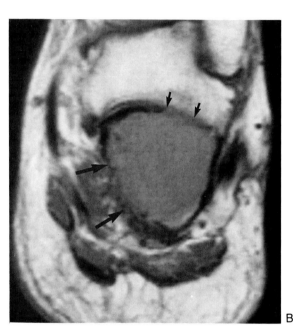

B

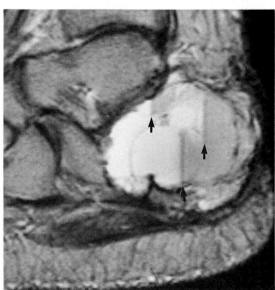

C

FIG. 9.38. Aneurysmal bone cyst. A: Lateral radiograph shows a trabeculated, expansile lytic lesion of the posterior calcaneus. B: Coronal MR TR/TE 600/20 image: the lesion reveals homogeneous intermediate signal intensity. There is erosion of medial cortex (*long arrows*) and of the subchondral bone plate of the posterior calcaneal facet (*short arrows*). C: Sagittal MR TR/TE: 1800/80 image. The lesion predominantly consists of multiple fluid-fluid levels (*arrows*). (Courtesy of D.M. Forrester, M.D., Los Angeles, CA.)

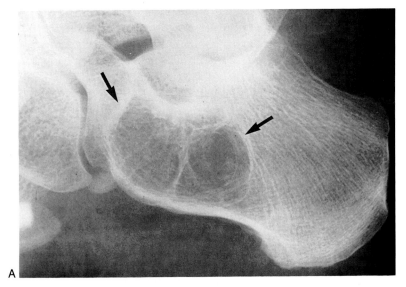

A

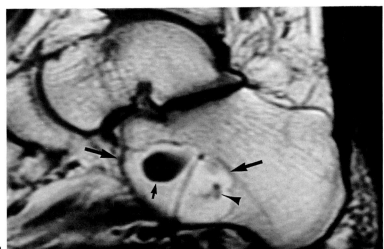

B

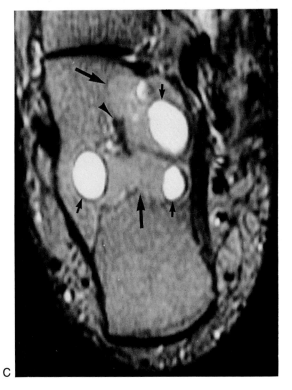

C

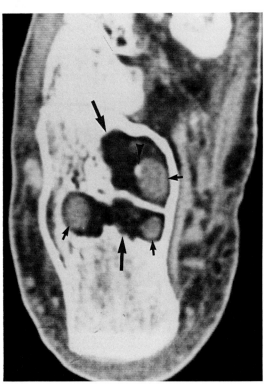

D

FIG. 9.39. Intraosseous lipoma. **A:** Lateral radiograph reveals a quadrangular, septated, lytic lesion (*long arrows*) with sclerotic margins. **B:** Sagittal MR TR/TE 500/15 image. **C:** Axial MR TR/TE 2700/80 image. The lesion (*long arrows*) reveals the signal intensity of fat. Intralesional cysts (*short arrows*) show low signal intensity in B and high signal intensity in C. Foci of calcification (*arrowheads*) are of low signal intensity in B and C. **D:** Axial CT reveals a fat-containing lesion (*long arrows*) with cysts (*short arrows*) and calcification (*arrowhead*).

260

metaphysis or diaphysis of a long tubular bone. Favored sites of involvement are the tibia, fibula, femur, and calcaneus. In the calcaneus, intraosseous lipoma arises in the same location as simple cysts: within the triangular zone between the major trabeculae in the anterior third. It has been suggested that the calcaneal lipoma may, in fact, represent a variant of a simple cyst (134).

Milgram has categorized intraosseous lipoma into three stages depending on the degree of involution (148). Stage I consists of viable fat cells without secondary necrosis; stage II is a transitional phase with viable fat cells interspersed with fat necrosis and calcifications; stage III consists of complete or near-complete secondary necrosis with necrotic fat, calcification, variable degrees of cyst formation, and reactive woven bone formation. Stage III lesions may be misdiagnosed histologically as bone infarcts and radiographically resemble an enchondroma with central calcified matrix.

Intraosseous lipoma demonstrates varying degrees of osteolysis and calcification, usually has a well-defined margin, and often expands the bony contour. Calcaneal lesions are characteristically osteolytic with a thin, sclerotic margin and often contain central calcification. Either CT or MRI may be used to confirm the fatty nature of intraosseous lipoma (151) (Fig. 9.39). MRI reveals a well-demarcated lesion with the signal characteristics of fat. Regions of signal void correspond to foci of calcification or ossification. Areas of necrosis or cyst formation have the signal characteristics of fluid, demonstrating low signal intensity on T1-weighted images and high signal intensity on T2-weighted images. Expansion of the bony contour may be appreciated on axial images.

Intraosseous Ganglion

Intraosseous ganglion is a subchondral lesion of bone that occurs in middle-aged adults. It is usually associated with mild intermittent localized pain made worse with activity. This lesion is histologically identical to a soft tissue ganglion. It has a predilection to involve the bones about the ankle, especially the distal tibia/medial malleolus. The pathogenesis of ganglion cysts of bone has not been established, although many theories abound (152–155). Recurrence is rare following curettage or excision.

On radiographs, an intraosseous ganglion usually appears as a subchondral, well-defined lytic lesion with a thin sclerotic margin. The lesion may appear multilocular but there is no expansion of the bony contour. Communication with the adjacent joint space is very rare (152,154). On MRI an intraosseous ganglion appears as a well-demarcated unilocular or multilocular

lesion with the signal characteristics of fluid and a low signal intensity margin (Fig. 9.40). Low signal intensity septations may be seen within the lesion (155).

Giant Cell Tumor

Giant cell tumor of bone is a benign, often locally aggressive tumor composed of multinucleated giant cells within a mononuclear stromal background. Roughly 75% of affected patients are between the ages of 20 and 40 years and this lesion is rare under the age of 15 and over age 60 (1,132). Giant cell tumor involves the end of a long tubular bone in 75% to 90% of cases and has a strong predilection for the bones about the knee (1,132). The bones of the foot and ankle are involved in 5% to 7% of cases (1,132,156). In this region, the distal tibia is most often involved, followed by the talus and calcaneus (157). When arising in the small bones of the hands and feet, giant cell tumor is more often multicentric and has a greater propensity for local recurrence (158).

The extent of surgical excision depends primarily on the pattern of growth. Curettage, coupled with cryosurgery, is adequate for lesions confined to bone. If tumor has penetrated cortical bone or extended into a joint a more aggressive approach, such as en bloc resection, is required (159).

On radiographs, giant cell tumor appears as a radiolucent, sometimes trabeculated lesion, producing cortical thinning and expansion, with a margin that is usually well defined but nonsclerotic (Fig. 9.41). The lesion usually involves the epiphysis and metaphysis, and characteristically extends to the subchondral bone. Cortical breakthrough with soft tissue extension may also be seen. Giant cell tumor in the small bones of the foot usually has a nonspecific appearance of an expansile, geographic, lytic lesion with variable trabeculation. On MRI, giant cell tumor may produce a heterogeneous pattern of signal intensity due to intralesional hemorrhage or cyst formation. Low to intermediate signal intensity on T1-weighted images and intermediate to high signal intensity on T2-weighted images is typical, and fluid-fluid levels may be seen (160). MRI may reveal cortical destruction and is useful in demonstrating soft tissue extension (Fig. 9.41). For tumors occurring in the distal tibia or fibula, coronal or sagittal MRIs provide optimal demonstration of the relation of tumor to the subchondral bone and joint space.

Enchondroma

Solitary enchondroma is a benign tumor that occurs between the ages of 10 and 50 years. The patient is usually asymptomatic or presents with painless swell-

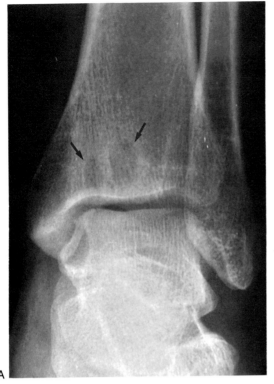

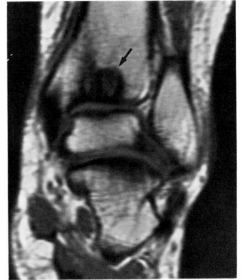

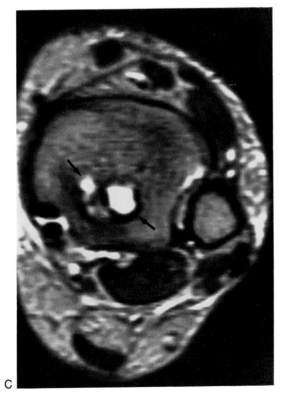

FIG. 9.40. Intraosseous ganglion. **A:** Anteroposterior radiograph demonstrates a lobulated, subchondral lytic lesion with faintly sclerotic margins within the distal tibia (*arrows*). **B:** Coronal MR TR/TE 800/20 image reveals a low signal intensity, lobulated lesion (*arrow*). **C:** Axial MR TR/TE 2000/80 image reveals a high signal intensity, septated lesion with a low signal intensity margin (*arrows*). (From ref. 155, with permission.)

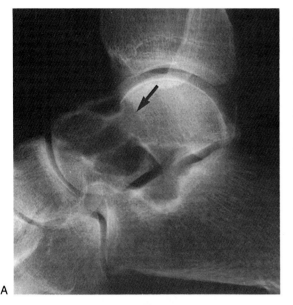

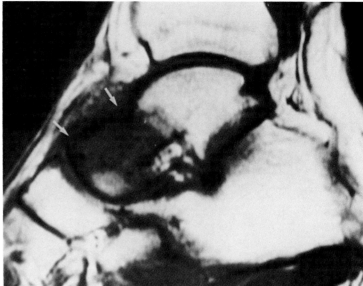

A

B

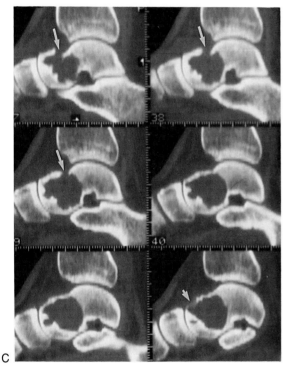

C

FIG. 9.41. Giant cell tumor. **A:** Lateral radiograph shows a lytic, trabeculated lesion of the distal talus (*arrow*). **B:** Sagittal MR TR/TE 500/20 image. The lesion reveals intermediate signal intensity and there is loss of dorsal cortical bone with soft tissue extension of tumor (*arrows*). **C:** Multiple sagittal reformatted CT images demonstrate a well-defined lytic lesion with destruction of dorsal cortical bone of talus at its proximal (*long arrow*) and distal (*short arrow*) aspects. (Courtesy of Mark D Murphey, M.D., Kansas City, KS.)

ing. Any bone may be affected but roughly one-half of solitary enchondromas occur in the metacarpals and phalanges of the hand (132). In the foot, the phalanges and metatarsals are usually involved. Treatment is usually not necessary for these lesions unless there is pain, pathologic fracture, or if the diagnosis is equivocal. Malignant transformation of solitary enchondroma oc-

curring in the small bones of the hand or foot is very rare (135).

Radiographically, enchondroma appears as a radiolucent, sometimes expansile lesion with a lobulated contour and endosteal erosion. A variable amount of intralesional calcification is usually present. Pathologic fracture is not uncommon. On MRI, an enchon-

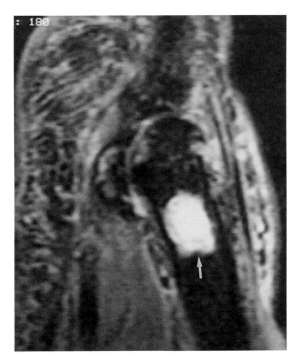

FIG. 9.42. Enchondroma. A sagittal STIR (2200/35/160) image reveals a lobulated, high signal intensity lesion within the first metatarsal (*arrow*).

droma demonstrates a homogeneous, lobular pattern of high signal intensity on T2-weighted or STIR images, reflecting its hyaline cartilage matrix (161) (Fig. 9.42). Calcified matrix appears as punctate or linear regions of low signal intensity.

Osteochondroma

Osteochondroma is a slow-growing, usually asymptomatic lesion and is the most common benign tumor

of bone. It is usually discovered in children and adolescents as a painless mass. It occurs in any bone that undergoes endochondral ossification and most often involves the long tubular bones. It is not uncommon in the distal tibia or fibula but rarely involves the bones of the foot (132,162,163). An osteochondroma arises from the surface of bone and is composed of cortex and spongiosa that are continuous with those of the native bone. The base of the lesion may be sessile or pedunculated and an osteochondroma always extends away from the adjacent joint. The lesion is covered by a cartilage cap that progressively ossifies with age. Growth of the tumor usually ceases when the epiphyses close; however, an unossified cartilage cap may persist into adulthood.

Surgical excision is performed for a variety of complications. Pain may be produced by impingement on neurovascular structures, due to fracture of the base of a pedunculated lesion or to formation of a bursa over the lesion. Correction of osseous deformity and malignant transformation are other surgical indications (135,162).

Osteochondroma has a characteristic radiographic appearance. It is typically metaphyseal and appears as a projection of bone that blends imperceptively with the underlying cortical and trabecular bone. MRI may be used to assess the relation of an osteochondroma to adjacent bone or to the neurovascular bundle or to demonstrate an associated bursa. MRI has been shown to be superior to CT in determining the size of an unossified cartilage cap (164). Accurate assessment of the cap thickness to within 2 mm has been documented with MRI (164). The unossified cap reveals low to intermediate signal intensity on T1-weighted and proton density images and very high signal intensity on T2-weighted images (Fig. 9.43). The overlying perichondrium is of low signal intensity on all pulse sequences.

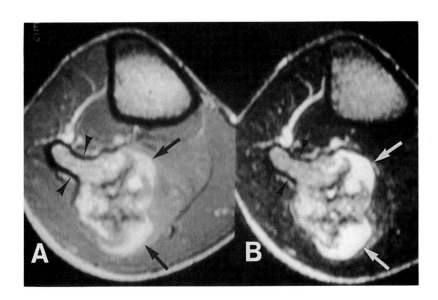

FIG. 9.43. Osteochondroma. **A:** Axial MR TR/TE 2000/20 and **B,** axial MR TR/TE 2000/80 images reveal a partially ossified osteochondroma of the proximal fibula. The base of the lesion is contiguous with the native cortex and spongiosa (*arrowheads*). The uncalcified cartilage cap (*arrows*) is slightly hyperintense to muscle in A and reveals very high signal intensity in B. (Courtesy of Donald Resnick, M.D., San Diego, CA.)

Although MRI can accurately assess the size of the cartilage cap, it is controversial whether an enlarged cap (one greater than 2 or 3 cm) correlates with development of chondrosarcoma (135).

Trevor Disease

Trevor disease (dysplasia epiphysealis hemimelica) is a congenital growth disorder characterized by cartilaginous overgrowth of a portion of one or more epiphyses (165). It is usually diagnosed between the ages of 2 and 14 years and predominantly involves the lower extremity, including the distal tibia and talus. There may be pain, swelling, and deformity. The radiographic appearance is characteristic, as multiple irregular ossification centers are seen to arise from one side of an epiphysis (166). These centers eventually fuse with the epiphysis and appear identical to an osteochondroma, both radiographically and histologically. MRI may be used to define the extent of the lesion and to demonstrate deformity of the adjacent articular surface (Fig. 9.44). Because MRI permits direct visualization of the unossified cartilage surface, it is likely to replace arthrography in assessing joint deformity in these patients (167).

Subungual Exostosis

Subungual exostosis has a similar radiographic appearance to osteochondroma but is believed to represent a posttraumatic lesion (168). It usually arises from the dorsal surface of the distal phalanx of the great toe and may cause pain, swelling, ulceration, and secondary infection. In many series, subungual exostosis is classified as an osteochondroma but, in fact, it is not a neoplasm and should not be considered to represent an osteochondroma (132).

Chondroblastoma

Chondroblastoma is a rare benign tumor that usually occurs in the second and third decades of life. In descending order, it most commonly involves the region of the knee, shoulder, hip, and foot/ankle (169,170). Chondroblastoma may exhibit an aggressive pattern of growth and may be accompanied by an aneurysmal bone cyst. Treatment is by curettage coupled with cryosurgery (132).

On radiographs, chondroblastoma typically appears as a lytic epiphyseal lesion with a thin sclerotic rim. It may traverse the open epiphysis into the metaphysis. Rarely, it may penetrate the subchondral bone and overlying articular cartilage or break through cortical bone. Calcification is observed in 30% to 50% of lesions (135). Chondroblastoma of the calcaneus tends to arise underneath the posterior talocalcaneal joint or posteriorly in the region of the apophysis (171). On MRI, chondroblastoma reveals predominant intermediate signal intensity on both T1- and T2-weighted images (161). Regions of high signal intensity may be seen on T2-weighted images and calcific regions of low signal intensity may be present. Cystic change or development of a secondary aneurysmal bone cyst may result in fluid-fluid levels (172).

Chondromyxoid Fibroma

Chondromyxoid fibroma is a rare benign lesion of cartilage that can involve any bone but tends to arise about the knee, foot, and ankle (173). It may occur at any age but most patients are between 5 and 30 years of age. Clinical symptoms tend to evolve slowly over months or years and consist of pain, swelling, and restriction of motion (132). In the foot, chondromyxoid fibroma most often involves the calcaneus, metatarsals, and phalanges. This tumor may be locally ag-

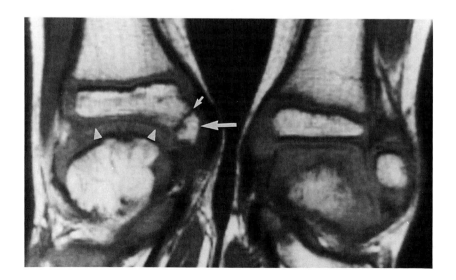

Fig. 9.44. Trevor disease. Coronal MR TR/TE 600/20 image demonstrates a partially mineralized epiphyseal osteochondroma arising from the medial distal tibial epiphysis (*long arrow*). A low signal intensity growth plate separates the lesion from the native epiphysis (*short arrow*). There is a rounded deformity of the articular surface of the unossified talar dome (*arrowheads*). (From ref. 214, with permission.)

gressive, with invasion of adjacent bones or extension along fascial planes (174). Thorough curettage and bone graft is usually adequate therapy.

Radiographically, chondromyxoid fibroma appears as a metaphyseal radiolucency with cortical expansion or destruction, coarse trabeculation, and a rounded or lobular sclerotic margin. This lesion may produce a "blowout" pattern of cortical destruction, although the surrounding periosteum is invariably found intact at surgery (173). The MRI features of chondromyxoid fibroma have not been established. For aggressive lesions, MRI is useful in documenting the intramedullary and soft tissue extent and in distinguishing between remodeling and invasion of bone (175) (Fig. 9.45).

Osteoid Osteoma

Osteoid osteoma is a common, benign osteoblastic lesion that has a distinctive histologic and radiographic appearance. Roughly 80% of affected patients are between the ages of 5 and 24 years (1). It most often involves the femur, tibia, humerus, and spine. Osteoid osteoma is relatively common in the foot and ankle, and usually involves the distal tibia or tarsal bones, especially the talus. In children, osteoid osteoma may be associated with premature closure of an epiphysis (176). Patients usually complain of pain, often worse at night or with activity, and often relieved by aspirin. Soft tissue swelling and tenderness may be present. On histologic examination osteoid osteoma is characterized by a central osteoid nidus, embedded in a highly vascularized connective tissue stroma. The

nidus may partially or completely calcify. The size of the nidus is used to distinguish osteoid osteoma from osteoblastoma; however, there is disagreement as to whether the upper limit of size for an osteoid osteoma is 1.5, 2.0, or 2.5 cm (132,134). The classical osteoid osteoma arises in cortical bone and incites a prominent sclerotic periosteal reaction. When the nidus arises in cancellous bone or in an intraarticular or subperiosteal location it elicits little or no sclerotic reaction and may be difficult to detect radiographically (177). Intraarticular lesions present with joint pain, synovitis, and effusion and the diagnosis is often delayed for months or years, as the patient is treated for arthritis (178–181). An early onset of osteoarthritis may ensue, further obscuring the diagnosis. Adequate treatment requires complete excision of the nidus. Intraoperative localization of the nidus may be accomplished with a 99mTc bone scan or preoperative labeling with tetracycline (182–184).

The classical radiographic appearance of osteoid osteoma is that of a rounded, 1- to 2-cm radiolucency surrounded by a broad, solid band of bone sclerosis. The nidus may be partially or completely calcified. As described above, reactive sclerosis is not a prominent feature in lesions that do not arise in cortical bone. This is particularly true of osteoid osteoma arising in the tarsal bones, wherein an intraarticular or subperiosteal location of the tumor is common. As a result, there is often a delay in diagnosis of osteoid osteoma in the foot (185,186). These lesions often appear as subtle or nonspecific lytic or sclerotic lesions and, when subperiosteal, may produce cortical scalloping.

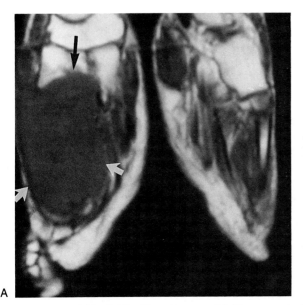
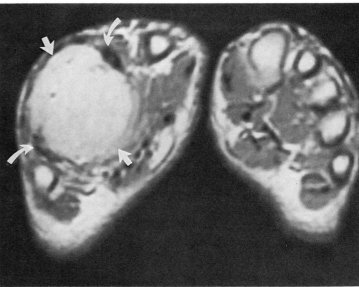

A
B

FIG. 9.45. Chondromyxoid fibroma. **A:** Axial MR TR/TE 600/20 image. There is a large, well-cicumscribed mass (*short arrows*), isointense with muscle, arising from the third metatarsal and invading the lateral cuneiform (*long arrow*). **B:** Coronal MR TR/TE 2000/20 image: The lesion (*arrows*) is hyperintense to muscle and is spreading apart the second and fourth metatarsals (*curved arrows*). The lesion revealed uniform high signal intensity on T2-weighted images. (From ref. 175, with permission.)

A bone scan may be useful in demonstrating abnormal uptake and is often useful in localizing the nidus. A bone scan, however, does not always reveal the typical pattern of focal abnormality that is classically seen in osteoid osteoma (187).

On MRI, the nidus of an osteoid osteoma appears as a region of low to intermediate signal intensity on both T1-weighted and T2-weighted images (188,189) (Fig. 9.46). Cortical osteoid osteomas reveal thickened, low signal intensity bone surrounding a nidus of

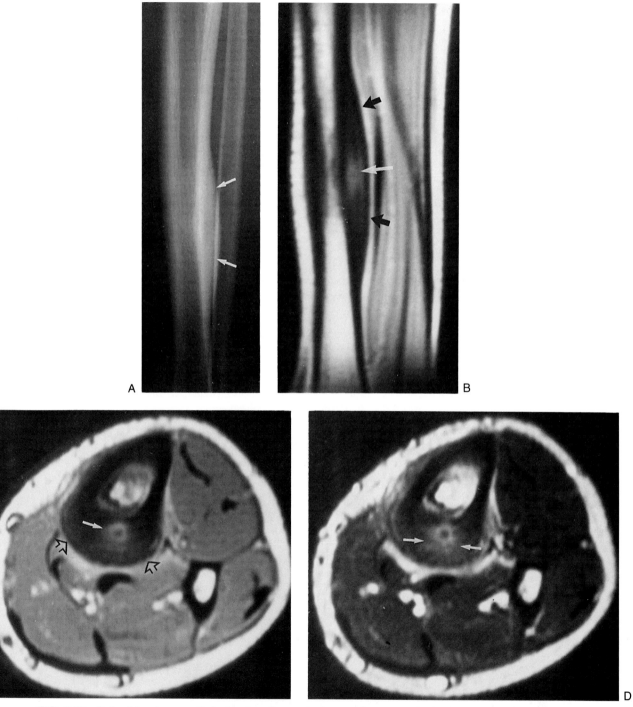

FIG. 9.46. Osteoid osteoma. **A:** Lateral radiograph demonstrates cortical thickening of the posterior tibia (*arrows*). **B:** Sagittal MR TR/TE 600/20 image reveals the intermediate signal intensity nidus (*white arrow*) within the low signal intensity reactive bone (*black arrows*). **C:** Axial MR TR/TE 2500/20 and **D,** axial MR TR/TE 2500/70 images. In C, the nidus appears as a halo of intermediate signal intensity (*arrow*) with central calcification and is embedded within dense cortical bone (*open arrows*). In D, there is a slight increase in signal intensity about the nidus (*arrows*). (Courtesy of Donald Resnick, M.D., San Diego, CA.)

low to intermediate signal intensity. Calcification within the nidus appears as a focal area of very low signal intensity. Intraarticular osteoid osteomas incite a broad zone of high signal intensity within the adjacent marrow on T2-weighted images, presumably reflecting an inflammatory response (Fig. 9.47). Proliferative synovitis and effusion may be seen in the adjacent joint.

The diagnosis of osteoid osteoma requires visualization of the nidus and is probably best accomplished with CT (190,191). It may be difficult with MRI to discern a partially calcified nidus embedded within reactive bone, especially if a small field-of-view, high-resolution examination is not performed. A cortical lesion with a completely calcified nidus may be difficult to diagnose by any imaging means, appearing as a diffusely sclerotic lesion on CT and revealing diffuse low signal intensity on MRI. It may be difficult to distinguish between osteoid osteoma and chronic osteomyelitis with a sequestrum with CT or MRI (187). This is especially true of lesions associated with prominent intramedullary reactive changes (Fig. 9.47). In such cases the "double-density sign" on a bone scan may

be useful for confirming the diagnosis of osteoid osteoma (187).

Osteoblastoma

Osteoblastoma is an uncommon benign tumor that is histologically related to osteoid osteoma but is characterized by a larger size and progressive growth (178,192). It most often occurs in the second and third decades of life and principally affects the spine and long tubular bones. Between 6% and 26% of osteoblastomas originate in the bones of the feet with a predilection for the talus (193). Dull pain is usually present and may persist for years before medical attention is sought.

Histologically, osteoblastoma consists of thick osteoid and woven bone in a vascularized connective tissue stroma. This tumor may be difficult to distinguish from osteosarcoma. "Aggressive osteoblastoma" is a form of this tumor characterized by locally aggressive growth and histologic features intermediate

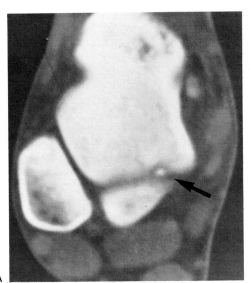

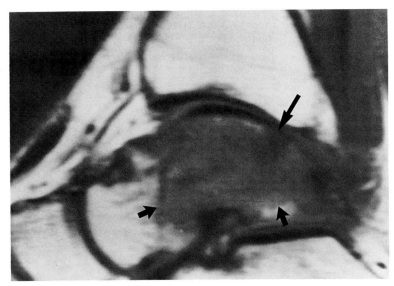

FIG. 9.47. Osteoid osteoma. **A:** Axial CT reveals calcification within the radiolucent nidus. **B:** Sagittal MR TR/TE 600/20 image shows a large region of low signal intensity in the talus (*short arrows*) and a small region of slightly lower signal intensity (*long arrow*). **C:** Sagittal MR TR/TE 2500/80 image demonstrates diffuse high signal intensity in the talus (*short arrows*). The partially calcified nidus shows persistent low signal intensity (*long arrow*). Note the high signal intensity joint effusion (*curved arrow*). (From ref. 189, with permission.)

between those of osteoblastoma and osteosarcoma. This lesion tends to extend into soft tissues and may cross the joint space and extend into adjacent bone (132). Osteoblastoma is treated by marginal resection, as curettage is associated with a high recurrence rate (178).

Osteoblastoma demonstrates a broad range of radiographic features. The typical lesion is an eccentric, expansile, radiolucent lesion with a variable degree of sclerosis and a well-defined margin. There is, however, considerable variation from this pattern and, as described above, this tumor may be quite aggressive. In the talus, osteoblastoma tends to arise at the dorsal neck and reveals a thin sclerotic intraosseous margin and expansive growth into the soft tissues (193). A thin shell of periosteal bone often surrounds this soft tissue component. Osteoporosis involving some or all of the bones of the feet and soft tissue swelling may also be present. In the metatarsals, osteoblastoma tends to have a delicate, trabeculated, soap bubble appearance (193).

As with osteoid osteoma, CT is useful in evaluating osteoblastoma because of its ability to detect calcification or ossification within the lesion and to reveal a thin shell of bone delineating a soft tissue component. This latter finding indicates the lesion is likely to be benign, even though there is cortical breakthrough. Although less sensitive to the detection of calcification, MRI may also be used to determine the extent of this lesion. The appearance of osteoblastoma on MRI will vary depending on the degree of sclerosis within the lesion. A combination of low and intermediate signal intensity is seen on T1-weighted images and mixed, intermediate and high signal intensity on T2-weighted images (193,194) (Fig. 9.48). MRI may be used to demonstrate subtle violation of cortical bone and extension into an adjacent joint (Fig. 9.48). A circumferential shell of bone may appear as a low signal intensity rim. Reactive edema and inflammation may be seen adjacent to the tumor within soft tissue or in the marrow space. In one reported case, reactive inflammation within adjacent bone and soft tissue obscured the tumor on MRI and CT was required for accurate localization (195).

MALIGNANT BONE TUMORS

Chondrosarcoma

Chondrosarcoma may arise *de novo* in a previously normal bone (primary form) or develop from a preexisting benign cartilage tumor such as an osteochondroma or enchondroma (secondary form). Chondro-

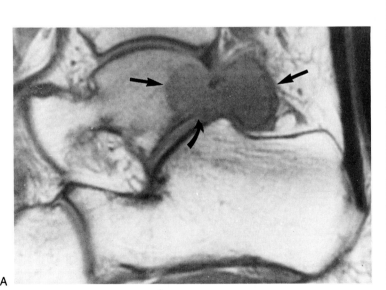
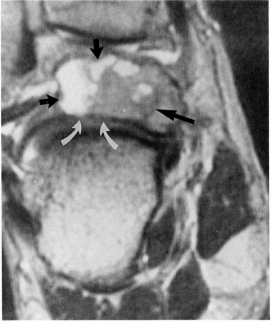

FIG. 9.48. Osteoblastoma. **A:** Sagittal MR TR/TE 800/20 image reveals an intermediate signal intensity mass within the posterior talus, extending into the posterior soft tissues (*arrows*). There is extension into the talocalcaneal joint with loss of the subchondral bone of the posterior talar facet (*curved arrow*). **B:** Coronal MR TR/TE 2100/80 image. Medially, the lesion is nearly isointense with the marrow space (*long arrow*). High signal intensity predominates at the lateral aspect of the lesion (*short arrows*). The subchondral bone of the posterior talar facet is eroded (*curved arrows*). (Courtesy of Lynne Steinbach, M.D., San Francisco, CA.)

A

B

sarcoma is categorized as "central" if it arises within the medullary space and "peripheral" if it arises near the bone surface. Chondrosarcoma may occur at any age but is most often diagnosed in patients between 30 and 60 years of age. The most frequent sites of involvement are the pelvis, femur, and shoulder girdle (132,134). Chondrosarcoma uncommonly affects the distal tibia and fibula, and is rare in the bones of the foot (196–198). The complaint of pain may be a useful sign, as uncomplicated, benign cartilage tumors are not painful. However, peripheral chondrosarcomas are often painless, and pelvic lesions often grow to a large size before becoming clinically evident. Recent enlargement of a previously stable osteochondroma is a useful sign of possible malignant transformation. The clinical behavior and radiographic appearance of chondrosarcoma vary greatly depending on both the histologic grade and location of the tumor. A low grade chondrosarcoma may appear benign radiographically and may be difficult to distinguish from enchondroma histologically (132). High grade chondrosarcomas tend to be locally aggressive and metastasize. The histologic grade of the tumor correlates well with the prognosis and determines whether a wide or radical excision is performed.

The radiographic appearance of chondrosarcoma varies widely depending on the grade of the tumor. It usually appears as a lobulated, lytic lesion and roughly two-thirds of chondrosarcomas contain calcification. Depending on the grade of the lesion, the margin may be poorly defined and there may be cortical destruction, soft tissue extension, or transarticular spread. Radiographic signs of a low grade chondrosarcoma include widespread or uniformly distributed rings or spicules of calcification. High grade lesions tend to contain faint, amorphous calcification and tend to be largely noncalcified (199).

On MRI, a well-differentiated chondrosarcoma reveals a lobular, fairly homogeneous pattern of low signal intensity on T1-weighted images and high signal intensity on T2-weighted images with intervening, low signal intensity fibrous septae (161) (Fig. 9.49). Higher grade chondrosarcomas contain less hyaline cartilage matrix and, as a result, may reveal a mixed pattern of intermediate signal intensity on both T1- and T2-weighted images. Areas of calcification may not be recognized on MRI.

Osteosarcoma

Osteosarcoma is a malignant tumor of bone in which the sarcomatous stromal tumor cells directly form os-

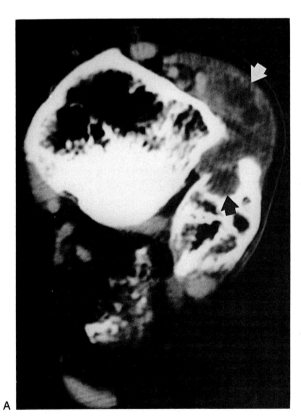 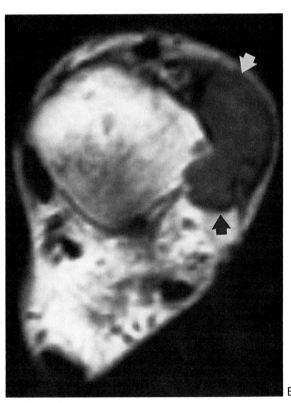

FIG. 9.49. Chondrosarcoma arising in patient with multiple enchondromas. **A:** Axial CT reveals a lytic lesion within the distal fibula, extending into the anterior soft tissues (*arrows*). **B:** Axial MR TR/TE 600/20 **(C)** TR/TE 2000/80 images reveal a lobulated mass with low signal intensity in **B** and high signal intensity in **C**, extending from the distal fibula into the adjacent soft tissues (*arrows*). (Courtesy of Daniel Vanel, M.D., Villejuif, France.)

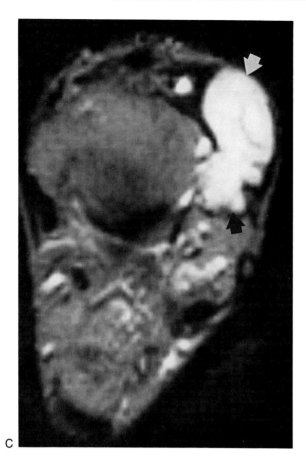

C

FIG. 9.49. (*Continued*)

teoid and immature bone. Its peak incidence is in the second decade of life and approximately one-half of osteosarcomas occur about the knee. Approximately 2% of osteosarcomas occur in the distal tibia or fibula, and roughly 1% arise in the bones of the foot (1,132,200). The tarsal and metatarsal bones are usually affected. Osteosarcoma occurs as a variety of intramedullary and juxtacortical forms, and is also classified into several histologic subtypes. The rate of tumor growth, degree of bone destruction, and clinical manifestations vary widely among these different forms. Whenever possible, patients are treated by limb salvage surgery or with a limited amputation (200,201). In the foot, a Syme amputation (disarticulation of the ankle joint) is performed if the fat pad of the heel and dorsal skin of the ankle are free of tumor. More distal lesions may be successfully managed with digital or transmetatarsal amputation. These procedures usually give excellent functional results (200).

On radiographs, intramedullary osteosarcoma usually appears as a sclerotic lesion with varying degrees of osteolysis. It should be noted that up to 13% of osteosarcomas may appear purely lytic, usually representing the telangiectatic variety (202). Staging of osteosarcoma is best accomplished with MRI (203–206). Intramedullary osteosarcoma usually reveals low signal intensity on T1-weighted images. High signal

intensity or a mixture of high and low signal intensity are seen on T2-weighted images. Osteoblastic lesions produce very low signal intensity on all pulse sequences due to the presence of tumor bone. Soft tissue extension of tumor usually reveals high signal intensity on T2-weighted images (205).

The intramedullary extent, soft tissue component, and relationship of tumor to the open epiphysis are most accurately delineated with MRI (203,204) (Fig. 9.50). The excellent accuracy of MRI is due to its high tissue contrast and multiplanar imaging capability. The extent of marrow involvement in osteosarcoma as revealed by MRI is accurate within several millimeters (203). Cortical involvement is best identified on cross-sectional images and may be evident on either T1- or T2-weighted images. Cortical bone may be difficult to evaluate, however, when it takes an angled or oblique course relative to the plane of section. Detection of soft tissue extent is important in staging, as the greatest longitudinal extension of an osteosarcoma may be its extraosseous component (203). When a long bone is involved, MRI is a sensitive means of detecting skip metastases. The direct longitudinal imaging capability of MRI is especially useful in assessing the relation of tumor to the epiphyseal plate or joint and in detecting unsuspected skip metastases in the proximal medullary space. The compartmental extent of tumor is best

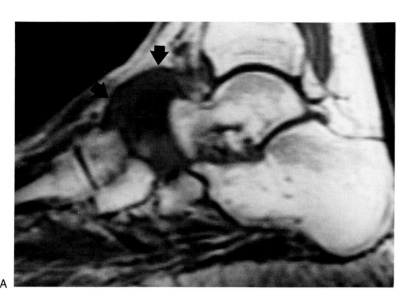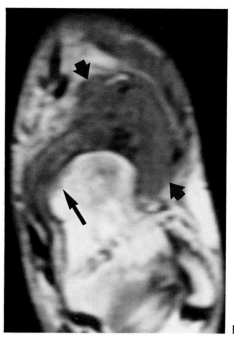

FIG. 9.50. Osteosarcoma. **A:** Sagittal MR, TR/TE 600/25 reveals a low signal intensity mass extending into the dorsal soft tissue from the navicular (*arrows*). **B:** Axial MR, TR/TE 600/25 image reveals the low signal intensity tumor (*short arrows*) and subtle extension into the head of the talus (*long arrow*). (Courtesy of Allan M. Haggar, M.D., Detroit, MI.)

shown on T2-weighted cross-sectional images (axial plane in the ankle, coronal plane in the foot) (204,205). CT is more sensitive in determining cortical disruption and in detecting calcification or ossification (205,206).

Ewing's Sarcoma

Ewing's sarcoma is a primitive malignant tumor of bone that predominantly occurs between the ages of 5 and 30 years. The bones of the lower extremity or pelvis are involved in roughly two-thirds of patients

(1,132). The foot and ankle are uncommon sites of involvement. In addition to local pain and swelling, patients often present with systemic signs and symptoms, including fever and leukocytosis. These clinical findings often suggest osteomyelitis. Advances in therapy have improved the prognosis in Ewing's sarcoma. A cure rate as high as 80% has been predicted in patients who have undergone surgical resection preceded by chemotherapy and irradiation (132). A poor prognosis is associated with metastatic disease and an inverse relationship has been postulated between tumor volume and prognosis (132). Those with localized lesions

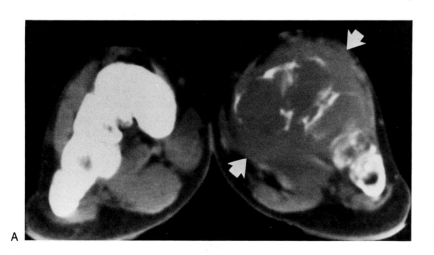

FIG. 9.51. Ewing's sarcoma. **A:** Coronal CT reveals a large soft tissue mass (*arrows*) associated with near complete destruction of the cuneiform bones and cuboid.

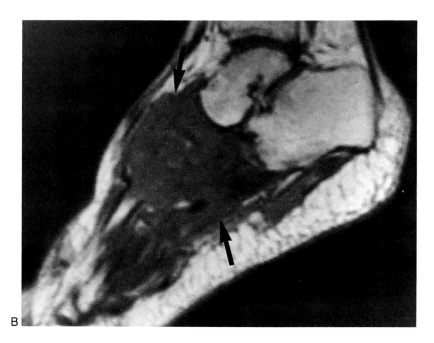

FIG. 9.51. (*Continued*) **B:** Sagittal MR TR/ TE 600/20, a low signal intensity mass (*arrows*) has destroyed the bones of the mid-foot.

and lesions involving the distal extremity usually have a more favorable course (132). For Ewing's sarcoma occurring in the foot, calcaneal lesions have a poor prognosis, whereas metatarsal lesions tend to fare well (207).

Radiographically, Ewing's sarcoma typically appears as a permeative, destructive lesion with periosteitis, poorly defined margins, and an associated soft tissue mass. This soft tissue mass is often quite prominent, as Ewing's sarcoma is a notoriously aggressive tumor with a propensity to invade local tissue (Fig.

9.51). This extraosseous component often undergoes hemorrhage and cystic degeneration (132). A sclerotic component is often present, representing reactive bone deposited on fragments of necrotic bone, perhaps related to the tumor outgrowing its blood supply (208). In some cases, a benign-looking honeycomb appearance may be seen.

On MRI, Ewing's sarcoma is capable of producing a variety of patterns of signal intensity depending on the presence of sclerosis or hemorrhage. MRI is superior to CT in documenting the extent of this aggres-

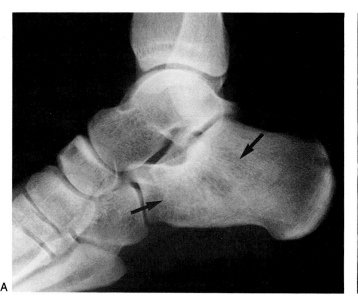

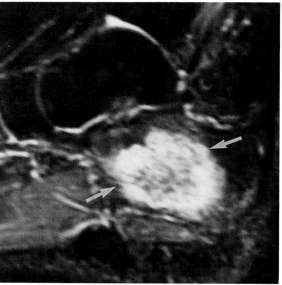

FIG. 9.52. Ewing's sarcoma. **A:** Lateral radiograph reveals a mixed lytic and sclerotic lesion of the calcaneus (*arrows*). **B:** Sagittal MR STIR (2000/43/160) image reveals a high signal intensity lesion with small foci of low signal intensity within the calcaneus (*arrows*). (*Figure continues on next page.*)

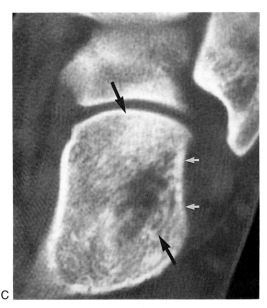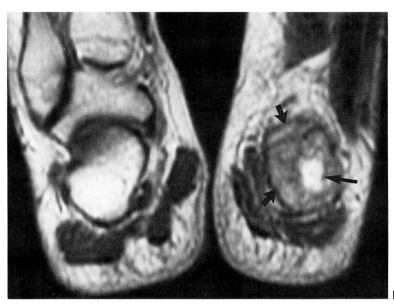

C   D

FIG. 9.52. (*Continued*) **C:** Coronal CT reveals a lytic/sclerotic lesion (*long arrows*) with partial resorption of the lateral cortex (*short arrows*). **D:** Coronal MR, TR/TE 2000/80 reveals a low signal intensity lesion filling the calcaneus (*short arrows*), with a focal region of high signal intensity (*long arrow*). There is no soft tissue extension. (Courtesy of Randall M. Patten, M.D., Kirkland, WA.)

sive tumor (209). Although CT is more sensitive to subtle cortical erosion, MRI is particularly useful in documenting the presence and extent of soft tissue involvement or in excluding soft tissue extension (209) (Fig. 9.52).

Metastatic Disease

Osseous metastases are rare in the foot. They are most commonly due to genitourinary, colorectal, and lung malignancies (210–212). The calcaneus, metatar-

sals, and phalanges are affected most often. Involvement of multiple bones has been reported in 32% of cases (211). Patients usually complain of pain, tenderness, and swelling. Metastases to the foot are usually associated with widespread metastatic disease and the average length of survival is between 10 and 15 months. Amputation of a phalanx, digit, or ray is recommended for solitary phalangeal or metatarsal lesions when the expected period of survival exceeds a few months (210).

On radiographs, an aggressive pattern of osteolytic destruction is typical (211). MRI is of limited value in

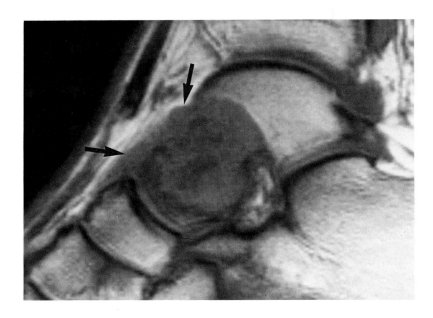

FIG. 9.53. Malignant melanoma metastatic to the talus. A sagittal MR, TR/TE: 500/20 image reveals a low signal intensity lesion of the talus with disruption of dorsal cortical bone and soft tissue extension (*arrows*).

these patients, although determination of lesion extent may be useful when amputation, local irradiation, or excision are planned The MRI characteristics of metastatic disease are nonspecific and lesions often demonstrate an aggressive pattern of growth (Fig. 9.53).

REFERENCES

1. Dahlin, DC and Unni, KK, *Bone Tumors. General Aspects and Data on 8,542 Cases.* 4th ed. 1986, Charles C. Thomas: Springfield, IL.
2. Enneking, WF, *Musculoskeletal Tumor Surgery.* 1983, Churchill Livingstone: New York.
3. Harrelson, JM, *Tumors of the foot,* in *Disorders of the Foot & Ankle,* MH Jahss, Editor. 1991, W.B. Saunders: Philadelphia. p. 1654–1677.
4. Bloem, JL, Bluemm, RG, Taminiau, AHM, et al., *Magnetic resonance imaging of primary malignant bone tumors.* Radiographics, 1987. 7: p. 425–445.
5. Bloem, JL, Taminiau, AHM, Eulderink, F, et al., *Radiographic staging of primary bone sarcoma: MR imaging, scintigraphy, angiography, and CT correlated with pathologic examination.* Radiology, 1988. 169: p. 805–810.
6. Bohndorf, K, Reiser M, Lochner B, et al., *Magnetic resonance imaging of primary tumours and tumour-like lesions of bone.* Skeletal Radiol, 1986. 15: p. 511–517.
7. Pettersson, H, Gillespy, TI, Hamlin, DJ, et al. *Primary musculoskeletal tumors: Examination with MR imaging compared with conventional modalities.* Radiology, 1987. 164: p. 237–241.
8. Tehranzadeh, J, Mnaymneh, W, Ghavam, C, et al., *Comparison of CT and MR imaging in musculoskeletal neoplasms.* J Comput Assist Tomogr, 1989. 13: p. 466–472.
9. Sundaram, M and McGuire, MH, *Computed tomography or magnetic resonance for evaluating the solitary tumor or tumor-like lesion of bone?* Skeletal Radiol, 1988. 17: p. 393–401.
10. Aisen, AM, Martel, W, Braunstein, EM, et al., *MRI and CT evaluation of primary bone and soft-tissue tumors.* AJR, 1986. 146: p. 749–756.
11. Demas, BE, Heelan, RT, Lane, J, et al., *Soft-tissue sarcomas of the extremities: Comparison of MR and CT in determining the extent of disease.* AJR, 1986. 150: p. 615–620.
12. Petasnick, JP, Turner, DA, Charters, JR, et al., *Soft-tissue masses of the locomotor system: Comparison of MR imaging with CT.* Radiology, 1986. 160: p. 125–133.
13. Sundaram, M, McGuire, MH, and Herbold, DR, *Magnetic resonance imaging of soft tissue masses: An evaluation of fifty-three histologically proven tumors.* Magn Reson Imaging, 1988. 6: p. 237–248.
14. Totty, WG, Murphy, WA, and Lee, JKT, *Soft-tissue tumors: MR imaging.* Radiology, 1986. 160: p. 135–141.
15. Shuman, WP, Patten, RM, Baron, RL, et al., *Comparison of STIR and spin-echo MR imaging at 1.5T in 45 suspected extremity tumors: Lesion conspicuity and extent.* Radiology, 1991. 179: p. 247–252.
16. Berquist, TH, Ehman, RL, King, BF, et al., *Value of MR imaging in differentiating benign from malignant soft-tissue masses: Study of 95 lesions.* AJR, 1990. 155: p. 1251–1255.
17. Kransdorf, MJ, Jelinek, JS, Moser, RPJ, et al., *Soft-tissue masses: Diagnosis using MR imaging.* AJR, 1989, 153: p. 541–547.
18. Reuther, G and Mutschler, W, *Detection of local recurrent disease in musculoskeletal tumors: Magnetic resonance imaging versus computed tomography.* Skeletal Radiol, 1990. 19: p. 85–90.
19. Vanel, D, Lacombe, MJ, Covanet, D, et al., *Musculoskeletal tumors: Follow-up with MR imaging after treatment with surgery and radiation therapy.* Radiology, 1987. 164: p. 243–245.
20. Holscher, HC, Bloem, JL, Nooy, MA, et al., *The value of MR imaging in monitoring the effect of chemotherapy on bone sarcomas.* AJR, 1990. 154: p. 763–769.
21. Lemmi, MA, Fletcher, BD, Marina, NM, et al., *Use of MR imaging to assess results of chemotherapy for Ewing sarcoma.* AJR, 1990. 155: p. 343–346.
22. Pan, G, Raymond, AK, Canasco, CH, et al., *Osteosarcoma MR imaging after preoperative chemotherapy.* Radiology, 1990. 174: p. 517–526.
23. Sanchez, RB, Quinn, SF, Walling, A, et al., *Musculoskeletal neoplasms after intraarterial chemotherapy: Correlation of MR images with pathologic specimens.* Radiology, 1990. 174: p. 237–240.
24. Erlemann, R, Reiser, MF, Peters, PE, et al., *Musculoskeletal neoplasms: Static and dynamic Gd-DTPA-enhanced MR imaging.* Radiology, 1989. 171: p. 767–773.
25. Erlemann, R, Sciuk, J, Bosse, A, et al., *Response of osteosarcoma and Ewing sarcoma to preoperative chemotherapy: Assessment with dynamic and static MR imaging and skeletal scintigraphy.* Radiology, 1990. 175: p. 791–796.
26. Sundaram, M, McGuire, MH, Herbold, DR, et al., *Magnetic resonance imaging in planning limb-salvage surgery for primary malignant tumors of bone.* J Bone Joint Surg, 1986. 68A: p. 809–819.
27. Sundaram, M and McLeod, RA, *MR imaging of tumor and tumor-like lesions of bone and soft tissue.* AJR, 1990. 155: p. 817–824.
28. Enneking, WF, Spanier, SS, and Goodman, MA, *A system for the surgical staging of musculoskeletal sarcoma.* Clin Orthop, 1980. 153: p. 106–120.
29. Kinsella, TJ, Loeffler, JS, Fraass, BA, et al., *Extremity preservation by combined modality therapy in sarcomas of the hand and foot: An analysis of local control, disease free survival and functional result.* Int J Radiat Oncol Biol Phys, 1983. 9: p. 1115–1119.
30. Owens, JC, Shiu, MH, Smith, R, et al., *Soft tissue sarcomas of the hand and foot.* Cancer, 1985. 55: p. 2010–2018.
31. Selch, MT, Kopald, KH, Ferreiro, GA, et al., *Limb salvage therapy for soft tissue sarcomas of the foot.* Int J Radiat Oncol Biol Phys, 1990. 19: p. 41–48.
32. Simon, MA and Enneking, WF, *The management of soft-tissue sarcomas of the extremities.* J Bone Joint Surg, 1976. 58A: p. 317–327.
33. Collin, C, Godbold, J, Hajdu, S, et al., *Localized extremity soft tissue sarcoma: An analysis of factors affecting survival.* J Clin Oncol, 1987. 5: p. 601–612.
34. Kirby, EJ, Shereff, MJ, and Lewis, MM, *Soft-tissue tumors and tumor-like lesions of the foot.* J Bone Joint Surg, 1989. 71A: p. 621–626.
35. Berlin, SJ, *A laboratory review of 67,000 foot tumors and lesions.* J Am Podiatr Assoc, 1984. 74: p. 341–347.
36. Richter, GM, Ernst, HU, Dinkel, E, et al., *Morphologie und diagnostik von knochen tumoren des fusses.* Radiologe, 1986. 26: p. 341–352.
37. McLeod, RA, *Bone and soft tissue neoplasms,* in *Radiology of the Foot and Ankle,* TH Berquist, Editor. 1988, Raven Press: New York.
38. Enzinger, FM and Weiss, SW, *Soft Tissue Tumors.* 2nd ed. 1988, CV Mosby: St. Louis.
39. Allen, PW and Enzinger, FM, *Hemangiomas of skeletal muscle: An analysis of 89 cases.* Cancer, 1972. 29: p. 8–22.
40. Tubiolo, AJ, Jones, RH, and Chalker, DK, *Cavernous hemangioma of the plantar forefoot. A literature review and case report.* J Am Podiatr Med Assoc, 1986. 76: p. 164–167.
41. Berlin, SJ, *Hemangioma of the foot. Report of four cases and review of the literature.* J Am Podiatr Assoc, 1970. 60: p. 63–75.
42. Borden, JI and Shea, TP, *Cavernous hemangioma of the foot. A case report and review.* J Am Podiatr Assoc, 1976. 66: p. 484–490.
43. Cohen, AJ, Youkey, JR, Clagett, GP, et al., *Intramuscular hemangiomas.* JAMA, 1983. 249: p. 2680–2683.
44. Buetow, PC, Kransdorf, MJ, Moser, RPJ, et al., *Radiologic appearance of intramuscular hemangioma with emphasis on MR imaging.* AJR, 1990. 154: p. 563–567.
45. Cohen, EK, Kressel, HY, Perosio, T, et al., *MR imaging of soft-tissue hemangiomas: Correlation with pathologic findings.* AJR, 1988. 150: p. 1079–1081.

46. Hawnaur, JM, Whitehouse, RW, Jenkins, JPR, *et al.*, *Musculoskeletal haemangiomas: Comparison of MRI with CT.* Skeletal Radiol, 1990. **19**: p. 251–258.

47. Kaplan, PA and Williams, SM, *Mucocutaneous and peripheral soft-tissue hemangiomas: MR imaging.* Radiology, 1987. **163**: p. 163–166.

48. Nelson, MC, Stull, MA, Teitelbaum, GP, *et al.*, *Magnetic resonance imaging of peripheral soft tissue hemangiomas.* Skeletal Radiol, 1990. **19**: p. 477–482.

49. Yuh, WTC, Kathol, MH, Sein, MA, *et al.*, *Hemangiomas of skeletal muscle: MR findings in five patients.* AJR, 1987. **149**: p. 765–768.

50. Steinhart, A, *Lower extremity soft-tissue tumors of adipose tissue,* in *Neoplasms of the Foot and Leg,* DR Cole and TM DeLauro, Editors. 1990, Williams & Wilkins: Baltimore. p. 143–149.

51. Booher, RJ, *Lipoblastic tumors of the hands and feet.* J Bone Joint Surg, 1965. **47A**: p. 727–740.

52. Nixon, HH and Scobie, WG, *Congenital lipomatosis: A report of four cases.* J Pediatr Surg, 1971. **6**: p. 742–745.

53. Kransdorf, MJ, Moser, RPJ, Meis, JM, *et al.*, *Fat-containing soft-tissue masses of the extremities.* Radiographics, 1991. **11**: p. 81–106.

54. Bush, CH, Spanier, SS, and Gillespy III, T, *Imaging of atypical lipomas of the extremities: Report of three cases.* Skeletal Radiol, 1988. **17**: p. 472–475.

55. Sundaram, M, Baran, G, Merenda, G, *et al.*, *Myxoid liposarcoma: Magnetic resonance imaging appearances with clinical and histologic correlation.* Skeletal Radiol, 1990. **19**: p. 359–362.

56. Allen, RA, Woolner, LB, and Ghormley, RK, *Soft tissue tumors of the sole. With special reference to plantar fibromatosis.* J Bone Joint Surg, 1955. **37A**: p. 14–26.

57. Aviles, E, Arlen, M, and Miller, T, *Plantar fibromatosis.* Surgery, 1971. **69**: p. 117–120.

58. Alexander, IJ, Johnson, KA, Shires, TC, *et al.*, *Aggressive fibromatosis of the plantar aspect of the foot. A case report.* Bull Hosp Joint Dis Orthop Instit, 1987. **47**: p. 103–108.

59. Wetzel, LH and Levine, E, *Soft-tissue tumors of the foot: Value of MR imaging for specific diagnosis.* AJR, 1990. **155**: p. 1025–1030.

60. Griffiths, HJ, Robinson, K, and Bonfiglio, TA, *Aggressive fibromatosis.* Skeletal Radiol, 1983. **9**: p. 179–184.

61. Hunt, RTN, Morgan, HC, and Ackerman, LV, *Principles in the management of extraabdominal desmoids.* Cancer, 1960. **13**: p. 825–836.

62. Rock, MG, Pritchard, DJ, Reiman, HM, *et al.*, *Extraabdominal desmoid tumors.* J Bone Joint Surg, 1984. **66A**: p. 1369–1374.

63. Sundaram, M, McGuire, MH, and Schajowicz, F, *Soft-tissue masses: Histologic basis for decreased signal (short T2) on T2-weighted MR images.* AJR, 1987. **148**: p. 1247–1250.

64. Kransdorf, MJ, Jelinek, JS, Moser, RPJ, *et al.*, *Magnetic resonance appearance of fibromatosis. A report of 14 cases and review of the literature.* Skeletal Radiol, 1990. **19**: p. 495–500.

65. Quinn, SF, Erickson, SJ, Dee, PM, *et al.*, *MR imaging in fibromatosis: Results in 26 patients with pathologic correlation.* AJR, 1991. **156**: p. 539–542.

66. Hawnaur, JM, Jenkins, JPR, and Isherwood, I, *Magnetic resonance imaging of musculoaponeurotic fibromatosis.* Skeletal Radiol, 1990. **19**: p. 509–514.

67. Stewart, D and Abrahamson, HF, *Fibrous tumors of the foot and leg,* in *Neoplasms of the Foot and Leg,* DR Cole and TM DeLauro, Editors. 1990, Williams & Wilkins: Baltimore. p. 120–143.

68. Chung, EB and Enzinger, FM, *Fibroma of tendon sheath.* Cancer, 1979. **44**: p. 1945–1954.

69. Das Gupta, TK, *Tumors of the Soft Tissues.* 1983, Appleton-Century-Crofts: Norwalk.

70. Mahajan, H, Kim, EE, Wallace, S, *et al.*, *Magnetic resonance imaging of malignant fibrous histiocytoma.* Magn Reson Imaging, 1989. **7**: p. 283–288.

71. Wetzel, LH, Levine, E, and Murphy, MD, *A comparison of MR imaging and CT in the evaluation of musculoskeletal masses.* Radiographics, 1987. **7**: p. 851–874.

72. Wu, K, *Fibrosarcoma of the foot.* J Foot Surg, 1987. **26**: p. 530–534.

73. Stull, MA, Moser, RPJ, Kransdorf, MJ, *et al.*, *Magnetic resonance appearance of peripheral nerve sheath tumors.* Skeletal Radiol, 1991. **20**: p. 9–14.

74. Das Gupta, TK Brasfield, RD, Strong, EW, *et al.*, *Benign solitary schwannomas (neurilemomas).* Cancer, 1969. **24**: p. 355–366.

75. Hennessee, MT, Walter, JHJ, Wallace, G, *et al.*, *Benign schwannoma. Clinical and histopathologic findings.* J Am Podiatr Med Assoc, 1985. **75**: p. 310–314.

76. Klatte, EC, Franken, EA, and Smith, JA, *The radiographic spectrum in neurofibromatosis.* Semin Roentgenol, 1976. **11**: p. 17–33.

77. Cohen, LM, Schwartz, AM, and Rockoff, SD, *Benign schwannomas: Pathologic basis for CT inhomogeneities.* AJR, 1986. **147**: p. 141–143.

78. Levine, E, Huntrakoon, M, and Wetzel, LH, *Malignant nerve-sheath neoplasms in neurofibromatosis: Distinction from benign tumors by using imaging techniques.* AJR, 1987. **149**: p. 1059–1064.

79. Sartoris, DJ and Resnick, D, *Magnetic resonance imaging of podiatric disorders: A pictorial essay.* J Foot Surg, 1987. **26**: p. 336–350.

80. Burk, DLJ, Brunberg, JA, Kanal, E, *et al.*, *Spinal and paraspinal neurofibromatosis: Surface coil MR imaging at 1.5T.* Radiology, 1987. **162**: p. 797–801.

81. Glazier, GM, Williamson, MR, and Lange, TA, *MRI or peripheral neurofibromas in children.* Orthopedics, 1989. **12**: p. 269–272.

82. Ducatman, BS, Scheithauer, BW, Piepgras, DG, *et al.*, *Malignant peripheral nerve sheath tumors. A clinicopathologic study of 120 cases.* Cancer, 1986. **57**: p. 2006–2021.

83. Sordillo, PP, Helson, L, Hajdu, SI, *et al.*, *Malignant schwannoma: Clinical characteristics, survival, and response to therapy.* Cancer, 1981. **47**: p. 2503–2509.

84. Storm, FK, Eilber, FR, Mirra, J, *et al.*, *Neurofibrosarcoma.* Cancer, 1980. **45**: p. 126–129.

85. Flandry, F and Hughston, JC, *Current concepts review: Pigmented villonodular synovitis.* J Bone Joint Surg, 1987. **69A**: p. 942–949.

86. Jaffe, HL, *Tumors and Tumorous Conditions of the Bones and Joints.* 1958, Lea & Febiger: Philadelphia.

87. Dorwart, RH, Genant, HK, Johnston, WH, *et al.*, *Pigmented villonodular synovitis of synovial joints: Clinical pathologic, and radiologic features.* AJR, 1984. **143**: p. 877–885.

88. Arthaud, JB, *Pigmented nodular synovitis: Report of 11 lesions in non-articular locations.* Am J Clin Pathol, 1972. **58**: p. 511–517.

89. Byers, PD, Cotton, RE, Deacon, OW, *et al.*, *The diagnosis and treatment of pigmented villonodular synovitis.* J Bone Joint Surg, 1968. **50B**: p. 290–305.

90. Rao, AS and Vigorita, VJ, *Pigmented villonodular synovitis (Giant-cell tumor of the tendon sheath and synovial membrane). A review of eighty-one cases.* J Bone Joint Surg, 1984. **66A**: p. 76–94.

91. Granowitz, SP, D'Antonio, J, and Mankin, HL, *The pathogenesis and long-term end results of pigmented villonodular synovitis.* Clin Orthop, 1976. **114**: p. 335–351.

92. Jelinek, JS, Kransdorf, MJ, Utz, JA, *et al.*, *Imaging of pigmented villonodular synovitis with emphasis on MR imaging.* AJR, 1989. **152**: p. 337–342.

93. Kottal, RA, Vogler, JBI, Matamoros, A, *et al.*, *Pigmented villonodular synovitis: A report of MR imaging in two cases.* Radiology, 1987. **163**: p. 551–553.

94. Spritzer, CE, Dalinka, MK, and Kressel, HY, *Magnetic resonance imaging of pigmented villonodular synovitis: A report of two cases.* Skeletal Radiol, 1987. **16**: p. 316–319.

95. Fletcher, AGJ and Horn, RCJ, *Giant cell tumors of tendon sheath origin.* Ann Surg, 1951. **133**: p. 374–384.

96. Jones, FE, Soule, EH, and Coventry, MO, *Fibrous histiocytoma of synovium.* J Bone Joint Surg, 1969. **51A**: p. 76–86.

97. Lisch, R and Marczak, L, *Giant cell tumors of the tendon sheath.* J Am Podiatr Med Assoc, 1986. **76**: p. 218–220.

98. Balsara, ZN, Stainken, BF, and Martinez, AJ, *Case report. MR image of localized giant cell tumor of the tendon sheath involving the knee.* J Comput Assist Tomogr, 1989. **13**: p. 159–162.

99. Sherry, CS and Harms, SE, *MR evaluation of giant cell tumors of the tendon sheath.* Magn Reson Imaging, 1989. **7**: p. 195–201.

100. Sundaram, M, McGuire, MH, Fletcher, J, et al., *Magnetic resonance imaging of lesions of synovial origin.* Skeletal Radiol, 1986. **15**: p. 110–116.

101. Lichtenstein, L, *Tumors of the synovial joints, bursae and tendon sheaths.* Cancer, 1955. **8**: p. 816–830.

102. Milgram, JW, *Synovial osteochondromatosis. A histopathological study of thirty cases.* J Bone Joint Surg, 1977. **59A**: p. 792–801.

103. Holm, CL, *Primary synovial chondromatosis of the ankle. A case report.* J Bone Joint Surg, 1976. **58A**: p. 878–880.

104. Karlin, CA, DeSmet, AA, Neff, J, et al., *The variable manifestations of extraarticular synovial chondromatosis.* AJR, 1981. **137**: p. 731–735.

105. Norman, A and Steiner, GC, *Bone erosion in synovial chondromatosis.* Radiology, 1986. **161**: p. 749–752.

106. Sim, FH, Dahlin, DC, and Ivins, JC, *Extra-articular synovial chondromatosis.* J Bone Joint Surg, 1977. **59A**: p. 492–495.

107. Milgram, JW, *Synovial osteochondromatosis in the foot.* Bull Hosp Joint Dis Orthop Inst, 1987. **47**: p. 245–250.

108. Murphy, FP, Dahlin, DC, and Sullivan, CR, *Articular synovial chondromatosis.* J Bone Joint Surg, 1962. **44A**: p. 77–85.

109. Feldman, F, Singson, RD, and Staron, RB, *Magnetic resonance imaging of para-articular and ectopic ganglia.* Skeletal Radiol, 1989. **18**: p. 353–358.

110. McEvedy, BV, *Simple ganglia.* Br J Surg, 1962. **49**: p. 585–594.

111. Soren, A, *Pathogenesis and treatment of ganglion.* Clin Orthop, 1966. **48**: p. 173–179.

112. Wenig, JA and McCarthy, DJ, *Synovial cyst of the hallux. A case report.* J Am Podiatr Med Assoc, 1986. **76**: p. 7–12.

113. Kliman, ME, and Freiberg, A, *Ganglia of the foot and ankle.* Foot Ankle, 1982. **3**: p. 45–46.

114. Burk, DLJ, Dalinka, MK, Kanal, E, et al., *Meniscal and ganglion cysts of the knee: MR evaluation.* AJR, 1988. **150**: p. 331–336.

115. Wright, PH, Sim, FH, Soule, EH, et al., *Synovial sarcoma.* J Bone Joint Surg, 1982. **64A**: p. 112–122.

116. Bernreuter, WK, Sartoris, DJ, and Resnick, D, *Magnetic resonance imaging of synovial sarcoma.* J Foot Surg, 1990. **29**: p. 94–100.

117. DeCostar, TA, Kamps, BS, and Crowen, JP, *Magnetic resonance imaging of a foot synovial sarcoma.* Orthopedics, 1991. **14**: p. 169–171.

118. Keigley, BA, Haggar, AM, Gaba, A, et al., *Primary tumors of the foot: MR imaging.* Radiology, 1989. **171**: p. 755–759.

119. Morton, MJ, Berquist, TH, McLeod, RA, et al., *MR imaging of synovial sarcoma.* AJR, 1991. **156**: p. 337–340.

120. Berthoty D, Haghighi P, Sartoris DJ, et al., *Osseous invasion by soft-tissue sarcoma seen better on MR than CT.* AJR.

121. Wu, KK, *Tumor review. Rhabdomyosarcoma of the foot.* J Foot Surg, 1988. **27**: p. 166–171.

122. Chung, EB and Enzinger, FM, *Chondroma of soft parts.* Cancer, 1978. **41**: p. 1414–1424.

123. Zlatkin, MB, Lander, PH, Begin, LR, et al., *Soft tissue chondromas.* AJR, 1985. **144**: p. 1263–1267.

124. Luger, AM, Ansbacher, L, Farrell, C, et al., *Case report 158. Extraskeletal myxoid chondrosarcoma.* Skeletal Radiol, 1981. **6**: p. 291–297.

125. Nakashima, Y, Unni, KK, Shives, TC, et al., *Mesenchymal chondrosarcoma of bone and soft tissue. A review of 111 cases.* Cancer, 1986. **57**: p. 2444–2453.

126. Enzinger, FM, *Clear cell sarcoma of tendons and aponeurosis. An analysis of 21 cases.* Cancer, 1965. **18**: p. 1163.

127. Pavlidis, NA, Fisher, C, and Wiltshaw, E, *Clear-cell sarcoma of tendons and aponeuroses: A clinicopathologic study. Presentation of six additional cases with review of the literature.* Cancer, 1984. **54**: p. 1412–1417.

128. Jahss, MH, *Disorders of the hallux and the first ray,* in *Disorders of the Foot & Ankle: Medical and Surgical Management.* MH Jahss, Editor. 1991, W.B. Saunders: Philadelphia, p. 943–960.

129. Craigen, MAC and Anderson, EG, *Traumatic epidermal inclusion cysts due to shoe impingement: A report of two cases.* Foot Ankle, 1991. **11**: p. 239–241.

130. Percy, EC, and Telep, GN, *Anomalous muscle in the leg: Soleus accessorium.* Am J Sports Med, 1984. **12**: p. 447–450.

131. Romanus, B and Lindahl, S, *Accessory soleus muscle. A clinical and radiographic presentation of eleven cases.* J Bone Joint Surg, 1986. **68A**: p. 731–734.

132. Huvos, AG, *Bone Tumors. Diagnosis, Treatment and Prognosis.* 2nd ed. 1991, WB Saunders, Philadelphia.

133. Norman, A and Schiffman, M, *Simple bone cysts: Factors of age dependency.* Radiology, 1977. **124**: p. 779–782.

134. Mirra, JM, *Bone Tumors. Clinical, Radiologic and Pathologic Correlations.* 1989, Lea & Febiger: Philadelphia.

135. Resnick, D and Niwayama, G, *Diagnosis of Bone and Joint Disorders.* 2nd ed. 1988, WB Saunders: Philadelphia.

136. Grumbine, NA and Clark, GD, *Unicameral bone cyst in the calcaneus with pathologic fracture. A literature review and case report.* J Am Podiatr Med Assoc, 1986. **76**: p. 96–99.

137. Smith, RW and Smith, CF, *Solitary unicameral bone cyst of the calcaneus.* J Bone Joint Surg, 1974. **56A**: p. 49–56.

138. Van Linthoudt, D and Lagier, R, *Calcaneal cyst: A radiological and anatomicopathological study.* Acta Orthop Scan, 1978. **49**: p. 310–316.

139. Tsai, JC, Dalinka, MK, Fallon, MD, et al., *Fluid-fluid level: A nonspecific finding in tumors of bone and soft tissue.* Radiology, 1990. **175**: p. 779–782.

140. Hudson, TM, *Radiologic-Pathologic Correlation of Musculoskeletal lesions.* 1987, Williams & Wilkins: Baltimore.

141. Erseven, A, Garti, A, and Weigl, K, *Aneurysmal bone cyst of the first metatarsal bone mimicking malignant tumor.* Clin Orthop, 1983. **181**: p. 171–174.

142. Hertzanu, Y, Mendelsohn, DB, and Gottschalk, F, *Aneurysmal bone cyst of the calcaneus.* Radiology, 1984. **151**: p. 51–52.

143. Soreff, J, *Aneurysmal bone cyst of the talus.* Acta Orthop Scand, 1976. **47**: p. 358–360.

144. Beltran, J, Simon, DC, Levy, M, et al., *Aneurysmal bone cysts: MR imaging at 1.5T.* Radiology, 1986. **158**: p. 689–690.

145. Cory, DA, Fritsch, SA, Cohen, MD, et al., *Aneurysmal bone cysts: Imaging findings and embolotherapy.* AJR, 1989. **153**: p. 369–373.

146. Hudson, TM, Hamlin, DJ, and Fitzsimmons, JR, *Magnetic resonance imaging of fluid levels in an aneurysmal bone cyst and in anticoagulated human blood.* Skeletal Radiol, 1985. **13**: p. 267–270.

147. Munk, PL, Helms, CA, Holt, RG, et al., *MR imaging of aneurysmal bone cysts.* AJR, 1989. **153**: p. 99–101.

148. Milgram, JW, *Intraosseous lipomas: Radiologic and pathologic manifestations.* Radiology, 1988. **167**: p. 155–160.

149. Ramos, A, Castello, J, Sartoris, DJ, et al., *Osseous lipoma: CT appearance:* Radiology, 1985. **157**: p. 615–619.

150. Reig-Boix, V, Guinot-Tormo, J, Risent-Martinez, F, et al., *Computed tomography of intraosseous lipoma of os calcis.* Clin Orthop, 1987. **221**: 286–291.

151. Dooms, GC, Hricak, H, Sollitto, RA, et al., *Lipomatous tumors and tumors with fatty component: MR imaging potential and comparison of MR and CT results.* Radiology, 1985. **157**: p. 479–483.

152. Feldman, F and Johnson, A. *Intraosseous ganglion.* AJR, 1973. **118**: p. 328–343.

153. Kambolis, C, Bullough, PG, and Jaffe, HJ, *Ganglionic cystic defects of bone.* J Bone Joint Surg, 1973. **55A**: p. 496–505.

154. Schajowicz, F, Sainz, MC, and Slullitel, JA, *Juxta-articular bone cysts (intra-osseous ganglia).* J Bone Joing Surg, 1979. **61B**: p. 107–116.

155. Dungan, DH, Seeger, LL, and Mirra, JM, *Case report 555. Intraosseous ganglion cyst of the distal end of the tibia.* Skeletal Radiol, 1989. **18**: p. 385–388.

156. Campanacci, M, Baldini, N, Boriani, S, et al., *Giant-cell tumor of bone.* J Bone Joint Surg, 1987. **69A**: p. 106–113.

157. Mechlin, MB, Kricun, ME, Stead, J, et al., *Giant cell tumor of tarsal bones. Report of three cases and review of the literature.* Skeletal Radiol, 1984. **11**: p. 266–270.

158. Wold, LE, and Swee, RG, *Giant cell tumor of the small bones of the hands and feet.* Semin Diagn Pathol, 1984. **1**: p. 173–184.

159. Eckardt, JJ and Grogan, TJ, *Giant cell tumor of bone.* Clin Orthop, 1986. **204**: p. 45–58.

160. Herman SD, Mesgarzadeh, M, Bonakdarpour A, et al., *The role of magnetic resonance imaging in giant cell tumor of bone.* Skeletal Radiol 1987. **16**: p. 635–643.

161. Cohen, EK, Kressel, HY, Frank, TS, et al., *Hyalin cartilage-origin bone and soft tissue neoplasms: MR appearance and histologic correlation.* Radiology, 1988. **167**: p. 477–481.

162. Fuselier, CO, Binning, T, Kushner, D, et al., *Solitary osteochondroma of the foot: An in-depth study with case reports.* J Foot Surg, 1984. **23**: p. 3–24.

163. Wu, KK, *Tumor Review. Large osteochondroma of the foot.* J Foot Surg, 1990. **29**: p. 88–93.

164. Lee, JK, Yao, L, and Wirth, CR, *MR imaging of solitary osteochondromas: Report of eight cases.* AJR, 1987. **149**: p. 557–560.

165. Azouz, EM, Slomic, AM, Marton, D, et al., *The variable manifestations of dysplasia epiphysealis hemimelica.* Pediatr Radiol, 1985. **15**: p. 44–49.

166. Kettelkamp, DB, Campbell, CJ, and Bonfiglio, M, *Dysplasia epiphysealis hemimelica. A report of fifteen cases and a review of the literature.* J Bone Joint Surg, 1966. **48A**: p. 746–766.

167. Ho, AMW, Blane, CE, and Kling, TFJ. *The role of arthrography in the management of dysplasia epiphysealis hemimelica.* Skeletal Radiol, 1986. **15**: p. 224–227.

168. Landon, GC, Johnson, KA, and Dahlin, DC, *Subungual exostoses.* J Bone Joint surg, 1979. **61A**: p. 256–259.

169. Bloem, JL and Mulder, JD, *Chondroblastoma: A clinical and radiological study of 104 cases.* Skeletal Radiol, 1985. **14**: p. 1–9.

170. Springfield, DS, Capanna, R, Gherlinzoni, F, et al., *Chondroblastoma. A review of seventy cases.* J Bone Joint Surg, 1985. **67A**: p. 748–755.

171. Kricun, ME, Kricun, R, and Haskin, ME, *Chondroblastoma of the calcaneus: Radiographic features with emphasis on location.* AJR, 1977. **128**: p. 613–616.

172. Kahmann, R, Gold, RH, Eckardt, JJ, et al., *Case report 337. Cystic chondroblastoma of calcaneus.* Skeletal Radiol, 1985. **14**: p. 301–304.

173. Gherlinzoni, F, Rock, M, and Picci, P, *Chondromyxoid fibroma. The experience at the Instituto Ortopedico Rizzoli.* J Bone Joint Surg, 1983. **65A**: p. 198–203.

174. Van Horn, JR, and Lemmens, JAM, *Chondromyxoid fibroma of the foot. A report of a missed diagnosis.* Acta Orthop Scand, 1986. **57**: p. 375–377.

175. Mitchell, MJ, Sartoris, DJ, and Resnick, D, *The foot and ankle.* Top Magn Reson Imag, 1989. **1**: p. 57–73.

176. Bordelon, RL, Cracco, A, and Booke, MK, *Osteoid-osteoma producing premature fusion of the epiphysis of the distal phalanx of the big toe.* J Bone Joint Surg, 1975. **57A**: p. 120–121.

177. Freiberger, RH, Loitman, BS, Helpern, M, et al., *Osteoid osteoma: A report on 80 cases.* Am J Roentgenol Radium Ther Nucl Med, 1959. **82**: p. 194–205.

178. Healey, JH and Ghelman, B, *Osteoid osteoma and osteoblastoma. Current concepts and recent advances.* Clin Orthop, 1986. **204**: p. 76–85.

179. Kattapuram, SV, Kushner, DC, Phillips, WC, et al., *Osteoid osteoma:: An unusual cause of articular pain.* Radiology, 1983. **147**: p. 383–387.

180. Norman, A, Abdelwahab, IF, Buyon J, et al., *Osteoid osteoma of the hip stimulating an early onset of osteoarthritis.* Radiology, 1986. **158**: p. 417–420.

181. Sherman, MS, *Osteoid osteoma associated with changes in adjacent joint.* J Bone Joint Surg, 1947. **29**: p. 483–490.

182. Ayala, AG, Murray, JA, Erling, MA, et al., *Osteoid-osteoma: Intraoperative tetracycline-fluorescence demonstration of the nidus.* J Bone Joint Surg, 1986. **68A**: p. 747–751.

183. Ghelman, B and Vigorita, VJ, *Postoperative radionuclide evaluation of osteoid osteomas.* Radiology, 1983. **146**: p. 509–512.

184. O'Brien, TM, Murray, TE, Malone, LA, et al., *Osteoid osteoma: Excision with scintimetric guidance.* Radiology, 1984. **153**: p. 543–544.

185. Shereff, MJ, Cullivan, WT, and Johnson, KA, *Osteoid osteoma of the foot.* J Bone Joint Surg, 1983. **65A**: p. 638–641.

186. Stapor, DJ and Jacobs, RL, *Osteoid osteoma of the talus. A case study.* Bull Hosp Joint Dis Orthop Inst, 1987. **47**: p. 273–277.

187. Helms, CA, Hattner, RS, and Vogler, JBI, *Osteoid osteoma: Radionuclide diagnosis.* Radiology, 1984. **151**: p. 779–784.

188. Glass, RBJ, Poznanski, AK, Fisher, MR, et al., *Case report. MR imaging of osteoid osteoma.* J Comput Assist Tomogr, 1986. **10**: p. 1065–1067.

189. Yeager, BA, Schiebler, ML, Wertheim, SB, et al., *Case report. MR imaging of osteoid osteoma of the talus.* J Comput Assist Tomogr, 1987. **11**: p. 916–917.

190. Aisen, AM and Glazer, GM, *Diagnosis of osteoid osteoma using computed tomography.* J Comput Assist Tomogr, 1984. **8**: p. 175–178.

191. Mahboubi, S, *CT appearance of nidus in osteoid osteoma versus sequestration in osteomyelitis.* J Comput Assist Tomogr, 1986. **10**: p. 457–459.

192. McLeod, RA, Dahlin, DC, and Beabout, JW, *The spectrum of osteoblastoma.* AJR, 1976. **126**: p. 321–335.

193. Kroon, HM and Schurmans, J, *Osteoblastoma: Clinical and radiologic findings in 98 new cases.* Radiology, 1990. **175**: p. 783–790.

194. Ellis, BI, Shier, CK, Gaba, AR, et al., *Case report 538: Osteoblastoma of the second metatarsal.* Skeletal Radiol, 1989. **18**: p. 228–232.

195. Crim, JR, Mirra, JM, Eckardt, JJ, et al., *Widespread inflammatory response to osteoblastoma: The flare phenomenon.* Radiology, 1990. **177**: p. 835–836.

196. Dahlin, DC and Salvador, AH, *Chondrosarcomas of bone of the hands and feet—A study of 30 cases.* Cancer, 1974. **34**: p. 755–760.

197. Lewis, MM, Marcove, RC, and Bullough, PG, *Chondrosarcoma of the foot. A case report and review of the literature.* Cancer, 1975. **36**: p. 586–589.

198. Wu, KK, *Tumor review: Chondrosarcoma of the foot.* J Foot Surg, 1987. **26**: p. 449–455.

199. Rosenthal, DI, Schiller, AL, and Mankin, HJ, *Chondrosarcoma: Correlation of radiological and histological grade.* Radiology, 1984. **150**: p. 21–26.

200. Wu, KK, *Tumor review: Osteogenic sarcoma of the foot.* J Foot Surg, 1987. **26**: p. 269–271.

201. Simon, MA, *Current concepts review. Limb salvage for osteosarcoma.* J Bone Joint Surg, 1988. **70A**: p. 307–310.

202. de Santos, LA and Edeiken, B, *Purely lytic osteosarcoma.* Skeletal Radiol, 1982. **9**: p. 1–7.

203. Gillespy, TI, Manfrini, M, Ruggieri, P, et al., *Staging of intraosseous extent of osteosarcoma: Correlation of preoperative CT and MR imaging with pathologic macroslides.* Radiology, 1988. **167**: p. 765–767.

204. Redmond, OM, Stack, JP, Dervan, PA, et al., *Osteosarcoma: Use of MR imaging and MR spectroscopy in clinical decision making.* Radiology, 1989. **172**: p. 811–815.

205. Sundaram, M, McGuire, MH, and Herbold, DR, *Magnetic resonance imaging of osteosarcoma.* Skeletal Radiol, 1987. **16**: p. 23–29.

206. Seeger, LL, Eckardt, JJ, and Bassett, LW, *Cross-sectional imaging in the evaluation of osteogenic sarcoma: MR and CT.* Semin Roentgenol, 1989. **24**: p. 174–184.

207. Reinus, WR, Gilula, LA, Shirley, SK, et al., *Radiographic appearance of Ewing sarcoma of the hands and feet: Report from the Intergroup Ewing Sarcoma Study.* AJR, 1985. **144**: p. 331–336.

208. Shirley, SK, Gilula, LA, Seigal, GP, et al., *Roentgenographic-pathologic correlation of diffuse sclerosis in Ewing sarcoma of bone.* Skeletal Radiol, 1984. **12**: p. 69–78.

209. Boyko, OB, Cory, DA, Cohen, MD, et al., *MR imaging of osteogenic and Ewing's sarcoma.* AJR, 1987. **148**: p. 317–322.

210. Healey, JH, Turnbull, ADM, Miedema, B, *et al., Acrometastases. A study of twenty-nine patients with osseous involvement of the hands and feet.* J Bone Joint Surg, 1986. **68A**: p. 743–746.

211. Libson, E, Bloom, RA, Husband, JE, *et al., Metastatic tumours of bone of the hand and foot. A comparative review and report of 43 additional cases.* Skeletal Radiol, 1987. **16**: p. 387–392.

212. Zindrick, MR, Young, MP, Daley, RJ, *et al., Metastatic tumors of the foot. Case report and literature review.* Clin Orthop, 1982. **170**: p. 219–225.

MRI of the Foot and Ankle,
edited by A.L. Deutsch, J.H. Mink, and R. Kerr,
Raven Press, Ltd., New York © 1992

CHAPTER 10

Muscle Injuries

Jerrold H. Mink

While great progress has been made in the understanding of the function, pathology, and repair processes of cartilage, bone, and ligamentous tissue, there is rather scant literature regarding similar properties of skeletal muscle. This is surprising in view of the fact that muscle injuries account for half of all injuries that occur in some sports, and that they are among the most common, lingering, and disabling conditions treated by orthopedic surgeons (1). Most muscle injuries, commonly known as muscle pulls or strains, result from rapid, violent contraction of the affected muscle during an excessively forceful stretch, and they frequently occur when exercise is intense, unaccustomed, and of long duration. Although injuries to muscles and tendons have been separated into different chapters in this and other books, one should be aware that muscles and tendons are so intimately related to one another that it is best to refer to them as a musculotendinous unit (2,3). The unit is composed of a contractile element, the muscle, and a passive element, the tendon. In fact, most injuries to muscle occur at the musculotendinous junction.

Individual muscle cells are known as muscle fibers, structures that are elongated multinucleated cells spanning up to 30 cm in length. These fibers originate and terminate in an attachment to a tendon or other connective tissue. The cytoplasm of a muscle cell is known as sarcoplasm, which is divided into longitudinal threads called myofibrils. They are crossed by striations known as A, I, H, and Z bands that differ in their chemical and optical properties.

Myofilaments are substructures of the myofibrils. The thicker myofilaments are called myosin; the thinner ones are known as actin. Both types of myofilaments are crossed by Z bands creating serially repeating regions known as sarcomeres. During muscle contraction, the actin filaments are seen to slide toward the center of the sarcomere in relation to the myosin. This action brings the Z bands closer together and produces shortening of the entire muscular unit. By actively shortening, muscle is able to produce force; by contracting and resisting lengthening, muscles serve to regulate movement or decelerate motion (4).

Two types of muscle fibers have been identified (1,4,5). These types, I and II, were initially distinguished from one another on the basis of color since type I fibers are red and type II are white. These fiber types are currently separable on the basis of histochemical differences. Type I fibers are characterized by the presence of low myofibrillar adenosine triphosphatase (ATPase) activity, whereas type II fibers have high ATPase activity. Histologic analysis reveals that type I fibers have abundant mitochondria and have bulky sarcomeres. Type II fibers have electron dense granules, composed of stores of glycogen throughout their sarcoplasm. Their sarcomeres are more streamlined and their membrane system is better developed for rapid transmission of nerve impulses into the fiber. Types I and II fibers show distinctly different physiologic properties reflecting their differing structure. Type I fibers are more resistant to fatigue than type II, and have a slower contraction time. Additionally, the force per unit in a type I fiber is much less than type II. Type I fibers are therefore best adapted for prolonged activity of relatively low intensity, those involving repetitive action, postural activity, or endurance-type activity. In contrast, type II fibers have a well-developed anaerobic energy system. They are best adapted for intense activities demanding speed and strength of short duration. They rapidly generate peak tension levels that fall back to baseline more quickly than type I fibers. Because of these properties, type I fibers have been designated as slow twitch, and type II as fast twitch fibers. Fast twitch fibers dominate

J. H. Mink: Tower Musculoskeletal Imaging Center, Los Angeles, California 90048.

in those human muscles that cross two joints, such as the hamstring muscles, rectus femoris, triceps, and biceps.

Since exercise is specific for muscle fiber type, and since individuals differ in their fiber type body composition, it is possible that people may be better suited for one type of activity rather than another (5). Biopsy studies of athletes have shown a significantly higher proportion of type I fibers in long distance runners and a higher proportion of type II fibers in sprinters; the muscle fiber composition of strength-trained athletes were mixed. It does not appear, however, that exercise, endurance, or strength training programs are capable of producing any significant change in the relative percentage of type I and II fibers in the adult population.

IMAGING OF MUSCLES

Before the advent of magnetic resonance imaging (MRI), nuclear medicine techniques, ultrasound, and computed tomography (CT) were used to assess muscle disorders (6–12). Technetium-99m is successful in localizing area of muscle damage by virtue of the deposition of the nuclide into areas of injured cell membranes and accumulation of intracellular calcium. The relative degree of deposition of the nuclear agent is proportional to the extent of muscle damage and the serum creatine phosphokinase. Scintigrams are abnormal within several hours of exercise-induced muscle injury. The pattern is most intense in 24 to 48 hr and within 1 week returns to normal (7,8,9). CT has been used extensively in assessment of soft tissue tumors, tumorlike conditions, and metabolic disorders such as the muscular dystrophies (10–15). There is, however, scant evidence of its use in evaluation of acute and chronic muscle injuries. Acute strains of the hamstring group are manifest on CT as focal areas of low attenuation, most commonly occurring in the long head of the biceps femoris. These areas are thought to represent edema and inflammation rather than blood, since hematomas are hyperdense on CT (12,16,17).

While still in a relative degree of infancy, MRI has rapidly established itself as the premier imaging modality for assessment of the full spectrum of muscle injuries, tumors, and infections (12,16–38).

Normal skeletal muscle is characterized by an intermediate to long T1 relaxation time and by a short T2 relative to other soft tissues. Muscle injuries are characterized by a long T2 relaxation time, but T1 values are quite similar to normal muscle; injuries are therefore most conspicuous on T2 and even more dramatically on inversion recovery (STIR) sequences, both of which optimize contrast between normal muscle and edema/hemorrhage (17,29,34,37). T2-weighted images (T2WI), however, may fail to distinguish edema from fatty infiltration of a muscle in those cases in which the degree of edema infiltration of the muscle is only moderate in degree (39). Normally, edema becomes brighter than fat on long TR sequences, but when the edema is "mingled" with the lower signal muscle fibers, the distinction between fat and edema may not be very evident. The T2 of fat is about 60 ms, which is about twice that of muscle (30 ms). When the degree of edema within a muscle is sufficient to lengthen the muscle T2 > 60 ms, edematous muscle is easily distinguished from fat. However, when there is mild or moderate edema so that the T2 of the edematous muscle is between 30 and 60 ms, it may be impossible to distinguish fatty infiltration from edema. Inversion recovery sequences by virtue of their high contrast, high conspicuity properties do not suffer from this difficulty (39). STIR sequences have the advantage that edema-associated increases in muscle T1 and T2 times are generally additive to signal intensity, as is spin density. Unfortunately, STIR sequences are characterized by decreased signal-to-noise ratios and heightened susceptibility to flow artifacts, and they provide only a limited number of slice locations/unit time (34). They must therefore must be performed in conjunction with T1 and/or proton density sequence images for optimal anatomic delineation.

We choose to examine a suspected muscle injury by means of an extremity coil, although the body coil is used to accommodate a larger body part (e.g., the upper thigh) and examine a larger field of view (when comparison with the opposite side is necessary). An oil marker is usually placed on the skin at the site of the "mass" or the point of maximal tenderness. The first sequence performed is a short repetition time (TR) study in the coronal plane. This sequence allows one to be certain of proper centering and to localize the superficial skin marker. Short TR sequences, although they are insensitive for detection of acute muscle injury and masses, are helpful for demonstrating atrophy, for detection of related osseous lesions, for quantification of muscle volumes, for detection of subacute hemorrhage, and for assessment of abnormal muscle architecture (29). An axial T2-weighted sequence is usually performed next, employing a TR = 2500–3500, echo time (TE) = 20/120. The axial plane is ideal for determination of (a) the transverse extent of a lesion, and (b) the relationship of the lesion to the surrounding muscle groups and the neurovascular bundle. Occasionally, a STIR axial sequence is substituted for the long TR sequence. Finally, a sagittal or coronal STIR sequence (depending on the location of the lesion) is performed to describe most graphically the longitudinal extent of the lesion (29,34).

HEMATOMA AND INTERSTITIAL HEMORRHAGE

In order to understand better the MR appearance of muscle injuries, it is important to distinguish between a hematoma and interstitial hemorrhage (2,16,37,40). A hematoma refers to a confluent collection of blood within a relatively restricted area; the lesion is well defined and has a distinctly masslike character. Interstitial hemorrhage refers to bleeding that insinuates itself between the fibers of the damaged connective tissue. The girth of the affected limb and the affected muscle is increased but there is no discrete mass.

The MR appearance of a hematoma is affected by both the field strength of the MR imager as well as the stage of evolution of the mass (37,41) (Fig. 10.1). On T1WI, a hematoma less than 48 hr old has a signal intensity similar to that of muscle; on STIR studies, it is usually dark. As the lesion ages, the water content decreases and the protein content increases. Both events tend to decrease the T1 and the T2 relaxation times moderately. Therefore, a subacute or chronic hematoma (7–300 days) usually has a signal intensity quite close to that of fat on a T1-weighted image. While the tissues are affected by the presence of oxyhemoglobin, deoxyhemoglobin, and intact red cells, the observed effect of T1 shortening is due predominantly to oxydative denaturation of hemoglobin, resulting in methemoglobin production (37,42,43). Methemoglobin, containing iron in a ferric form, is highly paramagnetic. The local concentration of methemoglobin increases over the 80 to 90 hr following injury; the T1

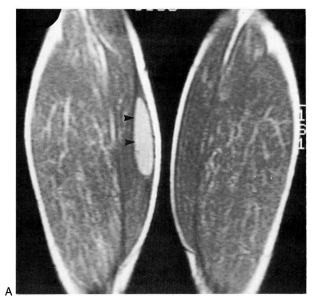

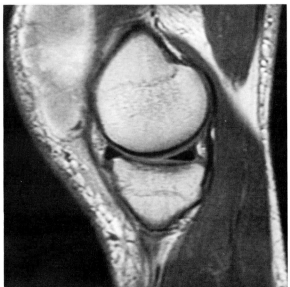

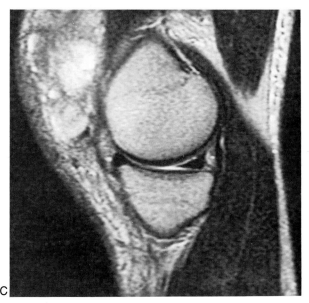

FIG. 10.1. Hemorrhage and hematoma. **A:** Coronal MR, TR/TE 300/15). This classic ovoid hematoma (*arrowheads*) in the medial head of the gastrocnemius is bright on T1WI, reflecting the characteristic short T1 of subacute lesions. **B:** Sagittal MR, TR/TE 2000/20. **C:** Sagittal MR, TR/TE 2000/80. These images are from another patient who suffered direct trauma to the leg 3 weeks prior. This hematoma has areas of high and low signal on both T1 and T2WI. The marked inhomogeneity, due to recurrent bleeding, is quite typical of a subacute hematoma. (*Figure continues on next page.*)

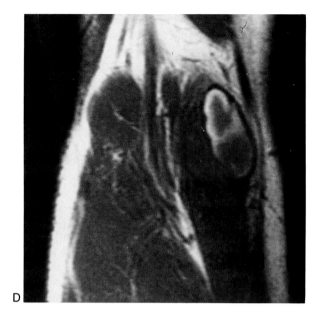

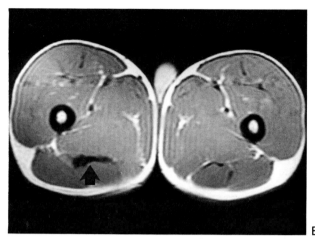

D   E

FIG. 10.1. (*Continued*) **D:** Axial MR, TR/TE 2500/80. In a different patient, another appearance of a subacute hematoma is identified. The mass in the gastrocnemius has a very dark rim due to deposition of hemosiderin. The lesion is predominantly bright, reflecting the long T2; the intermediate mass in the center represents intact red cells. **E:** Axial MR, TR/TE 2000/20. "Collapsed" hematoma following a muscle strain. The patient had suffered a muscle injury 6 months prior. In this case, the hematoma has largely resolved and the dark, hemosiderin-laden wall and fibrosis is all that remains.

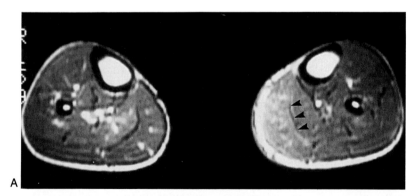

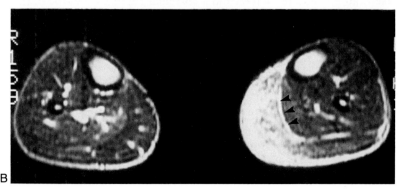

FIG. 10.2. Acute interstitial hemorrhage. **A:** Axial MR, TR/TE 2000/20. **B:** Axial MR TR/TE 2000/80. This professional football player was struck in the calf with a helmet incurring a painful, swollen calf. MR examination demonstrates abnormal signal in the medial head of the gastrocnemius (*arrowheads*). The intermediate signal on the proton density and the high signal on T2WI are consistent with edema fluid, yet the mechanism of injury and the marked discoloration of the skin that was present overwhelmingly suggests that significant blood must be present.

shortening of the hematoma parallels the time course of methemoglobin production.

While subacute hematomas characteristically demonstrate high signal on T1WI, especially along their rims, the appearance is not specific. A similar finding has been identified in some sarcomas and abscesses (33,44,45) (see Miscellaneous Muscle Disorders, below). On T2WI and occasionally T1WI, a central low intensity focus is commonly seen within a hematoma on images obtained at high field strengths. Its presence relates to preferential T2 shortening secondary to deoxyhemoglobin within intact red cells. This effect is 100 times stronger at high field strengths, and is no longer evident following lysis of the erythrocytes. Finally, the wall of a subacute/chronic hematoma is usually very dark, reflecting the presence of fibrosis and/or hemosiderin deposition (43). The residual of a long-standing hematoma whose liquid component has resorbed may be only a masslike region of decreased signal. In our experience, most hematomas do not demonstrate a "pure" appearance that precisely fits into one of the descriptions above. More commonly, considerable inhomogeneity of the lesion with a wide variety of signal intensities on both T1WI and T2WI is present, and is due to presumed repeated/continuing hemorrhage (Fig. 10.1).

The time-dependent effects of hemoglobin breakdown products on relaxation times, so important in determining the MR signal and image character in a hematoma, are much less significant in interstitial hemorrhage (16,37,40) (Fig. 10.2). In the latter, the dominant signal characteristic is one of edema rather than blood.

On a short TR sequence, interstitial hemorrhage has a signal character quite similar to that of muscle. In general, the T2 of oxygenated liquid blood is relatively long (100–200 ms) because of the high free water content relative to soft tissue. The precise reason why edema, rather than blood, dictates the signal character is unknown, but several postulates may be offered: (a) parenchymal blood incites a significant inflammatory response in adjacent tissues, quite different from a hematoma. The inflammatory reaction causes additional prolongation of T2 by further increasing the free water content (16,37). It is the inflammatory response and its attendant water increase that determines the signal, and (b) the existing cellular framework of the soft tissue alters the breakdown process and removal of blood products (37,40). MR signal in interstitial hemorrhage is affected more by the fluid than by the protein component. In summary, T1WI of both acute hematoma and acute interstitial/intraparenchymal hemorrhage demonstrates a signal similar to that of muscle. As a hematoma ages, its decreasing T1 value results in increasing signal on T1WI, whereas the T1 value for interstitial hemorrhage does not change. On T2WI, he-

matomas develop progressively decreasing T2 values, but the T2 remains sufficiently long that the lesion remains bright on T2WI. The signal of hemorrhage is not significantly affected by time; hemorrhage has an initially and persistently long T2, and remains bright on long TR sequences (17,40).

DIRECT MUSCLE INJURY

Laceration

Muscle lacerations result from penetrating injury. Although the wound itself heals rapidly, the site of the laceration is permanently characterized by a dense connective tissue scar. There is little true muscle regeneration across the scar site, and the muscle distal to the laceration shows little evidence of reinnervation (4,46). Therefore although the repair process results in reestablishment of structural continuity, restoration of function is incomplete. Only one-half of the ability of a lacerated muscle to generate tension, and two-thirds of its ability to shorten, are recovered (46). The MR appearance of a lacerated muscle is dictated by the extent of the injury (Fig. 10.3). There is typically a transverse defect in the continuity of the muscle, and the gap between the torn fibers usually fills with a combination of both blood and edema, creating a mass with mixed signal characteristics on both T1WI and T2WI. If the laceration has occurred near one end of the muscle, the tendon may also be lacerated, and in such cases the functional defect may be profound.

Contusion

A contusion of muscle is defined as a compressive- or concussive-type injury resulting from direct trauma by a blunt object. The term "charley horse" is synonymous with contusion. This type of injury is quite common in contact sports wherein the impact of one body part, often the knee, produces the injury in a large muscle, often the quadriceps. The blow results in capillary rupture and interstitial hemorrhage followed by edema and an inflammatory reaction. A contusion is differentiated from a muscular rupture by virtue of the uninterrupted ability of the muscle to function, and a contusion is differentiated from a strain by the mechanism of injury. Immediately following the injury, the affected individual may well continue to participate in the activity, but by the following day, muscle spasm sets in, leading to pain, swelling, disability, and stiffness. Contusions are graded in severity by the restriction in the range of motion of the adjacent joint (47). A mild contusion is one in which active or passive range of motion is limited by less than a third of normal. Affected patients have an average of 6 days of

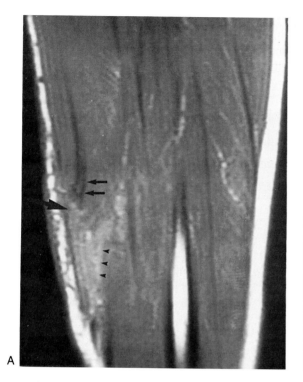

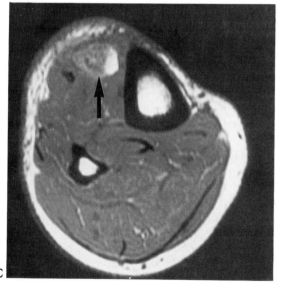

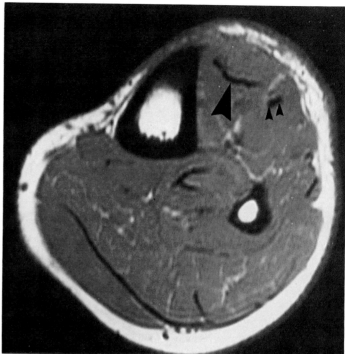

FIG. 10.3. Laceration of the anterior tibial muscle/tendon. **A:** Sagittal MR, TR/TE 600/20. There is a focal alteration in signal (*arrowheads*) of the tibialis anterior muscle. The tendon (*arrows*) is focally widened and is interrupted at the site of the laceration (*large arrow*). **B,C:** Axial MR, TR/TE 800/20; B is 2 cm above C. In B, the tibialis anterior tendon (*arrowhead*) is forming deep within the muscle on this image made above the level of the laceration. The extensor hallucis tendon (*arrowheads*) is also easily identified. In C, a mass of mixed signal (*arrow*) is seen replacing the normal tibialis anterior muscle/tendon; the mass is a mixture of blood and edema filling the site of the tear.

disability. A moderate contusion is one in which muscle spasm limits active motion to one-third to two-thirds of normal; these patients suffer disability for an average of 56 days. A severe contusion results in greater than two-thirds of loss of motion (3). Initial therapy should be directed toward limitation of the extent of the injury. Rest, ice, compression, and elevation are the mainstays of early therapy. Oral antiinflammatory agents, proteolytic agents, steroids, aspiration of the hematoma (if one has formed), ultrasound, short wave diathermy, and exercise have all been used in therapy with varying degrees of success, but the disability period does not appear to be significantly shortened in any case (47). Extended immo-

bilization is not necessarily beneficial, but the affected limb should be protected until a full range of motion is achieved. If unprotected, the individual may sustain a reinjury and further hemorrhage, and may potentially incur the development of myositis ossificans (3,46).

The MR appearance of a muscular contusion is a reflection of the composition of the inflammatory response which is edema, although surely blood, as evidenced by skin discoloration, is frequent (Fig. 10.2). It has been shown that the early posttraumatic change in muscle, caused by direct or stretch injury, is fiber swelling; the free water associated with this swelling causes the early diffuse increase in T2 (37). CT studies carried out in the hyperacute situation have confirmed this impression. The attenuation values of injured tissue are low relative to muscle, indicating that inflammation and/or edema is the major component of the muscle strain injury (12,37).

A contused muscle has four MRI characteristics: (a) the affected muscle is usually slightly increased in girth; (b) there is an increase is signal intensity within the muscle on a STIR or a long TR sequence. On short TR studies, the edema appears isointense or hypointense to muscle, and may be very difficult to distinguish from normal muscle; (c) because the inflammatory liquid is dispersed within and between the muscle fibers, the edema manifests a feathery, interstitial pattern; and (d) the integrity of the muscle is not violated; there are no significant areas of fiber disruption.

Myositis ossificans circumscripta (MO) is the localized formation of nonneoplastic heterotopic bone and cartilage in the soft tissues in proximity to bone (48). Histologically, there is rapidly proliferating mesenchymal tissue that may occasionally be mistaken for a sarcoma. Instead of orderly scar formation, osteogenesis occurs in the soft tissues. The classically described pattern of the "zoning" pattern of maturation of the cellular elements is the most important diagnostic feature. Ossification actually occurs in the interstitial blood rather than primarily in the muscle (2). The reasons proposed for the development of heterotopic ossification include unresolved blood clot, infection of the hematoma, tearing of the periosteum with seeding of cells into the hematoma, or a change in local pH. Symptoms of MO include pain, warmth, tenderness, loss of function out of proportion to the severity of the muscle contusion, and a tendency for symptoms to increase during the period in which one would expect them to decrease. Patients affected with MO present with a large firm tender mass within the contused muscle and restriction of motion of the adjacent joint. Flocculent calcification typical of MO can first be identified on conventional radiographs by 3 weeks postinjury, and by 6 weeks, structural organization is evident (Fig. 10.4). This calcification is predominantly along the periphery of the lesion. By 4 to 6 months, the bony mass will become mature, joint motion will be regained, and the mass of bone will begin to resorb (2,3). Rarely, resection of a symptomatic bony mass is necessary. Treatment consists of rest and immobilization to prevent further ossification. Proteolytic enzymes, intramuscular hyaluronidase, and radiotherapy are of little value.

The MR appearance of a muscle afflicted with MO is quite nonspecific, and has imaging characteristics quite similar to that of other types of muscle injury

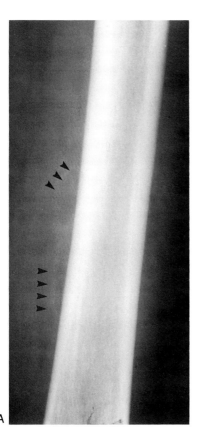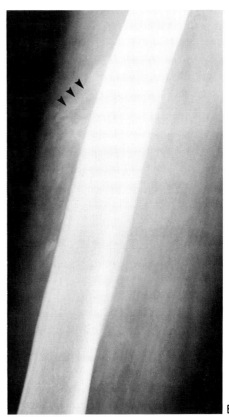

FIG. 10.4. Myositis ossificans. The patient, suffered a deep thigh bruise in a football game. **A** was made 1 month prior to **B**. Although the views are not precisely comparable, it is readily apparent that there has been a marked increase in the calcifications/ossification (*arrowheads*) occurring in the soft tissues during this rather short interval. (*Figure continues on next page.*)

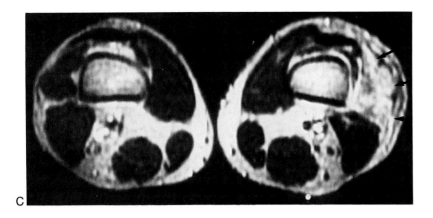

C

FIG. 10.4. (*Continued*) **C:** Axial MR, TR/TE 2000/80. This MR was obtained in another patient. The vastus lateralis muscle (*arrows*) is diffusely filled with high signal, which is mixed in character. The MR appearance of myositis ossificans is nonspecific; this biopsy-proved case of myositis ossificans has a similar appearance to that of other muscle injuries or even neoplasm. The conventional radiographs in this case showed calcifications at the time of the MR.

(Fig. 10.4). The affected muscle is often slightly enlarged in circumference, and demonstrates a diffuse increase in signal intensity on T2WI. There may be several areas of fluid confluence, suggesting hematoma formation. The conventional radiographically evident calcifications that are diagnostic of MO are generally not visible on MR.

INDIRECT MUSCLE INJURY: EXERCISE-INDUCED MUSCLE ALTERATIONS

Muscle pain is a frequent result of excessive exercise, especially following periods of relative inactivity. Several clinical syndromes characterized by muscle pain after exercise are differentiated by the time of onset of pain relative to the inciting event. Pain may begin during exercise (strain or muscle tear) or it may be delayed for 1 to 2 days (delayed onset muscle soreness).

In order to understand better exercise-related muscle injury, it is necessary to define the different types of muscle contractions. Isometric contraction produces tension without a change in length. Isotonic contraction is one in which the load is constant, and the muscle length changes during contraction. Two types of isotonic action are recognized. If the muscle shortens during contraction, a concentric action is said to have occurred; if the muscle lengthens during contraction, an eccentric action has occurred. An example of both types of isotonic muscle action can be found in the weightlifter performing a biceps-related exercise (Fig. 10.5). If a weight is placed in the hand while the arm is fully extended, and the hand is then brought up to the chest by flexing the arm at the elbow, the biceps muscle has actively shortened (concentric action). If the weight in the hand is then slowly lowered to the side, the biceps muscle is actively lengthening against resistance (eccentric action). Muscles produce greater tension when they stretch than when they shorten. Eccentric contractions are therefore capable of producing greater force than concentric actions, and are considered the primary cause of exertion-related sports injury (1,46,49). Additionally, eccentric actions, as opposed

to concentric actions, are associated with reduced oxygen consumption and less lactate production for the same power output. Eccentric muscle contractions require less energy than concentric actions for a given work load (50).

Injury prone muscles have three common characteristics: (a) they commonly perform eccentric actions. Eccentric actions of muscles are frequently those that limit, restrict, or regulate motion; for instance, some of the action of running is eccentric. Hamstring strains most frequently occur during intense bursts of speed when the hamstring is decelerating the rapidly extending knee. The muscle is therefore contracting while being forcefully lengthened; (b) they cross two joints, and they are subject to stretch at more than one site. The biceps brachii, the gastrocnemius, and the hamstring group are examples; and (c) strains are most likely to occur in those muscles used in sports or in activities requiring sudden increases or decreases in

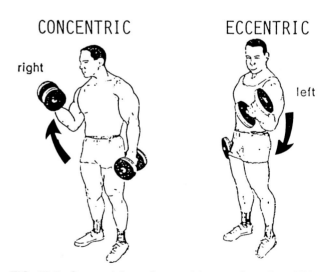

CONCENTRIC   ECCENTRIC

right

left

FIG. 10.5. Concentric and eccentric muscle action. This diagram depicts the two essential types of muscle action. In the right hand, the figure pulls the weight to his chest, and in doing so, shortens the biceps muscle. The action is termed concentric. In the left hand, the biceps lengthens while performing work, the essence of eccentric motion.

speed. These muscles commonly have a greater number of fast twitch type II fibers (49,51). While the hamstrings are the most frequently strained muscle group, the medial head of the gastrocnemius muscle, the rectus femoris, the hip adductors, and the hip flexors are commonly injured (6,46,51–59).

MRI of Physiologic Alterations in Muscle

The simplest type of exercise-induced change in muscle is found in a muscle that undergoes mild, nonexhaustive repetition (Fig. 10.6). Exercise is known to alter both the amount and distribution of water and

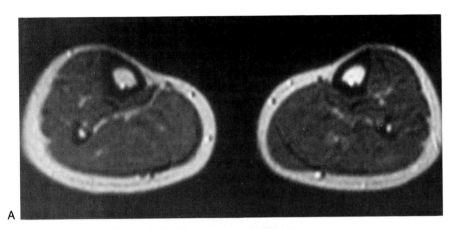

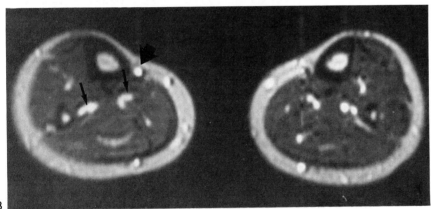

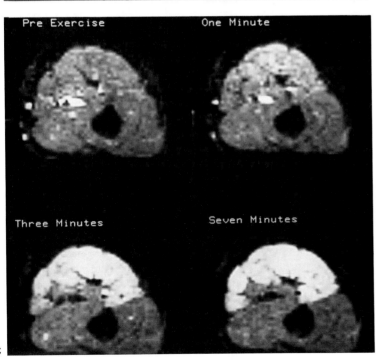

FIG. 10.6. Transient effects of exercise on muscle. **A, B:** Axial MR, TR/TE 2000/80. A is before, and B is made 5 min after jogging in place. The signal of the musculature is identical on A and B, although a "venogram effect" is identified; both the superficial (*large arrow*) and deep (*arrows*) veins become distended following exercise as seen in B. **C:** Axial MR TR/TE 2200/35/160. This patient performed a mild, nonexhaustive exercise of the biceps muscle. This case demonstrates the rapid (within 1 min) onset of signal increase (T2WI) within the muscle due to benign increases in local water concentrations. Intramuscular signal increases are transient and resolve quite quickly; imaging must be performed rapidly to detect these physiological changes.

electrolytes in muscle. Submaximal exercise transiently increases total muscle water content, and, subsequently, transient changes in tissue relaxation times can be detected by MRI in a forearm muscle that has performed as few as eight contractions (60). This initial increase in water content occurs primarily in the extracellular space, while more severe degrees of activity leads to increases in intracellular water and sodium (18,50,61). The water content in muscle increases as a result of the movement of water across the capillary wall, increased local tissue osmolality, and increased local blood flow.

Immediate postexercise T2 relaxation times increase regardless of the type of exercise (concentric vs. eccentric) that the individual performs, but T2 values for muscles that perform concentric actions are statistically significantly higher than those for muscles that perform eccentric actions (50,62). The changes in MR signal are readily detectable on images immediately following concentric, but not eccentric, muscle actions (50) (Fig. 10.7). These immediate postexercise T2 values and corresponding images of them are a reflection of the work done by muscle; MR signal increases on long TR/TE or STIR sequences correlate weakly with the level of exertion, but strongly with the mean force during exercise (18,61). In summary, the MR changes in muscle signal immediately following nonexhaustive exercise is a reflection of the work done by the muscle and the alterations in intra- and extracellular water content. The effect of local blood flow is not critical to the appearance of these changes; vascular occlusion does not prevent their appearance (18). If the exercise is submaximal and muscle damage does not occur, these transient physiologic changes, including venous dilatation, increase in muscle signal on contrast-oriented examinations and the increase in T2 values, reverts to normal within minutes of cessation of activity.

Strains

An acute strain of a muscle is defined as a painful stretch-induced injury resulting from a single applied violent force (2). An example of such an injury might be found in the sprinter who rapidly and forcefully contracts his quadriceps muscles as he pushes out from the blocks to start a race. Contusions and lacerations are a direct injury; strains have an indirect mechanism of production.

Muscle strains are typically divided into three grades that are distinguished from one another by the degree of disruption that occurs, but one should be clearly aware that it may be difficult to make this distinction reliably (2,3,29,53). A grade 1 strain is one in which there is a minor degree of tearing of the muscle fibers so that there is less than 5% of loss of motion distal to

the injury; there is no permanent defect. Pathologically, first degree strains are characterized by edema and low grade inflammation without significant muscle fiber disruption. Rest, ice, compression, and elevation are the mainstays of local therapy. A grade 2 strain is a more significant but still incomplete disruption of the muscle and is best classified as a partial tear. The clinical feature that distinguishes a first from a second degree strain is the loss of strength. Protection from further injury and proper therapy will nearly always result in rapid recovery with resolution by 10 to 14 days. A third degree strain, or complete rupture, is one in which there is extensive interruption of the muscle with a mop-end appearance of the torn edges. It is associated with a nearly complete loss of function, and therapy must be aimed at prompt restoration of the integrity of the musculotendinous unit. Spasm, retraction, and shortening occur immediately, and rapid contracture and necrosis make late repair unfeasible (2).

The direct mechanically induced injury effect of a strain on muscle is relatively minor (3,63,64). Rather, it is the subsequent biochemical response of the body to the injury that produces the histologic and clinical syndrome that is recognized as a strain. Following the injury, the affected cells self-destruct, releasing proteolytic enzymes; the exposed collagen fibers attract platelets that release further enzymes resulting in rapid breakdown of damaged muscle fibers by lysosomal proteases, free radicals, and other substances produced by macrophages. These events reach a peak several days following the exercise. Elevated temperatures, lowered pH, and other metabolic conditions further alter the situation. Eventually phagocytic inflammation, granulation tissue formation, revascularization, and complete restoration of functional myofibers occurs.

While contusions produce injury at the point of impact, strains produce a lesion at the histologic musculotendinous junction where injury to elastic, noncontractile tissue appears to be responsible for symptoms (1,46,65,66). Pain receptors are known to be most prevalent in the region of the tendon and related connective tissues; additionally, the muscle fibers nearest the tendon junction do not stretch exactly as the midportion of the muscle fiber does. It should be noted that when making reference to the musculotendinous junction, one is not referring to the macroscopic transition. In the biceps femoris, the proximal tendon and the muscle/tendon junction extend approximately 60% of the total length of the muscle; the distal tendon and muscle/tendon junction occupy 66% of the muscle length. Therefore, the anatomic and functional muscle tendon junction extend the entire length of the hamstring group, and injury can occur anywhere along the musculotendinous junction (12).

Following muscle strain, a predictable course of

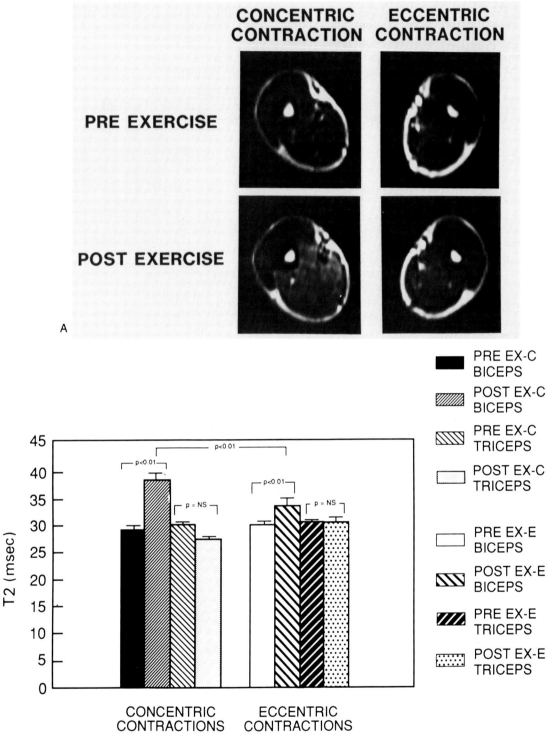

FIG. 10.7. Physiological increases in T2 following exercise. **A:** Axial MR, TR/TE 2000/80. These images are of the upper arms of a patient obtained before (*top row*) and immediately after (*bottom row*) the patient performed concentric (*left column*) and eccentric (*right column*) actions. The active muscles, the biceps and brachialis, that performed the concentric actions are differentiated easily on postexercise images by an increase in signal intensity. By comparison, little or no change occurs in signal intensity of active muscles that performed eccentric action. **B:** The graph shows T2 values of biceps and triceps measured before and after extremities performed concentric and eccentric actions (EX-C, concentric; EX-E, eccentric). (Courtesy of F. Shellock, Ph.D., Los Angeles, CA.) (From ref. 50, with permission.)

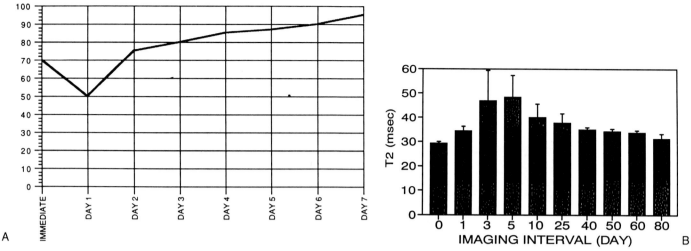

A

B

FIG. 10.8. Muscle strength and T2 after muscle strain. **A:** Muscle strain reduces muscle strength, which falls to its nadir on the first day. By the second week, function has returned to normal. **B:** The T2 of muscle following strain varies with the curve of the strength graph.

functional alterations occur (49,67,68) (Fig. 10.8). Strength decreases immediately following injury and the strained muscle is capable of generating only 70% of its normal force. At 24 hr, muscle function is at its lowest level (50% of control); recovery begins by 48 hr. The muscle is capable of generating 75% of its control contractile force by 2 days, and by 7 days, the muscle returns to near normal (90%) strength. Measurement of relaxation times of affected muscles in patients with acute strains reveal that both T1 and T2 values are prolonged to approximately two times normal. T2 values of injured muscles increase with increasing degrees of damage, perhaps related to a more extensive inflammatory/repair process and accompanying edema. The observed decrease in function is due to both an absolute decrease in the ability of the muscle to generate force and a voluntary patient component secondary to pain.

The ideal method of treating muscle strains is to prevent them, and a number of activities have been shown to decrease the incidence of such events. Proper warm-up and stretching exercises have been advocated as one method to reduce injury. Stretching increases flexibility in the lower extremity and warming up (isometric preconditioning) is of benefit in preventing muscular injury, increasing muscle contraction efficiency, and increasing the elasticity of the muscle tendon unit (46,69–71).

In contradistinction to the physiological pattern of the MR signal that accompanies exercise, patterns of injury to muscle make their appearance 24 to 48 hr after the event. The appearance of a muscle strain is dependent upon the degree of the injury and the time from injury that the MR is acquired. The MR appearance of a grade 1 strain of a muscle is similar to that of a contusion (Figs. 10.9, 10.10, 10.11). The slightly enlarged muscle has a feathery, interstitial increase in signal (long TR/TE or STIR sequence), due primarily to edema, and there is no interruption of muscle continuity (37,72). Perifascial fluid collections are com-

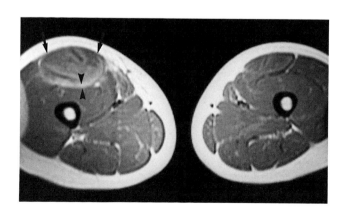

FIG. 10.9. Grade 1 strain of the rectus femoris. Axial MR, TR/TE 2000/20. This patient experienced pain in the right thigh after beginning a foot race, and underwent an MR the following morning. The rectus muscle (*arrows*) is enlarged and demonstrates a slight increase in signal. A bright perifascial rim (*arrowheads*) defines the boundary of the muscle.

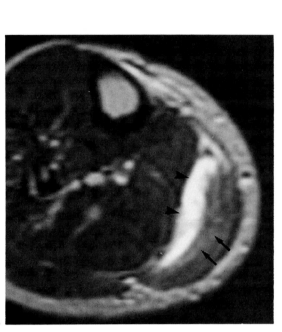
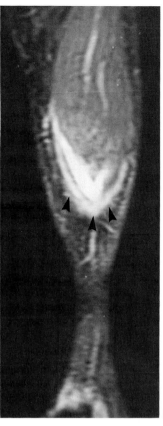

A
B

FIG. 10.10. Grade 1 muscle strain. **A:** Axial MR, TR/TE 2000/80. The gastrocnemius muscle demonstrates a mild increase in signal, but a perifascial fluid collection (*arrowheads*) is the most dramatic finding on the image. **B:** Coronal MR, TR/TE/TI 2200/35/160. *Arrowheads* define the fluid collection just deep to and distal to the gastrocnemius.

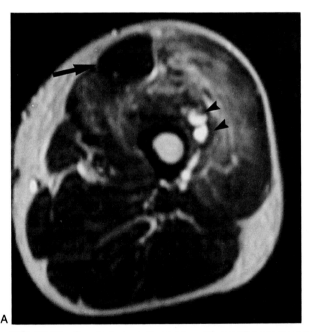
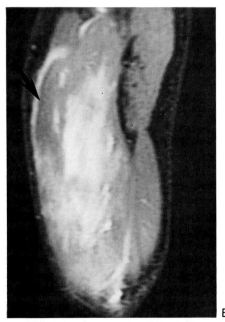

A
B

FIG. 10.11. Grade 1 muscle strain with small hematomas. **A:** Axial MR, TR/TE 2000/80. **B:** Sagittal STIR MR, TR/TE/TI 2200/35/160. This individual suffered repeated stretch injuries to the thigh. The entire vastus group is diffusely edematous. The rectus femoris (*large arrow*) is spared. Within the vastus intermedius is one, and perhaps several small focal fluid collections (*arrowheads*). These collections were bright on T1WI and are thought to represent hematomas from previous injuries. The STIR sequence is more dramatic than T2WI in demonstrating edema.

293

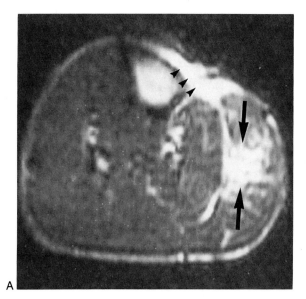
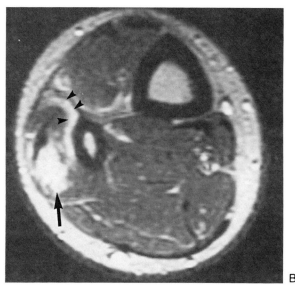

FIG. 10.12. Grade 2 strain of the gastrocnemius. **A:** This 26-year-old man suffered an acute muscle injury during a foot race. Axial MR, TR/TE 3000/80. The image demonstrates a focal stellate interruption (*arrows*) of the gastrocnemius. Focal interruption of the muscle fibers is characteristic of a grade 2 strain. A perifascial fluid collection is present just anterior to the muscle injury (*arrowheads*). **B:** Axial MR, TR/TE 2000/80. Another professional football player suffered a grade 2 strain (*arrows*) in the peroneal muscles, and there is an adjacent perifascial fluid collection (*arrowheads*).

mon. A grade 2 strain has an MR appearance that reflects the greater degree of injury (37) (Figs. 10.12, 10.13, 10.14). Physiologically, the primary difference between the grade 1 and 2 strains is the fact that in the latter, damage to the musculotendinous unit results in loss of function. The feathery MR appearance of in-

terstitial blood/edema typical of a grade 1 strain is present in the background, but additionally, a focal mass-like lesion and/or a stellate defect can inevitably be found within the injured muscle. While the MR signal character of this lesion is dictated primarily by the presence of water/edema, signal increases on short TR

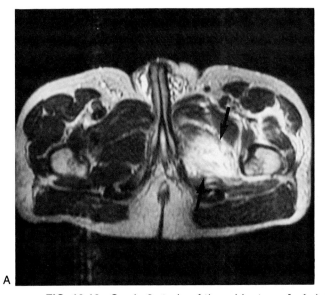
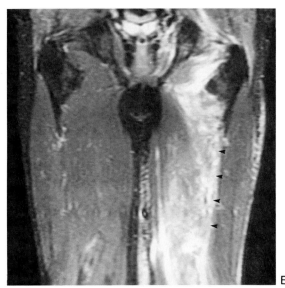

FIG. 10.13. Grade 2 strain of the adductors. **A:** Axial MR, TR/TE 2500/80. **B:** Coronal MR, TR/TE/TI 2200/35/160. This skier suffered abduction injury with the sudden onset of thigh pain. The obturator externus and the quadratus femoris (*arrows*) demonstrate diffuse edema within their substance with focal areas of apparent muscular discontinuity. The coronal sequence (B) demonstrates the full extent of the injury to the adductors (*arrowheads*).

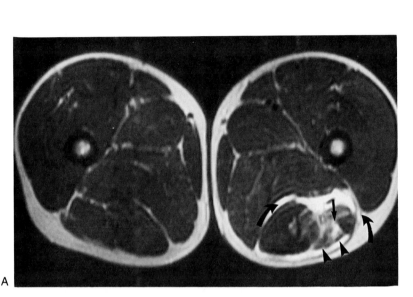

A

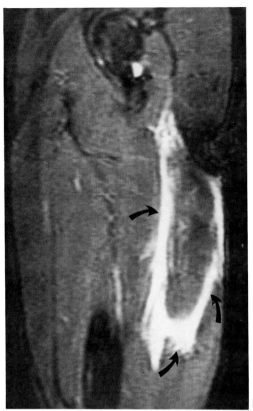

B

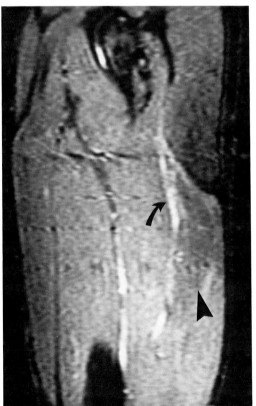

C

FIG. 10.14. Repetitive grade 2 hamstring strain. This professional football player suffered an acute hamstring strain during push-off from the line of scrimmage; the initial injury is depicted in **A** (axial MR TR/TE 2000/80) and **B** (sagittal MR, TR/TE/TI 2200/35/160). The biceps femoris muscle demonstrates edema throughout its substance (*arrowheads*) with several small focal areas perhaps representing limited muscle fiber interruption (*small arrow*) (grade 2 strain). Most striking however, is the ring of perifascial edema (*curved arrows*). **C:** Sagittal MR, TR/TE/TI 2200/35/160. Three weeks later, following conservative therapy and nearly complete rest, the ring of edema is virtually gone (*curved arrows*) and the patient was asymptomatic. The biceps muscle is slightly darker than the others, perhaps secondary to diffuse hemosiderin deposition. (*Figure continues on next page.*)

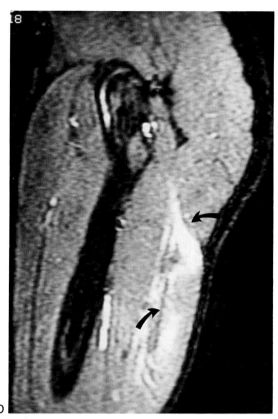 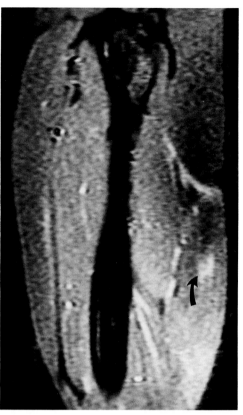

FIG. 10.14. (*Continued*) **D:** Sagittal MR, TR/TE 2200/35/160. Two weeks after C, the patient resumed working out, and again experienced the sudden onset of pain. The MR image again demonstrates intramuscular edema and perifascial fluid (*curved arrows*). **E:** Sagittal MR, TR/TE/TI 2200/35/160. The patient was again placed at rest, and 2 weeks later, a repeat MR demonstrates virtual resolution of the intramuscular and perifascial edema (*curved arrows*). While perifascial fluid collections may be rapidly mobilized if the part is protected, continued activity may lead to hematoma formation.

sequences, typical of blood, may rarely be seen (72). Depending on the age of the tear, there may either be a focal increase in the mass of the muscle, or if sufficient posttraumatic atrophy has occurred, the bulk may be decreased. Just as in the clinical situation, the imaging differentiation of grade 1 and 2 strains is often quite difficult.

Longitudinal MR examination of patients suffering first and second degree acute muscle strains reveals a predictable sequence of signal alterations (66,73). Soon after injury, there is a diffuse increase in signal within multiple muscles in the same compartment with the muscle that is in fact injured, but rapidly the pattern of injury becomes localized to those muscles that are actually injured. MR reveals that the signal increase is initially most evident within the center of the affected muscle. The signal abnormality spreads centrifugally to involve the entire muscle more homogeneously and becomes maximal by day 3 to 5. By 36 hr, a thin rim of increased signal (T2WI) appears in the perifascial space and intermuscular septa, closely applied to the injured muscle. Within the first week following injury, linear, streaky low signal alterations become evident in the fat adjacent to the injured muscle. The precise nature of these streaks is unknown, although similar lesions detected by CT have been attributed to myoglobin. If this supposition is true, the presence of these lines would indicate that the muscle injury is relatively acute. By 2 weeks, the abnormal signal within a strained muscle is often nearly resolved. However, the lesion will persist well beyond the time of clinical recovery (defined as pain-free motion). The clinical examination may therefore overestimate the degree of muscle recovery, an observation that could potentially have implications for rehabilitation programs.

The MR appearance of grade 3 strains is very striking. A definite interruption in the continuity of the entire muscle is evident. The torn edges of the muscle retract and assume a lobulated or serpiginous contour. The gap between the torn edges may fill in with blood in sufficient quantity that a true hematoma forms. Gross functional impairment necessitating surgical reconstruction usually makes MRI superfluous.

Delayed Onset Muscle Soreness

Delayed onset muscle soreness (DOMS) is defined as pain in skeletal muscle that occurs some time following unaccustomed muscular exertion (74). The clinical feature that distinguishes DOMS from strain is the time of onset of pain and dysfunction. The soreness progressively increases in intensity over the first 24 to 48 hr following exercise, peaks at 2 to 3 days, and usually resolves by 7 days (66,75). The most predictable method of producing DOMS is to have a muscle perform eccentric contractions. Although patients experience acute fatigue sooner after performing concentric rather than eccentric work, they will not develop DOMS (65,76,77).

DOMS is associated with a transient decrease in muscle performance (Fig. 10.15). This reduction is due both to reduced voluntary effort secondary to pain and a lowered inherent capacity of the muscle to produce force (68,74). There is no evidence that even repeated episodes of DOMS are associated with long-term loss of function or permanent muscle damage.

Although DOMS is quite prevalent and has been experienced by most adults on countless occasions, rather little is known about the basic cellular and biochemical mechanisms involved in its production. Possible explanations for the observed muscle soreness include accumulation of metabolic waste, structural damage, and elevated muscle temperatures (74). Muscle-based enzymes such as creatine phosphokinase (CPK) and lactic dehydrogenase (LDH) are routinely elevated in patients with DOMS, and the peak elevation of the enzymes occurs from 18 to 30 hr postexercise, the same time at which DOMS is maximal (75). Sequential muscle biopsies taken up to 1 week postexercise from the soleus muscle of individuals suffering from DOMS reveal no evidence of gross morphological fiber disruption or evidence of ischemic tissue injury. At the ultrastructural level, however, frequent myofibrillar disturbances and Z band streaming (a sign of muscle injury) is observed. Histologically, the pattern of injury and decrease in muscle function is evident immediately after exercise, when there is no soreness, but tissue damage increases over 24 to 48 hr (19,74). It remains unknown whether these findings reflect direct mechanical Z band disruption or whether they are a result of secondary activation of lysosomal enzymes producing inflammation and secondary injury, but it is clear that overloaded muscles do have their contractile machinery partially distorted. Biochemically, the injury manifests itself as an elevation of serum enzymes. Serum LDH, transaminases, and CPK activities increase in patients with DOMS, with the maximum values appearing at 8 to 24 hr postexercise (75,76). Finally, there does not appear to be any treatment for DOMS. Antiinflammatory medications, linaments, methanol, and camphor have little value in actually reducing soreness. Remarkably, performance of precisely the same motor task that caused the muscle soreness may temporarily result in alleviation of discomfort, but unfortunately, with cessation of exercise, the soreness returns.

Exertional rhabdomyolysis may be thought of as an extreme degree of DOMS that results in release of cellular contents into the general circulation (14,35,77). Pathologically, myocyte swelling, inflammation, and hyaline degeneration are present (35). Crush injuries, burns, prolonged muscular compression, toxin exposure, hypoxia, abnormalities of energy production, and extremely intense exercise, especially in hot climates, can be associated with rhabdomyolysis and even frank muscle necrosis. The diagnosis is confirmed by finding myoglobin in the urine. Patients with rhabdomyolysis experience intense pain and weakness following exercise. Acute renal failure, tetany, compartment syndromes, and disseminated intravascular coagulation may complicate rhabdomyolysis; while these complications may prove life-threatening, they fortunately are rare (74).

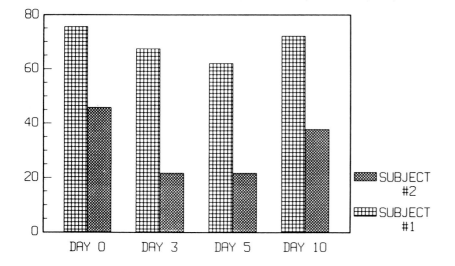

FIG. 10.15. Muscle strength during DOMS. The graph depicts the change in the ability of a muscle to produce force following DOMS. Both patients demonstrate maximal loss of muscle strength on days 3–5, and show a return to baseline strength by the second week.

The MR findings of postexercise soreness are similar to those described for grade 1 strains (Fig. 10.16). Edema within muscle bundles and perifascial fluid collections dominate the MRI. The similar appearance of muscle strains and DOMS makes it difficult to distinguish reliably between the two clinical syndromes on the basis of MR changes alone (73). Within 24 hr of exhaustive exercise, there is a predictable but transient increase in T1 and T2 relaxation times that can be visualized on STIR and long TR/TE sequences as an increase in signal intensity (29,66,73). This increase in signal is not initially limited to the muscles performing work, but rather extends over a more broad region. Patients do not generally experience soreness at this time. Within 48 to 72 hr, the signal changes become clearly demarcated, involving only those muscles that are sore. The MR signal intensity is proportional to the extent of ultrastructural myofibrillar alterations, and the volume of abnormal muscle on MR (32). The relative increase in T2 values correlates with the degree of functional impairment and pain, all of which become maximally severe by day 3 (29,68). T2 relaxation times remain statistically significantly increased for prolonged periods of time following the resolution of soreness. Shellock et al. longitudinally studied a group of patients that exercised to failure and ultimately developed soreness. While soreness, pain, and joint stiffness were present only in the first week following eccentric muscle actions, MRI showed subclinical signal abnormalities in the biceps muscle that lasted as long as 75 days after the disappearance of symptoms (66) (Fig. 10.16).

Correlation of serum creatine kinase (CK) and signal alterations seen on MRI demonstrate that whereas there was a positive correlation between the relaxation times, CK values, and pain, the MR signal abnormalities preceded and persisted longer than other commonly used indicators of injury (73,75). This finding may have an effect on the timing and the intensity of rehabilitation of athletes.

In patients with rhabdomyolysis, MRI reveals abnormal signal in the affected muscle. Both T1 and T2 values increase in muscles undergoing rhabdomyolysis; subsequently, there is an increase in signal on T2 and STIR sequences. It has been postulated that the signal alterations are secondary to the ubiquitous edema and inflammation that is present; the contribution of the macromolecular changes in damaged muscle is difficult to evaluate (14). MRI is extremely valuable in patients whose clinical syndrome suggests that decompressive fasciotomy is indicated; MRI can preoperatively localize the affected muscles. MRI cannot, at this time, be used to determine whether or not muscle is irreversibly damaged; preliminary evidence suggests that MR spectroscopy may be valuable in this regard (35).

The exquisite sensitivity of MRI to the detection of pathologic findings far exceeds it specificity. Changes on MRI due to exertional exercise are quite similar to those due to radiation, denervation, and infectious and inflammatory disorders such as polymyositis (29).

Compartment Syndromes

Compartment syndrome is a pathologic condition of skeletal muscle in which increased interstitial pressure within an anatomically confined space interferes with the function of the muscle and neurovascular components (4,37,78). The critical signs and symptoms of compartment syndrome are (a) pain out of proportion to the injury; (b) weakness and pain on passive stretch; (c) hypoesthesia in the distribution of the nerves traversing the affected compartment; and (d) tenseness of the boundaries of the compartment (79). In patients with compartment syndrome, nuclear medicine flow studies reveal a relative decrease in tracer activity in the affected compartment secondary to the decrease in capillary perfusion, although blood flow images do not demonstrate ischemia (36). The anterior and lateral compartments of the leg and the anterior (volar) compartment of the arm are the most frequently affected compartments. Common etiologies of acute compartment syndrome include hemorrhage, direct muscular trauma, nondisplaced tibial shaft fractures, intense muscular activity, and muscle rupture (4,78,80). The diagnosis is confirmed when intracompartmental pressures are 15 to 20 mm Hg at rest (normal = 0–4), rising to 75 mm Hg during exercise (normal = 50) (7). These elevated pressures compromise capillary perfusion but are not sufficient to occlude major arteries. Therefore, the pulse distal to the affected compartment is present until the very late stages of the syndrome. If sufficiently severe and untreated, an acute compartment syndrome may lead to muscle necrosis and fibrous contracture with permanent neurological damage (e.g., Volkmann's contracture). Therapy includes immediate decompression by means of fasciotomy and debridement of necrotic tissue.

Chronic exertional compartment syndromes (CCS) are more common than the acute variety. CCS is defined as a condition in which exercise-related pain interferes with the performance of recreational athletics (7,36). It is possible that either abnormal blood flow or buildup of noxious metabolites is responsible for symptoms. Patients present with deep pain over the anterior aspect of the leg which occurs after prolonged exercise; the pain is severe enough to limit the patient's activity. In CCS, the postexercise pressures remain abnormally elevated. At 1 min postexercise, intracompartmental pressures are 30 mm Hg and at 5 min postexercise, the value is at least 20 mm Hg (7,81). Treat-

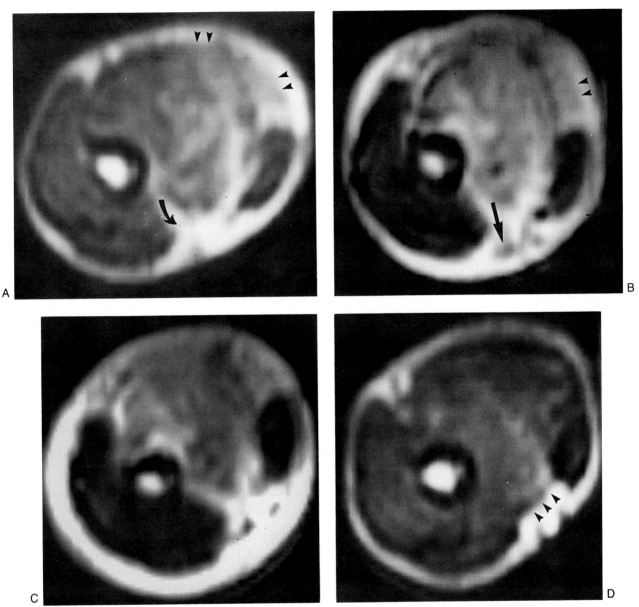

FIG. 10.16. DOMS. A–D: Axial MR, TR/TE 2000/80. This patient exercised to exhaustion by performing eccentric muscle contractions. Images of the biceps muscle were obtained on day 3 (A), 5 (B), 10 (C), and 25 (D) following exercise. On day 3, all of the muscles have a slight increase in signal intensity, with the biceps (*arrowheads*) revealing the most evident abnormality. By day 5, the signal alteration is confined to the symptomatic injured biceps muscle. There is a small fluid collection present (*curved arrow*) that is not optimally seen because of the windowing necessary to demonstrate the muscle abnormality best. Although the patient was asymptomatic by day 7, the abnormality can be identified on studies carried out on day 25. Several streaky low signal abnormalities (*large arrow*) are present in the subcutaneous tissue that are thought to represent myoglobin.

ment includes fasciotomy if activity alteration fails to relieve symptoms (79,82).

The MR findings in patients with acute compartment syndrome include swelling of the affected limb, resulting in increased girth, and an increase in signal intensity of muscle on contrast-oriented examinations (T2 or STIR sequences) (Fig. 10.17). Interestingly, the signal alteration may not always be limited to the one fascial compartment in which the pressures are elevated (35,37). In patients with symptoms suggestive of chronic compartment syndrome, transient increases in signal may be found within the muscle of one compartment postexercise. These foci often rapidly disappear concurrent with the resolution of symptoms. The signal alterations that are imaged in patients with CCS can be quantified by measurement of the T1 and T2 relaxation times. Both T1 and T2 values achieve a

peak immediately postexercise, and regression analysis of percent change in relaxation times versus time indicates that there is a relationship with recovery (36). The curves of T1 and T2 values versus time are similar to those curves generated by direct intracompartmental pressure measurements. It has been suggested that qualitative assessment of blood flow to injured muscle in patients with compartment syndrome may be evaluated using gadolinium (39).

Potential advantages of MRI over pressure measurements include the noninvasive nature of MRI and its ability to examine multiple compartments simultaneously. MRI has shown abnormalities in more than one compartment when the clinical situation suggested only a single compartment was affected; in those cases, surgical decompression was in fact necessary in more than one compartment (36).

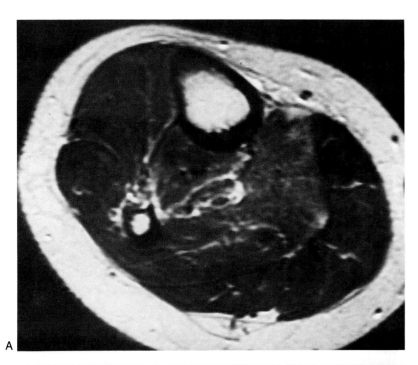

A

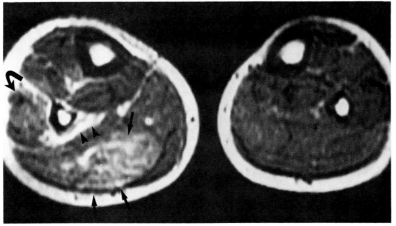

B

FIG. 10.17. Acute compartment syndrome. Both patients suffered injuries to the leg, and presented with severe leg pain and intact pulses. **A:** Axial MR, TR/TE 2000/80. There is a slight increase in signal in the deep posterior compartment. **B:** Axial MR TR/TE 2000/80. In this patient, there is increase in signal in the deep posterior compartment (*arrows*) and a slight increase in signal in the lateral compartment (*curved arrow*). A small perifascial fluid collection (*arrowheads*) is present. Involvement of multiple compartments often goes undiagnosed by interventional techniques.

MISCELLANEOUS MUSCLE DISORDERS

Atrophy

Muscle atrophy may result from either a lack of use (disuse atrophy) or from denervation (denervation atrophy) (41,43). Histologically, replacement of normal muscle by fat cells is identified (43). Following immobilization, muscle strength rapidly declines. This decrease is due to both a diminution in muscle size and a decrease in tension per unit of muscle cross-sectional area. The loss of mass is greatest soon after immobilization; atrophy begins after a lag of 1 to 3 days and is greatest during the next 5 days (83). After as little as 1 to 2 months, muscles may atrophy to one-half of their normal size, but disuse atrophy can be reversed if periods of immobilization are short. However, the longer the state of disuse atrophy is allowed to exist, the longer it takes to reverse the process. In fact, after

4 months, muscle atrophy from disuse may no longer be reversible.

Disuse atrophy with fatty replacement results in a diffuse marbling of increased signal intensity within the striated muscle (T1WI) (17) (Fig. 10.18). Most commonly there is a loss of muscle bulk. Muscle denervation results in detectable increases of both T1 and T2 values (41,43,84). The decrease in the size of the muscle fibers occurs concurrently with a relative shrinking of the myoplasm and a compensatory increase in the size of the extracellular fluid space; both of these events lead to an increase in the T2 values of the denervated tissues.

MRI has been used to assess and to characterize the nature and extent of benign and malignant soft tissue tumors (12,18–28,38). MRI is generally unable to distinguish benign from malignant lesions reliably, either by measurement of relaxation times or by imaging characteristics (17). While the overwhelming majority of neoplasms have decreased signal on T1WI, heman-

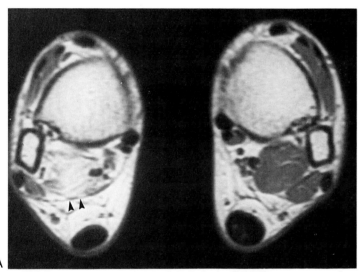

A

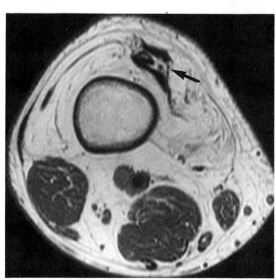

B

FIG. 10.18. Muscle atrophy. **A:** Atrophy of FHL. Axial MR, TR/TE 500/20. The FHL muscle (*arrowheads*) is diffusely infiltrated with fat. The extensor digitorum and extensor hallucis muscles and the peroneus brevis are also somewhat atrophic. Incidentally noted is bilateral Achilles tendonitis. **B:** Severe quadriceps atrophy. Axial MR, TR/TE 300/20. The quadriceps muscles are totally atrophic and blend nearly imperceptibly with the subcutaneous fat. The quadriceps tendon (*arrow*) is all that is visible in the extensor mechanism.

giomas are one notable exception (24,85) (Fig. 10.19). Vascular malformations are among the most common congenital abnormalities occurring in man. They are considered hamartomas rather than true neoplasms because of the frequent finding of vascular, adipose, and fibrous tissue, smooth muscle, and rarely bone within the lesion (28). While a variety of names have been suggested for these lesions (capillary hemangioma, cavernous hemangioma, venous malformation, angiolipoma, etc.), hemangioma is the single best term

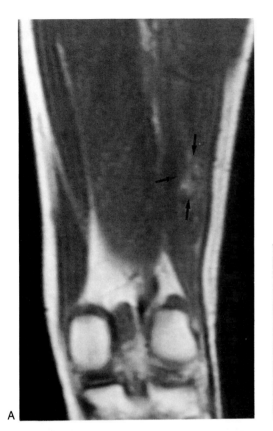

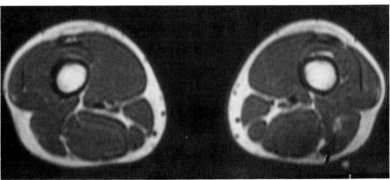

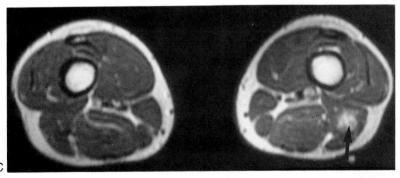

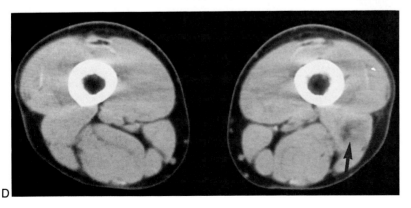

FIG. 10.19. Hemangioma of the biceps femoris muscle. This 17-year-old boy presented with a palpable mass in the back of the left leg. **A:** Coronal MR, TR/TE 500/20. A mass (*arrows*) is seen in the biceps femoris muscle. The lesion has both high and intermediate signal components. High signal on T1WI suggests the presence of fat; however, flowing blood and hemorrhage, both of which may be present in a hemangioma, also produce high signal on short TR studies. **B, C:** Axial MR, TR/TE 300/15 both before (B) and after (C) intravenous injection of gadolinium. The lesion (*arrow*) demonstrates unequivocal enhancement. On a CT scan (**D**), the low attenuation lesion is readily identified. The presence of an intramuscular mass that has fatty components, especially in the thigh of a young individual, must suggest the diagnosis of a hemangioma. **E:** Axial MR, TR/TE 2000/80. In another patient with a biopsy-proven hemangioma, the MR demonstrates the classic serpiginous character of the lesion (*arrowheads*); multiple fine septae (*tiny arrowheads*) are typical.

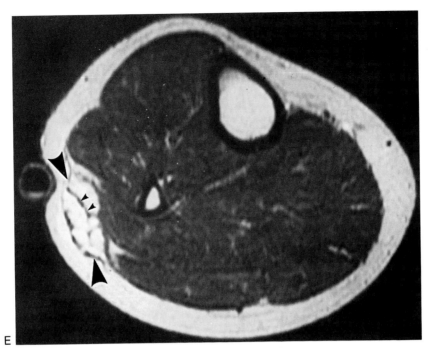

FIG. 10.19. (*Continued*)

for these benign growths characterized by an increased number of vascular channels and overgrowth of the endothelial lining cells. Skeletal muscle hemangiomas occur deep within striated muscle. Benign intramuscular hemangiomas have a fatty component within the tumor vascular matrix, a finding that may contribute to the high signal on T1WI. It is this property that may suggest the diagnosis of this benign lesion, and perhaps spare the patient biopsy; however, hemorrhage within a malignant lesion may also result in high signal on T1WI. Additionally, it is common to identify focal muscle atrophy adjacent to a hemangioma (24). This common tumor has a serpiginous configuration with high signal intensity on long TR/TE sequences due to

the presence of vascular-lined channels, a finding that is not found in soft tissue sarcomas.

High signal on T2WI may be found in otherwise normal skeletal muscle adjacent to malignant tumors of either bone or soft tissue (17,25). If the obvious tumor mass is well demarcated from the surrounding muscle, the increased signal intensity is most likely secondary to edema. If the distinction between muscle and tumor is not clear, abnormal signal in the adjacent muscle probably reflects local tumor infiltration. Extensive muscle edema associated with malignant musculoskeletal tumors is frequently an ominous finding (38).

Bacterial pyomyositis is an uncommon pyogenic disorder that is usually caused by *S. aureus* (45). While

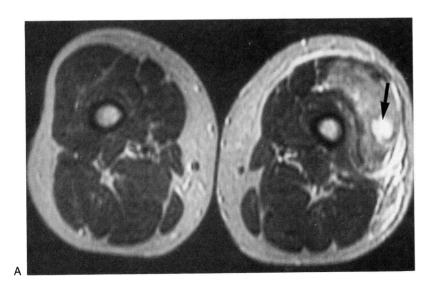

FIG. 10.20. Bacterial pyomyositis. **A:** Axial MR, TR/TE 2500/80. This immunologically normal woman developed subacute pain in the left thigh without a known injury. The MR demonstrates a diffuse increase in signal throughout the vastus lateralis with a focal area of fluid within the muscle (*arrow*). At surgery, an *S. aureus* abscess was drained. (*Figure continues on next page.*)

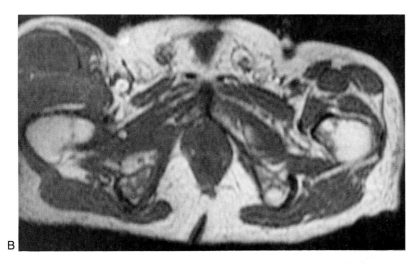

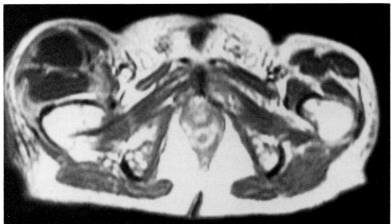

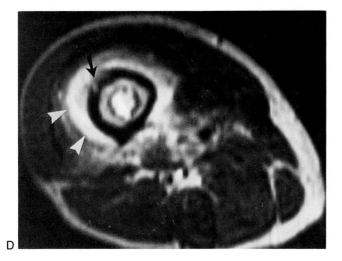

FIG. 10.20. (*Continued*) **B, C:** Pyomyositis in a patient with HIV. Axial MR, TR/TE 300/15 made before (B) and after (C) the intravenous administration of gadolinium. A large soft tissue mass is present anterior to the right hip. Following intravenous gadolinium injection, the rim is seen to markedly enhance (*arrows*). An *S. aureus* abscess was drained. **D:** Osteomyelitis. Axial MR, TR/TE 2200/80. In another patient, biopsy of the femur revealed an *S. aureus* infection in the medullary canal. The infection had spread to the adjacent musculature that was also (but secondarily) infected. The circumferential ring of edema/ pus, the cortical violation, and the medullary abscess distinguish this osteomyelitis from a primary pyomyositis.

patients infected with the human immunodeficiency virus (HIV) suffer from this disease, myositis occurs most frequently in normal men (86). The muscle of the thighs, calves, and buttocks are most commonly affected; multifocal disease is frequent. Low grade fever, weakness, and leukocytosis may be the only positive findings, but the affected skeletal muscle may be rapidly destroyed and replaced by pus. Prompt diagnosis is critical as bacterial myositis is one of the more read-

ily treatable complications of HIV. Nuclear medicine techniques, sonography, and CT scanning have all been used to diagnose pyomyositis, but MRI appears to be more sensitive and specific than these other modalities (Fig. 10.20). T1WI images of some patients with bacterial myositis demonstrate a rim of high signal intensity separating a central region that is isointense with the surrounding normal muscle (33,45). This finding is peculiar since it has not been recognized in ab-

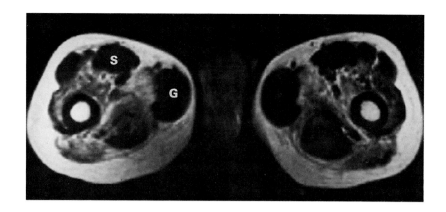

FIG. 10.21. Muscle atrophy and hypertrophy in Duchenne's muscular dystrophy. Axial MR, TR/TE 500/30. Symmetric proximal diminution in muscle volume is evident. The gracilis (*G*) and sartorius (*S*) muscles are spared. (Case courtesy of J. Fleckenstein, M.D., Dallas, TX) (From ref. 39, with permission.)

scesses in other locations. Potential etiologies for this high signal region include methemoglobin production as a result of subacute bleeding, or bacterial or macrophage sequestration of iron. In some patients with bacterial myositis, the abscess does not have this high intensity rim, although the entire mass has a slightly increased signal intensity when compared to normal skeletal muscle. On T2WI and STIR, all patients with bacterial myositis show large, well-defined central regions of markedly increased signal, surrounded by a broad zone of diffuse muscle edema. MRI is extremely valuable in helping to assess those patients presenting with fever, muscle pain, and a swollen limb. Differential considerations would include osteomyelitis, thrombophlebitis, septic arthritis, cellulitis, and pyomyositis. Osteomyelitis is distinguished by the significant and early involvement of the bone marrow. Thrombophlebitis shows marked signal alterations in the intermuscular fascia caused by obstructive edema with relative sparing of the muscles. Cellulitis should have rather little effect on the muscles themselves.

Rapid fatigueability, myalgia, and exercise-induced muscle contracture are characteristic of myophosphorylase deficiency (MPD) and phosphofructokinase deficiency (PFKD). Studies have shown a high prevalence of focal muscle abnormalities in patients with glycolytic myopathies and the ability of MRI to detect them (87). The coexistence of muscle edema, atrophy, and fatty infiltration should suggest a myopathic or neurogenic disorder (29). MRI has been successful in assessing the changes in muscles found in patients with Duchenne's muscular dystrophy, fascioscapulohumeral muscular dystrophy, and limb girdle muscular dystrophy (88) (Fig. 10.21). In the former, a pattern of pseudohypertrophy may be present, but all patients have decreased thigh muscle mass. Interestingly, the sartorius and gracilis muscles are relatively spared. In patients with limb girdle dystrophy, all have fatty replacement of the thigh. Disease duration does not correlate with severity as depicted by MRI (29).

Polymyositis, an idiopathic inflammatory myopathy, is a noninfectious disorder of muscle that may be associated with collagen vascular disease (89). Profound muscular weakness that is out of proportion to the degree of wasting is common; symmetric weakness of the limb girdle musculature and neck flexors, muscle tenderness, and ultimately atrophy characterize the disease.

Patients with chronic polymyositis have proximal and symmetric atrophy but highly focal involvement has been reported. The sartorius and gracilis are frequently spared. Although compensatory hypertrophy is characteristically found in patients with neurogenic muscle disorders, the same is not true for polymyositis, a fact that may be specific for this disease (39). Biopsy reveals necrosis of skeletal muscle fibers. MRI detects the foci of muscle inflammation as mottled or infiltrative increased signal intensity of T2WI (Fig. 10.22).

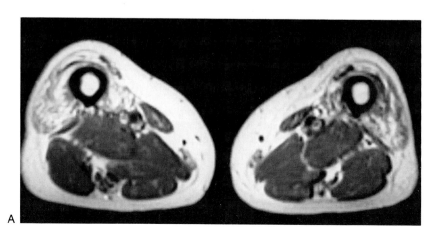

A

FIG. 10.22. Inclusion body myositis. **A:** Axial MR, TR/TE 700/20. (*Figure continues on next page.*)

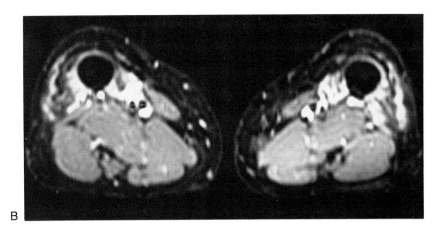

B

FIG. 10.22. (*Continued*) **B:** Axial MR, TR/TE/TI 2200/35/160. The T1WI reveals the marked degree of atrophy of the quadricep muscles that has occurred bilaterally; the STIR sequence most graphically depicts areas of active muscle inflammation that are intermingled with the atrophic zones. The anterior compartment predominance of the disease should suggest the specific diagnosis of inclusion body myositis.

The abnormalities are scattered and noncontiguous, a finding in direct contradistinction to the findings in neoplasms. MRI may be useful in following response to steroid administration (41).

MUSCLE SPECTROSCOPY

Magnetic resonance spectroscopy (MRS) is an important tool for the elucidation of the structure and function of macromolecules. More recently, attempts have been made to apply the same principles to biological systems.

An MRS spectrum is a representation of the intensity of energy released in the resonance process versus applied frequency (Fig. 10.23). The spectrum is usually depicted as a graph of resonant energy on the ordinate and frequency of resonance on the abscissa. Peaks on this graph represent frequencies where many nuclei within the sample resonate; troughs represent frequencies with a paucity of resonating nuclei. By observing the spectroscopic graph, detailed information about the structure of molecules within the sample can be determined.

In the absence of an applied magnetic field gradient, the hydrogen nuclei should resonate at a frequency specified by the strength of the main magnetic field, Bo, times the gyromagnetic ratio, g. However, in the presence of large molecules with many surrounding electrons, the precise magnetic field inside of the molecule's electron cloud is not identical to the main applied magnetic field. The electrons "screen" a portion of the magnetic field, so that the field in the midst of the electron cloud is lower than Bo. Hydrogen nuclei imbedded in a molecule's electron cloud will then resonate at a lower frequency than nuclei in an isolated small molecule, such as free water. This shift to lower frequencies is a sensitive and often specific indicator of the chemical environment surrounding the nucleus and can reveal a wealth of chemical information. Today, most investigations into the physiology of mus-

cle by means of MRS is being done by examination of phosphorus in its high energy forms, adenosine mono- (AMP), di- (ADP) and tri- (ATP) phosphate.

MRS is a noninvasive technique that can obtain detailed chemical information while cells are functioning. MRS has become preeminently important in the evaluation of muscle chemistry and metabolism (88,90–96). MRS's ability to determine chemical concentrations within living tissues has been instrumental in evaluating a variety of important chemical parameters. These include electrolyte shifts (97–100), intracellular

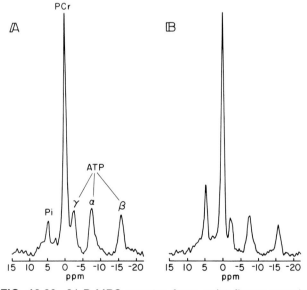

FIG. 10.23. 31-P MRS spectra from wrist flexor muscle of one patient before (**A**) and 24 hr after (**B**) 60 lengthening contractions. Each spectrum consists of 60 scans collected over 5 min. The five major peaks are (from *left* to *right*) inorganic phosphate (*Pi*), phosphocreatine (*PCr*), and the three peaks from ATP (*gamma, alpha,* and *beta*). For comparative purposes, the height of each spectrum was normalized to the same value of PCr. Compared with PCr, Pi is elevated and ATP is reduced following the eccentric action. (Case courtesy of K. McCully, Ph.D., Philadelphia, PA.) (From ref. 124, with permission.)

pH (101,102), body composition (103,104), energy metabolism (88,90–96), and inborn errors of metabolism (105–107).

Energy metabolism is critically important to the proper function of muscle. MRS allows *in vivo* monitoring of relative concentrations of high energy phosphate metabolites, such as phosphocreatine, ATP, ADP, and AMP. Quantitative analysis of 31-P spectra follows the bioenergetics of exercise response by using the fact that the concentration of phosphocreatine is relatively high in resting muscle but decreases rapidly with exercise (39). These metabolic changes are accompanied by a complementary increase in inorganic phosphate and a reduction in pH. Within minutes, all of these parameters return to their resting values. Changes in these and other high energy metabolites have proved helpful in evaluating normal muscle function (108), athletic conditioning (96,109–122), normal response to exercise (123), and muscle response to injury (124–126). The mechanisms of fatigue are complex and in addition to examination of high energy metabolites, changes in muscle response to electrical events may be important (123). Muscle metabolism is regulated by a variety of factors. The effects of hormonal influences are important and can be monitored with MRS (127). The detrimental effects of sepsis on muscle function can be quantitated and hopefully better understood with MRS (128). Nutritional effects can also be detected with spectroscopic methods (129).

Although MRS has proved useful in the evaluation of a broad spectrum of muscle function, chemistry, and disease, perhaps its greatest potential use is in the work-up of specific metabolic muscle diseases (130–132). Significant metabolic alterations have been detected in diabetes (133,134), fibromyalgia (135), and malignant hyperthermia (136,137). Molecular changes from denervation from multiple causes including trauma, congenital (21), amyotrophic lateral sclerosis (88,94), and poliomyelitis (94) have characteristic MRS signatures. In-born errors of muscle metabolism and other specific biomolecular abnormalities must be clearly differentiated and defined before specific therapy can be developed. Unfortunately, many of these conditions overlap in clinical presentations. MRS's specific ability to pinpoint abnormal biochemistry will be important to further advances in this field. MRS has been used in the evaluation of many of these diseases including paramyotonia congenita (105), mitochondrial cytopathy (106), McArdle's syndrome (107), Becker's dystrophy (138), rickets (139), PFKD (140,141), phosphoglycerate mutase deficiency (142), Duchenne's muscular dystrophy (143), limb-girdle muscular dystrophy (88), fascioscapulohumeral dystrophy (88), Kearn-Sayre mitochondrial muscle disease (88), mitochondrial myopathies (144), myotonic dystrophy (94,103), and Werdnig-Hoffmann disease (94,103).

This list will undoubtedly expand as activity in this field increases.

Muscle ischemia is a common clinical problem, especially in patients with peripheral vascular disease. There is currently tremendous interest in the use of MRS as a clinical tool in assessing this disorder; abnormal levels of phosphocreatine and inorganic phosphate have been associated with regions of ischemia (145–152). MRS may prove to be helpful in determining the significance of angiographically proven vascular lesions and may be helpful in determining location, timing, and extent of vascular interventions. The clinical response to vascular intervention may also be best determined by quantitating the metabolic response of ischemic muscle to attempted reperfusion. Compartment syndromes may involve similar pathophysiology and MRS has been used for evaluating this condition (153).

A recent area of research interest in MRS is the evaluation of inflammatory myopathies (30). The use of MRS in clinical decision making in this condition requires further evaluation (31,154).

MRI has revolutionized the detection and staging of soft tissue and muscle neoplasia (15,22,23,26,38, 155,156). MRI is highly sensitive in the detection of soft tissue and muscle neoplasia, but its specificity is usually not adequate for treatment planning. It is hoped that the ability of MRS for biochemical analysis will lead to accurate, noninvasive diagnostic criteria for clinical planning. MRI and MRS already show great promise in following neoplasm response to therapy (157,158).

Diagnosis and treatment planning would benefit by having the ability to monitor changes in metabolic parameters using a noninvasive method. The combination of MRI and multivoxel localized spectroscopy can be used to obtain images of the variations in distribution of both P-31 and proton metabolites. In this technique, spatial localization is provided by the same phase-encoding gradients as in MRI, thereby allowing direct comparison with the anatomic images. Because of the low signal to noise ratio of 31-P MRS, spatial resolution is limited. From a clinical point of view, it is essential that accurate methods of quantifying spectral data are available in a form readily interpreted by the clinician. The success of this technique remains to be documented.

Much of the initial enthusiasm for MRI in medicine in the 1970s and early 1980s was fueled by the prospects of using the rich biochemical information generated by MRS for medical diagnosis. MRS was heralded as the "noninvasive biopsy." While enthusiasm for MRS has waned in comparison to the revolution in medical diagnosis provided by MRI, the fundamental information obtainable by MRS continues to be profound. As experience is gained in this complicated field, it is likely that MRS will eventually play a more significant role in medicine than imaging.

REFERENCES

1. Garrett, WE, Safran, MR, Seaber, AV, *et al.*, *Biomechanical comparison of stimulated and nonstimulated skeletal muscle pulled to failure.* Am J Sports Med, 1987. **15**(5): p. 448–454.
2. O'Donoghue, DH, *Treatment of Injuries to Athletes.* 4th ed. 1984, W.B. Saunders: Philadelphia.
3. Zarins, B and Ciullo, JV, *Acute muscle and tendon injuries in athletes.* Clin Sports Med, 1983. **2**(1): p. 167–182.
4. Garrett, WEJ, *Basic science of musculotendinous injuries,* in *The Lower Extremity and Spine in Sports Medicine,* JA Nicholas and EB Hershman, Editors. 1986, CV Mosby: St Louis. p. 42–58.
5. Garrett, WE, Mumma, M, and Lucaveche, C, *Ultrastructural differences in human skeletal muscle fiber types.* Orthop Clin, 1983. **14**(2): p. 413–425.
6. Sutro, C and Sutro, W, *The medial head of the gastrocnemius. A review of the basis for partial rupture and for intermittent claudication.* Bull Hosp Jt Dis Orthop Inst, 1985. **45**(2): p. 150–157.
7. Matin, P, *Basic principles of nuclear medicine techniques for detection and evaluation of trauma and sports medicine injuries.* Semin Nucl Med, 1988. **18**(2): p. 90–112.
8. Valk, P, *Muscle localization of Tc-99m MDP after exertion.* Clin Nucl Med, 1984. **9**(9): p. 493–494.
9. Matin, P, Lang, G, Carretta, R, *et al.*, *Scintigraphic evaluation of muscle damage following extreme exercise: Concise communication.* J Nucl Med, 1983. **24**(4): p. 308–311.
10. Shirkhoda, A, Mauro, MA, Staab, EV, *et al.*, *Soft-tissue hemorrhage in hemophiliac patients. Computed tomography and ultrasound study.* Radiology, 1983. **147**: p. 811–814.
11. Termote, J, Baert, A, Crolla, D, *et al.*, *Computed tomography of the normal and pathologic muscular system.* Radiology, 1980. **137**: p. 439–444.
12. Garrett, WE, Rich, FR, Nikolaou, PK, *et al.*, *Computed tomography of hamstring muscle strains.* Med Sci Sports Exerc, 1989. **21**(5): p. 506–514.
13. Vukanovic, S and Wettstein, P, *CT localization of myonecrosis for surgical decompression.* AJR, 1980. **135**: p. 1298–1299.
14. Lamminen, AE, Hekali, PE, Tiula, E, *et al.*, *Acute rhabdomyolysis: Evaluation with magnetic resonance imaging compared with computed tomography and ultrasonography.* Radiology (Br), 1989. **62**: p. 326–331.
15. Aisen, AM, Martel, W, Braunstein, EM, *et al.*, *MRI and CT evaluation of primary bone and soft tissue tumors.* AJR, 1986. **146**: p. 749–756.
16. Dooms, GC, Fisher, MF, Hricak, H, *et al.*, *MR imaging of intramuscular hemorrhage.* J Comput Assist Tomogr, 1985. **9**: p. 908–913.
17. Fisher, MR, Dooms, GC, Hricak, H, *et al.*, *Magnetic resonance imaging of the normal and pathologic muscular system.* Magn Reson Imaging, 1986. **4**: p. 491–496.
18. Fleckenstein, JL, Canby, RC, Parkey, RW, *et al.*, *Acute effects of exercise on MR imaging of skeletal muscle in normal volunteers.* AJR, 1988. **151**: p. 231–237.
19. Newham, DJ, McPhail, G, Mills, KR, *et al.*, *Ultrastructural changes after concentric and eccentric contractions of human muscle.* J Neurol Sci, 1983. **61**: p. 109–122.
20. Milgram, JE, *Muscle ruptures and avulsions with particular reference to the lower extermities.* A.A.O.S. Instructional Course Lectures, 1953. **10**: p. 233–243.
21. Zochodne, DW, Thompson, RT, Driedger, AA, *et al.*, *Metabolic changes in human muscle denervation: Topical 31P NMR spectroscopy studies.* Magn Reson Med, 1988. **7**: p. 373–383.
22. Frank, JA, Ling, A, Patronas, NJ, *et al.*, *Detection of malignant bone tumors: MR imaging versus scintigraphy.* AJR, 1990. **155**: p. 1043–1048.
23. Wetzel, LH and Levine, E, *Soft-tissue tumors of the foot:*
Value of MR imaging for specific diagnosis. AJR, 1990. **155**: p. 1025–1030.
24. Yuh, WTC, Kathol, MH, Sein, MA, *et al.*, *Hemangiomas of skeletal muscle: MR findings in five patients.* AJR, 1987. **149**: p. 765–768.
25. Beltran, J, Simon, DC, Katz, W, *et al.*, *Increased MR signal intensity in skeletal muscle adjacent to malignant tumors: Pathologic correlation and clinical relevance.* Radiology, 1987, **162**: p. 251–255.
26. Sundaram, M and McLeod, RA, *Review article. MR imaging of tumor and tumorlike lesions of bone and soft tissue.* AJR, 1990. **155**: p. 817–824.
27. Hanna, SL, Fletcher, BD, Parham, DM, *et al.*, *Muscle edema associated with musculoskeletal tumors: MR imaging findings and clinical significance.* J Magn Reson Imaging, 1991. **1**(2): p. 194.
28. Kaplan, PA and Williams, SM, *Mucocutaneous and peripheral soft-tissue hemangiomas: MR imaging.* Radiology, 1987. **163**: p. 163–166.
29. Fleckenstein, JL and Shellock, FG, *Exertional muscle injuries: MRI evaluation.* Topics Magn Reson Imaging, 1991. **3**: p. 50–70.
30. Park, JH, Vansant, JP, Kumar, NG, *et al.*, *Dermatomyositis: Correlative MR imaging and P-31 MR spectroscopy for quantitative characterization of inflammatory disease.* Radiology, 1990. **177**(2): p. 473–479.
31. Fraser, DD, Frank, JA, and Dalakas, MC, *Inflammatory myopathies: MR imaging and spectroscopy.* Radiology, 1991. **179**(2): p. 341–342.
32. Giddings, CJ, Nurenberg, P, Stray-Gundersen, J, *et al.*, *Muscle injury assessed with magnetic resonance imaging and electronmicroscopy following downhill running in humans.* Med Sci Sports Exerc, 1991. **23 Suppl**(4).
33. Yuh, WTC, Schreiber, AE, Montgomery, WJ, *et al.*, *Magnetic resonance imaging of pyomyositis.* Skeletal Radiol, 1988. **17**: p. 190–193.
34. Greco, A, McNamara, M, Escher, R, *et al.*, *Spin-echo and STIR MR imaging of sports-related muscle injuries at 1.5T.* Radiology, 1990. **177** (P): p. 306–312.
35. Zagoria, RJ, Karstaedt, N, and Koubek, TD, *MR imaging of rhabdomyolysis.* J Comput Assist Tomogr, 1986. **10**: p. 268–270.
36. Amendola, A, Rorabeck, CH, Vellett, D, *et al.*, *The use of magnetic resonance imaging in exertional compartment syndromes.* Am J Sports Med, 1990. **18**(1): p. 29–34.
37. Ehman, RL and Berquist, TH, *Magnetic resonance imaging of musculoskeletal trauma.* Radiol Clin North Am, 1986. **24**(2): p. 291–319.
38. Hanna, S, Fletcher, B, and Parham, D, *Muscle edema in musculoskeletal tumors: MR imaging characteristics and clinical significance.* J Magn Reson Imaging, 1991. **1**: p. 441–449.
39. Fleckenstein, JL, Weatherall, PT, Bertocci, LA, *et al.*, *Locomotor system assessment by muscle magnetic resonance imaging.* Magn Reson Q, 1991. **7**: p. 79–103.
40. Swensen, SJ, Keller, PL, Berquist, TH, *et al.*, *Magnetic resonance imaging of hemorrhage.* AJR, 1985. **145**: p. 921–927.
41. *MRI of the Musculoskeletal System. A Teaching File.* JH Mink and AL Deutsch, Editors. 1990, Raven Press; New York.
42. Unger, EC, Glazer, HS, Lee, JKT, *et al.*, *MRI of extracranial hematomas: Preliminary observations.* AJR, 1986. **146**: p. 403–407.
43. Deutsch, AL and Mink, JH, *Magnetic resonance imaging of musculoskeletal injuries.* Radiol Clin North Am, 1989. **27**(5): p. 983–1002.
44. Sundaram, M, McGuire, MH, Herbold, DR, *et al.*, *High signal intensity soft tissue masses on T1 weighted pulsing sequences.* Skeletal Radiol, 1987. **16**: p. 30–36.
45. Fleckenstein, JL, Burns, DK, Murphy, FK, *et al.*, *Differential diagnosis of bacterial myositis in AIDS: Evaluation with MR imaging.* Radiology, 1991. **179**: p. 653–658.
46. Garrett, WEJ, *Injuries to the muscle-tendon unit.* Instr Course Lect, 1988. **37**: p. 275–282.
47. Jackson, DW and Feagin, JA, *Quadriceps contusions in young adults. Relationship of severity of injury to treatment and prognosis.* J Bone Joint Surg (Am), 1973. **55**: p. 95–105.

48. Amendola, M, Glazer, GM, Agha, Z, et al., *Myositis ossificans circumscripta: Computed tomographic diagnosis*. Radiology, 1983. **149**: p. 775–779.

49. Garrett, WE, *Muscle strain injuries: Clinical and basic aspects*. Med Sci Sports Exerc, 1990. **22**(4): p. 436–443.

50. Shellock, FG, Fukunaga, T, Mink, JH, et al., *Acute effects of exercise on MR imaging of skeletal muscle: Concentric vs eccentric actions*. AJR, 1991. **156**: p. 765–768.

51. Garrett, WE, Califf, JC, and Bassett, FH, *Histochemical correlates of hamstring injuries*. Am J Sports Med, 1984. **12**(2): p. 98–103.

52. Anzel, SH, Covey, KW, Weiner, AD, et al., *Disruption of muscles and tendons an analysis of 1,014 cases*. Surgery, 1959. **45**(3): p. 406–414.

53. Baker, BE, *Current concepts in the diagnosis and treatment of musculotendinous injuries*. Med Sci Sports Exerc, 1984. **16**(4): p. 323–327.

54. Burkett, LN, *Causative factors in hamstring strains*. Med Sci Sports Exerc, 1970. **2**(1): p. 39–42.

55. Arner, O and Lindholm, A, *What is tennis leg?* Acta Chir Scand, 1958. **116**: p. 73–75.

56. Miller, WA, *Rupture of the musculotendinous juncture of the medial head of the gastrocnemius muscle*. Am J Sports Med, 1977. **5**(5): p. 191–193.

57. Miller, AP, *Strains of the posterior calf musculature ("tennis leg")*. Am J Sports Med, 1979. **7**(3): p. 172–174.

58. Burkett, LN, *Investigation into hamstring strains: The case of the hybrid muscle*. J Sports Med, 1976. **3**(5): p. 228–231.

59. Symeonides, PP, *Isolated traumatic rupture of the adductor longus muscle of the thigh*. Clin Orthop, 1973. **88**: p. 64–66.

60. Peshock, RM, Fleckenstein, JL, Malloy, CR, et al., *Echoplanar imaging in the evaluation of skeletal muscle exercise*. J Magn Reson Imaging, 1991. **1**(2): p. 149.

61. Fisher, MJ, Meyer, RA, Adams, GR, et al., *Direct relationship between proton T2 and exercise intensity in skeletal muscle MR images*. Invest Radiol, 1989. **25**: p. 480–485.

62. Cohen, MS, Shellock, FG, Nadeau, KA, et al., *Acute Muscle T2 Changes During Exercise*. SMRM Book of Abstracts, 1991. p. 107.

63. Fisher, BD, Baracos, VE, Shnika, TK, et al., *Ultrastructural events following acute muscle trauma*. Med Sci Sports Exerc, 1990. **22**: p. 185–193.

64. Armstrong, RB, *Initial events in exercise-induced muscular injury*. Med Sci Sports Exerc, 1990. **22**(4): p. 429–435.

65. Newham, DJ, Mills, KR, Quigley, BM, et al., *Pain and fatigue after concentric and eccentric muscle contractions*. Clin Sci, 1983. **64**: p. 55–62.

66. Shellock, FG, Fukunaga, T, Mink, JH, et al., *Exertional muscle injury: Evaluation of concentric versus eccentric actions with serial MR imaging*. Radiology, 1991. **179**: p. 659–664.

67. Nikolaou, PK, MacDonald, BL, Glisson, RR, et al., *Biomechanical and histological evaluation of muscle after controlled strain injury*. Am J Sports Med, 1987. **15**(1): p. 9–14.

68. Shellock, FG, Fukunaga, T, Day, K, et al., *Serial MRI and cybex testing evaluations of exertional muscle injury: Concentric vs eccentric actions*. Med Sci Sports Exerc, 1991. **23**: p. S110.

69. Wikorsson-Moller, M, Oberg, B, Ekstrand, J, et al., *Effects of warming up, massage, and stretching on range of motion and muscle strength in the lower extremity*. Am J Sports Med, 1983. **11**(4): p. 249–252.

70. Safran, MR, Garrett, WE, Seaber, V, et al., *The role of warmup in muscular injury prevention*. Am J Sports Med, 1988. **16**(2): p. 123–128.

71. Taylor, DC, Dalton, JC, Seaber, AV, et al., *Viscoelastic properties of muscle-tendon units. The biomechanical effects of stretching*. Am J Sports Med, 1990. **18**(3): p. 300–309.

72. De Smet, AA, Heiner, JP, et al., *Magnetic resonance imaging of muscle tears*. Skeletal Radiol, 1990. **19**: p. 283–286.

73. Fleckenstein, JL, Weatherall, PT, Parkey, RW, et al., *Sports-related muscle injuries: Evaluation with MR imaging*. Radiology, 1989. **172**: p. 793–798.

74. Armstrong, RB, *Mechanisms of exercise-induced delayed onset muscular soreness: A brief review*. Med Sci Sports Exerc, 1984. **16**(6): p. 529–538.

75. Tiidus, PM and Ianuzzo, CD, *Effects of intensity and duration of muscular exercise on delayed soreness and serum enzyme activities*. Med Sci Sports Exerc, 1983. **15**: p. 461–465.

76. Schwane, JA, Johnson, SR, Vandenakker, CB, et al., *Delayed-onset muscular soreness and plasma CPK and LDH activities after downhill running*. Med Sci Sports Exerc, 1983. **15**: p. 51–56.

77. Zabetakis, P, *Muscle soreness and rhabdomyolysis*, in *The Lower Extremity and Spine in Sports Medicine*, JA Nicholas and EB Hershman, Editors. 1986, CV Mosby: St Louis. p. 59–71.

78. Anouchi, YL, Parker, RD, and Seitz, WH, *Posterior compartment syndrome of the calf resulting from misdiagnosis of a rupture of the medial head of the gastrocnemius*. J Trauma, 1987. **27**(6): p. 678–680.

79. Matsen, FA, Winquist, RA, Krugmire, RB, et al., *Diagnosis and management of compartmental syndromes*. J Bone Joint Surg (Am), 1980. **62**: p. 286–291.

80. Arciero, RA, Shishido, NS, and Parr, TJ, *Acute anterolateral compartment syndrome secondary to rupture of the peroneus longus muscle*. Am J Sports Med, 1984. **12**(5): p. 366–367.

81. Pedowitz, RA, Hargens, AR, Mubarak, SJ, et al., *Modified criteria for the objective diagnosis of chronic compartment syndrome of the leg*. Am J Sports Med, 1990. **18**(1): p. 35–40.

82. Rorabeck, CH, *The diagnosis and management of chronic compartment syndrome*. Instr Course Lect, 1989. **38**: p. 466–472.

83. Booth, FW, *Physiologic and biomechanical effects of immobilization on muscle*. Clin Orthop, 1987. **219**: p. 15–20.

84. Polak, JF, Jolesz, FA, and Adams, DF, *Magnetic resonance imaging of the skeletal muscle prolongation of T1 and T2 subsequent to denervation*. Invest Radiol, 1988. **23**: p. 365–369.

85. Cohen, EK, Kressel, HY, Perosio, T, et al., *MR imaging of soft-tissue hemangiomas: Correlation with pathologic findings*. AJR, 1988. **150**: p. 1079–1081.

86. Scott, JA, Palmer, EL, and Fischman, AJ, *HIV-associated myositis detected by radionuclide bone scanning*. J Nucl Med, 1989. **30**(4): p. 556–558.

87. Fleckenstein, JL, Peshock, RM, Lewis, SF, et al., *Magnetic resonance imaging of muscle injury and atrophy in glycolytic myopathies*. Muscle Nerve, 1989. **12**: p. 849–855.

88. Murphy, WA, Totty, WG, and Carroll, JE, *MRI of normal and pathologic skeletal muscle*. AJR, 1986. **146**: p. 565–574.

89. Plotz, PH, Dalakas, M, Leff, RL, et al., *Current concepts in the idiopathic inflammatory myopathies: Polymyositis, dermatomyositis, and related disorders*. Ann Intern Med, 1989. **111**: p. 143–157.

90. Achten, E, Van, CM, Willem, R, et al., *31P-NMR spectroscopy and the metabolic properties of different muscle fibers*. J Appl Physiol, 1990. **68**(2): p. 644–649.

91. McCully, KK, Kent, JA, and Chance, B, *Muscle injury and exercise stress measured with 31-P magnetic resonance spectroscopy*. Prog Clin Biol Res, 1989. **315**(1): p. 197–207.

92. Chance, B, Younkin, DP, Kelley, R, et al., *Magnetic resonance spectroscopy of normal and diseased muscles*. Am J Med Genet, 1986. **25**(4): p. 659–679.

93. Vock, P, Hoppeler, H, Hartl, W, et al., *Combined use of magnetic resonance imaging (MRI) and spectroscopy (MRS) by whole body magnets in studying skeletal muscle morphology and metabolism*. Invest Radiol, 1985. **20**(5): p. 486–491.

94. Barany, M, Siegel, IM, Venkatasubramanian, PN, et al., *Human leg neuromuscular diseases: P-31 MR spectroscopy*. Radiology, 1989. **172**(2): p. 503–508.

95. Barany, M, Langer, GB, Glick, RP, et al., *In vivo H-1 spectroscopy in humans at 1.5 T*. Radiology, 1988. **167**(3): p. 839–844.

96. Edwards, RH, *New techniques for studying human muscle function, metabolism, and fatigue*. Muscle Nerve, 1984. **7**(8): p. 599–609.

97. Naritomi, H, Kanashiro, M, Sasaki, M, et al., *In vivo measurements of intra- and extracellular Na+ and water in the brain and muscle by nuclear magnetic resonance spectroscopy with shift reagent*. Biophys J, 1987. **52**(4): p. 611–616.

98. Syme, PD, Dixon, RM, Allis, JL, et al., *A non-invasive method of measuring concentrations of rubidium in rat skeletal muscle*

in vivo by 87Rb nuclear magnetic resonance spectroscopy: Implications for the measurement of cation transport activity in vivo. Clin Sci, 1990. **78**(3): p. 303–309.

99. Higgins, RM, Richardson, AJ, Endre, ZH, *et al., Hypophosphataemia after renal transplantation: Relationship to immunosuppressive drug therapy and effects on muscle detected by 31P nuclear magnetic resonance spectroscopy.* Nephrol Dial Transplant, 1990. **5**(1): p. 62–68.

100. Le Rumeur, E, Le Moyec, L, Yvin, JC, *et al., Assessment of intracellular magnesium depletion in rat striated muscle by in vivo 31P NMR.* Magn Reson Med, 1990. **13**(3): p. 504–506.

101. Wray, S, *Regulation of intracellular pH in rat uterine smooth muscle, studied by 31P NMR spectroscopy.* Biochim Biophys Acta, 1988. **972**(3): p. 299–301.

102. Victor, RG, Bertocci, LA, Pryor, SL, *et al., Sympathetic nerve discharge is coupled to muscle cell pH during exercise in humans.* J Clin Invest, 1988. **82**(4): p. 1301–1305.

103. Barany, M, Venkatasubramanian, PN, Mok, E, *et al., Quantitative and qualitative fat analysis in human leg muscle of neuromuscular diseases by 1H MR spectroscopy in vivo.* Magn Reson Med, 1989. **10**(2): p. 210–226.

104. Leroy, WA, Duboc, D, Bittoun, J, *et al., Spectroscopic MRI: A tool for the evaluation of systemic lipid storage disease.* Magn Reson Imag, 1990. **8**(4): p. 511–515.

105. Lehmann, HF, Hopfel, D, Rudel, R, *et al., In vivo P-NMR spectroscopy: Muscle energy exchange in paramyotonia patients. Muscle Nerve, 1985.* **8**(7): p. 606–610.

106. Narayana, PA, Slopis, JM, Jackson, EF, *et al., In vivo muscle magnetic resonance spectroscopy in a family with mitochondrial cytopathy: A defect in fat metabolism.* Magn Reson Imaging, 1989. **7**(2): p. 133–139.

107. Argov, Z, Bank, WJ, Maris, J, *et al., Muscle energy metabolism in McArdle's syndrome by in vivo phosphorus magnetic resonance spectroscopy.* Neurology, 1987. **37**(11): p. 1720–1724.

108. Dawson, MJ, *The relation between muscle contraction and metabolism: Studies by 31P nuclear magnetic resonance spectroscopy.* Adv Exp Med Biol, 1988. **226**(1): p. 433–448.

109. Fleckenstein, JL, Bertocci, LA, Nunnally, RL, *et al., Exercise-enhanced MR imaging of variations in forearm muscle anatomy and use: Importance in MR spectroscopy.* AJR, 1989. **153**(4): p. 693–698.

110. Shenton, DJ, Heppenstall, RB, Chance, B, *et al., Electrical stimulation of human muscle studied using 31P-nuclear magnetic resonance spectroscopy.* J Orthop Res, 1986. **4**(2): p. 204–211.

111. Park, JH, Brown, RL, Park, CR, *et al., Energy metabolism of the untrained muscle of elite runners as observed by 31P magnetic resonance spectroscopy: Evidence suggesting a genetic endowment for endurance exercise.* Proc Natl Acad Sci USA, 1988. **85**(23): p. 8780–8784.

112. McCully, KK, Kent, JA, and Chance. B, *Application of 31P magnetic resonance spectroscopy to the study of athletic performance.* Sports Med, 1988. **5**(5): p. 312–321.

113. McCully, KK, Boden, BP, Tuchler, M, *et al., Wrist flexor muscles of elite rowers measured with magnetic resonance spectroscopy.* J Appl Physiol, 1989. **67**(3): p. 926–932.

114. Boicelli, CA, Baldassarri, AM, Borsetto, C, *et al., An approach to noninvasive fiber type determination by NMR.* Int J Sports Med, 1989. **10**(1): p. 53–54.

115. Park, JH, Brown, RL, Park, CR, *et al., Functional pools of oxidative and glycolytic fibers in human muscle observed by 31P magnetic resonance spectroscopy during exercise.* Proc Natl Acad Sci USA, 1987. **84**(24): p. 8976–8980.

116. Sapega, AA, Sokolow, DP, Graham, TJ, *et al., Phosphorus nuclear magnetic resonance: A non-invasive technique for the study of muscle bioenergetics during exercise.* Med Sci Sports Exerc, 1987. **19**(4): p. 410–420.

117. Inch, WR, Serebrin, B, Taylor, AW, *et al., Exercise muscle metabolism measured by magnetic resonance spectroscopy.* Can J Appl Sport Sci, 1986. **11**(2): p. 60–65.

118. Taylor, DJ, Styles, P, Matthews, PM, *et al., Energetics of human muscle: Exercise-induced ATP depletion.* Magn Reson Med, 1986. **3**(1): p. 44–54.

119. Kuno, S, Akisada, M, Katsuta, S, *et al., Evaluation of exercise muscle energetics by NMR.* Ann Physiol Anthropol, 1990. **9**(2): p. 235–239.

120. Lopata, M, Onal, E, Aronson, R, *et al., Effects of inspiratory loading on 31 phosphorus magnetic resonance (PMR) spectroscopy of the inspiratory intercostal muscles in normal humans.* Chest, 1990. **3**(1): p. 97.

121. Helpern, JA, Kao, W, Gross, B, *et al., Interleaved 31P NMR with transcutaneous nerve stimulation (TNS): A method of monitoring compliance-independent skeletal muscle metabolic response to exercise.* Magn Reson Med, 1989. **10**(1): p. 50–56.

122. Clark, BJ, Acker, MA, McCully, K, *et al., In vivo 31P-NMR spectroscopy of chronically stimulated canine skeletal muscle.* Am J Physiol, 1988. **254**(2): p. 258–266.

123. Le Rumeur, E, Le Moyec, L, Toulouse, P, *et al., Muscle fatigue unrelated to phosphocreatine and pH: An " in vivo" 31-P NMR spectroscopy study.* Muscle Nerve, 1990. **13**(5): p. 438–444.

124. McCully, K, Argov, Z, Boden, B, *et al., Detection of muscle injury in humans with 31-P magnetic resonance spectroscopy.* Muscle Nerve,1988. **11**(3): p. 212–216.

125. Kariya, Y, Itoh, M, Nakamura, T, *et al., Magnetic resonance imaging and spectroscopy of thigh muscles in cruciate ligament insufficiency.* Acta Orthop Scand, 1989. **60**(3): p. 322–325.

126. Taylor, DJ, Brosnan, MJ, Arnold, DL, *et al., Ca^{2+}-ATPase deficiency in a patient with an exertional muscle pain syndrome.* J Neurol Neurosurg Psychiatry, 1988. **51**(11): p. 1425–1433.

127. Argov, Z, Renshaw, PF, Boden, B, *et al., Effects of thyroid hormones on skeletal muscle bioenergetics. In vivo phosphorus-31 magnetic resonance spectroscopy study of humans and rats.* J Clin Invest, 1988. **81**(6): p. 1695–1701.

128. Jacobs, DO, Maris, J, Fried, R, *et al., In vivo phosphorus 31 magnetic resonance spectroscopy of rat hind limb skeletal muscle during sepsis.* Arch Surg, 1988. **123**(11): p. 1425–1428.

129. Pichard, C, Vaughan, C, Struk, R, *et al., Effect of dietary manipulations (fasting, hypocaloric feeding, and subsequent refeeding) on rat muscle energetics as assessed by nuclear magnetic resonance spectroscopy.* J Clin Invest, 1988. **82**(3): p. 895–901.

130. Sugie, H, Tsurui, S, Sugie, Y, *et al., Study of metabolic myopathies using 1H NMR spectroscopy—analysis of muscle metabolites and muscle autolytic change.* Rinsho Shinkeigaku, 1990. **30**(3): p. 320–323.

131. Challiss, RA, Blackledge, MJ, and Radda, GK, *Spatial heterogeneity of metabolism in skeletal muscle in vivo studied by 31P-NMR spectroscopy.* Am J Physiol, 1988. **3**(1): p. 1–11.

132. Meyer, RA, Kuchmerick, MJ, and Brown, TR, *Application of 31P-NMR spectroscopy to the study of striated muscle metabolism.* Am J Physiol, 1982. **242**(1).

133. Challiss, RA, Vranic, M, and Radda, GK, *Bioenergetic changes during contraction and recovery in diabetic rat skeletal muscle.* Am J Physiol, 1989. **1**(1): p. 1: 29–37.

134. Challiss, RA, Blackledge, MJ, and Radda, GK, *Spatially resolved changes in diabetic rat skeletal muscle metabolism in vivo studied by 31P-n.m.r. spectroscopy.* Biochem J, 1990. **268**(1): p. 111–115.

135. Kushmerick, MJ, *Muscle energy metabolism, nuclear magnetic resonance spectroscopy and their potential in the study of fibromyalgia.* J Rheumatol Suppl, 1989. **19**(1): p. 40–46.

136. Kozak, RG, Gascard, JP, and Redouane, BK, *Detection of peranesthetic malignant hyperthermia by muscle contracture tests and NMR spectroscopy.* Ann Fr Anesth Reanim, 1986. **5**(6): p. 584–589.

137. Foster, PS, Hopkinson, K, and Denborough, MA, *31P-NMR spectroscopy: The metabolic profile of malignant hyperpyrexic porcine skeletal muscle.* Muscle Nerve, 1989. **12**(5): p. 390–396.

138. Newman, RJ, *An in vivo study of muscle phosphate metabolism in Becker's dystrophy by 31P NMR spectroscopy.* Metabolism, 1985. **34**(8): p. 737–740.

139. Mize, CE, Corbett, RJ, Uauy, R, *et al., Hypotonia of rickets: A sequential study by P-31 magnetic resonance spectroscopy.* Pediatr Res, 1988. **24**(6): p. 713–716.

140. Argov, Z, Bank, WJ, Maris, J, *et al., Muscle energy metabolism in human phosphofructokinase deficiency as recorded by 31P nuclear magnetic resonance spectroscopy. Ann Neurol, 1987. 22*(1): p. 46–51.

141. Giger, U, Argov, Z, Schnall, M, *et al., Metabolic myopathy in canine muscle-type phosphofructokinase deficiency.* Muscle Nerve, 1988. **11**(12): p. 1260–1265.

142. Argov, Z, Bank, WJ, Boden, B, *et al., Phosphorus magnetic resonance spectroscopy of partially blocked muscle glycolysis. An in vivo study of phosphoglycerate mutase deficiency.* Arch Neurol, 1987. **44**(6): p. 614–617.

143. Newman, RJ, Bore, PJ, Chan, L, *et al., Nuclear magnetic resonance studies of forearm muscle in Duchenne dystrophy.* Br Med J [Clin Res], 1982. **284**(6322): p. 1072–1074.

144. Arnold, DL, Taylor, DJ, and Radda, GK, *Investigation of human mitochondrial myopathies by phosphorus magnetic resonance spectroscopy.* Ann Neurol, 1985. **18**(2): p. 189–196.

145. Authier, B, Rossi, A, Albrand, JP, *et al., Effects of acute arterial occlusion on muscle energy metabolism. An experimental model using phosphorus NMR spectroscopy in the rat.* J Mal Vasc, 1987. **12**(4): p. 323–328.

146. Williams, DM, Fencil, L, and Chenevert, TL, *Peripheral arterial occlusive disease: P-31 MR spectroscopy of calf muscle.* Radiology, 1990. **175**(2): p. 381–385.

147. Hands, LJ, Bore, PJ, Galloway, G, *et al., Muscle metabolism in patients with peripheral vascular disease investigated by 31P nuclear magnetic resonance spectroscopy.* Clin Sci, 1986. **71**(3): p. 283–290.

148. Heppenstall, RB, Scott, R, Sapega, A, *et al., A comparative study of the tolerance of skeletal muscle to ichemia. Tourniquet application compared with acute compartment syndrome.* J Bone Joint Surg (Am), 1986. **68**(6): p. 820–828.

149. Keller, U, Oberhansli, R, Huber, P, *et al., Phosphocreatine content and intracellular pH of calf muscle measured by phosphorus NMR spectroscopy in occlusive arterial disease of the legs.* Eur J Clin Invest, 1985. **15**(6): p. 382–388.

150. Balschi, JA, Bittl, JA, Springer, CJ, *et al., 31P and 23Na NMR spectroscopy of normal and ischemic rat skeletal muscle. Use of a shift reagent in vivo.* Nmr Biomed, 1990. **3**(2): p. 47–58.

151. Rexroth, W, Semmler, W, Guckel, F, *et al., Assessment of muscular metabolism in peripheral arterial occlusive disease using 31P nuclear magnetic resonance spectroscopy. Comparison with metabolite concentrations in femoral blood.* Klin Wochenschr, 1989. **67**(16): p. 804–812.

152. Blum, H, Schnall, MD, Chance, B, *et al., Intracellular sodium flux and high-energy phosphorus metabolites in ischemic skeletal muscle.* Am J Physiol, 1988. **3**(1): p. 1–8.

153. Heppenstall, RB, Sapega, AA, Scott, R, *et al., The compartment syndrome. An experimental and clinical study of muscular energy metabolism using phosphorus nuclear magnetic resonance spectroscopy.* Clin Orthop, 1988: p. 138–155.

154. Park, JH, Gibbs, SJ, Price, RR, *et al., Inflammatory myopathies: MR imaging and spectroscopy.* Radiology, 1991. **179**(2): p. 343–344.

155. Berquist, TH, Ehman, RL, King, BF, *et al., Value of MR imaging in differentiating benign from malignant soft-tissue masses: Study of 95 lesions.* AJR, 1990. **155**: p. 1251–1255.

156. Pettersson, H, Eliasson, J, Egund, N, *et al., Gadolinium-DTPA enhancement of soft tissue tumors in magnetic resonance imaging—Preliminary clinical experience in five patients.* Skeletal Radiol, 1988. **17**: p. 319–323.

157. Karczmar, GS, Meyerhoff, DJ, Boska, MD, *et al., P-31 spectroscopy study of response of superficial human tumors to therapy.* Radiology, 1991. **179**(1): p. 149–153.

158. Lemmi, MA, Fletcher, BD, Marina, NM, *et al., Use of MR imaging to assess results of chemotherapy for Ewing sarcoma.* AJR, 1990. **155**: p. 343–346.

MRI of the Foot and Ankle,
edited by A.L. Deutsch, J.H. Mink, and R. Kerr,
Raven Press, Ltd., New York © 1992

CHAPTER 11

MR Angiography

Fred L. Steinberg, Charles L. Dumoulin, and Andrew L. Deutsch

Magnetic resonance angiography (MRA) represents a rapidly developing area within the field of magnetic resonance imaging (MRI) that exploits the properties of moving blood during MRI acquisition to produce images of the vascular system (1–18). MRA developed as an outgrowth of the early work in MRI that dealt with reduction of image artifacts arising from motion. Mechanisms that degraded conventional MRIs were eventually identified and modifications in imaging techniques were introduced to circumvent the undesirable effects of vascular flow and motion, allowing clinical images to be obtained with marked artifact reduction. Several research groups recognized, however, the potential of exploiting these very artifact-producing phenomena. Instead of trying to control or eliminate these phenomena, they designed MRI strategies that took advantage of the phenomena to generate flow-sensitive images. From the inception of this work, the potential value of MRA to the diagnostic imaging armamentarium was recognized.

The earliest acceptance of clinical MRA in the diagnosis and staging of vascular diseases has occurred for applications in the brain and extracranial carotid arteries (19–25). Neurovascular applications of MRA have grown during the past few years as the rapid pace of research has produced a variety of new techniques and instrumentation. MRA of the intracranial arterial as well as venous circulation provides the prototype for MRA of the peripheral arterial and venous circulation of the extremities, for which considerably less experience has been reported. Differences in anatomy and blood flow physiology, however, have necessitated the development of new methods specifically tailored for assessment of the peripheral vascular system (26–28). The potential for future development in this area represents the rationale for inclusion of this section in a book devoted to imaging of the lower extremity musculoskeletal system. This chapter provides the interested reader with a basic primer of the physical principles underlying vascular MRI as well as an overview of present and potential future applications as they relate to the lower extremity and foot and ankle.

HISTORICAL PERSPECTIVE

Early work by Singer (29) and Hahn (30) explored the relationships of flow phenomena in the context of nonimaging applications of magnetic resonance. In 1982, Moran first introduced the basic tenets for the detection of motion with MR (31). Wedeen and colleagues created the first set of MRA images on normal volunteers as early as 1984 (32). Employing cardiac-gated spin-echo techniques that depended on phase differences in arterial blood flow signal intensity between systole and diastole, Wedeen was able to create images of arterial flow in the lower extremities and extracranial carotid arteries. His technique required two sets of acquired images to be subtracted from one another to produce MR angiograms. Due to the duration of the exam and its insensitivity to smaller vessels, particularly those with only slightly pulsatile or steady flow, the technique was not considered clinically viable. Independent of Wedeen's work, Dumoulin and Hart designed a gradient-echo technique that relied on additional gradient pulses to create velocity-induced phase shifts (9). This technique, called phase-contrast MRA, reduced the imaging time to only a few minutes and allowed for more precise detection of blood flow within a range of velocities and flow directions. Subsequent

F. L. Steinberg: Center for Vascular and Advanced Body MRI, Roxsan Radiology Medical Group, Beverly Hills, California 90048.

C. L. Dumoulin: General Electric Research and Development Center, Schenectady, New York 12301.

A. L. Deutsch: Tower Musculoskeletal Imaging Center, Los Angeles, California 90048, and Department of Radiology, University of California, San Diego, California.

developments in phase-contrast MRA by this group have included time-resolved (33,34) and three-dimensional imaging procedures (35).

During the early days of MRI, several groups investigated the complicated behavior of contrast relating to blood flow in conventional MRIs (36,37). Particularly intriguing was the relatively bright appearance of blood as it entered the imaged region when scanning was performed rapidly (2). Laub and colleagues recognized the potential for an angiographic representation of these data and developed the method that has become known as three-dimensional time-of-flight angiography (19). Masaryk et al. reported the first clinical evaluations of MRA with this technique in 1988 (20,21). A second class of time-of-flight MRA based on two-dimensional rather than three-dimensional data acquisition was demonstrated by Gullberg et al. in 1987 (12). This technique overcame some of the limitations of three-dimensional data acquisition, and has proven particularly useful for imaging venous structures in the legs.

THE PHYSICS OF MR ANGIOGRAPHY

Users of MR angiography should be aware of several physical aspects of the technique to have a fuller ap-

preciation of its strengths and limitations. This is particularly true considering the complexity of the methods and the importance of proper diagnosis.

PHYSIOLOGICAL FLOW

The nature of flow within a blood vessel depends heavily on the velocity, pulsatility, and physical properties and shape of the vessel (38). Consequently, flow patterns found in arteries are very different from those found in veins. In addition, flow in a curved or branched vessel differs from that in a straight vessel. Also, when a blood vessel has a narrowing, or stenosis, flow can become complex, particularly if the narrowing is irregular in shape.

If one constructs a large tank, such as the one shown in Fig. 11.1, and drains that tank through a relatively small tube having a circular cross-section, the profile of velocity at the entrance to the tube will be uniform (i.e., all the fluid traveling through the tube at that point will be traveling at the same velocity). This uniform distribution of velocities is called plug flow. As the fluid moves down the tube, however, the viscous nature of the fluid causes the layer of fluid closest to the wall of the tube to slow down. This in turn slows down the adjacent fluid until a new flow profile is estab-

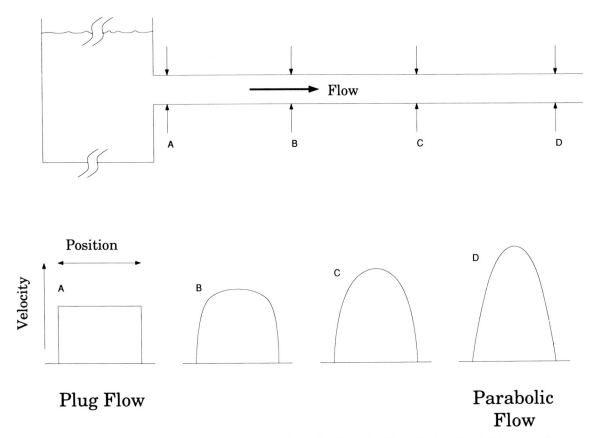

FIG. 11.1. The development of parabolic flow in a circular tube. Note that as the fluid enters the tube from the large reservoir, the velocity distribution is uniform. This is called plug flow. As the fluid moves down the tube, however, the velocity profile changes to a parabola.

lished. This new profile has a parabolic distribution and is characterized by zero velocity at the wall of the tube and a velocity in the center of the tube that is twice that of the average velocity. It is important to note that as the fluid moves down the tube, the plug flow profile cannot be maintained, but parabolic flow, once established, is maintained indefinitely.

Frequently, it is convenient to think of the flow within a blood vessel as being uniform across the vessel. Unfortunately, this assumption is often erroneous since plug flow is rarely found *in-vivo* except during periods of acceleration and deceleration. Frequently, an assumption of parabolic flow is more appropriate, but this too is not always correct.

Parabolic fluid flow within a tube is changed if the tube curves or bifurcates (Fig. 11.2). In the curved tube, the parabolic flow is skewed toward the outer wall by inertial effects. As the fluid hits the outer wall

of the vessel, secondary motions in the flow are created. In the case of a bifurcation, the flow is split between two paths. As in the curved tube, inertial effects skew the flow profile toward the inner walls of the bifurcation and a region of flow separation can arise. This region is characterized by slow flow and can contain flow moving in the opposite direction.

In all the flow examples that have been discussed so far, the fluid flow is assumed to be nonturbulent. Turbulent flow can arise if the fluid is made to go through a relatively small opening, such as a stenosis, or if the flow velocity is suddenly changed. The turbulence or nonturbulence of flow is determined by the viscosity and velocity of the fluid and the diameter of the vessel. This state is characterized by a unitless quantity called the Reynolds number. Turbulence occurs when the Reynolds number of the fluid flow exceeds 2000 to 2500.

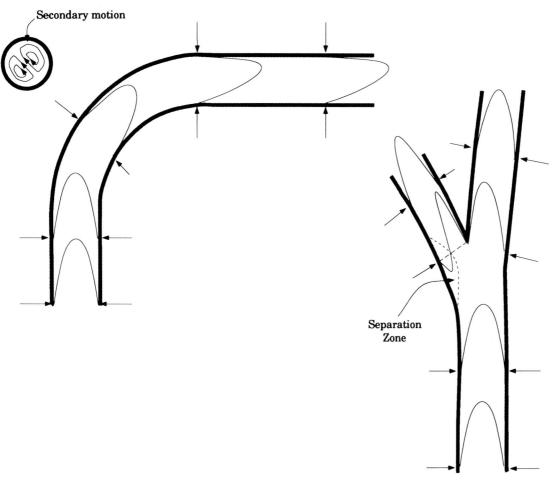

FIG. 11.2. Changes in a parabolic flow profile induced by (**left**) a curve in the tube and (**right**) a bifurcation. Note that as the parabolic flow profile enters the curved section of the tube it is skewed toward the outer wall. This happens because the inertia of the moving fluid carries it away from the midline of the tube. As the fluid moves toward the wall, it displaces the fluid already there and secondary motions in the fluid are created. Secondary motions are also created in a bifurcation. Frequently this motion leads to a reversal of the flow in part of the tube. This separation of the flow profile occurs in a region called the separation zone. Separation zones are frequently seen in the bifurcation of the carotid (and other) arteries in the body.

When complex or turbulent flow is present, unstable eddies of all sizes are spontaneously created and destroyed. This is frequently seen with Doppler ultrasound in high-grade stenoses and in flow associated with aneurysms. With MR, complicated and unstable flow profiles arising from turbulent and near-turbulent flow frequently causes signal loss, leading to apparent discontinuity in vessels and overestimation of the severity and length of stenoses. These problems have proven difficult to overcome with MRA techniques, but improvements in imaging methods and hardware are making MRA more robust.

If blood vessels were perfectly rigid, the acceleration of blood flow by the heart in each cardiac cycle would be propagated through the arterial system at the speed of sound (assuming that blood behaves as an incompressible fluid). Blood vessels are compliant, however, and the increase in arterial blood pressure at the beginning of the cardiac cycle causes the arteries to expand. This expansion slows the propagation of the pressure wave. As the blood flows down the aorta,

much of it enters relatively large branches of the arterial tree such as the brachiocephalic arteries, the celiac trunk, and the renal arteries. In a normal individual, these branches offer little resistance to the blood flow and the temporal profile of blood flow in the aorta is not substantially altered. Distal to the renal arteries, however, blood flow profiles change. In a normal individual, flow becomes triphasic. During systole it flows forward and then reverses direction momentarily before flowing forward once again. During most of diastole, however, the flow actually stops. In individuals with stenotic lesions this flow pattern is changed. Flow distal to a stenosis tends to be more constant over time and flow reversal does not occur. Several temporal flow profiles are shown in Fig. 11.3.

THE SOURCE OF THE MR SIGNAL

From the point of view of an MR scanner, the human body is nothing more than a collection of hydrogen

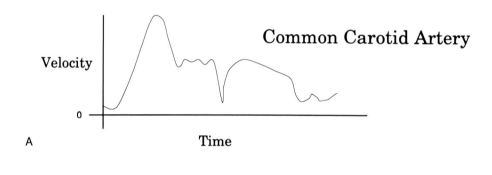

A

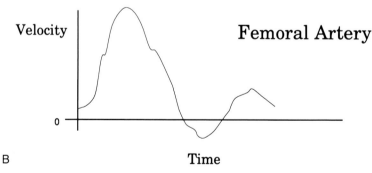

B

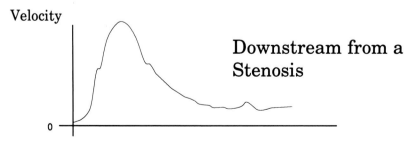

C

FIG. 11.3. Velocity as a function of time during the cardiac cycle in the common carotid artery (**A**) and femoral artery (**B**) of a healthy individual. **C:** The velocity profile distal to a stenosis.

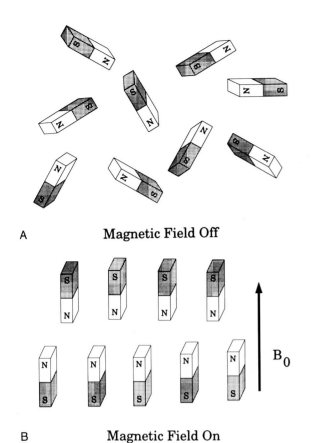

A   **Magnetic Field Off**

B_0

B   **Magnetic Field On**

FIG. 11.4. Bar magnet representation of the nuclei in the body in the absence of an external magnetic field (**top**) and in the presence of an external magnetic field (**bottom**).

atoms, most of which are part of water molecules. The nuclei of these hydrogen atoms have a property called spin, which causes them to behave as tiny bar magnets. Since there are many hydrogen atoms within the body, and since the bar magnets are orientated in all directions, there is no net magnetic field created in the body, as seen in Fig. 11.4A. When this collection of atoms is placed in a large magnet, however, the bar magnet within each hydrogen nucleus aligns with or against the main magnetic field (Fig. 11.4B). Since the nuclei aligned with the field are at a lower energy state than their counterparts aligned against the field, there is a slight excess in the population in the lower energy state. Consequently, there is a net magnetic field generated in the body by the excess population. This net magnetic field is called longitudinal magnetization and it is aligned with the main magnetic field. It is worth noting that the strength of the longitudinal magnetization is directly proportional to the strength of the main magnetic field. Consequently, stronger magnets generate more longitudinal magnetization.

It is convenient to portray the net magnetic field generated by the hydrogen nuclei in the body as a single vector as shown in Fig. 11.5A. This vector actually represents many bar magnets, all aligned in the same direction.

One attribute of longitudinal magnetization is that it cannot be directly observed. It can be influenced, however, by a second magnetic field. This can be done by applying an rf pulse of an appropriate strength and fre-

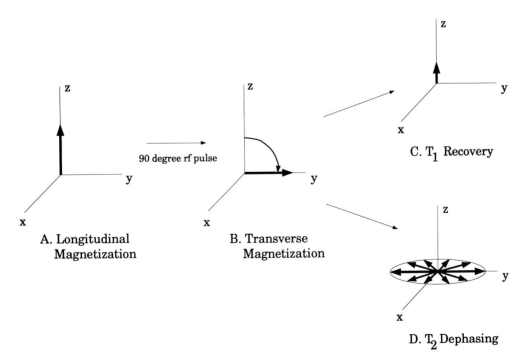

90 degree rf pulse

C. T_1 Recovery

A. Longitudinal Magnetization

B. Transverse Magnetization

D. T_2 Dephasing

FIG. 11.5. Once the body is placed in the magnetic field, the hydrogen nuclei develop longitudinal magnetization (**A**). This magnetization can be converted to transverse magnetization with an rf pulse (**B**). The magnetization returns to its equilibrium state through the T1 mechanism (**C**) and the T2 mechanism (**D**).

quency to nutate the longitudinal magnetization into the transverse plane, as shown in Fig. 11.5B. The degree of rotation imparted to the magnetization is called the flip angle, and stronger rf pulses give larger flip angles. Note that the maximum amount of transverse magnetization is generated when the flip angle is 90°. Unlike longitudinal magnetization, transverse magnetization can induce a signal that can be detected in a receiver coil. It is this signal that is used to build an MR image.

Amplitude is the only parameter that is needed to describe the state of longitudinal magnetization. Two parameters, however, are needed to describe transverse magnetization. These are amplitude and phase. In a vector model of magnetization, the amplitude is represented as the length of the vector. The phase of the magnetization, on the other hand, is represented as the angle of rotation of the vector in the transverse plane. This rotation angle can be expressed in radians or degrees with respect to a reference. This reference phase (i.e., the angle that is considered to be zero) is typically chosen to be the phase of the transverse magnetization immediately after it has been created by the rf pulse.

After an rf pulse two processes occur to return the magnetization into alignment with the main magnetic field. The first process is the gradual reestablishment of longitudinal magnetization (Fig. 11.5C). This occurs exponentially with a time constant called T1. The second process occurs because the net magnetization arises from a large number of nuclei. Since each component of the net magnetization is in a unique environment, the individual components of the magnetization eventually lose phase coherence with one another as shown in Fig. 11.5D. This loss of phase coherence also occurs exponentially, but with a time constant called T2. By necessity T1 is always greater than or equal to T2.

Coherent changes in the phase of transverse magnetization are an essential part of conventional MRI and of MR angiography. Several processes can lead to a coherent change in phase, but the most important process is the temporary change in magnetic field that occurs with the application of a magnetic field gradient pulse.

Unlike the static magnetic field, the gradients have a spatial dependence in which the exact field at a given location is proportional to its position along the direction of the gradient. Gradient pulses generated in an MRI system typically last for a few milliseconds and cause relatively small changes in the magnetic field. Nevertheless, the pulses are powerful enough to change the phase of transverse magnetization and the size of this change is proportional to the change in magnetic field (and hence the location of the magnetization along the gradient).

IMAGE FORMATION WITH MR

In the creation of a conventional MRI, spatial information is encoded by the application of magnetic field gradients. These gradients cause the strength of the magnetic field to vary in a linear fashion across a selected direction of the body. Changing the strength of the magnetic field changes the frequency of the signal created by the transverse spin magnetization. This change in frequency can be detected and interpreted as positional information.

In a conventional image, two or three dimensions of data are typically acquired. The first dimension is determined by the application of a magnetic field gradient during the acquisition of the signal. Since transverse magnetization at different points along this magnetic field gradient resonate at different frequencies, the detected signal contains many different frequencies, each from a unique point along the gradient. These frequency components are easily resolved by the application of a linear mathematical process called a Fourier transformation. This first dimension is usually called the readout or frequency-encoded dimension.

Resolution of spatial information in the second dimension occurs through a similar mechanism. The application of a second magnetic field gradient, however, cannot be made simultaneously with the frequency-encoding gradient because the two gradients would merely combine to give a gradient in an oblique direction. Rather, spatial encoding in the second dimension is accomplished with a short magnetic field gradient pulse applied before the data detection. This pulse induces a phase shift in the signal that is proportional to the location of the transverse magnetization in the second gradient dimension. As subsequent data are collected, this gradient pulse is varied in amplitude to cause the phase of the signals to change in a linear fashion. Application of a Fourier transformation in this phase-encoded dimension resolves data as it does in the frequency-encoded dimension. Resolution of data in the third dimension is easily accomplished by using an additional phase-encoding dimension.

PHYSICS OF FLOW-RELATED ENHANCEMENT

Longitudinal magnetization, although not directly observable, determines the maximum amount of transverse magnetization that can be generated. If we apply an rf pulse infrequently and allow the longitudinal magnetization to return to its equilibrium (or fully relaxed state) between pulses, each rf pulse will generate a large amount of transverse magnetization. If the same rf pulse is applied more frequently, however, insufficient time exists for the reestablishment of a fully relaxed longitudinal state, and subsequent rf pulses nutate a smaller longitudinal vector. If this is carried further with more frequent rf pulses, the longitudinal magnetization reaches a state of saturation and very little transverse magnetization is generated after each rf pulse.

In modern time-of-flight MR angiography procedures, a region of interest is subjected to frequent rf pulses designed to saturate the longitudinal magnetization. Consequently, tissue in this region of interest generates little detectable signal. Blood that enters the region of interest, however, has not been subjected to the nutation effects of the rf pulses, and thus is in a fully relaxed state. Since this blood is fully relaxed, its signal is relatively strong. This is illustrated in Fig. 11.6.

There are several important aspects of in-flow–enhanced angiography. First is that the blood is fully relaxed only before it reaches the region of interest. Once the blood is in the region of interest it is subjected to

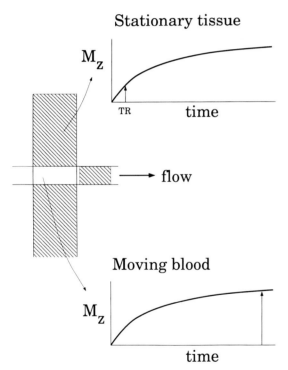

Stationary tissue

Moving blood

FIG. 11.6. Penetration of fully relaxed blood into a region being subjected to frequent rf pulses. In this figure a thick slab is excited by the rf pulses with a repetition time called TR. The region of the slab excitation is denoted by the cross-hatching. A vessel carrying flowing blood enters the slab from the left and exits to the right. After each rf pulse the longitudinal magnetization attempts to return with time to its equilibrium value in an exponential fashion, as illustrated in the two curves. The tissue surrounding the vessel gives an attenuated signal because its longitudinal magnetization is not allowed to return to a fully relaxed state by the frequent application of rf pulses. The blood that enters the region of interest, on the other hand, gives an intense signal because it has not experienced any rf pulses.

the same saturation effects that are suppressing the signals from the surrounding tissue. This causes blood to lose its contrast after it has experienced several rf pulses. Consequently, the penetration of detectable blood into the region of interest is limited by the velocity of the blood, the repetition rate of the rf pulses, the flip angle of the rf pulses, and the T1 of blood.

The contrast mechanism of in-flow–enhanced angiography is not flow. Rather, it is the different levels of saturation that can be obtained between flowing and nonflowing tissue. A compromise must be made to maximize the signal from blood and minimize the signal from the surrounding tissue. Consequently, surrounding tissue is difficult to suppress fully since the steps taken to suppress the tissue also act to limit the penetration of visible blood into the region of interest.

If all tissue in the body had the same T1 the contrast generated by in-flow effects would be unambiguous. Unfortunately, tissues having a short T1, can appear artifactually bright in these images. For example, thrombus and mucus can appear isointense with flowing blood in some imaging protocols. Care should be taken to avoid interpreting these tissues as patent vascular structures.

THE PHYSICS OF VELOCITY-INDUCED PHASE SHIFTS

Time-of-flight effects arise from the movement of longitudinal magnetization during a relatively long period. A second flow phenomenon occurs when transverse magnetization moves in the direction of a magnetic field gradient. This effect can be the source of image artifacts in conventional MRI, and it can be exploited to form angiographic images.

A fundamental aspect of MR is that nuclei resonate at a frequency that is exactly proportional to the strength of the magnetic field. Consequently, when a magnetic field gradient is applied, the magnetic field is changed and transverse magnetization at different locations resonate at different frequencies. If the duration of the gradient is finite, a phase shift in the transverse magnetization directly proportional to position is induced. This phase shift is proportional to position, and thus encodes position.

The position-dependent phase shifts generated by a gradient pulse can be undone by applying a second gradient pulse of equal duration but opposite polarity. If the nuclei move during the interval between the first and second gradient pulses, however, the phase shifts induced by the first pulse will not be exactly canceled by those of the second pulse. The residual phase shift will be directly proportional to the distance that the nuclei traveled in the interval between the gradient pulses, and thus it will also be proportional to the flow

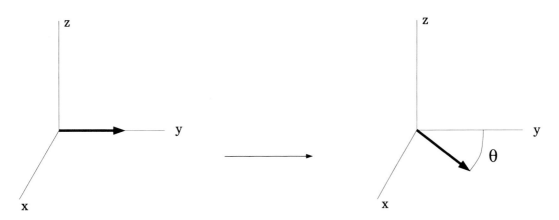

1. Generate Transverse
   Magnetization

2. Apply Flow-Encoding
   Gradient Pulses

3. Phase shift now proportional
   to Velocity

FIG. 11.7. Velocity-induced phase shifts in transverse spin magnetization. In the first step, transverse spin magnetization is created by nutating longitudinal spin magnetization with an rf pulse (see Fig. 11.5). This transverse magnetization is represented as a vector in the XY plane. Then a flow-encoding gradient pulse is applied. Details of flow-encoding pulses are described later in the text. This flow-encoding pulse induces a phase shift that is independent of the location of the spin within the magnet, but is proportional to velocity. This phase shift, denoted as θ in step 3 is the angle of rotation that has been induced in the vector representing the transverse magnetization. It can be expressed as either radians (i.e., a number between $-\pi$ and π) or as degrees (-180.0 to 180.0). Note that this effect is the fundamental phenomenon of phase-sensitive MRA methods.

velocity. This phase change, illustrated in Fig. 11.7, is the key to phase sensitive flow imaging procedures such as phase-contrast MRA.

As blood moves in the body, its position as a function of time is determined not only by its velocity but also by its acceleration and higher order terms of motion. Motion-induced phase shifts can be made proportional to any combination of these terms by appropriately designed gradient waveforms. The most common flow-encoding gradient waveform is the simple bipolar gradient pulse described above and shown in Fig. 11.8. This waveform induces a phase shift that is independent of position, but is proportional to velocity and all higher orders of motion.

In modern phase-sensitive MRA, velocity-induced phase shifts are used to discriminate signals arising from flowing blood from that arising from stationary tissue. Signals obtained in this way are detected only by virtue of their motion. Consequently, suppression of background tissue in an ideal instrument is complete and artifactually bright signals from short T1 tissue does not occur. Furthermore, since the induced phase shift is directly proportional to velocity, quantitative flow information can be extracted.

Phase-sensitive MRA methods have a few limitations that should be recognized by the clinician. First, phase-sensitive methods are very demanding on the quality of the instrument, and phase stability is essen-

tial. Fortunately, most modern MR scanners, when within their specifications, are adequate. A second limitation is that only a single flow dimension is obtained in each measurement. Consequently, a phase-sensitive acquisition has the potential to be longer than an equiv-

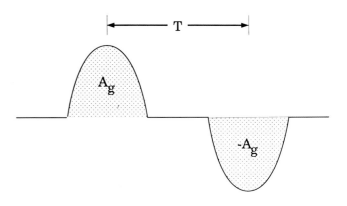

$$\theta = \gamma VTA_g$$

FIG. 11.8. The bipolar flow-encoding gradient pulse. The first lobe dephases transverse magnetization by an amount proportional to position. The second lobe rephases the magnetization. If the magnetization moves in the interval between the pulses, however, the cancellation of the induced phase shift is incomplete. The residual phase shift is proportional to velocity.

alent time-of-flight acquisition, but this is not always the case. An additional point that must be considered is the choice of the velocity sensitivity. Stronger flow-encoding gradient pulses induce larger phase shifts for lower velocities, but at the risk of aliasing phase shifts induced by higher velocities.

MRA TECHNIQUES

MRA is not a single technique. Rather, it is a collection of methods, each having some unique features and limitations. Because of the relative strengths and weaknesses of each method and the complicated nature of flow in the body, different clinical applications are best served by different imaging protocols.

In general there are two broad classes of MRA defined by the fundamental phenomena that give contrast in each case. These are (a) time-of-flight methods in which movement of longitudinal magnetization is detected, and (b) phase-sensitive methods in which phase shifts induced by movement of transverse magnetization in the presence of a field gradient are detected. Many variations of both types of MRA have been described in the literature. Only a few of these, however, are widely used. These methods are described below.

Time-of-flight MRA

In time-of-flight MRA, the contrast between blood and stationary tissue is determined by the inflow of unsaturated spins into the imaging volume and the saturation of stationary tissue in that same volume. Two methods are currently in use. These are three-dimensional time-of-flight (3D-TOF) and two-dimensional time-of-flight (2D-TOF) angiography. A new method, multislab three-dimensional time-of-flight angiography (18), combines the best aspects of the two- and three-dimensional methods and will also be discussed.

3D-TOF

With 3D-TOF MRA, a three-dimensional image is acquired in a single scan as shown in Fig. 11.9. A limited volume, closely matched to the acquired field-of-view, is excited by the rf pulses. This excitation volume is typically several centimeters thick. Blood from outside the excited volume enters the volume and initially gives a strong signal. Rapidly flowing unsaturated blood penetrates deeply into the volume and may traverse it entirely if the vessel is relatively straight. Slowly moving blood, on the other hand, is easily saturated and quickly becomes invisible in the angiogram. Blood flowing in tortuous vessels is forced to spend substantial time in the imaging volume and is also at risk of becoming saturated.

The choice of imaging parameters with 3D-TOF angiography is a compromise between the need to have strong blood signals in the volume of interest and the need to suppress the background as well as possible. Typical parameters used in neurovascular applications

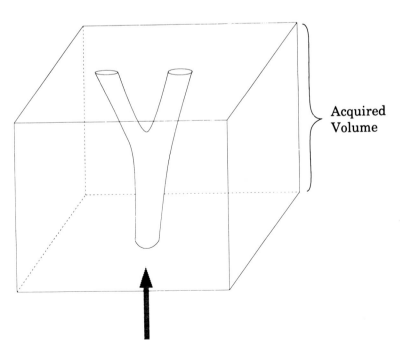

Acquired Volume

Inflow of unsaturated blood

FIG. 11.9. Geometry of a typical three-dimensional time-of-flight procedure. In this procedure the entire volume of interest is subjected to the rf pulses and a full three-dimensional image is acquired. The frequent rf pulses cause the entire region to reach a state of partial saturation. Consequently, the saturated magnetization gives only a weak signal. Blood flowing into the region, on the other hand, has not experienced the rf pulses and is in a fully relaxed state. This causes the blood to give a relatively strong signal. Unfortunately, once the blood has experienced several rf pulses, it too becomes saturated and contrast between blood and the surrounding tissue is lost.

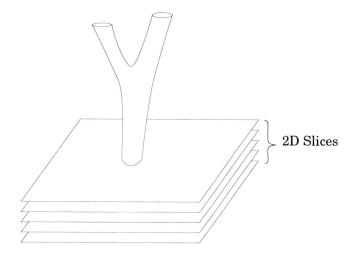

2D Slices

FIG. 11.10. Geometry of a typical two-dimensional time-of-flight procedure. In this procedure only the tissue in a thin slice is excited by the rf pulses. Consequently, the saturation region is limited to the slice. Blood entering the slice is not saturated and appears bright. A three-dimensional angiogram is generated by sequentially acquiring the slices until a full three-dimensional matrix is collected. Since the saturation region in this technique is much smaller than it is for a three-dimensional time-of-flight procedure, penetration of fully relaxed blood is more efficient and the contrast between blood and surrounding tissue is usually better. Image resolution in the third (i.e., vertical) dimension, however, is usually less than with true three-dimensional methods due to instrument limitations.

of 3D-TOF include:

TR = 40–50 ms
TE = minimum
Flip angle = 30°
FOV = as small as practical
Slice thickness = 0.7–1.5 mm

Since lower extremity MRA frequently requires imaging long lengths of blood vessels, standard 3D-TOF techniques are not practical and have not been widely used for the lower leg, foot, and ankle.

2D-TOF

The penetration problem in 3D-TOF procedures can be lessened by decreasing the acquisition volume. This is accomplished in the 2D-TOF procedure by acquiring data in thin planes perpendicular to the blood vessel as shown in Fig. 11.10. Data from each plane are collected in a single scan. Additional planes are acquired on subsequent scans until a full three-dimensional matrix is obtained. Note that here the term "two-dimensional" refers to a single scan and not to the final data matrix.

2D-TOF procedures are much more sensitive to slow flow than 3D-TOF procedures because of the decreased sensitivity to the penetration effect. An additional benefit is that the flip angle can be increased to saturate the stationary tissue more efficiently. Furthermore, increasing the field-of-view in the slice direction carries no penalty and long vessels are relatively straightforward to image. While 2D-TOF methods are much less sensitive to penetration effects than 3D-TOF methods, blood flow in vessels lying in the plane of data acquisition can be more difficult to image because of the more aggressive use of saturation.

Gradient and rf power limitations make the excitation of a slice thinner than about 2.0 mm difficult. Consequently, 2D-TOF procedures typically have poorer resolution in the slice dimension than 3D-TOF procedures. Fortunately, this is rarely a problem for applications in the lower extremities.

Typical parameters used in both neurovascular and

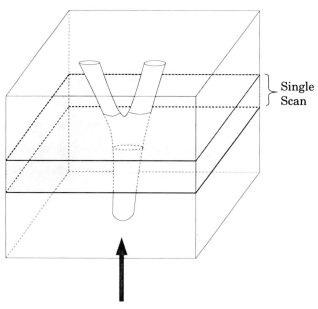

Single Scan

Inflow of unsaturated blood

FIG. 11.11. Geometry of a typical multislab three-dimensional time-of-flight procedure. This method is a hybrid of three-dimensional and two-dimensional time-of-flight angiography. In this technique three-dimensional time-of-flight MRA images are collected at several locations over the region of interest. This minimizes the loss of contrast that occurs as the fully relaxed blood enters the region of the rf pulses and becomes saturated, without loss of resolution in the third dimension.

lower extremity applications include:

TR = 40–50 ms
TE = minimum
Flip angle = 50–90°
FOV = as small as practical
Slice thickness = 1.5–2.0 mm

Since 2D-TOF procedures work best for flow that is perpendicular to the acquired image planes, acquisition of 2D-TOF angiograms in the lower extremity is usually best achieved by straightening the foot by plantar flexion and scanning in the axial plane.

Multislab 3D-TOF

The primary shortcoming of 3D-TOF procedures is the penetration problem experienced by slowly moving blood. The primary shortcoming of 2D-TOF procedures (at least in neurovascular procedures), on the other hand, is the limited resolution in the third dimension. A hybrid technique, shown in Fig. 11.11, overcomes both problems by stacking adjacent volumes of 3D-TOF data. This technique is relatively

new, but appears promising for neurovascular work. Its potential for applications of the lower extremities is less certain, but worth investigating.

Phase Contrast MRA

Phase contrast MRA procedures are techniques that are sensitive to velocity-induced phase shifts in transverse magnetization. In these procedures, data are acquired first with flow-encoding gradients of one polarity and then with flow-encoding gradients of the opposite polarity. The complex difference of the acquired data is then taken. Signals from stationary tissue have no velocity-induced phase shift, and thus cancel upon subtraction. Signals from moving spins, however, combine additively and are preserved as illustrated in Fig. 11.12.

The velocity sensitivity of a phase contrast angiogram is determined by the amplitude and duration of the flow-encoding gradient pulse. Since it is the phase shift that is proportional to velocity, the signal that is presented in a phase contrast angiogram is approximately proportional to velocity only if the velocity in-

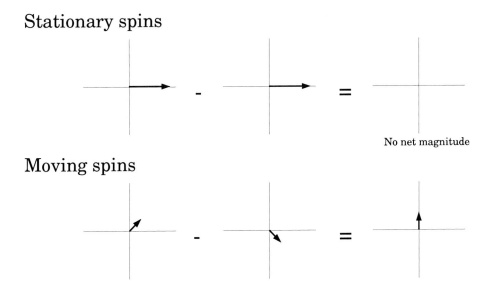

FIG. 11.12. Vector representation of the suppression of stationary tissue and the preservation of moving blood in phase-contrast angiography. In a phase-contrast procedure two sets of data are collected. The first data set is collected with a bipolar gradient pulse (e.g., a positive lobe followed by a negative lobe) that induces a phase shift that is proportional to velocity (see Fig. 11.8). The second data set is collected in an identical fashion except that the polarity of the bipolar gradient is reversed (e.g., a negative lobe followed by a positive lobe). The difference of these two data sets is then calculated. Most of the transverse magnetization in the body is stationary and is not affected by the flow-encoding pulses since the flow-encoding pulses induce a phase shift that is proportional to velocity and the velocity of stationary tissue is zero. Consequently, the signals from stationary tissue are cancelled upon subtraction of the detected signals as illustrated in the top row of the figure. Signals from moving blood, on the other hand, undergo a phase shift that is proportional to the blood's velocity and has a mathematical sign that is controlled by the gradient polarity. Consequently, when the difference is calculated, the signals from moving blood add constructively and appear in the angiogram.

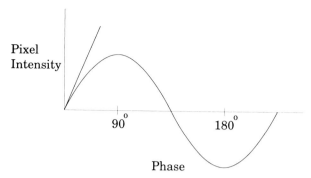

Pixel Intensity

90° 180°

Phase

FIG. 11.13. The relationship between motion-induced phase shifts (and hence velocity) and image pixel intensity in phase-contrast angiography. As the velocity of blood increases, the phase shift induced by a flow-encoding gradient increases. Unfortunately, if the phase shift increases too much it becomes indistinguishable from a smaller phase shift. For example, blood moving at a given velocity might induce a 45° phase shift. Blood moving three times faster would induce a 3 × 45 = 135° phase shift. When the MRI is formed, this 135° phase shift gives a signal intensity that is identical to the intensity generated by the 45° phase shift. To avoid this problem, the phase shift for the largest expected velocity should be limited to 90°. If the phase shift of the largest velocity is limited to about a radian (i.e., 57°), the pixel intensity in the angiographic image is approximately proportional to velocity. If it were exactly proportional to velocity, the signal intensity would be given by the straight line.

duces a phase shift less than about 1 radian (i.e., 57.29°). The velocity at which the pixel intensity is maximized, or in other words, the velocity giving a 90° phase shift, is frequently referred to as Venc~. The relationship between image pixel intensity and velocity is shown in Fig. 11.13.

The ability to select the flow-encoding strength gives the operator a great deal of power. By the judicious choice of gradients the flow sensitivity can be set to detect very slow flow or very high flow velocities. Another advantage is that the detected phase shifts carry directional information that frequently proves to be diagnostically useful. Unlike TOF methods, phase contrast methods are equally sensitive to flow in all directions and do not suffer from the penetration effect.

Several phase contrast MRA methods have proven useful for neurovascular, abdominal, and extremity applications. These are described below.

2D Phase Contrast Angiography

Phase contrast MRA procedures are created by incorporating flow-encoding gradient pulses into conventional gradient-recalled imaging procedures. Images containing only signals from flowing blood can be

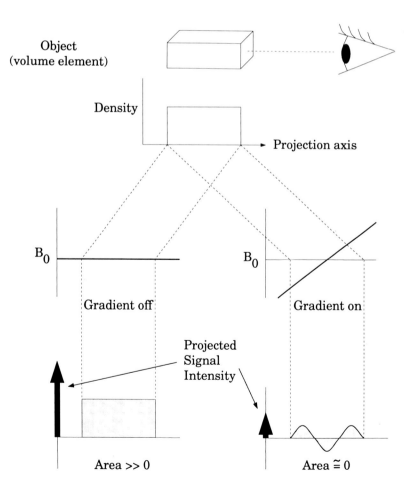

Object (volume element)

Density

Projection axis

B_0 B_0

Gradient off   Gradient on

Projected Signal Intensity

Area >> 0   Area ≅ 0

FIG. 11.14. The effect of projection dephasing on a large object. In this figure an observer (the eye) is using MR to look at an object. The density of the object is uniform as shown in the second row of the figure. This object can be examined in the absence of a magnetic field gradient (*left*) or in the presence of a magnetic field gradient (*right*). Without the gradient, all the detected signals from each part of the object occur at the same frequency and phase. Consequently, when the signals are detected, they add constructively and give a relatively large signal intensity. If the object is detected in the presence of a magnetic field gradient applied in the direction of the projection, however, spins at different locations along the gradient resonate at different frequencies and have different phase shifts. This results in destructive interference of signals from the various parts of the object and a much weaker signal intensity. Signals from small objects, such as blood vessels, are unaffected since the strength of the dephasing gradient is chosen so that small objects have only a small frequency distribution along the projection direction.

obtained using the same scan orientations and fields-of-view found in conventional MRI. Because the phase contrast mechanism efficiently suppresses signals from stationary tissue, angiographic images obtained from much larger volumes are possible. Thus, full projection angiograms can be obtained in the same scan time as a conventional image.

Subtraction of complex data to suppress stationary tissue is limited by the dynamic range of the data. If the stationary signal component is substantially larger than the signals from flowing blood, inaccuracies in the subtraction may leave residual stationary tissue signal that is comparable in amplitude to the flow signal. One method that has proven useful to overcome this problem is to intentionally introduce a small magnetic field inhomogeneity along the direction of the projection, as shown in Fig. 11.14. This dephases the transverse magnetization of large features such as stationary tissue, but leaves the magnetization in small features such as vessels relatively undisturbed.

One problem with any projection technique is that the image voxel is highly anisotropic. The in-plane resolution of the image may be high, but each voxel has a depth that can be as large as the thickness of the anatomy being imaged. Overlapping vessels in a projection angiogram can share image voxels yet be physically in regions having different magnetic field strengths. If this happens, the signals from each vessel may have different absolute phases, and destructive interference of signals in the overlapping region is possible. Similarly, if overlapping vessels have very different flow or if a vessel is large enough to have a substantial variation of flow velocities in its projection, anomalous loss of signal is possible.

Cine Phase Contrast Angiography

Cine phase contrast MRA is a variant of 2D phase contrast angiography in which images from many points in the cardiac cycle are obtained, as illustrated

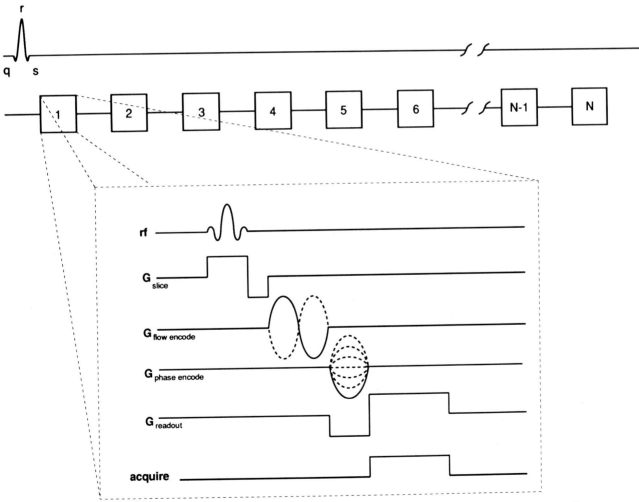

FIG. 11.15. Time-resolved or cine 2D phase-contrast angiography pulse sequence. The pulse sequence includes an rf excitation pulse and gradient pulses for slice selection, flow encoding, and image formation. The sequence is repeated N times for each cardiac cycle.

in Fig. 11.15. This technique has proven particularly useful for applications in the pelvis and extremities where blood flow is highly dynamic.

In normal blood flow in the extremities, there is a triphasic pattern of flow that has a rapid forward flow component in systole, a slow reverse flow component at the beginning of diastole and either stagnant flow or slow forward flow for the duration of diastole. Consequently, in nongated techniques, approximately two-thirds of the data acquisition occurs when there is no significant flow. Cardiac-gated cine angiograms, on the other hand, acquire images at multiple points during the cardiac cycle, and some images are guaranteed to be acquired entirely during periods of flow. Because dynamic flow is found primarily in arteries rather than veins, it can be used to differentiate arteries from veins.

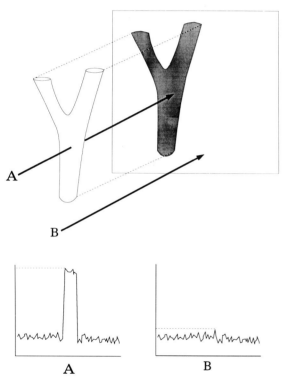

FIG. 11.16. Projection of the maximum intensity pixel to extract a two-dimensional image from a three-dimensional data set. In this procedure "rays" are cast through the three-dimensional object. A two-dimensional projection is created by reducing the data encountered by each "ray" to a single value. With the Maximum Intensity Pixel (*MIP*) algorithm, the value of the most intense pixel is chosen for the projection image. In this illustration two "rays" are highlighted. The first "ray" encounters the bright signal in a vessel and selects the most intense pixel. Likewise the most intense pixel encountered by the second "ray" is selected, but this pixel contains noise. More sophisticated algorithms have been developed, but are not in widespread use.

3D Phase Contrast MRA

Many of the problems of two-dimensional projection angiography can be overcome by obtaining the data directly in three dimensions. Unlike a projection angiogram, a typical 3D angiogram has approximately isotropic voxels. Phase variations across a voxel are minimized because the voxel dimensions are small. Perhaps the most significant advantage, however, is that the data can be analyzed retrospectively in a number of ways. For example, subvolumes of the acquired data set can be extracted to enhance the presentation of features of interest and cross-sections of vessels can be generated.

3D phase contrast MRA is now widely used for neurovascular and abdominal applications. It has not yet been applied extensively in the lower extremities, however, because the dynamic nature of arterial flow has been better imaged with the cine 2D phase contrast procedure.

Strategies for Vessel Selectivity

Vessel selectivity with x-ray angiography is usually straightforward and is controlled by the placement of the catheter. Veins are separated from arteries by simply waiting for the contrast media to pass from the arterial to the venous system. Selective MR angiography, on the other hand, is more difficult since vascular structures are detected by virtue of blood motion rather than the selective replacement of a bolus of blood. Nevertheless, several strategies have been developed to isolate selected structures in MR angiograms. Some of these strategies are applied during data acquisition and others are applied during postprocessing. These techniques select vessels by virtue of location, flow direction, mean velocity, and flow dynamics.

Saturation

Saturation of longitudinal magnetization adjacent to the imaged volume is a widely used method to suppress the appearance of undesired vessels. With this method, extra rf pulses are applied in a volume adjacent to the region of interest. These rf pulses typically have a flip angle between 90° and 120°. Since these pulses are applied frequently, longitudinal spin magnetization in this region does not have time to recover, and is destroyed. As blood moves through this volume, it too becomes saturated. Consequently, as it moves into the imaged region, it is invisible. Blood flowing into the imaged region from the opposite direction, however, does not experience the saturating pulse and is unaffected.

Saturation can be used to select vessels with all MRA procedures. In a 3D-TOF procedure the saturation volume is placed next to the imaged volume. In a 2D-TOF procedure, the saturation volume is always adjacent to the imaged slice and is moved with the slice on subsequent scans.

Suppression of selected blood vessels by saturation relies on the time-of-flight phenomenon. As the saturated blood moves into the region of interest, it is no longer subjected to the saturation pulses and may eventually reach a new steady state determined by the rf pulses in the imaging volume. In a time-of-flight procedure, this new steady state is still somewhat saturated and the blood remains poorly contrasted. With phase contrast procedures, however, the contrast mechanism is motion rather than saturation and when the saturated blood reaches its new steady state, enough magnetization may exist to make the vessel visible.

Use of Phase Information

Phase contrast MRA procedures collect data that contain information about the direction as well as speed of blood flow. Although the speed is typically displayed as a pixel intensity, alternate displays in which the phase of the moving blood is displayed are usually available. Such a presentation makes the direction of flow in a vessel immediately obvious.

Relaxation Contrast Agents

Intravenous injections of relaxation agents, such as gadolinium (Gd)-DTPA, are widely used to alter the T1 of selected tissues. For example, in neurological applications of MRI, Gd-DTPA injections highlight breakdown of the blood–brain barrier. In addition, many neoplasms become more visible in MRIs with the injection of a relaxation contrast agent.

Contrast agents are also beginning to find use in MRA since they shorten the T1 of blood. For time-of-flight procedures this makes the blood more difficult to saturate, and thus increases the penetration of relaxed blood into the imaged volume. Slowly moving blood such as that found in many veins becomes more readily detected. Unfortunately, tissues such as mucous membranes, neoplasms, and regions of hemorrhage are also highlighted and become more readily visible. For phase contrast procedures, the penetration problem and the reduced T1 of some tissues are not an issue and the primary benefit of a contrast injection is an increase in the signal-to-noise ratio. In general, contrast agents make certain vascular structures easier to image, but are of limited usefulness in selectively highlighting a given vascular feature.

MRA POSTPROCESSING TECHNIQUES

Most of the MRA techniques in use for applications of the extremities acquire three dimensions of data. In 2D-TOF, 3D-TOF, and 3D-phase contrast methods the three dimensions are spatial. In cine 2D phase contrast, however, only two dimensions are spatial and the third is temporal. The reduction of these data into a two dimensional format suitable for filming is an important aspect of the MRA process and is described below.

Maximum Intensity Projection

Once three spatial dimensions of data are created, computational steps are necessary to reformat the data into two-dimensional images. Filming thin slice extractions of the three-dimensional data set is straightforward and occasionally useful. The creation of projections in which one of the spatial dimensions is collapsed, however, is usually more helpful. The simplest and most commonly used algorithm that accomplishes this is called the maximum intensity projection (MIP) method. With this technique a ray is traced through the three-dimensional data set for each pixel in the resulting two-dimensional projection. The maximum pixel value found by each ray determines the pixel value in the projection image as shown in Fig. 11.16. This is a highly nonlinear algorithm in which all depth information is lost. In other words, vessels close to the viewer are indistinguishable from vessels farther away. A simple means to recover this depth information is to display several MIP projections sequentially at a variety of view angles on a display monitor. This creates an illusion of the three-dimensional object. More advanced algorithms in which the nearest local maximum is projected are currently under development.

Subvolume Reconstruction

In ideal MR angiograms the contrast between the bright blood and suppressed stationary tissue is sufficient to guarantee that only the vessels are detected in the MIP algorithm. Unfortunately, suppression of stationary tissue is frequently incomplete, particularly for time-of-flight procedures, and the MIP algorithm projects the most intense pixels of the stationary tissue background. This problem is minimized by applying the MIP algorithm only over a selected subvolume of data. In addition to improving the contrast of the projection, subvolume reconstructions can be used to remove overlapping blood vessels to enhance the appearance of the vessels of interest. This effectively allows the operator to perform selective MR angiography. The overall image quality as well as the detection of small blood vessels and vessels with slow flow is greatly enhanced with this technique.

Temporal Filtering

Temporally resolved data such as that obtained with cine 2D phase contrast angiography can also be subjected to projection procedures. The appearance of all vessels can be maximized by applying an MIP algorithm in the temporal dimension. An alternative projection algorithm frequently useful is the calculation of the standard deviation, rather than the maximum pixel, along the ray. This highlights those features that are most dynamic (typically arteries) and suppresses those features that are constant during the cardiac cycle (i.e., veins and background). In cases of arterial blood flow downstream from occlusions and high grade stenoses, however, the arterial flow may no longer be pulsatile and a standard deviation projection may suppress rather than enhance the appearance of the vessel.

CLINICAL APPLICATIONS

The role of MRA in clinical assessment of the vascular system is in a state of rapid evolution. The majority of the reported experience to date has been in applications relating to both the extracranial carotid and intracranial circulation (13,20–25). As significant differences between the intracranial and peripheral circulation exist, the reported experience to date in cerebrovascular imaging may not be directly applicable to MR evaluation of the lower extremities (6,7,15, 26,39). Additionally, it is recognized that MRA significantly differs from conventional arteriography in its ability to depict vascular features such as microvascularity, tumor blush, and arteriovenous circulation time (40). As such, its ultimate role compared to arteriography remains to be established. It is clear, however, from our own as well as other groups reported experience, that MRA can provide a clinically useful roadmap of the arterial and venous anatomy of the lower extremity and reliably demonstrate a variety of vascular abnormalities (4,6,8,16,39,41–49). This section will endeavor to review the capability of MRA to depict normal vascular anatomy as well as consider the present and likely emerging applications for MRA as they pertain to the peripheral circulation with particular reference to most common abnormalities affecting the lower extremities.

Lower Extremity Flow Considerations

As previously discussed, the first investigations regarding the clinical utility of MRA were directed at investigations of the carotid arteries and intracranial circulation. The extra- and intracranial circulation is characterized by a large component of diastolic as well as systolic flow. In the high resistance peripheral circulation, however, a completely different pattern of blood flow is evident. In the normal popliteal artery, for example, there is a triphasic waveform of high systolic forward flow followed by a small phase of reverse flow and then a very slow forward flow component (42). Forward flow only occurs during one-third of the cardiac cycle. As such, with techniques designed to image continuously throughout the cardiac cycle, two-thirds of the phase-encoding steps will be acquired when there is no flow information present. As a consequence of such differences in flow physiology, specific stragegies need to be adopted in order to image the normal triphasic flow pattern of the lower extremities successfully.

A number of other additional considerations present challenges for lower extremity imaging compared to evaluation of the cranial circulation. Principal among these is the wide field of view necessary for global imaging (up to 40 cm), as well as the need for sensitivity to a broad range of blood flow velocities and blood vessel diameters that range from 1 cm in diameter iliac arteries where flow velocities are seen on the order of 100 cm/s, to the 3-mm tibial arteries with diastolic flow velocities under 20 cm/s. These large differences make it difficult to select a single velocity sensitivity that is sufficient to image the entire leg without encountering phase wrap and/or undersensitivity to velocity difficulties (17,26–28,33,34,44,50). The orientation of the flowing blood also represents an important consideration in designing an imaging strategy. In addition, there are complex flow direction considerations to be contended with in the pelvis and at other sites, including the tibial trifurcation. Another challenge for optimal image interpretation is a need for suppression of signal from overlapping vascular structures such as veins as well as from background tissue. All of these concerns need to be addressed for clinically useful MRA examinations to be accomplished.

Lower Extremity MRA Techniques

Two primary techniques have been used for assessment of the lower extremity (11,41,47). These include 2D-TOF and cine phase contrast techniques. 2D-TOF techniques with slices acquired perpendicular to direction of blood flow are capable of covering a wide field of view as they are less susceptible than 3D-TOF to problems of saturation and signal loss as the flow penetrates the imaging volume. With 2D-TOF techniques, we most commonly employ a 32-cm field of view. A tracking saturation pulse is employed to eliminate venous flow (11,13,18,51). A TR time of 50 ms is chosen and the TE set with flow compensation to the minimum value (approximately 7.4 ms on our system). A set of 5-mm contiguous sections are obtained using a 256 × 128 matrix with each section requiring approximately 6 s for acquisition. To image a 30-cm field approximately 6 min is required. To evaluate smaller vessels, changes in voxel size must be made. For assessment of arterial structures below the knee, 3-mm sections are obtained using a 256 × 192 matrix for tibial vessels and 1.5-mm sections and 256 × 192 matrix for evaluation of the small vessels in the foot (50).

The cine phase contrast technique require cardiac gating and acquisition of a set of images throughout the cardiac cycle. Prior to the scan, a velocity-encoding sensitivity is preselected, which controls the duration of the flow-encoding gradients. Coronal projections rather than slices are acquired with infinite thickness. This reduces problems relating to the vessel wandering in and out of the imaging slice. Each 40-cm acquisition is dependent on the heart rate, but a 256 × 128 image can be acquired in as fast as 2 min of imaging time. Therefore, it is possible to cover the four stations from the aortic bifurcation to the foot in as little as 10 min if the proper flow encoding is performed. If a suboptimal flow encoding is selected, artifacts including nonvisualization of arteries and pseudostenoses can be produced. By interrogating the selected anatomy with a range of flow encodings, the incidence of these artifacts can be controlled.

For depiction of normal anatomy, cine phase contrast performs better than time-of-flight techniques, particularly in the pelvis and femoral arteries (6,26,50). In certain situations, unsuppressed stationary tissue in the tibia and fibula create suboptimal images in 2D-TOF techniques whereas this is usually not a problem with cine phase contrast MRA. In the evaluation of slow flow in the foot, however, shorter TEs are currently available using time-of-flight techniques, leading to better overall image quality. This remains a difficult area to achieve consistently high quality images. To increase slow flow sensitivity in a phase contrast acquisition necessitates longer TE times. This may lead to uncontrolled background dephasing with poor stationary tissue suppression for short acquisitions.

Vascular Anatomy

Arterial

The lower extremities are supplied by a system of branching arteries that can provide alternate pathways

of arterial flow in the case of possible obstruction (52,53) (Fig. 11.17). The common femoral artery is the blood vessel that continues from the external iliac artery below the inguinal ligament. There usually is a bifurcation into a superficial femoral artery and profunda femoral artery. The profunda femoral artery divides into several branches including the medial circumflex femoral, lateral circumflex femoral, and perforating and muscular branches, which provide flow to the muscles of the thigh. This major branch is also the chief source of collaterals to the lower leg when the superficial femoral artery is occluded (52). The superficial femoral artery is the direct continuation of the common femoral artery to the lower leg and continues to the adductor canal where it becomes the popliteal artery with four main branches to the knee called the geniculate branches. Below the knee, the vessels trifurcate into the anterior tibial, posterior tibial, and peroneal arteries. There is usually a short segment where the posterior tibial and peroneal arteries are joined before dividing, called the tibioperoneal trunk. The anatomy of the trifurcation can be readily depicted using MRA (Fig. 11.17). The anterior tibial artery continues into the ankle as the dorsalis pedis artery, which then divides into a metatarsal branch and a medial tarsal artery. The posterior tibial artery continues into the posterior plantar arch of the foot and divides into a lateral tarsal and a distal metatarsal branch. Communicating arches on the plantar aspect of the foot are frequent and serve to prevent ischemic foot changes (52,53).

The plantar arch of the foot is formed by the lateral plantar artery and the deep plantar branch of the dorsalis pedis artery (53) (Fig. 11.18). The course of the plantar arch is deep to the metatarsal bones from the base of the fifth metatarsal bone to the proximal third of the first metatarsal bone. The arch gives off four plantar metatarsal branches and several perforating vessels. These perforators anastomose with the dorsal metatarsal arteries. Paired plantar digital arteries arise via the metatarsal arteries. There is an extensive collateral network around the ankle and the calcaneus that is similar to the complex around the knee (52,53).

Venous Anatomy

The venous anatomy of the lower extremity is divided into a dual system: the superficial and the deep system: (53,54). In the lower extremity, the venous anatomy generally contains paired blood vessels in the deep system with an extensive networklike pattern of vessels in the superficial system. There are three pairs of deep calf veins that ascend in correspondingly adjacent locations to the anterior tibial, peroneal, and posterior tibial veins. These veins merge to form the popliteal vein, which continues into the thigh as the

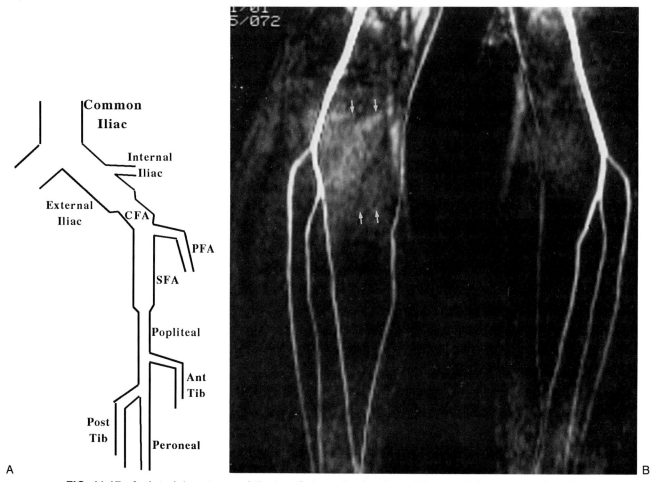

A

B

FIG. 11.17. A: Arterial anatomy of the leg. Schematic drawing of the arterial anatomy of the leg and pelvis. **B:** Cine phase contrast MRA of the normal popliteal artery and trifurcation. This image is the postprocessed standard deviation collapse view obtained from a coronal cardiac-gated cine phase-contrast projection MRA acquisition of the lower leg. Sixteen frames during the cardiac cycle were obtained with effective TR = 22 ms, TE = 12 ms, and 20° flip angle. Superior/inferior single flow direction sensitivity, velocity encoding of approximately 40 cm/s, and inferior presaturation to eliminate venous flow were employed. The approximate time of acquisition was determined by the heart rate and was about 2½ min. The visualized arterial anatomy reflects flow that is superior-inferior in direction. Note the lack of flow in the horizontally oriented vessels such as the middle geniculate arteries due to the direction selectivity of this technique. The bright background signal (*arrows*) is due to unsuppressed stationary tissue. This occurs primarily as a consequence of variable TR during the cardiac cycle.

FIG. 11.18. Arterial anatomy of the foot and ankle. **A:** Schematic drawing of the arterial anatomy of the foot and ankle. **B:** 2D time-of-flight MRA of normal foot and ankle arteries. Sagitally reformatted axial GRE with TR/TE 45 ms/7.4 ms, 60° flip angle, 1.5-mm slice thickness, and inferior presaturation. The exam was acquired with an extremity coil. Postprocessing using a maximum intensity projection algorithm was performed. The foot and ankle were flexed to align arterial flow in the slice direction. Note the excellent depiction of the anterior tibial, dorsalis pedis artery, and posterior tibial arteries. The apparent luminal irregularities (*small arrows*) are caused by slice thickness artifacts of the maximum intensity projection algorithm. This artifact can be suppressed

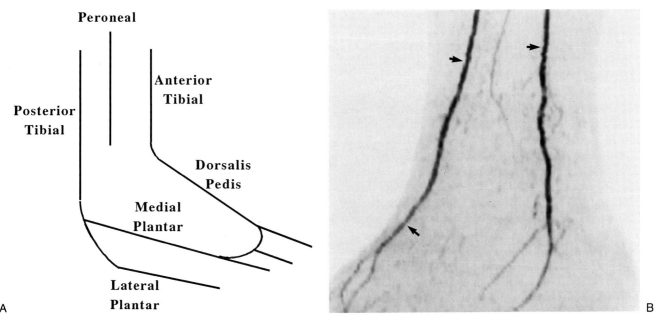

A

B

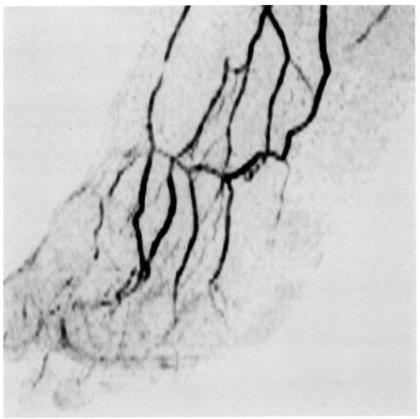

C

by acquiring thinner slices with the trade-off of limiting coverage per unit of time. **C:** 2D time-of-flight MRA of the normal forefoot arteries. Oblique sagittally reformatted axial GRE with TR/TE 45 ms/7.4 ms, 60° flip angle, 1.5-mm slice thickness. Inferior presaturation is used to suppress signal from venous flow and thus produce predominantly arterial images. This image was obtained with an extremity coil and postprocessed using the maximum intensity projection algorithm. The foot and ankle were flexed to align arterial flow perpendicular to the acquistion plane to maximize sensitivity to slow flow. Note the ability of this technique to image the intrinsic small vessels of the foot.

superficial femoral vein. Frequent duplication in the popliteal and superficial femoral vein occur. This can lead to errors in diagnosis of thrombosis if only one of the limbs is affected (54). Additional deep veins drain into the popliteal vein via the soleus and gastrocnemius veins. The profunda femoris vein, saphenous vein, and superficial femoral vein join to form the common femoral vein, which enters the pelvis beneath the inguinal ligament as the external iliac vein (Fig. 11.19).

The plantar venous arch is the largest deep vein in the foot. Since there is enormous variability in the rest of the veins of the foot, it is usually best to leave them unnamed until they merge at the ankle. The superficial venous drainage complex includes the greater saphenous vein and the lesser saphenous vein, which lie in the subcutaneous tissues. The lesser saphenous vein is found on the lateral aspect of the calf and merges with the popliteal vein while the great saphenous vein empties into the common femoral vein at the groin. There may be multiple duplications of these veins as well as several tributaries and perforating collaterals. An important aspect of the venous circulation is the fact that it is a low pressure, high capacitance system

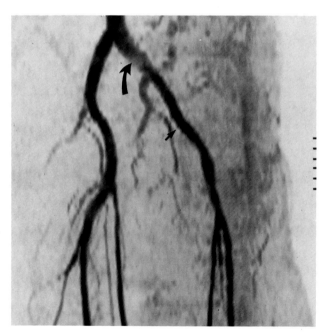

FIG. 11.19. Normal MRA of pelvic veins. 2D TOF MRA demonstrating excellent depiction of the normal pelvic and proximal femoral venous anatomy. The image represents an oblique coronally reformatted axial GRE with TR/TE 45 ms/7.4 ms, 60° flip angle, and 3-mm slice thickness. Superior presaturation was employed and the study obtained in the body coil. Note that small gradations in venous flow signal do not indicate eccentric clots (*curved arrow*), but reflect variations in venous flow during the respiratory cycle. The apparent blood vessel discontinuities (*arrow*) are slice thickness artifacts produced by the maximum intensity projection algorithm.

that contains valves. Since the flow characteristics may be very sluggish or even stagnant, muscular contraction is required to propel blood in an antegrade fashion, and the valves prevent retrograde flow in the presence of gravity (53).

The venous circulation of the lower extremities can be divided into two zones: the upper zone including the popliteal vein and the lower zone including the tibial veins and veins of the feet. The upper zone is well suited to imaging by MRA since there is relatively constant flow in a velocity range that both TOF and phase contrast can detect. In the lower zone, however, the flow is somewhat stagnant and in the prone position may be very low velocity, below the sensitivity of both TOF and phase contrast. In fact, the flow is usually intermittent due to muscular contractions in the calf. If the imaging is performed under these circumstances frequently vessels are then absent by MRA. Another consideration is the soft tissue compression of various venous compartments due to positioning and compression by pillows and sponge pads. This is particularly evident in the popliteal space.

Atherosclerotic Peripheral Vascular Disease

Atherosclerotic disease is the most common disease affecting the arterial side of the circulation in the United States (52,55–57). It is a diffuse progressive process that involves the wall of blood vessels in the peripheral arterial circulation. Symptoms are frequently due to focal lesions that produce hemodynamically significant alterations in pressure and blood flow. Atherosclerosis may lead to aneurysm formation, vessel wall rupture, dissection, arterial embolization, ischemic stenosis, and hypertension due to loss of elasticity in the wall of the aorta (55). Currently, the diagnosis and staging of atherosclerotic disease is done by contrast angiography. Contrast angiography estimates the hemodynamic significance of an arterial stenosis by two methods: percent lumen stenosis and residual lumen diameter (53,58). Accurate staging for purposes of diagnosis and therapy planning requires lesion identification and grading, and assessment of the inflow and outflow circulation. Lesion grading relates to the assessment of both the severity of a stenotic or occlusive arterial lesion as well as its length.

Assessment of arterial peripheral vascular disease is well accomplished by conventional arteriographic methods (52,53). The noninvasive nature of MRA and the lack of need for contrast material, however, makes this technique highly attractive as a possible alternative to conventional arteriography. To compete as a diagnostic modality, however, MRA must meet several critical challenges. The technique must be able to display the vascular anatomy in a clinically useful and understandable manner, and be able to depict reliably not only the presence of a stenotic lesion but also grade its severity in order to allow the most optimal determination of the type of therapy (26).

Several recent studies have attested to both the future potential as well as current difficulties in the use of various MRA techniques in the evaluation of peripheral vascular disease (6,14,32,41,43,48,59,60). In early MRA trials using a pulsatile blood flow technique first described by Wedeen et al., MRA was compared to angiography in 35 patients with aortoiliac and lower extremity vascular disease (32). Pulsatile MRA tended to overestimate the degree and length of focal stenoses (32). Pulsatile MRA performed better in the assessment of total arterial occlusions in the peripheral vascular system than on focal stenoses with detection rates ranging from 100% for common iliac occlusions to 81% for below-knee arterial occlusions (32). There were, however, relatively high rates of false positive occlusions detected (e.g., 20% common iliac, superficial femoral 17%). The factors that determine blood flow detection by pulsatile MRA are the size of the artery, the orientation of blood flow, and the nature of disease in the arteries upstream. If the inflow vessels are occluded or severely stenotic, then the pulsatile nature of blood flow is decreased and the ability to detect blood flow is consequently decreased. Pulsatile MRA has tended to overestimate the degree of stenoses and occlusions, and the distal runoff has not reliably imaged in the setting of proximal disease. As a result, pulsatile MRA is currently considered to be suboptimal in the clinical assessment of peripheral vascular disease (32).

Since 1988, essentially two MRA techniques have evolved for clinical use: (a) phase contrast MRA and (b) 2D-TOF MRA (see previous discussion). Cine MRA holds several distinct advantages in comparison to 2D-TOF MRA. Wide fields of view up to 40 cm and short imaging times in the range of 2 min per acquisition allow an entire study of the pelvic and lower extremity arteries to be acquired in between 20 and 40 minutes (Fig. 11.20). Another major advantage of cine MRA is elimination of artifacts due to motion during the acquisition. Current cine MRA techniques are able to freeze respiratory motion and bowel motion. Since the cine MRA is a direct projection technique, no additional computer postprocessing is required after image reconstruction. This eliminates artifacts due to computer reformatting and reprojection algorithms and suboptimal slice thickness (45,61). By adjusting the velocity-encoding gradients, cine phase contrast MRA is more sensitive to slow arterial flow and yields better suppression of stationary tissue as well as elimination of pulsatile artifacts. This allows visualization

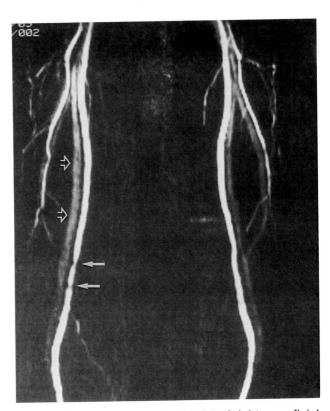

FIG. 11.20. Cine phase contrast MRA of right superficial femoral artery focal stenosis. This MRA image is the post-processed standard deviation collapse view obtained from a cardiac-gated cine phase contrast MRA acquisition of the lower leg. This postprocessing technique suppresses signal from nonpulsatile flow. Sixteen frames during the cardiac cycle were obtained with effective TR = 22 ms, TE = 12 ms, 20° flip angle, superior/inferior single flow direction sensitivity, velocity encoding of approximately 40 cm/s, and inferior presaturation to eliminate venous flow. Using cine phase contrast MRA in the leg, a short segmental tight stenosis (*arrows*) was identified with good runoff via the popliteal artery. The cine phase contrast MRA technique as contrasted to the 2D-TOF MRA technique has been shown to depict accurately the severity and length of focal stenoses. Note the companion femoral venous flow (*open arrows*) indicating a component of transmitted pulsatility. The status of the inflow vessels was accurately determined by MRA and the patient underwent percutaneous balloon angioplasty. The MRA obviated the need for conventional angiography in this patient with renal insufficiency.

of arterial flow distal to high grade stenoses and occlusions (Fig. 11.21). Because of the wide range of velocity sensitivities and the temporal resolution of cine MRA, this technique does not overestimate the severity or length of stenoses or occlusions. Dynamic information in the cardiac cycle is available from cine MRA studies that is not present from time-of-flight images (26,33).

As previously discussed, 2D-TOF techniques can also be used to assess the peripheral vasculature. 2D-

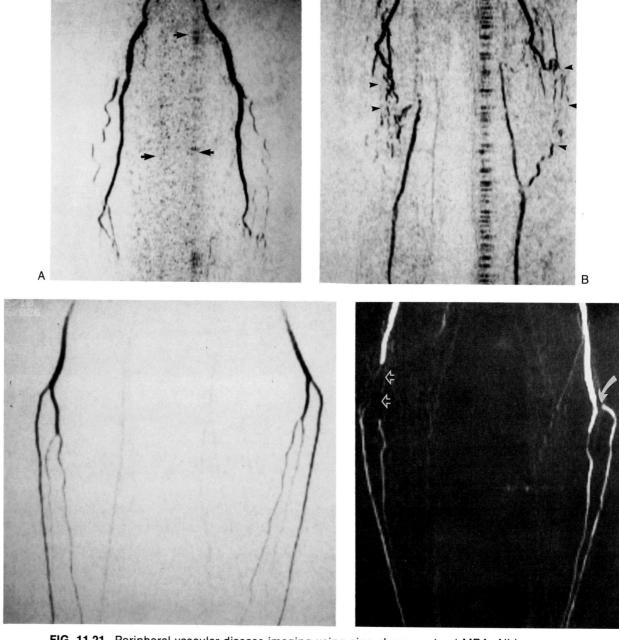

FIG. 11.21. Peripheral vascular disease imaging using cine phase contrast MRA. All images reflect postprocessed standard deviation collapse views obtained from a cardiac-gated cine phase contrast MRA acquisition of the lower leg. Sixteen frames during the cardiac cycle were obtained with effective TR = 22 ms, TE = 12 ms, 20° flip angle, superior/inferior single flow direction sensitivity, velocity encoding of approximately 40 cm/s, and inferior presaturation to eliminate venous flow. The approximate time of acquisition was determined by the heart rate and was about 2½ min for each 40-cm station. **A:** Bilateral long segment superficial femoral artery occlusions starting at their origins are seen. The zipperlike artifact (*arrow*) is caused by a phase-encoding artifact of arterial pulsatility transmitted from the abdominal aorta. **B:** Reconstitution of the distal SFA is seen bilaterally. Note the excellent depiction of the collateral flow from the profunda arteries to the reconstituted superficial femoral arteries (*arrowheads*). **C:** MRA demonstrating patent popliteal arteries and three vessel runoff bilaterally. This case illustrates the ability of cine phase contrast MRA to visualize arterial flow distal to occlusions. **D:** Cine phase contrast MRA of a different patient demonstrates right popliteal artery occlusion (*open arrows*) with visualization of anterior tibial, peroneal, and dorsalis pedis arteries distally. The apparent stenosis at the trifurcation on the left (*curved arrow*) is caused by the insensitivity of this technique to flow in the horizontal direction and represents an artifact.

TOF MRA does not require cardiac gating or MRI devices with shielded gradients. Another major advantage of 2D-TOF MRA is the acquisition of a three dimensional data set from which MRAs at any oblique angulation can be created. In a recent study, Owen et al. found MRA using 2D-TOF techniques to be quite capable of demonstrating small peripheral vessels in both normal and diseased patients (59). Excellent arterial signal enhancement, stationary spin suppression, and venous flow suppression were obtained. MRA studies correlated well with conventional angiograms. Obstructed vascular segments were reliably identified and extensive collateral flow was easily appreciated (59). Identification of exactly which vessel reconstituted distally was readily accomplished using axial images, whereas similar determinations often required multiple injections with conventional angiography (59). Focal stenoses, however, were not well visualized (59). Mulligan and Lanzer in reporting their results

comparing 2D-TOF MRA with angiography found that this MRA technique tended to overestimate the severity and length of a stenosis or occlusion and that the pelvic arteries were difficult to visualize (15,62). The tendency for 2D-TOF techniques to confuse moderate multifocal stenoses with intermediate length occlusions has been a common pitfall in our experience (Fig. 11.22). Yucel et al., however, report using 2D-TOF with increasingly high degrees of success in detecting target arteries distal to proximal occlusions (50).

MRA can be used as a problem-solving technique in patients with peripheral vascular disease. In patients considered at high risk for evaluation with conventional angiography because of concerns for renal insufficiency, MRA can be used successfully to evaluate the status of their peripheral vasculature. The distinction between long and short segment occlusive disease can be accomplished and patients effectively evaluated

A

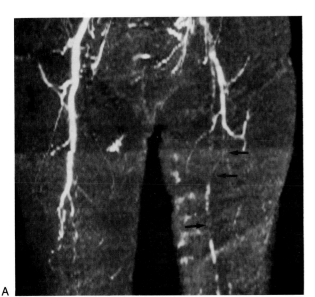
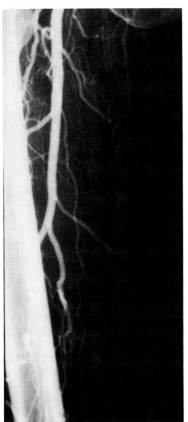
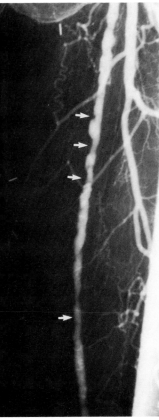

B,C

FIG. 11.22. Overestimation of arterial stenosis by 2D-TOF MRA. **A:** Coronally reformatted axial GRE obtained with TR/TE 45 ms/7.4 ms, 60° flip angle, 5-mm slice thickness, inferior presaturation, body coil, and postprocessed using a maximum intensity projection algorithm. There is complete occlusion of the right SFA at its origin with visualization of the right profunda femoris artery. On the left, there is an apparent long segment occlusion of the SFA (*arrows*). In reality, there were multiple mild stenoses without occlusion. This case illustrates the tendency for overestimation of severity and length of stenoses using 2D-TOF MRA techniques. **B:** The conventional angiogram confirms complete right SFA occlusion with visualization of the profunda femoris artery. **C:** The conventional angiogram more accurately depicts the status of multiple left SFA stenoses (*arrows*).

with regard to candidacy for percutaneous angioplasty. Koch et al. found MRA to depict reliably the length and degree of atherosclerotic lesions with less than 80% diameter reduction (46). In this study, however, short (<1 cm) and high-grade stenoses (>80%) often could not be distinguished from occlusions in MRA (46). Similar difficulties were encountered, however, with color Duplex ultrasound in this study. MRA can also be used in the noninvasive monitoring of patients following prior vascular interventional procedures (46).

Aneurysms

Peripheral aneurysms are a common complication of atherosclerotic disease (39,56,63). In contrast to aortic and thoracic aneurysms in which rupture is the major danger, peripheral aneurysms principally cause disability secondary to distal embolization or thrombosis with resultant ischemia and gangrene of the extremity.

The popliteal artery is the most common site of peripheral atherosclerotic aneurysms (63). As with other

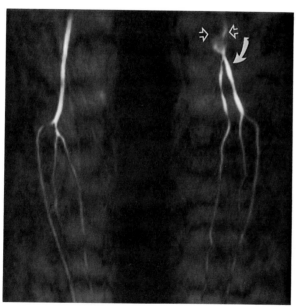
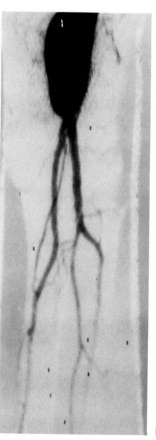

FIG. 11.23. Left popliteal artery aneurysm. This elderly male patient presented with a pulsatile mass behind the knee. Axial GRE MR images determined that an aneurysm without thrombus in the lumen was present. **A:** Single frame from a 16-frame cardiac-gated cine phase contrast MRA. Effective TR/TE was 24 ms/13 ms, 20° flip angle, superior/inferior flow sensitivity, velocity sensitivity approximately 40 cm/s, and inferior presaturation to suppress venous flow. Approximate image acquisition time was 4 min. An aneurysm of the left popliteal artery is detected. The popliteal aneurysm itself is not well depicted due to unrecoverable signal dropout (*open arrows*) from intravoxel phase dispersion related to complex flow in the aneurysm. MRA detected an important arterial anomaly; a high posterior tibial artery (*curved arrow*) arising from the popliteal artery aneurysm itself. This had important implications in the surgical planning of an arterial reconstruction that would incorporate flow to both the medial and lateral compartments of the lower leg and foot. Note the background signal intensity from unsuppressed stationary tissue in the lower leg. The black and white alternating pattern is due to the background phase variation in signal intensity. **B:** Confirmatory contrast intraarterial digital subtraction angiogram of left popliteal artery aneurysm.

peripheral aneurysms secondary to atherosclerosis, men are more commonly affected than woman and typically are in the sixth and seventh decades of life. Popliteal aneurysms are bilateral in at least 25% of cases and are commonly associated with aneurysms of the abdominal aorta (63). Popliteal aneurysms are insidious in their nature and are most commonly asymptomatic When symptomatic, most patients present with signs of ischemia due to thrombosis and distal embolization. Popliteal aneurysms also may present with calf vein thrombosis due to compression of the popliteal vein (63).

Femoral artery aneurysms are virtually all atherosclerotic in origin and again are seen most commonly in elderly men (52,56). The usual course of femoral artery aneurysms is to thrombose with subsequent ischemia of the extremity. Ischemia from peripheral embolization of thrombotic material in the aneurysm is less common than thrombosis and rupture is unusual (52). The existence of additional aneurysms (e.g., aortoiliac or popliteal) is seen in most patients with femoral aneuryms and detection of associated aneurysms represents an important aspect of the work-up of these patients. Associated aortoiliac aneurysms are detected in about 85% of patients: 70% have bilateral femoral aneurysms and 45% have popliteal aneurysms (56).

While conventional angiography has an essential role in preoperative planning, certain aspects of combined MRA and MRI may provide more information than arteriography, which has significant limitations with regard to the detection of aneurysms related to its depiction of only the intraluminal extent of lesions.

This may contribute to significantly underestimating the size of an aneurysm because of organized thrombus along the wall. Angiography has been used most commonly for assessment of the distal arteries for the presence of emboli and their capacity to be used as target vessels in surgical bypass. Cross-sectional imaging methods including ultrasound, x-ray, CT, and most recently MRI are more effective for aneurysm detection as a consequence of their ability to image the arterial wall, thrombus, and lumen (26,64).

Certain aspects of combined MRI and MRA in particular may provide more information than other techniques. Specifically, MRI will more accurately size the aneurysm and detect the presence of intraluminal thrombus. It may also be more accurate at detecting subacute and chronic leaking aneurysms than angiography due to the presence of characteristic MR signal intensities indicating the presence of hemorrhage (65). We have studied four patients with suspected popliteal aneurysms using MR projection angiography in combination with cross-sectional thin section imaging. (Figs. 11.23, 11.24) An advantage of MRA over other noninvasive techniques relates to its ability to evaluate the status of the inflow and outflow vessels. Both cine phase contrast MRA and 2D-TOF MRA have been employed with success in the evaluation of the tibial vessels and the more proximal femoral arteries (26,39,45,47,48,50). MRA is able to depict accurately the arterial anatomy with respect to distal occlusions, anatomic variants, and proximal stenoses (4,26,46,66). MRA has proven valuable in both detection of femoral artery aneurysms as well as in assess-

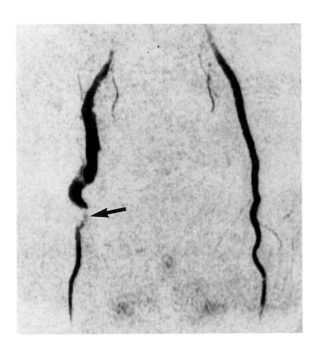

FIG. 11.24. MRA of right femoral artery aneurysm with stenosis in the femoral artery distal to the aneurysm. Postprocessed cardiac-gated cine phase contrast MRA. Effective TR/TE was 22 ms/12 ms, 20° flip angle, superior/inferior flow sensitivity, velocity sensitivity approximately 60 cm/s, inferior presaturation to suppress venous flow. Approximate image acquisition time was 4 min. Note almost complete background signal intensity suppression. The MRA shows the patent lumen of the artery, but underestimates the true width of the aneurysm due to laminated thrombus along the wall. In this respect it is similiar to conventional angiography. Note the signal dropout in the stenosis just distal to the aneurysm (*arrow*). This stenosis was confirmed during surgical repair.

ment of complications of the aneurysms and related inflow and outflow anatomy (63) (Fig. 11.25).

Acute arterial embolic disease represents a common complication of atherosclerotic peripheral vascular disease and aneuryms. MRA techniques can identify the level of vascular occlusions, but like conventional angiography, frequently cannot adequately detect flow in vessels distal to the occlusion. This is because initially there may be no collateral flow during the acute phase and that it takes several hours for this flow to develop (56,67). In current clinical practice, contrast arteriography remains the examination of choice for assessment of acute arterial emboli. A possible use for MRA in lower extremity embolic disease, however, may be in the noninvasive monitoring of patients undergoing thrombolytic therapy.

Diabetic Foot Ulcers

An initial traumatic insult to the subcutaneous tissues of the foot in the setting of a compromised vascular supply is considered to represent the most common etiology for cutaneous ulcers in the diabetic foot (68). The incapacity of the arterial system to provide adequate tissue perfusion leads to the failure to heal the ulcer. Once the ulcer has formed it has a high likelihood of infection and this further impairs the healing

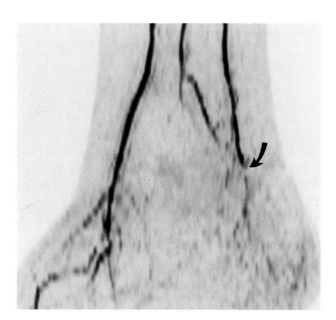

FIG. 11.25. 2D time-of-flight MRA of diabetic foot. Sagittally reformatted axial GRE with TR/TE 45 ms/7.4 ms, 60° flip angle, 1.5-mm slice thickness, inferior presaturation obtained with an extremity coil and postprocessed using a maximum intensity projection algorithm. MRA in this elderly diabetic patient with a nonhealing foot ulcer demonstrates arterial flow in the foot distal to proximal occlusions. There is occlusion of the posterior tibial artery at the ankle (*arrow*). The peroneal, anterior tibial, and dorsalis pedis arteries are patent.

process (68). Severe tibial trifurcation disease with sparing of the iliac and femoral arteries frequently characterizes diabetic vascular disease. The surgical treatment frequently targets vessels that are not detected by conventional angiography. In most series, the 2-year patency of these surgical bypasses range from 50% to 95% (68–70). As for other forms of occlusive arterial disease, the goal of conventional angiography is to assess the inflow vessels, identify the lesion, and assess the outflow vessels. For the diabetic, target vessels in the distal tibial distribution or even the foot need to be identified for surgical planning. While the velocity of blood flow in these vessels may be low, high-resolution 2D-TOF MRA frequently can detect the reconstituted dorsalis pedis artery and plantar arch vessels, but may not see flow more distally due to in-plane saturation (see Fig. 11.25). Cine phase contrast MRA, even with strong velocity encoding, may not detect some of the target vessels due to unsuppressed stationary tissue signal, but in general has a greater sensitivity to detecting small vessels in the foot. One caveat in regard to imaging of these patients is the possible difficulty for MRA in the vicinity of prior implanted metallic surgical clips either for saphenous vein harvesting or other surgical procedures. MRA is sensitive to the artifacts produced by metal and may not detect normal flow in the vicinity of these artifacts. These artifacts tend to contribute to the overestimation of lesions.

Vascular Surgical Reconstructions

There are a number of common vascular surgical procedures that are encountered in the population of patients with peripheral vascular disease. These bypass grafts are commonly divided into inflow procedures and outflow procedures (52,53). The most common inflow procedure is the aortobifemoral bypass graft that frequently uses a synthetic material as opposed to native vein. The other frequently encountered bypass grafts are the cross femoral bypass graft, which represents an extraanatomic bypass graft from the nondiseased common femoral artery tunneled under the skin across the pelvis and anastomosed to the corresponding common femoral artery or possibly profunda femoris artery. The third inflow procedure is called the axillofemoral bypass graft, which carries blood flow from the distal subclavian or axillary artery to the leg via a skin tunnel through the lateral chest and abdominal wall. The outflow procedures are generally characterized as a femoropopliteal bypass graft and femoro or popliteal artery distal bypass graft with the target vessel usually being a tibial or peroneal artery. In the setting of distal tibial artery occlusion, bypass to the dorsalis pedis and the posterior plantar arch are not infrequently attempted.

Routine evaluation of peripheral bypass surgery is currently most commonly accomplished using conventional arteriography, digital subtraction angiography (DSA), and Doppler ultrasound. While experience is limited, MRA appears capable of providing sufficient and reliable information in assessing peripheral bypass grafts (66,71) (Fig. 11.26). Although the spatial resolution of MRA is less than that of conventional arteriography, this does not appear to be a critical limitation as the caliber of the bypass graft and of the lower extremity leg vessels is above the threshold of resolution with MRA and the important question relates to the patency of the bypass graft and distal vessels (66,71). The detection of relevant associated pathology such as aneurysm, stenosis, or occlusion at the anastamosis or periphery, information essential to therapeutic decision making, can be detected by MRA with an accuracy competitive with that of DSA (66,71).

Traumatic Occlusions

In the current state of the art, there is little role for the initial diagnosis of traumatic occlusions of the ar-

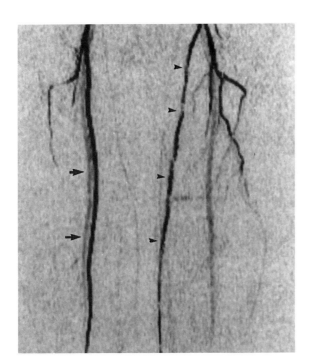

FIG. 11.26. MRA of left femorotibial bypass graft to above the ankle with occluded native femoral, popliteal, and tibial arteries due to thromboemboli. Postprocessed cardiac-gated cine phase contrast projection MRA. Effective TR/TE was 22 ms/12 ms, 20° flip angle, superior/inferior flow sensitivity, velocity sensitivity approximately 60 cm/s, inferior presaturation to suppress venous flow. Approximate image acquisition time was 4 min. MRA depicts flow in the bypass graft (*arrowheads*). No graft pulse could be palpated. Despite the use of presaturation, there is visualization of veins (*arrows*) due to rapid venous flow.

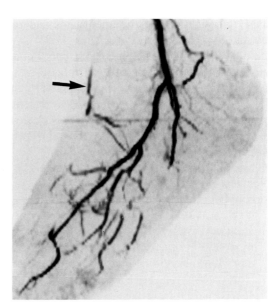

FIG. 11.27. MRA of traumatic occlusion of anterior tibial artery. Sagittally reformatted axial GRE with TR/TE 45 ms/7.4 ms, 60° flip angle, 1.5-mm slice thickness, inferior presaturation obtained with an extremity coil and postprocessed using a maximum intensity projection algorithm. The patient sustained a laceration to the foot during a motorboat accident. The anterior tibial artery is occluded with reconstitution of an isolated segment of the dorsalis pedis artery (*arrow*). The MRA shows patent posterior tibial artery and plantar arch supplying metatarsal branches.

teries of the lower extremities by MRA, especially in the setting of acute ischemia. It is important to remember, in addition, that in the setting of arterial injury, arterial extravasation cannot be detected by MRA. It is also questionable whether intimal injuries can be identified in the setting of acute trauma. Therefore, at this time MRA is not recommended as a primary imaging modality in the setting of acute trauma. The technique, however, is clearly capable of depicting arterial occlusions and may be used in the subacute and chronic setting (66) (Fig. 11.27).

Arteriovenous Malformations and Tumor Vascularity

Vascular malformations are classified into two primary types; high flow and low flow lesions (52,53,72). Angiography and color flow ultrasound have been used to distinguish between the two. High flow lesions are characterized by enlarged inflow arteries and dilated draining veins. The actual nidus may be difficult to identify. Doppler waveform analysis of the AVM may show a low resistance pattern of pulsatile flow with significant diastolic arterial flow. Flow on the venous side may have pulsatile characteristics and behave like an arteriovenous (AV) fistula. In low-flow lesions, the arteries have normal high resistance triphasic waveforms and flow within the lesion may be difficult to identify. On MRI, high-flow lesions may produce a signal void on spin-echo images (72).

Vascular malformations cause different symptoms depending on their size. The purpose of MRA and MRI is to give the surgeon an idea of the extent of the lesion and the involvement of underlying tissues. Specifically, MRI must determine whether there is involvement of underlying muscle, bones, subcutaneous fat, and dermis. The role of imaging is to determine the overall arterialization of the lesion because this will determine the behavior of the AVM as well as predict the success of a surgical or endovascular intervention (Fig. 11.28).

Currently, the role of MRA in the work-up of AVMs and tumor vascularity remains investigational. While MRA can yield images of dilated arteries supplying abnormal tissue, it does not have the spatial resolution or velocity sensitivity to image neovascularity or small arterial feeders. It is important to remember that MRA cannot see tumor blush or capillary filling in the same fashion as contrast angiography. In a preliminary study, however, Swan et al. found MRA useful in the evaluation of the vascularity surrounding musculo-skeletal masses (73). MRA provided multiplane evaluation of vessel localization and patency and identified feeder vessels and neovascularity (73). The MRA ex-

aminations correlated well with conventional arteri-ography. 2D-TOF was found to be the most flexible sequence allowing multiplane reconstruction from a single acquisition (73). A collapsed axial view provided unique spatial localization not available with conventional angiography (73). Two-dimensional phase contrast imaging was found to be most valuable in this study in areas where vessel geometry causes TOF signal loss or when hemorrhage was present obscuring the vasculature (73). This study certainly suggests an enlarging role for MRA in the preoperative planning for musculoskeletal neoplasms.

Arteriovenous Fistula

An arteriovenous fistula is a short communication between an artery and a nearby vein. This condition is usually acquired by a penetrating wound that creates the connection. In rare circumstances, this condition may lead to profound hemodynamic consequences. Angiographic assessment of AV fistula is essential for preoperative surgical planning in order to identify the following: (a) the size and number of feeding arteries, (b) the collateral circulation, (c) the venous circulation distal to the fistula, (d) possible associated aneurysms both arterial and venous, and (e) the status of the arterial circulation distal to the fistula (52,53).

Reported experience with MRA of AV fistulas is quite limited. Yucel et al. have reported depicting a case by 2D-TOF MRA that was subsequently confirmed by conventional arteriography (50). To have demonstrated this lesion using 2D-TOF techniques, the flow must have been extremely rapid in order to overcome the effect of the tracking saturation pulse that was used to suppress the normal venous flow. Rak et al., in reporting on 30 symptomatic vascular malformations, found MRI capable of consistently distinguishing between high-flow lesions (AV malformations and AV fistulas) from low-flow lesions (venous malformations) (40). In this study, MRI was found to complement angiography by depicting anatomic relationships of the lesions to organs, nerves, tendons, and muscles. Following treatment, MRI was an effective means for evaluating the efficacy and permanence of therapy (40). It is likely that MRA may complement colorflow ultrasound in detection and characterization of AV fistula and associated vascular lesions. The ability of MRA to yield an angiographic type projection may eventually obviate the need for conventional angiography (74).

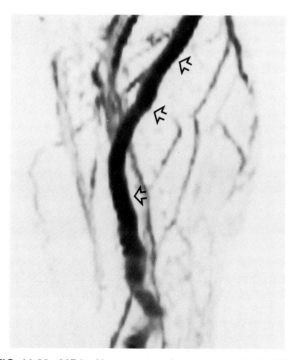

FIG. 11.28. MRA of lower extremity venous varix draining an AVM in the ankle. Sagittally reformatted axial GRE with TR/TE 45 ms/7.4 ms, 60° flip angle, 1.5-mm slice thickness, obtained with an extremity coil and postpro-cessed using a maximum intensity projection algorithm. Note the enlarged subcutaneous varicosity of the saphe-nous vein (*arrows*). No presatuation was used in order to detect in-plane flow. Since no presaturation was used, this image contains both arteries and veins.

VENOUS DISEASE OF THE LOWER EXTREMITY

Thrombophlebitis is an inflammatory reaction of the wall of a vein to a thrombus. The etiology of thrombophlebitis is multifactorial and may be due to one of a number of factors including problems with coagulation, the wall of the affected vessel, and the circulating cellular elements within the blood. The clinical syndrome consists of pain, swelling, and redness. The significance of the deep venous thrombosis (DVT) is determined by its location. If the DVT involves the calf vessels, it may progress to involve more proximal vessels such as the popliteal vein. Injury to the venous valves in the popliteal vein has been associated with chronic recurrent thrombophlebitis and DVT above the level of the popliteal vein has been associated with life-threatening pulmonary emboli (40). The treatment of DVT consists primarily of anticoagulation. Rarely is thrombolytic therapy employed except in severe cases such as phlegmasia cerulia dolens or venous ischemia of the lower extremities due to venous outflow obstruction (41).

MRA has been employed in the diagnosis and staging of venous occlusions with great success. Spritzer et al. have reported a high accuracy finding DVT using a 2D-TOF technique (75,76). In general, MRA is very sensitive for detecting venous flow in the politeal vein and above, but is less sensitive for flow in the tibial veins and veins of the calf. The reasons for this relate to a number of factors. The first relates to the large number of vessels, their relative small size, and their tortuous course. The second principle consideration is that flow in the tibial veins may be relatively stagnant and intermittently propelled by muscular contractions in the calf. Both 2D-TOF and phase contrast techniques tend to suffer from the same consequences in the lower leg due to this complex constellation of blood vessels and flow.

From the popliteal vein to the femoral vein and iliac veins in the pelvis, MRA is the only noninvasive imaging modality that can reliably identify pelvic vein DVT. In clinical practice, patients with suspected DVT are evaluated primarily by colorflow ultrasound and Doppler of the legs. If iliac vein thrombosis is still in question, an MR venogram is performed. We use a combination of 2D phase contrast projections and 2D-TOF techniques as well as thin-slice 2D phase contrast to evaluate for the presence of DVT. Although the slices are reformatted into venogram equivalent images, it is important to see the raw data images to find intraluminal nonoccluding thrombi. Rarely, a bright T1-weighted clot may fill the lumen of a vein and appear completely normal on time-of-flight images. In these circumstances, a 2D phase contrast image is invaluable in preventing a false positive interpretation. For the evaluation of DVT, Spritzer et al. have reported the accuracy of MRA in detecting DVT of the lower extremity including calf, thigh, and pelvis as essentially 100%. In their institution MRA has replaced venography for assessment of suspected deep vein thrombosis (75). It has been our experience, however, that flow in the tibial veins may be stagnant or at least slower than the prescribed MRA velocity sensitivity and that the tibial veins are frequently not visualized. In addition, occasionally patient position and external compression either at the popliteal space or the groin may cause loss of flow signal from the veins. Given these technical limitations, combined with a consideration of the cost of MRA compared to colorflow ultrasound, it is difficult, in our opinion, to justify offering MRA as the primary imaging modality in the evaluation of DVT. The present role for MRA in the detection of venous disease at our institution is reserved for the evaluation of pelvic vein DVT and in those cases where ultrasound or venography are indeterminate (Figs. 11.29).

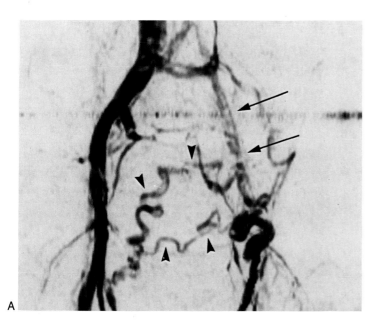

A

FIG. 11.29. MRA of pelvic vein occlusions. **A:** 2D phase-contrast MRA using TR/TE 22 ms/12ms, 20° flip angle, sensitive to flow in all three orthogonal directions, velocity sensitivity approximately 40 cm/s. Approximate imaging time was 3 min. This MRA shows complete occlusion of the left femoral vein and left iliac venous system with transabdominal (*arrowheads*) and transperineal venous collaterals draining blood from the left leg to the right side. Note the flow signal in the suboptimally suppressed left iliac artery (*arrows*). This vessel is easily identified since it arises from an aortic bifurcation, and not the inferior vena cava. Flow within the collateral vessels was not seen on axial 2D-TOF MRA due to in-plane saturation of slow flow. (*Figure continues on next page.*)

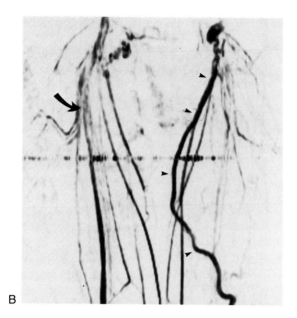

B

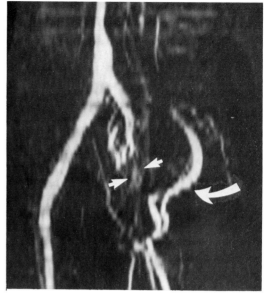

C

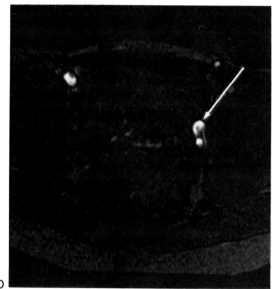

D

FIG. 11.29. (*Continued*) **B:** Note the dilated left saphenous vein (*arrowheads*) draining the leg. Also note the proximal right femoral vein signal loss due to velocity aliasing (*curved arrow*). **C:** Pelvic venous occlusion in a different patient using 2D-TOF MRA. Oblique coronally reformatted axial GRE with TR/TE 45 ms/7.4 ms, 60° flip angle, 5-mm slice thickness, superior presaturation obtained and postprocessed using a maximum intensity projection algorithm. The left common iliac vein is seen, but the left external iliac vein is missing (*arrows*). Collaterals from the left common femoral vein (*curved arrow*) are seen. **D:** Axial flow-sensitive GRE image shows the collateral vessel in the obturator region. Time-of-flight MRA preprocessed raw data cross-sectional images show that the enlarged vessel (*arrow*) was an enlarged transobturator collateral vein. Both of these cases illustrate different strengths of their respective techniques. Specifically, the 2D phase-contrast MRA was sensitive to flow in all directions and was able to detect right to left flow that was not seen on 2D time-of-flight MRA. The second case illustrates the importance of conventional MRI in conjunction with MRA images in order to determine the relationship of flow in blood vessels to adjacent viscera and anatomic landmarks.

CONCLUSIONS

This chapter has provided a brief overview of the physical principles of blood flow and the present techniques available to image flowing blood using MRI. Research and development in the area of MRA represents one of the most active areas of investigation in diagnostic imaging. Future developments in pulse sequence design and computer postprocessing are promising to allow even greater utilization of MRA. The clinical future of MRA in the diagnostic imaging evaluation of peripheral vascular disease, however, awaits further clinicopathological correlation. It ap-

pears unlikely at present, however, that MRA will ever replace all the information obtained by conventional angiography. Early clinical studies have established its value in selected settings and as an adjunctive procedure for assessing lesions of the musculoskeletal system.

REFERENCES

1. Axel, L, *Blood flow effects in magnetic resonance imaging.* AJR, 1984. **143**: p. 1157–1166.
2. Bradley, WG, Jr., *Flow phenomena in MR imaging.* AJR, 1988. **150**: p. 983–994.

3. Chakeres, DW, Schmalbrock, P, Brogan, M, *et al.*, *Normal venous anatomy of the brain: Demonstration with gadopentetate dimeglumine in enhanced 3-D MR angiography.* AJR, 1991. **156**: p. 161–172.

4. Cramer, BM, Schlegel, EA, Boos, M, *et al.*, *MR angiography for follow-up after percutaneous vessel recanalization and surgery.* Radiology, 1990. **177(P)**: p. 144–145.

5. Crawley, AP, Cohen, MS, Yucel, EK, *et al.*, *Single-shot MR imaging: Applications to angiography.* Cardiovasc Int Radiol, In press. .

6. Davis, VA, Bennett, JBW, and Schmalbrock, P, *Comparison of methods for lower extremity MR angiography* in *SMRM, Ninth Annual Scientific Meeting and Exhibition.* 1990. New York.

7. de Graaf, RG and Groen, JP, *MR angiography with pulsatile blood flow,* in *SMRM, Ninth Annual Scientific Meeting and Exhibition.* 1990. New York.

8. Ducksoo, K, Edelman, RR, Kent, KC, *et al.*, *Abdominal aorta and renal artery stenosis: Evaluation with MR angiography.* Radiology, 1990. **174**: p. 727–731.

9. Dumoulin, CL and Hart, HR, Jr., *Magnetic resonance angiography.* Radiology, 1986. **161**: p. 717–720.

10. Dumoulin, CL, Souza, SP, and Feng, H, *Multiecho magnetic resonance angiography.* Magn Reson in Med, 1987. **5**: p. 47–57.

11. Dumoulin, CL, *Magnetic resonance angiography.* Persp Radiol, 1989. **2**: p. 1.

12. Gullberg, GT, Wehrli, FW, Shimakawa, A, *et al.*, *MR vascular imaging with a fast gradient refocusing pulse sequence and reformatted images from transaxial sections.* Radiology, 1987. **165**: p. 241–246.

13. Keller, PJ, Drayer, BP, Fram, EK, *et al.*, *MR angiography with two-dimensional acquisition and three-dimensional display.* Radiology, 1989. **173**: p. 527–532.

14. Kugel, KB, Friedmann, G, Bunke, J, *et al.*, *MR angiography of vascular occlusive disease—experimental studies and clinical examinations of the aortoiliac and the femoral arteries,* in *SMRM, Tenth Annual Scientific Meeting and Exhibition.* 1991. San Francisco.

15. Lanzer, P, Bohning, D, Groen, J, *et al.*, *Aortoiliac and femoropopliteal phase-based NMR angiography: A comparison between FLAG and RSE.* Magn Reson Med, 1990. **15**: p. 372–385.

16. Meuli, RA, Wedeen, VJ, Geller, SC, *et al.*, *MR gated subtraction angiography: Evaluation of lower extremities.* Radiology, 1986. **159**: p. 411–418.

17. Pelc, NJ, Shimakawa, A, and Glover, GH, *Phase contrast CINE MRI,* in *8th Annual Meeting Society of Magnetic Resonance in Medicine.* 1989. Amsterdam.

18. Lenz, GW, Haacke, EM, Masaryk, TJ, *et al.*, *In-plane vascular imaging: Pulse sequence design and strategy.* Radiology, 1988. **166**: p. 875–882.

19. Ruggieri, PM, Laub, GA, Masaryk, TJ, *et al.*, *Intracranial circulation: Pulse-sequence considerations in three-dimensional (volume) MR angiography.* Radiology, 1989. **171**: p. 785–791.

20. Masaryk, TJ, Modic, MT, Ruggieri, PM, *et al.*, *Three-dimensional (volume) gradient-echo imaging of the carotid bifurcation: Preliminary clinical experience.* Radiology, 1989. **171**: p. 801–806.

21. Masaryk, TJ, Modic, MT, Ross, JS, *et al.*, *Intracranial circulation: Preliminary clinical results with three-dimensional (volume) MR angiography.* Radiology, 1989. **171**: p. 793–799.

22. Pernicone, JR, Siebert, JE, Potchen, EJ, *et al.*, *Three-dimensional phase-contrast MR angiography in the head and neck: Preliminary report.* AJR, 1990. **155**: p. 167–176.

23. Wagle, WA, Dumoulin, CL, Souza, SP, *et al.*, *3DFT MR angiography of carotid and basilar arteries.* AJNR, 1989. **10**: p. 911–919.

24. Pernicone, JR, Siebert, JE, Potchen, EJ, *et al.*, *Three-dimensional phase-contrast MR angiography in the head and neck: Preliminary report.* AJNR, 1990. **11**: p. 457–466.

25. Ross, JS, Masaryk, TJ, Modic, MT, *et al.*, *Magnetic resonance angiography of the extracranial carotid arteries and intracranial vessels: A review.* Neurology, 1989. **39**: p. 1369–1376.

26. Steinberg, FL, Yucel, EK, Dumoulin, CL, *et al.*, *Peripheral vascular and abdominal applications of MR flow imaging techniques.* Magn Reson Med, 1989. **14**: p. 315–320.

27. Steinberg, FL, Yucel, EK, Dumoulin, CL, *et al.*, *Cardiac gated phase contrast MR angiography of the lower extremities,* in *SMRM Eighth Annual Meeting.* Amsterdam, 1989.

28. Souza, SP, Steinberg, FL, Caro, C, *et al.*, *Velocity- and cardiac phase-resolved MR flow imaging,* in *SMRM, Eighth Annual Meeting.* 1989.

29. Singer, JR, *Blood flow rates by nuclear magnetic resonance.* Science, 1959. **130**: p. 1652–1653.

30. Hahn, EL, *Detection of sea-water motion by nuclear precession.* J Geophys Res, 1960. **65**: p. 776–783.

31. Moran, PR, *A flow velocity zuegmatographic interlace for NMR imaging in humans.* Magn Reson Imaging, 1982. **1**: p. 197–203.

32. Wedeen, VJ, Meuli, RA, Edelman, RR, *et al.*, *Projective imaging of pulsatile flow with magnetic resonance.* Science, 1985. **230**: p. 946.

33. Dumoulin, CL, Souza, SP, Walker, MF, *et al.*, *Time-resolved magnetic resonance angiography.* Magn Reson Med, 1988. **6**: p. 275–286.

34. Souza, SP and Dumoulin, CL, *Dynamic magnetic resonance angiography.* Dynamic Cardiovasc Imaging, 1987. **1**: p. 126.

35. Dumoulin, CL, Souza, SP, Walker, MF, *et al.*, *Three-dimensional phase contrast angiography.* Magn Reson Med, 1989. **9**: p. 139–149.

36. Crooks, LE, Mills, CM, Davis, PL, *et al.*, *Visualization of cerebral and vascular abnormalities by NMR imaging: The effects of imaging parameters on contrast.* Radiology, 1982. **144**: p. 843.

37. Wehrli, FW, Shimakawa, A, MacFall, JR, *et al.*, *MR imaging of venous and arterial flow by a selective saturation-recovery spin echo (SSRSE) method.* J Comp Asst Tomogr, 1985. **9**: p. 537–545.

38. Caro, CG, Parker, KH, Fish, PJ, *et al.*, *Blood flow near the arterial wall and arterial disease.* Clin Hemorheol, 1985. **5**: p. 849–871.

39. Dousset, V, Wehrli, RW, Louie, A, *et al.*, *Popliteal artery hemodynamics: MR imaging-US correlation.* Radiology, 1991. **179**: p. 437–441.

40. Rak, KM, Yakes, WF, Ray, RL, *et al.*, *Therapeutic implications of MR imaging of symptomatic vascular malformations.* Radiology, 1991. **181(P)**: p. 228.

41. Steinberg, FL, Wedeen, V, Geller, S, *et al.*, *Peripheral vascular disease: Comparison of multiphase cardiac gated gradient echo MR projection angiograms with contrast angiography,* in *Seventh Annual Meeting of Society of Magnetic Resonance in Medicine.* San Francisco, 1988.

42. Masui, T, Caputo, GR, Chang, J, *et al.*, *MR angiography and blood flow measurements in the popliteal artery and trifurcation arteries,* in *SMRM, Ninth Annual Scientific Meeting and Exhibition.* 1990. New York.

43. Steinberg, FL, Wedeen, VJ, Geller, SC, *et al.*, *Abdominal aortic aneurysms: Comparison of multiphase cardiac gated gradient echo MR projection angiography with contrast angiography,* in *7th Annual Meeting Society of Magnetic Resonance in Medicine.* San Francisco, 1988.

44. Steinberg, FL, Wedeen, VJ, Geller, SC, *et al.*, *Multiphase cardiac gated gradient echo MR projection angiography of lower extremity occlusive disease.* Radiology, 1988. **169 (P)**: p. 109.

45. Grisham, JP, Steinberg, FL, Yucel, EK, *et al.*, *MR angiography of pelvic blood vessels by coronal reconstruction.* Magn Reson Imag, 1989. **7(S1)**: p. 185.

46. Koch, M, Maier, SE, Baumgartner, I, *et al.*, *Magnetic resonance angiography and flow quantification in peripheral vessel disease before and after percutaneous transluminal angioplasty (PTA),* in *SMRM, Tenth Annual Scientific Meeting and Exhibition.* 1991. San Francisco.

47. Lanzar, P, Gross, G, Keller, F, *et al.*, *Sequential 2D inflow NMR anteriography: Quantitation of peripheral vascular lesions,* in *SMRM, Ninth Annual Scientific Meeting and Exhibition.* 1990. New York.

48. Krug, B, Kugel, H, Friedmann, G, *et al.*, *MR angiography of vascular occlusive disease—experimental studies and clinical examinations of the aortoiliac and the femoral arteries,* in *SMRM, Tenth Annual Scientific Meeting and Exhibition.* 1991. San Francisco.

49. Bretzman, PA, Manaster, BJ, Davis, WL, *et al.*, *MR angio-*

graphic evaluation of the trifurcation vessels in vascularized fibular graft candidates. Radiology, 1991. **181(P):** p. 228.

50. Yucel, EK, Hansen, ME, Egglin, TE, *et al.*, *MR angiography of lower-extremity arterial disease.* J Magn Reson Imaging, 1991. **1:** p. 177.

51. Doyle, M, Matsuda, T, and Pohost, GM, *A new acquisition mode for 2D inflow refreshment angiography.* Magn Reson Med, 1991. **18:** p. 51–62.

52. Bron, KM, *Femoral Arteriography,* in *Abrams Angiography: Vascular and Interventional Radiology,* H Abrams, Editor. 1983, Little-Brown: Boston.

53. Kadir, S, *Arteriography of the lower extremity vessels,* in *Diagnostic Angiography,* S Kadir, Editor. 1986, W.B. Saunders: Philadelphia. p. 254–307.

54. Rabinov, K and Paulin, S, *Venography of the lower extremities,* in *Abrams Angiography: Vascular and Interventional Radiology,* H Abrams, Editor. 1983, Little, Brown: Boston. p. 1877–1921.

55. Haimovici, H, *Anatomic distribution of aortoiliac and infrainguinal atherosclerosis,* in *Current Therapy in Vascular Surgery,* CB Ernst and JC Stanley, Editors. 1991, B.C. Decker Inc: Philadelphia. p. 361–365.

56. Graham, LM, Zelenock, GB, Whitehouse, WM, Jr., *et al.*, *Clinical significance of arteriosclerotic femoral artery aneurysms.* Arch Surg, 1980. **115:** p. 502–507.

57. Ross, R and Glomset, JA, *The pathogenesis of atherosclerosis.* N Engl J Med, 1976. **295:** p. 369–377.

58. Wong, WH, Kirkeeide, RL, and Goulde, KL, *Computer applications in angiography,* in *Cardiac Imaging and Image Processing,* SM Collins and DJ Skorton, Editors. 1986, McGraw-Hill: New York.

59. Owen, RS, Sheline, M, Listerud, J, *et al.*, *Lower leg MR angiography in healthy and diseased subjects,* in *SMRM, Tenth Annual Scientific Meeting and Exhibition.* 1991. San Francisco.

60. Mohiaddin, RH, Sampson, C, Firmin, DN, *et al.*, *MR morphological and flow imaging in peripheral vascular disease.* Magn Reson Imaging, 1990. **8 (Supp 1):** p. 312.

61. Anderson, CM, Saloner, D, Tsuruda, JS, *et al.*, *Artifacts in maximum-intensity-projection display of MR angiograms.* AJR, 1990. **154:** p. 623–629.

62. Mulligan, SA, Matsuda, T, Lanzer, P, *et al.*, *Peripheral arterial occlusive disease: Prospective comparison of MR angiography and color duplex US with conventional angiography.* Radiology, 1991. **178:** p. 695–700.

63. Abbott, WM, *Popliteal artery aneurysm,* in *Current Therapy in Vascular Surgery,* CB Ernst and JC Stanley, Editors. 1991, B.C. Decker Inc: Philadelphia. p. 357–360.

64. Jager, KA, Ricketts, HJ, and Strandness, DE, Jr., *Duplex scanning for the evaluation of lower limb arterial disease,* in *Non Invasive Diagnostic Techniques in Vascular Disease,* EF Bernstein, Editor. 1985, CV Mosby: St. Louis.

65. Higgins, CB, Herfkens, RJ, Hricak, H, *et al.*, *Nuclear magnetic resonance imaging of atherosclerosis.* Radiographics, 1984. **4:** p. 137–149.

66. Fillmore, DJ, Yucel, EK, Briggs, SE, *et al.*, *Magnetic resonance angiography of pediatric vascular grafts.* ATR, 1991. **157:** 1069–1071.

67. Kaufman, JL, Shah, DM, Chang, BD, *et al.*, *Spontaneous atheroembolism,* in *Current Therapy in Vascular Surgery,* CB Ernst and JC Stanley, Editors. 1991, B.C. Decker Inc: Philadelphia. p. 587–590.

68. Anderson, CB and Munn, JS, *Cutaneous ulcers in the diabetic foot,* in *Current Therapy in Vascular Surgery,* CB Ernst and JC Stanley, Editors. 1991, B.C. Decker Inc: Philadelphia. p. 580–584.

69. Hurley, JJ, Aver, AI, Hershey, FB, *et al.*, *Distal arterial reconstruction: Patency and limb salvage in diabetics.* J Vasc Surg, 1987. **5:** p. 796–802.

70. Ascer, E, Veith, FJ, Gupta, SK, *et al.*, *Short vein grafts: A: superior option for arterial reconstructions to poor or compromised outflow tracts.* J Vasc Surg, 1988. **7:** p. 370–378.

71. Ostertun, B, Keller, E, van Dijk, P, *et al.*, *Magnetic resonance angiography in postoperative control of peripheral bypass surgery,* in *SMRM, Tenth Annual Scientific Meeting and Exhibition.* 1991.

72. Cohen, JM, Weinreb, JC, and Redman, HC, *Arteriovenous malformations of the extremities: MR imaging.* Radiology, 1986. **158:** p. 475–479.

73. Swan, JS, De Smet, AA, Heiner, JP, *et al.*, *Applications of MR angiography in preoperative musculoskeletal tumor planning.* Radiology, 1991. **181(P):** p. 228.

74. Pearce, WH, Rutherford, RB, Whitehill, TA, *et al.*, *Nuclear magnetic resonance imaging: Its diagnostic value in patients with congenital vascular malformations in the limbs.* J Vasc Surg, 1988. **8:** p. 64–70.

75. Spritzer, CE, Sussman, SK, Blinder, RA, *et al.*, *Deep venous thrombosis evaluation with limited flip-angle, gradient-refocussed MR imaging: Preliminary experience.* Radiology, 1988. **166:** p. 371–375.

76. Spritzer, CE, Pelc, NJ, and Lee, JN, *Rapid MR imaging of blood flow with a phase sensitive, limited flip angle, gradient recalled pulse sequence: Preliminary experience.* Radiology, 1990. **176:** p. 255–262.

MRI of the Foot and Ankle,
edited by A.L. Deutsch, J.H. Mink, and R. Kerr,
Raven Press, Ltd., New York © 1992

CHAPTER 12

Spectrum of Disorders

Roger Kerr

This chapter describes the use of magnetic resonance imaging (MRI) in three groups of disorders. Entrapment neuropathies may be difficult to diagnose clinically and have a variety of causes. Plantar heel pain is a common problem and may be caused by osseous or soft tissue disorders. Articular disease is common in the foot and ankle and MRI shows promise as a means to assess disease severity and response to treatment.

ENTRAPMENT NEUROPATHIES

Several entrapment neuropathies have been described in the foot and ankle (1–3). There is usually an insidious onset of intermittent pain referred to the distribution of the involved nerve (Fig. 12.1). This is followed by sensory or motor deficits (4). Nerve injury is usually due to compression or stretching of the nerve and may occur secondary to a variety of processes (Table 12.1). The most common mechanism is an increase in pressure on the nerve within a closed space. This may occur due to constriction by a tight overlying retinaculum or due to compression of the nerve by a mass lesion. Signs and symptoms may be subtle, intermittent, or poorly localized and may require physical exertion in order to be elicited. As a result, this group of disorders is often underdiagnosed (3). Electromyography and nerve conduction studies may be diagnostic; however, a negative test does not preclude the diagnosis of entrapment neuropathy (3). Radiographs may be used to demonstrate a bony spur or other osseous abnormality but are usually of limited value. MRI has considerable potential in contributing to the care of patients with symptoms of an entrapment

TABLE 12.1. *Causes of entrapment neuropathy*

Normal anatomic structure
  e.g., flexor retinaculum, extensor retinaculum, accessory or hypertrophied muscle
Postural deformity
  e.g., hindfoot valgus, excessive pronation
Tumor or tumorlike lesion
  e.g., ganglion, peripheral nerve sheath tumor
Inflammation
  e.g., synovial hypertrophy, tenosynovial effusion
Degenerative disease
  e.g., osteophyte formation
Trauma
  e.g., displaced fracture, edema, hematoma, fibrous scar
Metabolic
  e.g., diabetic neuropathy

neuropathy. In patients with tarsal tunnel syndrome, for example, MRI has been used to determine the site and extent of nerve entrapment and is useful in determining the extent of surgical decompression required (5,6). It is likely to be useful in selected patients with other forms of entrapment neuropathy.

INTERDIGITAL NEUROMA

The interdigital neuroma (also known as Morton's neuroma and plantar neuroma) is not a tumor but a degenerative, fibrosing process occurring in and about the plantar digital nerve (7–9). It is the most common nerve entrapment in the foot and ankle (10,11). Interdigital neuroma is most frequent between the ages of 25 and 50 years and 80% of cases occur in women (7,8). It is usually unilateral but bilaterality has been reported in up to 27% of patients (8). Patients typically complain of pain at the distal metatarsal interspace, radiating distally and transversely through the toes. A palpable mass is often not detected and, in some cases, the pain is poorly localized. The pain may have a throbbing,

R. Kerr: Musculoskeletal Imaging, Department of Radiology, Cedars–Sinai Medical Center, Los Angeles, California 90048; USC School of Medicine, Los Angeles, California.

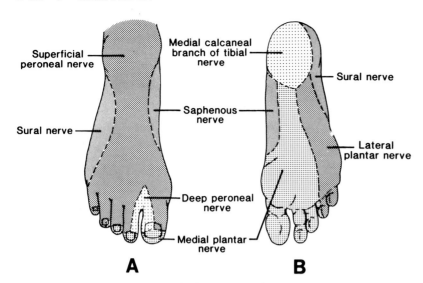

FIG. 12.1. The peripheral nerve sensory distribution of (**A**) the dorsum and (**B**) the plantar surface of the foot.

burning, or "electric" character and is typically made worse with ambulation and relieved by removing the shoe and massaging the affected area. The interdigital neuroma most often arises at the third intermetatarsal space between the metatarsophalangeal joints and plantar to the deep transverse metatarsal ligament. The etiology of interdigital neuroma is unproved but it is currently considered as an entrapment neuropathy that develops secondary to repetitive trauma and fibrous degeneration of the nerve (4). It has been postulated that dorsiflexion of the toes, a cavus arch, and walking in high-heeled shoes cause the interdigital nerve to be caught under the distal edge of the transverse ligament (2) (Fig. 12.2). A distended intermetatarsal bursa may also be contributory (10). The third nerve is the most vulnerable to compression because it is larger, formed by a conjunction of the medial and lateral plantar nerves, and is relatively fixed in position (4) (Fig. 12.3).

Repeated trauma produces inflammation and fibrosis of the nerve and of the digital vessels (7–9). Surgery is often performed when conservative measures fail; however, surgery is often not completely curative. Minimal or no improvement has been reported postoperatively in 13% to 14% of patients and residual tenderness and numbness were identified in roughly two-thirds of patients following surgical excision (8,11).

The MR diagnosis of interdigital neuroma is best accomplished in the coronal or axial plane using a small

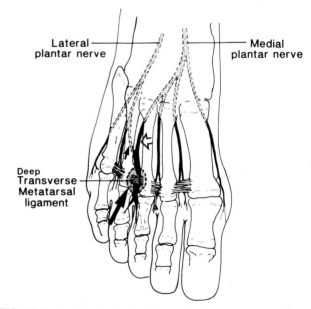

FIG. 12.3. Anatomic basis of interdigital neuroma at third interspace. The third digital branch of the medial plantar nerve (*open arrow*) and a communicating branch of the common digital nerve (*small arrow*) merge to form the third digital nerve. Increased size and lack of mobility predispose this nerve to development of inter-digital neuroma (*large arrow*) under the deep transverse metatarsal ligament. (Adapted from ref. 77, with permission.)

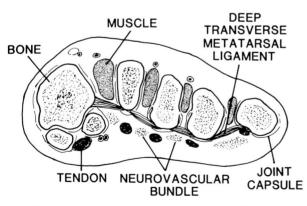

FIG. 12.2. Coronal diagram at the level of the metatarsophalangeal joints. The deep transverse metatarsal ligament blends with the plantar metatarsophalangeal joint capsules and forms a septum between the metatarsal heads and the plantar compartment. With dorsiflexion of the toes, the digital nerve may be compressed between the ligament and the plantar surface.

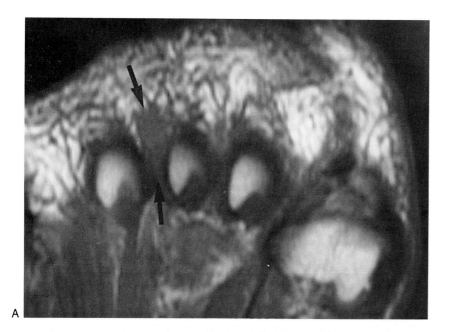

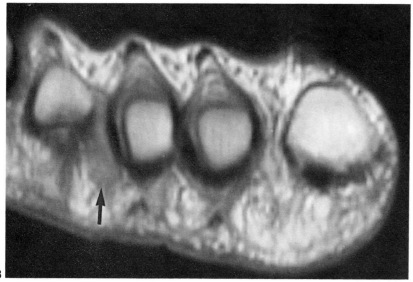

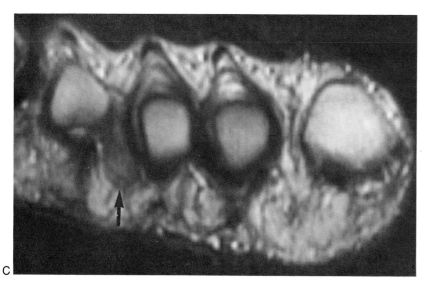

FIG. 12.4. Interdigital neuroma. **A**: Axial MR, TR/TE 500/25 image through the plantar aspect of the forefoot demonstrates a low signal intensity mass (*arrows*) between the third and fourth metatarsal heads. **B**: Coronal MR, TR/TE 3000/20 and **C**, coronal MR, TR/TE 3000/1000 images reveal a low signal intensity mass (*arrow*) between the plantar aspects of the third and fourth metatarsal heads. More proximal images revealed a distended intermetatarsal bursa in this interspace, possibly contributing to development of this lesion.

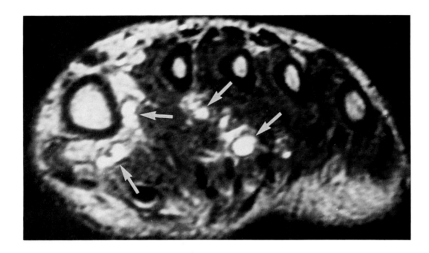

FIG. 12.5. Plantar neuromas. Axial MR, TR/TE 2500/80 image reveals multiple rounded, high signal intensity lesions (*arrows*) within the intermediate plantar compartment and adjacent to the first metatarsal. These lesions were isointense with muscle on T1-weighted and proton-density images.

(10–14 cm) field of view. The lesion demonstrates low to intermediate signal intensity on T1-weighted and proton density images and low signal intensity on T2-weighted images, reflecting its densely fibrous composition (Fig. 12.4).

Interdigital neuroma should be distinguished from true plantar neuromas as their MRI characteristics are quite different. Plantar neuromas are isointense with muscle on T1-weighted images and uniformly bright on T2-weighted images (Fig. 12.5).

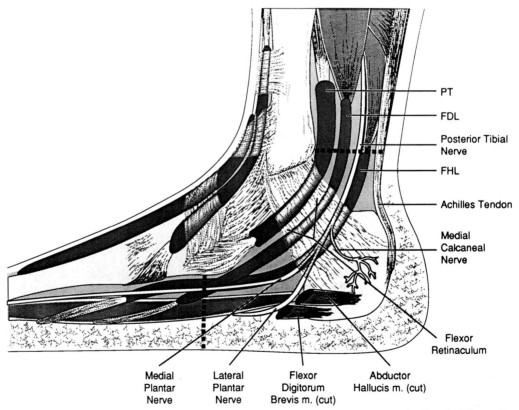

FIG. 12.6. The tarsal tunnel. A sagittal diagram of the medial ankle and hindfoot/midfoot demonstrates the medial tendons and the posterior tibial nerve and its branches coursing under the flexor retinaculum. Posterior tibial vessels (*not shown*) run adjacent to the nerve and its branches. Distal to the flexor retinaculum, the abductor hallucis muscle (cut in this diagram) overlies the medial and lateral plantar nerves. Dotted lines indicate the proximal and distal borders of the tarsal tunnel. (PT, posterior tibial tendon; FDL, flexor digitorum longus tendon; FHL, flexor hallucis longus tendon.) (From ref. 6, with permission.)

TARSAL TUNNEL SYNDROME

Normal Anatomy

The tarsal tunnel is a passageway through which the medial ankle tendons and posterior tibial neurovascular bundle pass. Its proximal and distal borders are often difficult to define but, in general, it extends from the level of the medial malleolus to the level of the tarsal navicular (12). It occupies the medial-posterior aspect of the ankle and extends into the medial-plantar aspect of the foot (Fig. 12.6). The tunnel has an osseous floor formed, from proximal to distal, by the tibia, talus, sustentaculum tali, and medial wall of the calcaneus. The roof is formed by the deep fascia of the leg, the flexor retinaculum, and distally by the abductor hallucis muscle (Fig. 12.7).

The flexor retinaculum is a thickened continuation of the deep aponeurotic fascia of the leg and extends in a fanlike manner from the medial malleolus to the medial surface of the calcaneus and the proximal as-pect of the abductor hallucis muscle. Its proximal and distal margins are not well defined. The tarsal tunnel is compartmentalized by several deep fibrous septae that extend from the undersurface of the flexor retinaculum to the medial malleolus. These septae run between the tendons and the neurovascular bundle and enclose them in separate small tunnels. Some of these septae are attached to the neurovascular bundle, thereby causing it to be relatively immobile and quite vulnerable to traction forces or space-occupying lesions. Consequently, even mild compression or traction forces may elicit the sensory symptoms of tarsal tunnel syndrome.

From anterior to posterior, the contents of the tarsal tunnel include the posterior tibial tendon, flexor digitorum longus tendon, posterior tibial neurovascular bundle, and flexor hallucis longus tendon. A variety of branching patterns of the posterior tibial nerve have been described (13,14). Bifurcation into the medial and lateral plantar nerves usually occurs beneath the flexor retinaculum but rarely occurs proximal to it. The me-

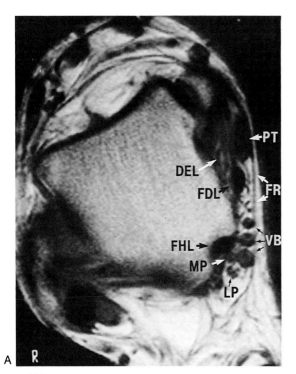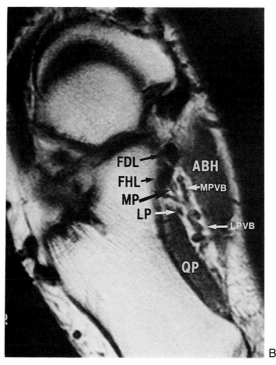

FIG. 12.7. The tarsal tunnel. Axial SE 600/20 MR images through (A) the tibiotalar and (B) tal-ocalcaneal portions of the tarsal tunnel. Note that the nerves lie deep to the vascular bundles. The medial plantar nerve is always in close proximity to the flexor hallucis longus tendon. The roof of the tarsal tunnel is formed in A by the flexor retinaculum and in B by the abductor hallucis muscle. (ABH, abductor hallucis muscle; DEL, deltoid ligament; FDB, flexor digitorum brevis muscle; FDL, flexor digitorum longus muscle; FHL, flexor hallucis longus tendon; FR, flexor retinaculum; LP, lateral plantar nerve; LPNVB, lateral plantar neurovascular bundle; LPVB, lateral plantar vascular bundle; MP, medial plantar nerve; MPNVB, medial plantar neurovascular bundle; MPVB, medial plantar vascular bundle; NVB, posterior tibial neurovascular bundle; PT, posterior tibial tendon; QP, quadratus plantae muscle.) (From ref. 6, with permission.)

dial calcaneal nerve arises beneath the flexor retinaculum or proximal to it with equal frequency. It may arise from the posterior tibial nerve or the lateral plantar nerve and may divide into multiple branches.

The medial and lateral plantar nerves are located deep to their accompanying vessels (15). Within the distal aspect of the tarsal tunnel, upper and lower chambers are formed for the medial and lateral neurovascular bundles, respectively, by the transverse interfascicular septum (Fig. 12.8). This structure extends from the medial surface of the calcaneus to the deep fascia of the abductor hallucis muscle. The upper chamber is limited medially by the flexor retinaculum and laterally by the flexor hallucis longus tendon. The medial plantar nerve is always in close proximity to the flexor hallucis longus tendon, coursing posteromedial to it. The lower chamber is limited medially by the abductor hallucis muscle and laterally by the quadratus plantae muscle. Distally, the lateral plantar nerve extends laterally along the sole of the foot between the quadratus plantae and flexor digitorum brevis muscles. The medial plantar nerve provides sensory innervation to most of the plantar surface of the foot and innervates the abductor hallucis, flexor digitorum brevis, flexor hallucis brevis, and first lumbrical muscles (Fig. 12.1). The lateral plantar nerve provides sensory innervation to the lateral plantar aspect of the foot and innervates the remaining intrinsic muscles of the foot (Fig. 12.1).

Pathologic Findings

Tarsal tunnel syndrome is an entrapment neuropathy of the posterior tibial nerve or of its branches (16–23). It is characterized by burning pain and paresthesias along the plantar surface of the foot and in the toes, made worse with weightbearing. Pain may also localize to the medial plantar aspect of the heel or radiate proximally along the medial calf. Sensory deficits are common but muscle weakness is a late infrequent finding. The main physical finding is a positive percussion sign (distal paresthesia produced by percussion over the affected portion of the nerve). The nerve may also be tender at and proximal to the site of compression. There are a variety of etiologies of tarsal tunnel syndrome (Table 12.2). It may be caused by processes that place increased tension on the nerve (such as valgus or varus deformities or scar formation), or by compression or constriction of the nerve. Tarsal tunnel syndrome has also been reported in association with rapid weight gain, fluid retention, and chronic thrombophlebitis (23).

Diagnosis of tarsal tunnel syndrome may be difficult as the physical findings are often poorly localized. Electromyography and nerve conduction studies may be useful in confirming the diagnosis. Variable results have been reported with these techniques, however, with the sensitivity ranging from 65% to 90% (20,24,25). A normal nerve conduction study, therefore, does not exclude the diagnosis.

Most patients with tarsal tunnel syndrome eventually require surgical decompression (26–28). The results of surgery are variable, and between 10% and 30% of patients report little or no relief postoperatively (21,26,29). Treatment failure may be due to an incomplete release of the flexor retinaculum or to failure to identify and remove a compressing lesion.

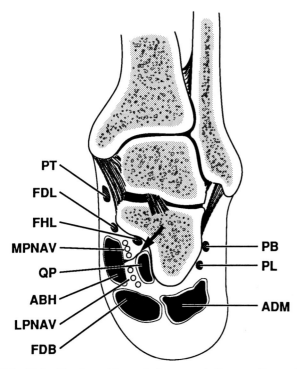

FIG. 12.8. The tarsal tunnel. A coronal diagram through the distal aspect of the tarsal tunnel reveals the medial and lateral neurovascular bundles, separated by the transverse interfascicular septum (*arrow*).

TABLE 12.2. *Common causes of tarsal tunnel syndrome*

Idiopathic—"tight flexor retinaculum"
Posttraumatic
Valgus or varus hindfoot
Dilated or varicose veins
Tenosynovitis with effusion
Tumor or tumorlike lesion
Accessory or hypertrophied abductor hallucis muscle
Rheumatoid arthritis with synovial hypertrophy
Diabetic neuropathy

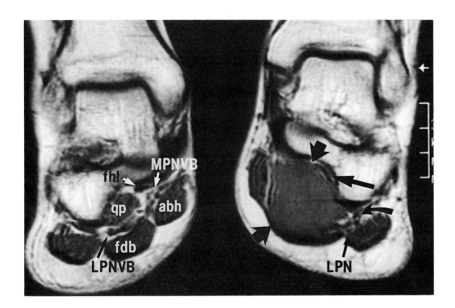

FIG. 12.9. Malignant peripheral nerve sheath tumor. A large mass (*short arrows*) of intermediate signal intensity on a coronal SE 760/20 MR image underlies the abductor hallucis muscle. The mass compresses and displaces the medial plantar neurovascular bundle (*long arrow*) and the lateral plantar neurovascular bundle (*curved arrow*). See Fig. 12.7 legend for abbreviations. (From ref. 6, with permission.)

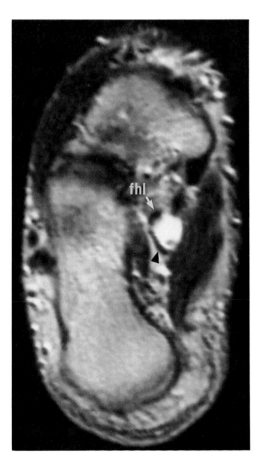

FIG. 12.10. Neurilemoma. Axial MR, TR/TE 1900/80 image reveals a high signal intensity mass (*arrow*) adjacent to the flexor hallucis longus (*fhl*), compressing the medial plantar neurovascular bundle (*arrowhead*). Also see Fig. 9.14. (From ref. 6, with permission.)

MRI is an accurate means of demonstrating the presence and extent of lesions causing tarsal tunnel syndrome. It is particularly well suited to evaluating this disorder because similar signs and symptoms may be produced by lesions located anywhere from several centimeters proximal to the ankle joint to the plantar soft tissues of the midfoot. With MRI, the contents of the tarsal tunnel are clearly visualized, including the neurovascular bundles. The most common causes of tarsal tunnel syndrome are well shown with MRI and include ganglion cysts, venous varicosities, neoplasms such as malignant peripheral nerve sheath tumor (Fig. 12.9), neurilemoma (Fig. 12.10), hemangioma (Fig. 12.11), tenosynovitis, posttraumatic fracture deformity (Fig. 12.12), fluid collections (Fig. 12.13), fibrous scar (Fig. 12.14), abductor hallucis muscle hypertrophy, and valgus hindfoot.

DEEP PERONEAL NERVE ENTRAPMENT

The deep peroneal nerve is located within the dorsal soft tissues of the ankle and foot and may become entrapped in several locations (Fig. 12.15). Above the level of the ankle joint, the deep peroneal nerve lies between the extensor hallucis longus (EHL) and tibialis anterior tendons as these structures pass under the superior extensor retinaculum. The EHL tendon crosses over the nerve at the level of the superior band of the inferior extensor retinaculum. The nerve then travels distally between the EHL and extensor digitorum longus (EDL) tendons, passing over the talonavicular joint and giving off a lateral branch as it passes distal to the inferior extensor retinaculum. The medial

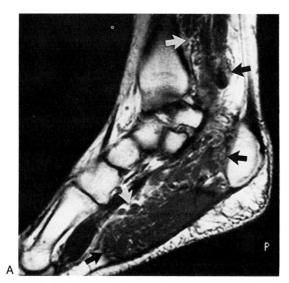
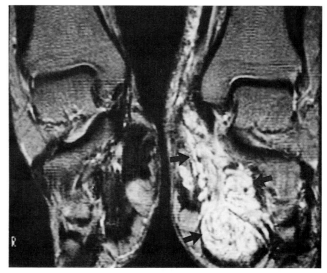

FIG. 12.11. Hemangioma. **A**: Sagittal MR, TR/TE 600/20 image demonstrates a mass composed of multiple rounded and tubular intermediate signal intensity structures that extends from the posterior ankle, through the tarsal tunnel, into the plantar soft tissues of the forefoot (*arrows*). **B**: Coronal MR, TR/TE 2000/80 image. A septated, high signal intensity mass fills the distal tarsal tunnel (*arrows*). Note atrophy of all the medial plantar muscles in B. (From ref. 6, with permission.)

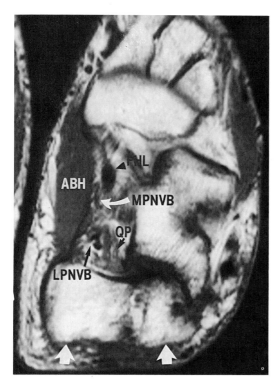

FIG. 12.12. Posttraumatic tarsal tunnel syndrome. An axial MR, TR/TE 600/20 image reveals non-union of a calcaneal fracture with 90° rotation of the calcaneal tuberosity (*arrows*). The lateral plantar neurovascular bundle is entrapped between the abductor hallucis muscle, the quadratus plantae muscle, and the malaligned calcaneus. (From ref. 6, with permission.)

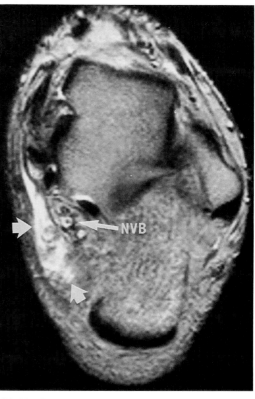

FIG. 12.13. Posttraumatic tarsal tunnel syndrome. In a patient with recent blunt trauma and a calcaneal contusion (*not shown*) an axial MR, TR/TE 1800/80 image reveals fluid filling the tarsal tunnel (*arrows*) (NVB, neurovascular bundle). (From ref. 6, with permission.)

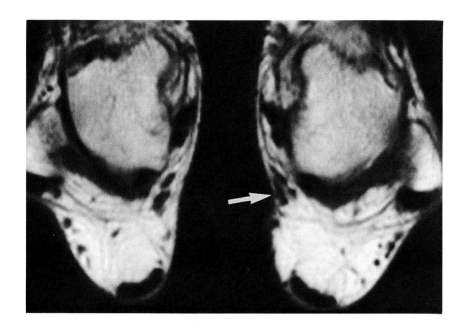

FIG. 12.14. Tarsal tunnel syndrome secondary to posttraumatic scar. An axial MR, TR/TE 600/20 image at the ankle level demonstrates tethering of the neurovascular bundle (*arrow*) with loss of the overlying subcutaneous fat (compare with opposite side). (From ref. 6, with permission.)

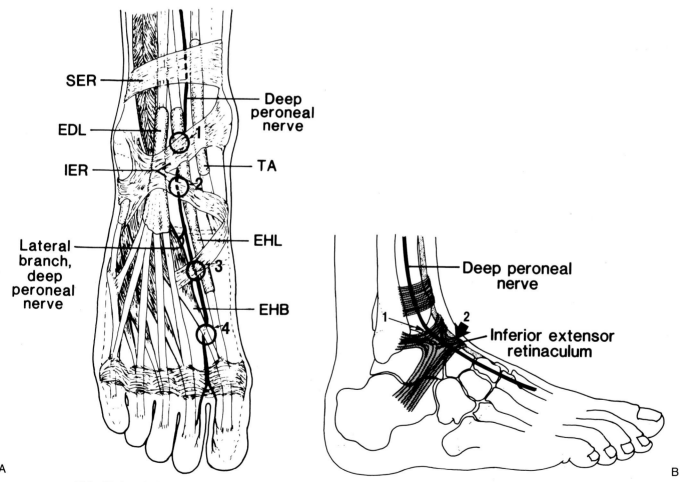

FIG. 12.15. A, B: Deep peroneal nerve entrapment. Points of enlargement include (1) under the leading edge of the inferior extensor retinaculum; (2) by talonavicular osteophytes, (3) by cuneiform-metatarsal osteophytes or an os intermetatarseum; and (4) where the nerve passes under the extensor hallucis brevis tendon.

branch of the deep peroneal nerve then courses distally between the extensor hallucis brevis (EHB) muscle/tendon and the EHL tendon, passing over the medial cuneiform and over the space between the first and second metatarsals. The nerve passes underneath the EHB tendon and then pierces the dorsal aponeurosis of the foot. It provides sensation to the first web space and the adjacent surfaces of the first and second toes.

In patients with entrapment of the deep peroneal nerve, discomfort is produced at the site of nerve compression and there is pain, numbness, or paresthesia at the dorsal aspect of the first interspace (3,30,31,32). The deep peroneal nerve innervates the extensor digitorum brevis and first and second dorsal interosseous muscles, and weakness or atrophy is a late manifestation of nerve compression. The nerve may be compressed anywhere along its course (Fig. 12.15). The most common site of entrapment is under the taut inferior extensor retinaculum and is referred to as "anterior tarsal tunnel syndrome" (3,31). The nerve is prone to entrapment under the superior edge of the inferior retinaculum where the extensor hallucis longus tendon crosses over it. More distal entrapment may occur due to dorsal osteophytes from the talonavicular, naviculocuneiform, or cuneiform-metatarsal joints or due to compression by an os intermetatarsium. The nerve may also be entrapped distally where the EHB tendon passes over it. A ganglion is a common source of nerve compression and may arise at any location. Deep peroneal nerve entrapment may also occur due to tight-fitting shoes or ski boots, and in soccer players who kick the ball with the dorsum of the foot (3). A lateral radiograph is useful to exclude the presence of dorsal osteophytes and an os intermetatarsium is best identified on a dorsoplantar radiograph. MRI may be used to demonstrate soft tissue mass lesions, such as a ganglion, in patients with this disorder (Fig. 12.16).

SURAL NERVE ENTRAPMENT

The sural nerve arises from the tibial nerve 3 cm above the knee joint. It descends between the heads of the gastrocnemius and pierces the deep fascia at the middle third of the leg. Above the ankle, the sural nerve courses along the lateral border of the Achilles tendon and is anterolateral to the short saphenous veins. At the ankle it lies posterior to the peroneal tendons, giving lateral calcaneal branches to the ankle and heel. The nerve passes 1.0 to 1.5 cm below the tip of the lateral malleolus, behind the peroneal tendons, into the foot. Distally, the nerve divides into two terminal branches that provide sensation to the lateral aspect of the fifth toe and the fourth web space (12).

Sural nerve entrapment produces numbness and paresthesia on the lateral aspect of the foot with local

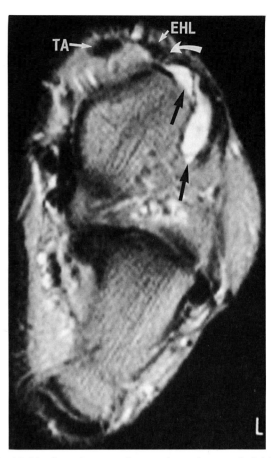

FIG. 12.16. Anterior tarsal tunnel syndrome. Axial MR, TR/TE 1800/80 image demonstrates a high signal intensity ganglion (*arrows*) pushing the deep peroneal nerve (*curved arrow*) against the overlying inferior extensor retinaculum and extensor hallucis longus (EHL) tendon. (TA, tibilias anterior tendon.)

tenderness and a positive percussion sign (33,34). Although entrapment may occur anywhere along the course of the nerve, it is most often found at the ankle. Fibrosis due to recurrent ankle sprains is a common cause of sural nerve compression (33). Fibrous compression of the nerve compression has also been described following a displaced calcaneal fracture, a fracture of the base of the fifth metatarsal and Achilles tendon rupture (33,35). A ganglion is a common etiology. Sural nerve dysfunction is also observed in association with diabetes. With MRI, the sural nerve is identified within the posterolateral soft tissues of the ankle and hindfoot, adjacent to the short saphenous vein. Nerve compression by a mass lesion, such as a ganglion, or by fibrous scar is well demonstrated (Fig. 12.17).

SUPERFICIAL PERONEAL NERVE ENTRAPMENT

The superficial peroneal nerve pierces the deep fascia in the anterolateral leg 10 to 12 cm proximal to the

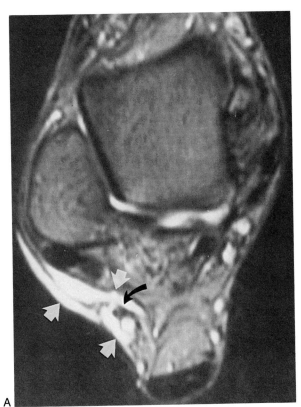 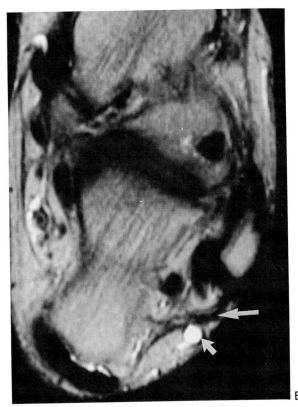

FIG. 12.17. Sural nerve entrapment. **A**: Axial MR, TR/TE 2500/80 image. A septated, high signal intensity ganglion (*arrows*) surrounds the sural nerve (*curved arrow*). **B**: In another patient, axial TR/TE 3200/100 image reveals a linear fibrous scar (*long arrow*) adjacent to the small saphenous vein (*short arrow*) in the expected location of the sural nerve.

tip of the lateral malleolus and then becomes subcutaneous. It divides into two cutaneous branches 6 cm above the lateral malleolus that provide sensation to the dorsum of the ankle and foot, except for the first web space. Entrapment produces pain with variable numbness and paresthesia along the nerve distribution. The nerve is most commonly entrapped as it emerges from under the deep fascia in the distal leg and patients may complain only of pain at this site. Fibrosis secondary to chronic ankle sprains is another common etiology (1–3).

PLANTAR HEEL PAIN

Heel pain may be classified as plantar, medial, posterior, or lateral. A plantar or medial distribution of heel pain is most often encountered (36,37). Lateral pain is often due to peroneal tendon dysfunction. Posterior heel pain relates to abnormalities of the Achilles tendon or the adjacent bursae. Medial heel pain usually derives from posterior tibial tendon disorders or tarsal tunnel syndrome. Tendon abnormalities associated with these forms of heel pain are described in the chapter by Mink on Tendons. Plantar heel pain may originate from several structures but most often is secondary to abnormality of the plantar fascia (36) (Table 12.3).

Plantar heel pain is a common problem and is most often seen in the middle-aged and elderly population and in athletes, especially runners (38). It is bilateral in 10% to 30% of patients and may be associated with obesity (39,40). In one study, 90% of the female and 40% of the male patients with a painful heel were obese (41). Among athletes heel pain is seen most frequently in long distance runners (37,42). Some of the causes

TABLE 12.3. *Causes of plantar heel pain*

Plantar fasciitis
Inflammation at plantar fascia origin
Plantar fascia rupture
Entrapment of first branch of lateral plantar nerve
Tarsal tunnel syndrome
Fat pad atrophy/inflammation
Flexor hallucis longus tenosynovitis
Calcaneal stress fracture/stress reaction
Heel spur fracture
Inflammatory arthritis

of plantar heel pain may be distinguished by the site of maximal plantar tenderness (Fig. 12.18).

Many patients with plantar heel pain have an abnormality at the origin or within the substance of the plantar fascia. The plantar fascia is a multilayered fibrous aponeurosis that has a medial, central, and lateral component. The central portion is largest and originates from the medial calcaneal tuberosity. The deep layer of the aponeurosis divides into five tracts distally that insert on the proximal phalanges. The flexor digitorum brevis muscle also arises from the medial calcaneal tuberosity as well as from the proximal aspect of the plantar aponeurosis. With extension of the metatarsophalangeal joints during gait, the plantar fascia is elongated and tightens and functions to elevate the longitudinal arch in a manner analogous to a windlass (43). This subjects the plantar fascia to a tensile force and places a traction stress at its origin.

Plantar fasciitis may occur on a mechanical basis due to increased strain associated with a pronation or cavus deformity. A more common cause is repetitive trauma. In both situations, microtears occur in the origin of the plantar fascia and elicit a local inflammatory reaction (44–46). Biopsy of patients with chronic plantar fasciitis reveals findings of collagen degeneration consisting of collagen necrosis, angiofibroblastic hyperplasia, chondroid metaplasia, and matrix calcification (42,43,47). This process is believed to begin at the origin of the plantar fascia from the medial tuberosity and, in the chronic phase, to extend distally along the course of the plantar fascia (48). A similar inflammatory process at the origin of the flexor digitorum brevis muscle probably leads to the development of a plantar calcaneal spur (36). Plantar fascial degeneration and inflammation may also occur in association with rheumatoid arthritis, the seronegative spondyloarthropathies, gout, and systemic lupus erythematosus.

Plantar and medial heel pain may develop secondary to entrapment of the first branch of the lateral plantar nerve (49). This nerve courses vertically along the medial wall of the calcaneus and then takes a horizontal course along the inferior boarder of the calcaneus, just distal to the medial calcaneal tuberosity. Entrapment of the nerve occurs as it changes from a vertical to a horizontal direction and is caught between the abductor hallucis muscle and medial head of the quadratus plantae muscle. Entrapment may also occur adjacent to the medial calcaneal tuberosity secondary to a bony spur or soft tissue inflammation at the origin of the flexor digitorum brevis muscle and plantar fascia (49).

A stress reaction at the medial calcaneal tuberosity has also been postulated as a cause of medial plantar heel pain (46,50). There is increased uptake of radionuclide on a delayed bone scan and periostitis may be identified on an oblique radiograph. Bone fatigue probably does not occur as an isolated finding but, more likely, accompanies inflammatory and degenerative changes within the plantar fascia, adjacent to the medial calcaneal tuberosity.

There is disagreement with regard to the appropriate usage of the term "plantar fasciitis." Most authors use this term to refer to all forms of plantar heel pain related to inflammatory or degenerative changes within the plantar aponeurosis (40). In the acute phase inflammation is localized to the origin of the plantar fascia and maximal tenderness is elicited at this site (42,48). In the chronic phase, pain extends distally along the entire course of the fascia and the fascia may appear thickened or nodular on physical examination. Patients with this chronic form are maximally tender along the midportion of the plantar fascia and symptoms are exacerbated by dorsiflexion of the toes. Morning pain and stiffness are common (42).

Other authors reserve the term "plantar fasciitis" for the chronic form described above and use the term "heel pain syndrome" for all sources of medial plantar heel pain localized to the origin of the plantar fascia and flexor digitorum brevis muscle or the medial calcaneal tuberosity (36). These patients may be distinguished clinicallly from "plantar fasciitis" by the location of the point of maximal tenderness and by the absence of pain with dorsiflexion of the toes in heel pain syndrome.

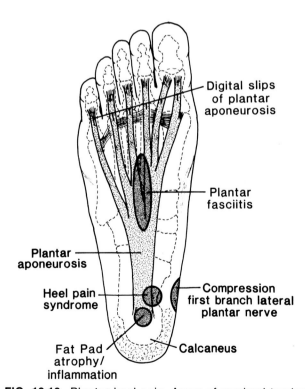

FIG. 12.18. Plantar heel pain. Areas of maximal tenderness in patients with plantar heel pain of varied etiologies. (Adapted from ref. 36, with permission.)

Most patients with plantar heel pain respond to conservative management. Patients with recalcitrant pain may respond to surgical release of the origin of the plantar fascia with decompression of the first branch of the lateral plantar nerve. In one study this resulted in complete relief of symptoms in 82% of patients (44).

Conventional radiography is usually of limited value in evaluating patients with plantar heel pain. Radiographs are useful to demonstrate a fracture, bone or soft tissue neoplasm, or evidence of arthritis. However, a specific cause of heel pain is rarely identified. Several studies have documented that a plantar heel spur is not necessarily a significant finding. A heel spur may be seen in 16% (51) to 63% (41) of nonpainful heels. In one study 50% of patients with heel pain had a plantar spur (51). In another study only 10% of patients with heel spurs were symptomatic (52). A plantar spur may be symptomatic when there is atrophy of the fat pad and with hind foot valgus: situations in which it is subjected to an increased mechanical load. An increased prevalence of spurs has been reported in obese patients (41,45). Sclerosis or periosteal thickening in the region of the medial calcaneal tuberosity may represent a stress reaction. This finding, however, may also be seen in asymptomatic patients and may represent a normal variant (41). Radiographs may reveal increased thickness of the heel fat pad and of the proximal plantar fascia in patients with plantar heel pain (50). A concave osseous defect at the base of a plantar heel spur may be a sign of bony fatigue (50).

A bone scan is frequently abnormal in patients with heel pain. In one study, increased radionuclide uptake was observed on delayed images and on immediate blood pool images in 21% of affected patients (41). The appearance ranged from a focal abnormality of the medial calcaneal tuberosity to a diffuse increased uptake within the calcaneus. It probably reflects periosteal inflammation accompanying an inflammatory or degenerative enthesopathy at the origin of the plantar fascia (53). It is likely that bone injury (periostitis/stress reaction) occurring adjacent to the origin of the plantar fascia reflects a reaction to an inflammatory or degenerative enthesopathy (53). As such, it is best considered as a secondary sign of an active soft tissue process rather than as a primary osseous lesion.

MRI is a sensitive means of demonstrating the soft tissue and osseous abnormalities associated with plantar fasciitis or heel pain syndrome (54). In patients with plantar heel pain a routine imaging protocol consists of sagittal T1-weighted, sagittal STIR, and coronal dual echo pulse sequences. A 12- or 14-cm field of view should be used to optimize anatomic definition. The plantar fascia appears as a 3- to 4-mm thick, well-defined, low signal intensity structure on sagittal and coronal MR images (54). In symptomatic feet the plantar fascia is thickened to 7 to 8 mm and, instead of appearing black, reveals intermediate signal on T1-weighted and proton density images. Various-sized regions of high signal intensity are observed within the thickened fascia on T2-weighted or STIR images. These abnormalities predominate within the proximal portion of the plantar fascia (Fig. 12.19). High signal

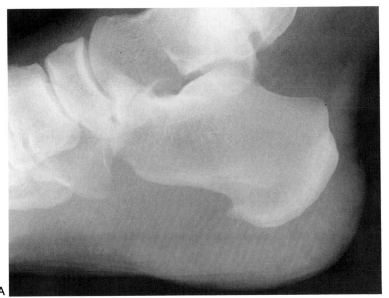
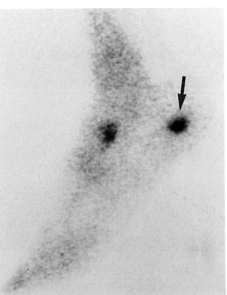

A   B

FIG. 12.19. Heel pain syndrome. **A:** A lateral radiograph demonstrates a small, well-defined calcaneal spur. The subcalcaneal fat pad appears somewhat radiodense. **B:** A delayed ^{99}mTc bone scan reveals focal increased radionuclide uptake at the medial posterior calcaneus (*arrow*) and at the distal talus. (*Figure continues on next page.*)

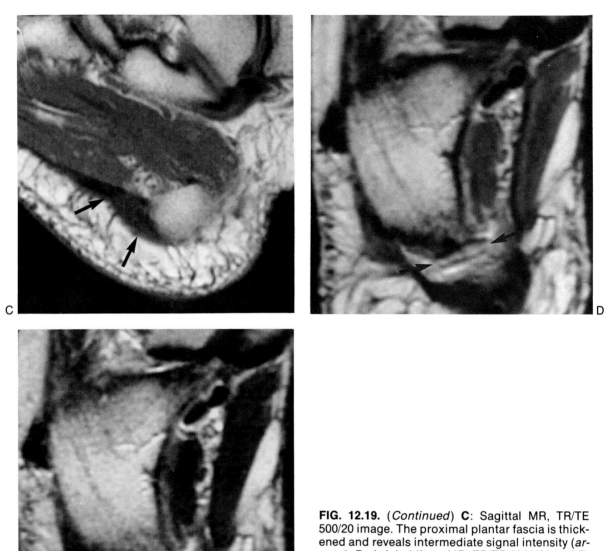

FIG. 12.19. (*Continued*) **C**: Sagittal MR, TR/TE 500/20 image. The proximal plantar fascia is thickened and reveals intermediate signal intensity (*arrows*). **D**: Axial oblique MR, TR/TE 3200/20 and **E**, 3200/100 images demonstrate a bandlike region with the signal characteristics of fluid (*arrows*) at the origin of the plantar fascia from the calcaneus. CT showed no osseous abnormality. Abnormal bone scan is presumably due to periosteal irritation of calcaneus at origin of plantar fascia.

intensity is often seen in the adjacent soft tissue and the plantar fat pad. Focal increased signal intensity may be observed within the calcaneus, adjacent to the origin of the plantar fascia, presumably reflecting a localized mechanical or inflammatory reaction (Fig. 12.20). Soft tissue and intraosseous regions of high signal intensity are often more prominent on STIR images than on T2-weighted images. Relatively focal (Fig. 12.21) or diffuse (Fig. 12.22) patterns of involvement of the plantar fascia may also be observed, beginning

several centimeters distal to its origin. Focal increased uptake may be noted within the calcaneus on bone scan in the absence of an identifiable calcaneal abnormality on MRI or CT, presumably reflecting periosteal reaction to the adjacent soft tissue process (Fig. 12.19). The role of MRI in evaluating patients with plantar heel pain has not been established. MRI may be used to confirm an abnormality within the plantar fascia and to exclude other potential causes of heel pain. It may also be used to assess the response to therapy. It is

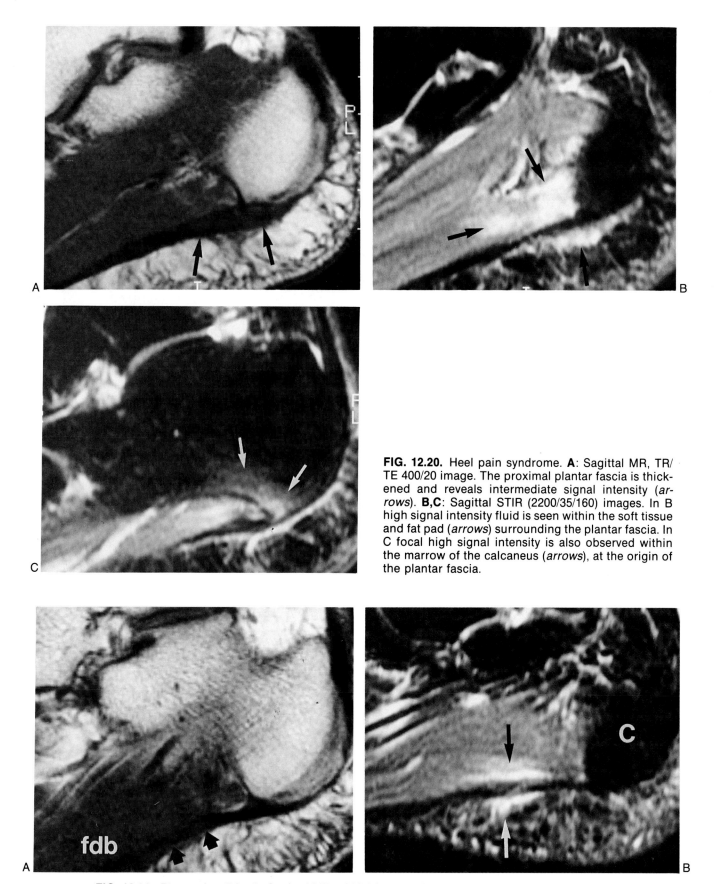

FIG. 12.20. Heel pain syndrome. **A**: Sagittal MR, TR/ TE 400/20 image. The proximal plantar fascia is thickened and reveals intermediate signal intensity (*arrows*). **B,C**: Sagittal STIR (2200/35/160) images. In B high signal intensity fluid is seen within the soft tissue and fat pad (*arrows*) surrounding the plantar fascia. In C focal high signal intensity is also observed within the marrow of the calcaneus (*arrows*), at the origin of the plantar fascia.

FIG. 12.21. Plantar fasciitis. **A**: Sagittal MR, 500/20 image. Distal to its origin from the calcaneus the plantar aponeurosis reveals intermediate signal intensity (*arrows*) and blends in with the flexor digitorum brevis muscle (*fdb*). **B**: Sagittal STIR (2200/35/160) image reveals focal regions of high signal intensity (*arrows*) dorsal and plantar to the plantar aponeurosis. (C, calcaneus.)

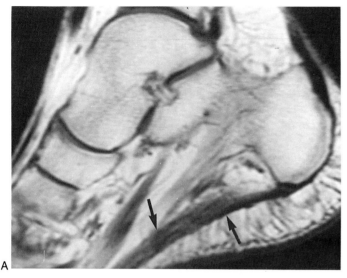

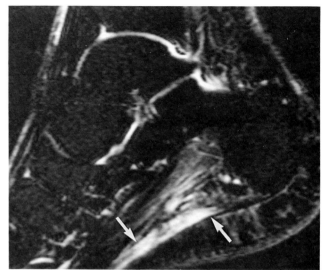

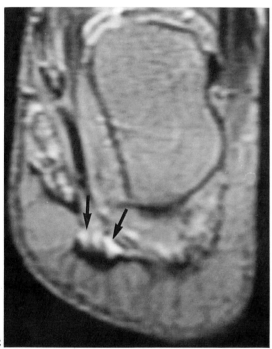

FIG. 12.22. Plantar fasciitis. **A**: Sagittal MR, TR/TE 350/15 images. **B**: Sagittal STIR. The mid-to-distal aspect of the plantar aponeurosis reveals a thickened band of intermediate signal intensity (*arrows*) in A that converts to high signal intensity (*arrows*) in B. **C**: A coronal MR, TR/TE 2600/80 image reveals high signal intensity fluid (*arrows*) within the dorsal aspect of the plantar aponeurosis.

probably most useful in patients with poorly localized signs or symptoms and in those who do not respond to conservative management.

ARTICULAR DISEASE

The role of MRI in evaluating articular disorders is still evolving. The use of extremity coils that permit improved spacial resolution, the development of new pulse sequences, and the application of gadolinium-enhanced imaging have dramatically improved the ability of MRI to detect articular abnormalities. Based on studies done to date, it appears that MRI will be

most useful in detecting early findings of arthritis, assessment of disease activity, evaluating the efficacy of therapy, and in detecting the complications of disease or complications of its treatment.

In recent years a more aggressive treatment approach has been used in patients with rheumatoid arthritis (RA). Individuals with early or mild disease are being treated with a variety of drugs (55). A valid measure of the efficacy of drug treatment, however, does not currently exist. Various quantitative techniques have been devised to assess the activity of RA in the hand and wrist. However, these methods are tedious and time consuming. More importantly, these techniques are not sufficiently sensitive to the small changes that occur over the short period of time of a typical drug study (56–59). A recent review concluded that neither the traditional and laboratory measurements of inflammation nor radiologic analysis are able to guide therapy or provide accurate assessment of the long-term outcome (55).

In patients with RA, MRI can demonstrate cartilage loss and bone erosions earlier than conventional radiography (60–62). Associated tenosynovial effusions are also well shown. In patients with juvenile RA, MRI is more sensitive than radiography for detection of cartilage loss, synovial inflammation, or avascular necrosis (Fig. 12.23) (61,62). In order to distinguish acutely inflamed synovium from joint effusion, MRI with intravenous gadolinium is required. Joint fluid and inflamed synovium both reveal low signal intensity on T1-weighted images and high signal intensity on T2-weighted images. Although the synovial tissue may appear somewhat more heterogeneous than fluid, it is usually not possible to distinguish one from another. Following the intravenous administration of gadolinium (Gd)-DTPA, acutely inflamed synovium reveals high signal intensity on T1-weighted images, reflecting diffuse enhancement (63–65). A joint effusion remains low in signal intensity on T1-weighted Gd-DTPA–enhanced images. Chronic fibrotic synovial inflammation reveals minimal enhancement and, in some patients, cannot be distinguished from joint effusion on T1-weighted Gd-DTPA–enhanced images (66–68). Initial results indicate that in patients undergoing drug therapy, clinical symptoms correlate well with changes in synovial thickness and synovial enhancement with Gd-DTPA and with the extent of joint effusion as shown by MRI (66).

MRI may also be of value in evaluating patients with hemophilic arthropathy. Although the ankle is the third most common site of hemarthrosis in hemophilia, it is the most commonly affected joint during the second decade of life (69). Hemarthrosis incites an intense inflammatory reaction that leads to a hypervascular synovial proliferation. If the process is not controlled, recurrent episodes lead to articular cartilage destruction, synovial fibrosis, and equinus, varus, or cavus deformity (70). Synovectomy is sometimes performed to halt the progression of hemophilic arthropathy, but is only effective if the articular cartilage is intact (71).

MRI may be used to demonstrate the presence of intraarticular fluid, the extent of synovial hypertrophy, and to detect cartilage loss (Fig. 12.24) (72,73). As discussed above, synovial hypertrophy is best evaluated with intravenous Gd-DTPA MRI. Because MRI can reveal small areas of cartilage destruction before joint space narrowing becomes radiographically evident, it may be useful in selecting patients for synovectomy. MRI may also reveal intraosseus hemorrhage not evident on radiographs (74). The presence and extent of soft tissue hemophilic pseudotumors is also well shown with MRI (75).

In patients with degenerative arthritis, MRI may be used to demonstrate cartilage loss and bony impingement related to osteophyte formation (Fig. 12.25). Masslike, periarticular exostoses may also be shown with MRI (Fig. 12.26).

In patients with gout, the extent of cartilage loss,

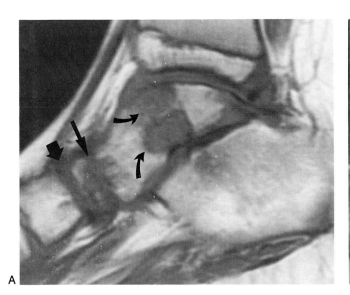
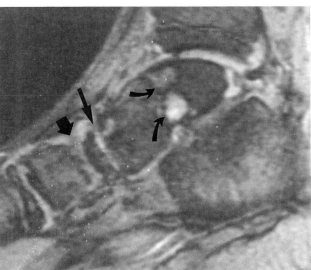

A   B

FIG. 12.23. Juvenile rheumatoid arthritis. **A**: Sagittal MR, TR/TE 600/20. **B**: Sagittal MR, T2* gradient-echo images reveal subchondral cysts (*curved arrows*) within the talus bordering the tibiotalar and posterior talocalcaneal articulations. The articular cartilage of the tibiotalar joint is intact. There is involvement of the talonavicular (*long arrow*) and naviculocuneiform joints (*short arrow*) with partial collapse of the navicular.

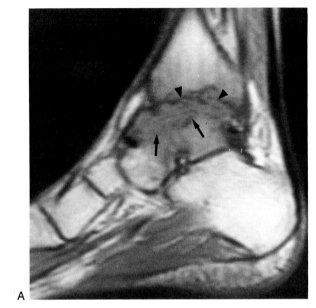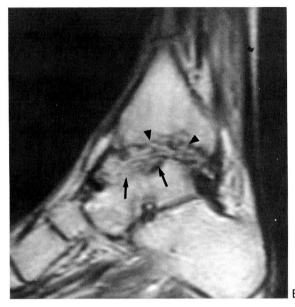

A B

FIG. 12.24. Hemophilic arthropathy. **A:** Sagittal MR, TR/TE 2000/120 and **B,** 2000/70 images demonstrate erosion of the talar dome (*arrows*) and erosion of the distal tibial articular surface (*arrowheads*). In B, the joint is filled with material of heterogeneous signal intensity consistent with hypertrophied synovium, fluid, inflammation, and hemosiderin.

osseous destruction, and soft tissue tophus are well demonstrated with MRI (Fig. 12.27). A gouty tophus may reveal low to intermediate signal intensity on both T1-weighted and T2-weighted images.

MRI may be of value in evaluating patients with suspected tarsal coalition. Although this disorder is well demonstrated with CT, MRI is potentially useful in determining the type of coalition. An osseous coalition will demonstrate continuity of the marrow space across the articulation whereas fibrous or cartilaginous coalitions reveal a low signal intensity band at the joint (76).

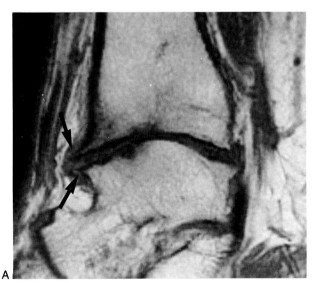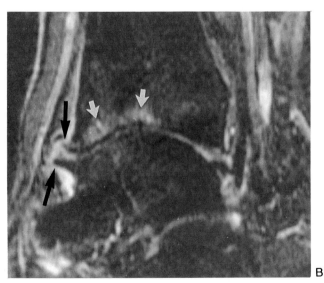

A B

FIG. 12.25. Degenerative arthritis with osteophytosis. **A:** Sagittal MR, TR/TE 600/20 images and **B,** sagittal STIR 2200/35/160 images reveal diffuse cartilage loss. In B, edema is noted within the subchondral marrow of the distal tibia (*short arrows*). Dorsiflexion was limited by large dorsal osteophytes (*long arrows*).

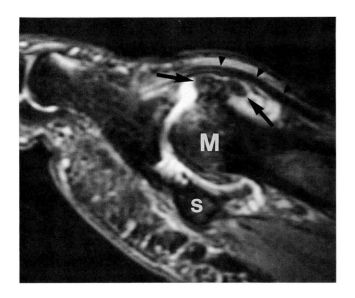

FIG. 12.26. Dorsal exostosis. Sagittal STIR 2200/35/160 image of the first metatarsophalangeal joint reveals a large dorsal exostosis (*arrows*) protruding under the extensor tendon (*arrowheads*) and a high signal intensity joint effusion. (M, metatarsal head; s, sesamoid bone.)

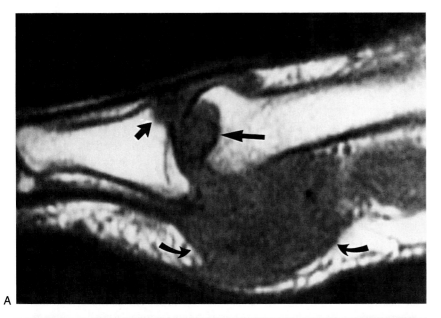

A

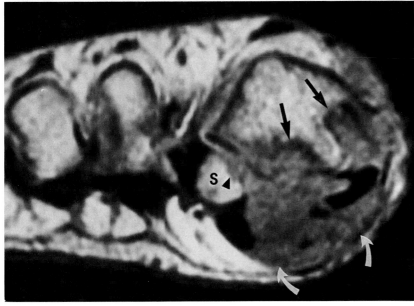

B

FIG. 12.27. Gout. **A**: Sagittal 650/20 image reveals erosion of the first metatarsal head (*long arrow*) and of the base of the first proximal phalanx (*short arrow*) and a large, exophytic, low signal intensity tophus (*curved arrows*). **B**: Axial 2500/20 and **C**, axial TR/TE 2500/70 MR images reveal erosions of the first metatarsal head (*arrows*) and of the lateral sesamoid (*arrowhead*) and a low signal intensity tophus (*curved arrows*). Note that the medial sesamoid has been destroyed by the tophus. (S, lateral sesamoid.) (*Figure continues on next page.*)

363

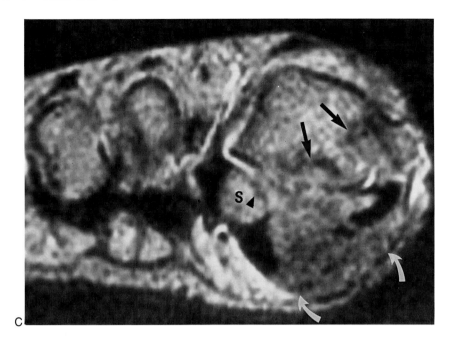

FIG. 12.27. (*Continued*)

REFERENCES

1. Dawson, DM, Hallett, M, and Millender, LH, *Entrapment Neuropathies*. 2nd ed. 1990, Little, Brown: Boston.
2. Kopell, HP and Thompson, WAL, *Peripheral entrapment neuropathies of the lower extremity*. N Engl J Med, 1960. **262**: p. 56–60.
3. Schon, LC and Baxter, DE, *Neuropathies of the foot and ankle in athletes*. Clin Sports Med, 1990. **9**: p. 489–509.
4. Lusskin, R and Battista, A, *Peripheral neuropathies affecting the foot: Traumatic, ischemic and compressive disorders*. In *Disorders of the Foot and Ankle. Medical and Surgical Management*, MH Jahss, Editor. 1991, W.B. Saunders: Philadelphia. p. 2089–2124.
5. Erickson, SJ, Quinn, SF, Kneeland, JB, *et al.*, *MR imaging of the tarsal tunnel and related spaces: Normal and abnormal findings with anatomic correlation*. AJR, 1990. **155**: p. 323–328.
6. Kerr, R, and Frey, C, *MR imaging in tarsal tunnel syndrome*. J Comput Assist Tomogr, 1991. **15**: p. 280–286.
7. Addante, JB, Peicott, PS, Wong, KY, *et al.*, *Interdigital neuromas. Results of surgical excision of 152 neuromas*. J Am Podiatr Med Assoc, 1986. **76**: p. 493–495.
8. Bradley, N, Miller, WA, and Evans, JP, *Plantar neuroma: Analysis of results following surgical excision in 145 patients*. South Med J, 1976. **69**: p. 853–854.
9. Reed, RJ and Bliss, BO, *Morton's neuroma*. Arch Pathol, 1973. **95**: p. 123–129.
10. Alexander, IJ, Johnson, KA, and Parr, JW, *Morton's neuroma: A review of recent concepts*. Orthopedics, 1987. **10**: p. 103–106.
11. Mann, RA and Reynolds, JC, *Interdigital neuroma—a critical clinical analysis*. Foot Ankle, 1983. **3**: p. 238–243.
12. Sarrafian, SK, *Anatomy of the Foot and Ankle. Descriptive, Topographic, Functional*. 1983, JB Lippincott: Philadelphia. p. 118–128.
13. Dellon, AL and Mackinnon, SE, *Tibial nerve branching in the tarsal tunnel*. Arch Neurol, 1984. **41**: p. 645–646.
14. Havel, PE, Ebraheim, NA, Clark, SE, *et al.*, *Tibial nerve branching in the tarsal tunnel*. Foot Ankle, 1988. **9**: p. 117–119.
15. Zeiss, J, Fenton, P, Ebraheim, N, *et al.*, *Normal magnetic resonance anatomy of the tarsal tunnel*. Foot Ankle, 1990. **10**: p. 214–218.
16. Edwards, WG, Lincoln, CR, Bassett, FH, III, *et al.*, *The tarsal tunnel syndrome. Diagnosis and treatment*. JAMA, 1969. **207**: p. 716–720.

17. Janecki, CJ and Dovberg, JL, *Tarsal tunnel syndrome caused by neurilemoma of the medial plantar nerve*. J Bone Joint Surg, 1977. **59A**: p. 127–128.
18. Keck, C, *The tarsal tunnel syndrome*. J Bone Joint Surg (Am), 1962. **44**: p. 180–182.
19. Lam, SJS, *A tarsal tunnel syndrome*. Lancet, 1962. **2**: p. 1354–1355.
20. Linscheid, RL, Burton, RC, and Fredericks, EJ, *Tarsal-tunnel syndrome*. South Med J, 1970. **63**: p. 1313–1323.
21. Radin, EL, *Tarsal tunnel syndrome*. Clin Orthop, 1983. **181**: p. 167–170.
22. Sammarco, GJ and Stephens, MM, *Tarsal tunnel syndrome caused by the flexor digitorum accessorius longus. A case report*. J Bone Joint Surg (Am), 1990. (**72**): p. 453–454.
23. Wilemon, WK, *Tarsal tunnel syndrome. A 50-year survey of the world literature and a report of two new cases*. Orthop Rev, 1979. **8**: p. 111–117.
24. Irani, KD, Grabois, M, and Harvey, SC, *Standardized technique for diagnosis of tarsal tunnel syndrome*. Am J Phys Med, 1982. **61**: p. 26–31.
25. Oh, SJ, Sarla, PK, Kuba, T, *et al.*, *Tarsal tunnel syndrome: Electrophysiological study*. Ann Neurol, 1979. **5**: p. 327–330.
26. Mann, R, *Tarsal tunnel syndrome*. In *Surgery of the Musculoskeletal System*, CM Evarts, Editor. 1990, Churchill Livingstone: New York. p. 4059–4064.
27. Jackson, DL and Haglund, B, *Tarsal tunnel syndrome in athletes. Case reports and literature review*. Am J Sports Med, 1991. **19**: p. 61–65.
28. O'Malley, GM, Lambdin, CS, and McCleary, GS, *Tarsal tunnel syndrome. A case report and review of the literature*. Orthopedics, 1985. **8**: p. 758–760.
29. Cimino, WR, *Tarsal tunnel syndrome: A review of the literature*. Foot Ankle, 1990. **11**: p. 47–52.
30. Borges, LF, Halle, HM, Selkoe, DJ, *et al.*, *The anterior tarsal tunnel syndrome: Report of two cases*. J Neurosurg, 1981. **54**: p. 89–92.
31. Dellon, AL, *Deep peroneal nerve entrapment on the dorsum of the foot*. Foot Ankle, 1990. **11**: p. 73–79.
32. Zongzhao, L, Jiansheng, Z, and Li, Z, *Anterior tarsal tunnel syndrome*. J Bone Joint Surg, 1991. **73B**: p. 470–473.
33. Pringle, RM, Protheroe, K, and Mukherjee, SK, *Entrapment neuropathy of the sural nerve*. J Bone Joint Surg, 1974. **56B**: p. 465–468.
34. Raynor, KJ, Raczka, EK, Stone, PA, *et al.*, *Entrapment of the sural nerve*. J Am Podiatr Med Assoc, 1986. **76**: p. 401–403.

35. Gould, N and Trevino, S, *Sural nerve entrapment by avulsion fracture at the base of the fifth metatarsal bone.* Foot Ankle, 1981. 2: p. 153–155.
36. Pfeffer, GB and Baxter, DE, *Surgery of the adult heel.*, In *Disorders of the Foot & Ankle*, MH Jahss, Editor. 1991, W.B. Saunders: Philadelphia. p. 1396–1416.
37. Sundberg, SB and Johnson, KA, *Painful conditions of the heel.*, In *Disorders of the Foot & Ankle*, MH Jahss, Editor. 1991, W.B. Saunders: Philadelphia, p. 1382–1395.
38. Lapidus, PW and Guidotti, FP, *Painful heel: Report of 323 patients with 364 painful heels.* Clin Orthop, 1965. 39: p. 178–186.
39. DuVries, HL, *Heel spur (calcaneal spur).* Arch Surg, 1957. 74: p. 536–542.
40. Schepsis, AA, Leach, RE, and Gorzyca, J, *Plantar fasciitis. Etiology, treatment, surgical results, and review of the literature.* Clin Orthop Rel Res, 1991. 266: p. 185–196.
41. Williams, PL, Smibert, JG, Cox, R, *et al.*, *Imaging study of the painful heel syndrome.* Foot Ankle, 1987. 7: p. 345–349.
42. Clancy, WG, Jr, *Tendinitis and plantar fasciitis in runners.* Orthopedics, 1983. 6: p. 217–233.
43. Hicks, JH, *The mechanics of the foot. II. The plantar aponeurosis and the arch.* J Anat, 1954. 88: p. 25–30.
44. Baxter, DE and Thigpen, CM, *Heel pain—operative results.* Foot Ankle, 1984. 5: p. 16–25.
45. Furey, JG, *Plantar fasciitis. The painful heel syndrome.* J Bone Joint Surg, 1975. 57A: p. 672–673.
46. Graham, CE, *Painful heel syndrome: Rationale of diagnosis and treatment.* Foot Ankle, 1983. 3: p. 261–267.
47. Snider, MP, Clancy, WG, Jr, and McBeath, AA, *Plantar fascia release for chronic plantar fasciitis in runners.* Am J Sports Med, 1983. 11: p. 215–219.
48. Kwong, PK, Kay, D, Voner, RT, *et al.*, *Plantar fasciitis: Mechanics and pathomechanics of treatment.* Clin Sports Med, 1988. 7: p. 119–126.
49. Kenzora, JE, *The painful heel syndrome: An entrapment neuropathy.* Bull Hosp Jt Dis Orthop Inst, 1987. 47: p. 178–189.
50. Amis, J, Jennings, L, Graham, D, *et al.*, *Painful heel syndrome: Radiographic and treatment assessment.* Foot Ankle, 1988. 9: p. 91–95.
51. Tanz, SS, *Heel pain.* Clin Orthop, 1963. 28: p. 169–177.
52. Rubin, G and Witton, M, *Plantar calcaneal spurs.* Am J Orthop, 1963. 5: p. 38–41.
53. Sewell, JR, Black, CM, Chapman, AH, *et al.*, *Quantitative scintigraphy in diagnosis and management of plantar fasciitis (calcaneal periostitis): Concise communication.* J Nucl Med, 1980. 21: p. 633–636.
54. Berkowitz, JF, Kier, R, and Rudicel, S, *Plantar fasciitis: MR imaging.* Radiology, 1991, 179: p. 665–667.
55. Gabriel, SE, and Luthra, HS, *Rheumatoid arthritis: Can the long-term outcome be altered.* Mayo Clin Proc, 1988. 63: p. 58–68.
56. Brower, AC, *Use of the radiograph to measure the course of rheumatoid arthritis.* Arthritis Rheum, 1990. 33: p. 316–324.
57. DeCarvalho, A, *Discriminative power of Larsen's grading system for assessing the course of rheumatoid arthritis.* Acta Radiol (Diagn), 1981. 22: p. 77–80.
58. Kaye, JJ, Callahan, LF, Nance, EP, Jr, *et al.*, *Rheumatoid arthritis: Explanatory power of specific radiographic findings for patient clinical status.* Radiology, 1987. 165: p. 753–758.
59. Kaye, JJ, *Arthritis: Roles of radiography and other imaging techniques in evaluation.* Radiology, 1990. 177: p. 601–608.
60. Beltran, J, Caudill, JL, Herman, LA, *et al.*, *Rheumatoid arthritis: MR imaging manifestations.* Radiology, 1987. 165: p. 153–157.
61. Senac, MO, Jr, Deutsch, D, Bernstein, BH, *et al.*, *MR imaging in juvenile rheumatoid arthritis.* AJR, 1988. 150: p. 873–878.
62. Yulish, BS, Lieberman, JM, Newman, AJ, *et al.*, *Juvenile rheumatoid arthritis: Assessment with MR imaging.* Radiology, 1987. 165: p. 149–152.
63. Bjorkengren, AG, Geborek, P, Rydholm, U, *et al.*, *MR imaging of the knee in acute rheumatoid arthritis: Synovial uptake of gadolinium-DOTA.* AJR, 1990. 155: p. 329–332.
64. Demsar, F, Jevtic, V, Kos-Golja, M, *et al.*, *MR imaging of hand joints in patients with rheumatoid arthritis: Use of Gd-DTPA.*, in *1991 meeting of the Society of Magnetic Resonance in Medicine.* San Francisco.
65. Kursunoglu-Brahme, S, Riccio, T, Weisman, MH, *et al.*, *Rheumatoid knee: Role of gadopentetate-enhanced MR imaging.* Radiology, 1990. 176: p. 831–835.
66. Kaminsky, S, Hauer, R, and Felix, R, *Rheumatoid arthritis of the hip: Gadopentetate enhanced MR-imaging: Sensitivity, long-term follow-up and histopathologic correlation.*, in *1991 meeting of the Society of Magnetic Resonance in Medicine.* San Francisco.
67. Konig, H, Sieper, J, and Wolf, KJ, *Rheumatoid arthritis: Evaluation of hypervascular and fibrous pannus with dynamic MR imaging enhanced with Gd-DTPA.* Radiology, 1990. 176: p. 473–477.
68. Lang, P, Stevens, M, Vahlensieck, M, *et al.*, *Rheumatoid arthritis of the hand and wrist: Evaluation of soft tissue inflammation and quantification of inflammatory activity using unenhanced and dynamic Gd-DTPA enhanced MR imaging.*, in *1991 meeting of the Society of Magnetic Resonance in Medicine.* San Francisco.
69. Gamble, JG, Bellah, J, Rinsky, LA, *et al.*, *Arthropathy of the ankle in hemophilia.* J Bone Joint Surg, 1991, 73A: p. 1008–1015.
70. Zimbler, S, McVerry, B, and Levine, P, *Hemophilic arthropathy of the foot and ankle.* Orthop Clin North Am, 1976. 7: p. 985–997.
71. Arnold, WD and Hilgartner, MW, *Hemophilic arthropathy: Current concepts of pathogenesis and management.* J Bone Joint Surg, 1977. 59A: p. 287–305.
72. Kulkarni, MV, Drolshagen, LF, Kaye, JJ, *et al.*, *MR imaging of hemophilic arthropathy.* J Comput Assist Tomogr, 1986. 10: p. 445–449.
73. Yulish, BS, Lieberman, JM, and Strandjord, SE, *Hemophilic arthropathy: Assessment with MR imaging.* Radiology, 1987. 164: p. 759–762.
74. Kerr, R, *Magnetic resonance imaging.*, In *Imaging of the Foot and Ankle*, DM Forrester, ME Kricun, and R Kerr, Editors. 1988, Aspen Publishers, Inc.: Rockville, p. 283–316.
75. Wilson, DA and Prince, JR, *MR imaging of hemophilic pseudotumors.* AJR, 1988. 150: p. 349–350.
76. Graham, JL, *Adult foot disorders.*, in *Radiology of the Foot and Ankle*, TH Berquist, Editor. 1989, Raven Press: New York. p. 349–401.
77. Mann, RA, Editor, *DuVries' Surgery of the Foot.* CV Mosby: St. Louis. 1978.

Subject Index